The Cardiac Rhythms

A Systematic Approach to Interpretation

The Cardiac Rhythms

A Systematic Approach to Interpretation

Third Edition

RAYMOND E. PHILLIPS, M.D., F.A.C.P.

Attending Physician, Phelps Memorial Hospital, North Tarrytown,
New York; Attending Physician, St. Agnes Hospital, White Plains, New York;
Associate Professor of Medicine, New York Medical
College, Valhalla, New York.

MARY K. FEENEY, R.N., M.N.

Staff Nurse, Telemetry Unit, St. Joseph's Hospital; formerly
Critical Care Clinical Nurse Specialist, St. Joseph's Hospital,
Milwaukee, Wisconsin.

W.B. SAUNDERS COMPANY
Harcourt Brace Jovanovich, Inc.
Philadelphia · London · Toronto · Montreal · Sydney · Tokyo

W. B. SAUNDERS COMPANY

Harcourt Brace Jovanovich, Inc.

The Curtis Center

Independence Square West

Philadelphia, PA 19106-3399

Library of Congress Cataloging-in-Publication Data

Phillips, Raymond E.
    The cardiac rhythms : a systematic approach to interpretation /
Raymond E. Phillips, Mary K. Feeney. — 3rd ed.
        p.   cm.
    ISBN 0-7216-2427-8
    1. Arrhythmia—Diagnosis.   2. Electrocardiography.   I. Feeney,
Mary K.   II. Title.
    [DNLM: 1. Arrhythmia.   2. Electrocardiography.   3. Heart—
physiology.   4. Heart Rate.   WG 202 P362c]
RC685.A65P46   1990
616.1′2807′547—dc20
DNLM/DLC   90-8315

Editor: Michael Brown

Developmental Editor: Robin Richman

Designer: Bill Donnelly

Production Manager: Linda R. Turner

Manuscript Editor: Wendy Andresen

Illustration Coordinator: Peg Shaw

Indexer: Nancy Matthews

Cover Designer: W. B. Saunders Staff

The Cardiac Rhythms: A Systematic Approach to Interpretation   ISBN 0-7216-2427-8

Printed in the United States of America

Last digit is the print number: 9   8   7   6   5   4   3   2

Preface

The Cardiac Rhythms presents a method for learning the disorders of the heartbeat from the electrocardiogram. The subject matter is introduced on an elementary level and developed to an intermediate degree of complexity. It is oriented in particular to preparing the reader for experience in the Critical Care Unit.

This book has been designed as a primer for self-study, using a large number of examples to develop the skills of interpretation. It also serves as an illustrative outline and exercise supplement for a formal course or for group instruction.

The text has been integrated into a stylized pictorial framework with a step-by-step exposition of the basic determinants of heart rate and rhythm. The dynamics of the normal heartbeat are given considerable attention to establish a sound working knowledge of physiological principles before proceeding to the more difficult abnormal rhythms. Pertinent effects of the autonomic nervous system and the cardiac drugs are introduced early in the text and are integrated throughout into the learning experience. Anatomical and electrophysiological details are included only to the depth that is essential for the interpretation of the cardiac rhythms.

Although all disturbances of the heartbeat fall within a relatively few basic types, they appear in endless variation for any given type and in combinations of patterns. Because of this diversity, multiple examples of each class of arrhythmia are provided. Numerous clinical sequences are included to demonstrate the transitions of rhythms and the effects of treatment. A workbook format is followed so that readers may actively participate in problem solving while developing the practice of careful search and accurate diagnosis. Emphasis is placed on the use of descriptive terminology and comprehensive interpretation. At various stages in the book, test electrocardiograms are presented (with answers provided) to give readers further practice and an opportunity to evaluate their progress.

In this, the third edition, the text has been rewritten to accommodate a profoundly expanding knowledge of the cardiac arrhythmias. Those areas undergoing the most substantial revision are rhythms caused by reentrant mechanisms and electronic pacemaker rhythms. In addition, selected cardiac drugs, including those that have only recently become available, are presented in a format that allows easier reference. Information on important cardiac entities has been extended somewhat to acquaint readers with general electrocardiography, but the focus remains on disorders of the rhythms.

We wish to thank collectively our many professional colleagues who have contributed clinical material for this edition, as well as those individuals who have provided continual encouragement.

RAYMOND E. PHILLIPS
MARY K. FEENEY

Acknowledgments

We appreciate the enormous efforts of many in the publication of this book. Wendy Andresen provided careful editing and constructive comments throughout its writing. Of the staff at W. B. Saunders Company, Robin L. Richman, Developmental Editor, integrated countless details, and Linda R. Turner, Production Manager, orchestrated the many stages of publication with great skill and graciousness. We thank Michael Brown, Editor-in-Chief, for his patience and guidance throughout the long preparation. The encouragement and critiques of many colleagues are highly valued, as are their contributions of special electrocardiograms used in this book.

R.E.P.
M.K.F.

Contents

1   The Heartbeat 1

    ANATOMY 1
    THE MYOCARDIUM 12
    THE SARCOMERE 13
        The Resting Sarcomere 16
        The Activated Sarcomere 17

2   The Electrocardiogram 22

    ELECTROCARDIOGRAPHIC PAPER 24
    COMPONENTS OF THE CARDIAC CYCLE 25
    ELECTROCARDIOGRAPHIC COMPONENTS 32
        Review 42
    STANDARDIZATION MARKERS 42
    DETERMINATION OF RATE 45
        The Ruler Method 45
        The Grid Method 47
        The Scan Method 50
    THE STANDARD ELECTROCARDIOGRAM 51
        Bipolar Limb Leads 53
        Unipolar Limb Leads 56
        Unipolar Precordial Leads 57
    COMPONENT ABNORMALITIES 60
        Chamber Enlargement 60
        ST Segment Deviation 61
        Q Wave Changes 65
        T Wave Changes 65
        QRS Axis Deviation 67
    ARTIFACTS 70
    CARDIAC RHYTHM MONITORING 72
    ELECTRODE PLACEMENT FOR MONITORING 74
        Suggested Electrode Placement 74
        Alternative Systems for Monitoring 76
        Automatic Warning Systems 77

3   The Sinus Node 80

    IMPULSE FORMATION 80
        Action Potential 82
        Normal Sinus Rhythm 84

AUTONOMIC NERVOUS SYSTEM 91
    Structure of the Autonomic Nervous System 92
    Physiology of the Autonomic Nervous System 93
    Regulatory Mechanisms of the Autonomic Nervous System .. 95
SINUS NODE: IMPULSE FORMATION 96
    Excitation 96
    Sinus Tachycardia 96
SINUS NODE: IMPULSE FORMATION 105
    Depression 105
    Sinus Bradycardia 106
    Sinus Pause 111
    Sinus Arrest 113
    The Vasovagal Reflex 114
    Carotid Hypersensitivity 115
DYNAMIC RHYTHM PROFILE 116
SINUS NODE DYSFUNCTION 118
    Etiologies of Sinus Node Dysfunction 119
    Characteristics of Sinus Node Dysfunction 119
SINUS NODE: IMPULSE CONDUCTION 123
    Depression 123
    Sinoatrial Block 123
PREPARATION OF A CARDIAC RHYTHM NOTEBOOK 128

4   The Atria 129

IMPULSE FORMATION 129
    Atrial Escape Complex 130
    Atrial Escape Rhythm 131
    Wandering Atrial Pacemaker 133
ATRIUM: IMPULSE FORMATION 133
    Excitation 133
    Atrial Premature Complex 133
    Blocked Atrial Premature Complexes 142
    The Refractory Period 144
    Multifocal Atrial Premature Complexes 146
    Atrial Tachycardia 147
    Electrocardioversion 164
    Atrial Tachycardia with Atrioventricular Block 166
ATRIAL FLUTTER 172
    Treatment of Atrial Flutter 183
ATRIAL FIBRILLATION 187
    Treatment of Atrial Fibrillation 195
SELF-EVALUATION: STAGE 1 205

5   The Atrioventricular Node 212

FUNCTIONS 212
ANATOMICAL COMPONENTS 214
RECORDING ATRIOVENTRICULAR NODAL ACTIVITY 215
    Electrocardiogram—PR Interval 215
    His Bundle Electrogram 217
ATRIOVENTRICULAR NODE: IMPULSE CONDUCTION 219
    Excitation 219
    Ventricular Preexcitation 220

ATRIOVENTRICULAR NODE: IMPULSE CONDUCTION 235
Depression 235
First-Degree Atrioventricular Block 236
Second-Degree Atrioventricular Block 244
Third-Degree Atrioventricular Block 262

6   The Atrioventricular Junction 266

IMPULSE FORMATION 266
Atrioventricular Junctional Escape Complex 267
Atrioventricular Junctional Rhythms with Decreased
Impulse Formation 268
Atrioventricular Junctional Rhythms with
Atrioventricular Block 275
ATRIOVENTRICULAR JUNCTION:
IMPULSE FORMATION 283
Excitation 283
Atrioventricular Junctional Premature Complex 283
Retrograde Block 286
Atrioventricular Junctional Tachycardia 287
Enhanced Automaticity 288
Reentrant Tachycardias 296
Supraventricular Tachycardia 306
Variant Accessory Pathway Tachycardia 309
Treatment of Atrioventricular Junctional Tachycardias 310
SELF-EVALUATION: STAGE 2 312

7   The Bundles 321

IMPULSE CONDUCTION 321
Depression 323
Right Bundle Branch Block 326
Left Bundle Branch Block 332
The Hemiblocks 335
Combined Conduction Defects 337

8   The Ventricles 340

IMPULSE FORMATION 340
Ventricular Escape Beat 341
Idioventricular Rhythm 344
Ventricular Rhythm in Complete Atrioventricular Block 346
Ventricle: Impulse Formation 348
Excitation 348
Ventricular Premature Complexes 349
Ventricular Tachycardia 377
Ventricular Flutter 398
Ventricular Fibrillation 399
VENTRICLE: IMPULSE FORMATION 405
Depression 405
Ventricular Bradycardia 405
Ventricular Pause 409
DIFFERENTIATION OF SUPRAVENTRICULAR RHYTHMS
WITH ABERRANT VENTRICULAR CONDUCTION FROM
VENTRICULAR RHYTHMS 411

1. Relationship Between Atrial Beats and
   Ventricular Beats 412
2. QRS Complex Morphology 414
3. Post-Extrasystolic Pause 418
4. Regularity of Rhythm 418
5. Onset of a Tachycardia 419
6. Captured Beat 420
7. Fusion Beat 420
8. The Ashman Phenomenon 421
9. T Waves 421
10. Rate Change 422
11. Preexcitation Syndrome 423
12. Atrial Fibrillation 424
SELF-EVALUATION: STAGE 3 425

9   The Electronic Pacemaker 433
ELECTRONIC IMPULSE FORMATION 434
   Excitation 434
ELECTRONIC PACEMAKER COMPONENTS 435
   Energy Source 435
   Conductor Lead 435
   Electrode 436
ELECTRONIC PACEMAKER RHYTHM 437
METHODS OF APPLYING AN
ELECTRONIC PACEMAKER 442
   Transvenous Approach 442
   Transthoracic Approach 443
   External Approach 444
BRADYCARDIC INDICATIONS FOR THE ELECTRONIC
PACEMAKER 445
   Rhythms of Depressed Impulse Formation 445
   Rhythms of Depressed Impulse Conduction 446
ASSESSING ELECTRONIC PACEMAKER CAPTURE 448
   Pulse Generator 448
   The Electrodes 452
   Myocardial Response 452
ELECTRONIC PACEMAKER LEAD PATTERNS 452
THE ASYNCHRONOUS ELECTRONIC PACEMAKER 453
   The Ventricular-Inhibited Electronic Pacemaker 456
ASSESSING ELECTRONIC PACEMAKER SENSING 458
   Oversensing 465
   Failure to Sense 467
   Testing the Ventricular-Inhibited Pacemaker 468
THE ELECTRONIC PACEMAKER CODE 476
   Chamber Paced 477
   Chamber Sensed 477
   Sensing Response 477
THE ATRIAL PACEMAKER 478
PHYSIOLOGICAL PACEMAKERS 480
   The Atrial Synchronous Pacemaker 480
   The Noncardiac Rate-Responsive Pacemaker 485
   The Atrioventricular Sequential Pacemaker 488
   The Universal Pacemaker 496

PACEMAKER-MEDIATED TACHYCARDIA 507
TACHYCARDIC INDICATIONS FOR THE
ELECTRONIC PACEMAKER 510
    The Atrial Overdrive Pacemaker 510
    The Ventricular Overdrive Pacemaker 512
THE EXPANDED ELECTRONIC PACEMAKER CODE 512
AUTOMATIC IMPLANTABLE CARDIOVERTER-
DEFIBRILLATOR 513
SELF-EVALUATION: STAGE 4 515

10   **The Cardiac Drugs** 523
DRUGS OF EXCITATION 524
    Sympathetic Nervous System: Stimulation 524
    Parasympathetic Nervous System: Inhibition 528
DRUGS OF DEPRESSION 529
    Sympathetic Nervous System: Inhibition 529
    Parasympathetic Nervous System: Stimulation 530
    Drugs that Affect the Cell Membrane 530
DIGITALIS 552
    Myocardium 552
    Vasomotor Tone 552
    Electrophysiology 552
    Digoxin (Lanoxin) 555
GENERAL PRECAUTIONS WHEN ADMINISTERING
CARDIAC DRUGS 556

Glossary 557

Abbreviations in Common Use 566

Answer Section 567

Index 581

1 The Heartbeat

ANATOMY
THE MYOCARDIUM
THE SARCOMERE

The Resting Sarcomere
The Activated Sarcomere

The heart is a fist-sized organ consisting of four muscular walled chambers. To perform their function as a pump effectively, these chambers must contract in a synchronized pattern and at an appropriate rate. In effect, each heartbeat is the result of a complex sequence of activation of many components, each governed by electrochemical events. The strength of each beat and the rate of the beats must be sensitively matched to the ever-changing demands of the circulatory system. Ordinarily, all these factors are smoothly integrated to meet the variations of cardiac output required by physical activity, emotional stress, digestion, and ambient temperature. Disturbances in the rate and the synchronization of cardiac contraction—generally termed **arrhythmias**—are the subject of this book.

ANATOMY

Although the spatial relationships of the cardiac chambers may be difficult to envision, the heart can be represented in an easily understood model (Fig. 1–1). Two of the four chambers form the overlying dome, the thin-walled **atria**. The other two chambers, the **ventricles**, form the tapered body of the heart and have much thicker walls.

The atrium and the ventricle on each side act as a functional unit. The right atrium and the right ventricle receive blood from the body as a whole by way of the **systemic venous system**. Blood is pumped from the right side to the lungs via the **pulmonary arterial system**. The chambers on the left side receive blood from the lungs by the **pulmonary venous system** and propel it to the body through the **systemic arterial system**, thus completing the circuit. The actual arrangements of these structures and their sequence of action can be better appreciated from the perspective of developmental anatomy.

In an embryo, the heart first forms as a bulge in the midline, a primitive circulatory tube in which muscle cells develop prodigiously in the wall (Fig. 1–2). During the fourth week of life, peristaltic waves appear sporadically along the thickened muscular wall, moving from the hind end to the fore end, and so constituting the basic heartbeat. In

1

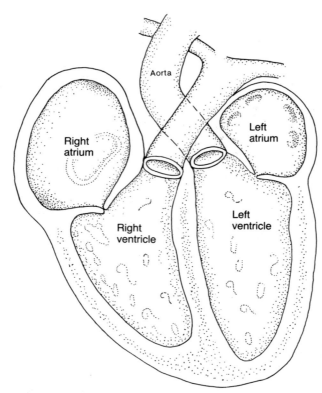

Figure 1–1. The cardiac chambers.

time, these waves occur with increasing frequency and with greater regularity. Vessels that deliver blood to the heart make up the **venous** circulation, and those into which the heart ejects blood compose the **arterial** circulation.

Having once established a pumping action, this specialized segment of the primitive circulatory tube undergoes rapid enlargement, elongating and thickening at the same time. These changes result in sharp convolutions in which an S-shaped loop is formed (Fig. 1–3). The loop brings forward the hind end of the cardiac tube, and this venous section is destined to become the atria. Note that this portion of the cardiac tube now lies **forward** of the arterial portion, which will eventually form the ventricles.

Meanwhile, the walls of the future ventricles become greatly thickened with dense muscular tissue (Fig. 1–4). The future atria balloon out around the root of the arterial trunk. Thus, the basic structure of the heart is now established, with the atria lying above the ventricles (really, cephalad or toward the head). Even with such drastic changes in anatomical relationships, the original peristaltic sequence is maintained, although through a more circuitous pathway. In other words, for each heartbeat, the atria contract first, propelling blood received from the venous circulation into the ventricles. Ventricular contraction then follows, and blood is pumped into the arterial circulation.

Even as the convolutions and the expansions of the primitive heart are evolving, partitions appear within the heart. One set of partitions forms longitudinally in the middle of the cardiac tube (Fig. 1–5). It becomes the intraatrial and the intraventricular septa, separating the chambers into a right and a left series. It further divides the arterial trunk into the aorta and the pulmonary artery.

In addition, mobile partitions develop across the cardiac tube (Fig. 1–6). These thin, fibrous structures become the cardiac valves, serving to direct blood flow only in one direction. Two of these partitions are interposed between the chambers of the

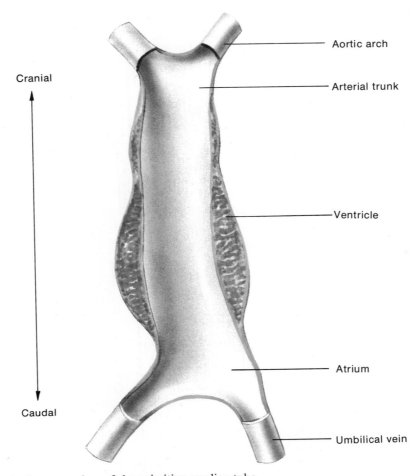

Figure 1–2. Cutaway view of the primitive cardiac tube.

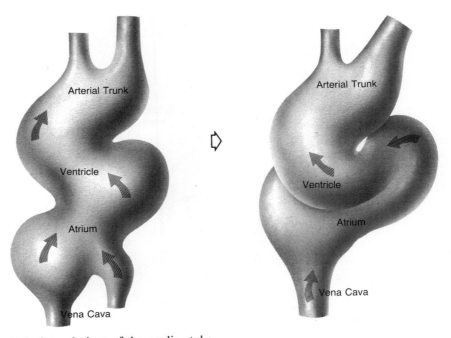

Figure 1–3. Convolutions of the cardiac tube.

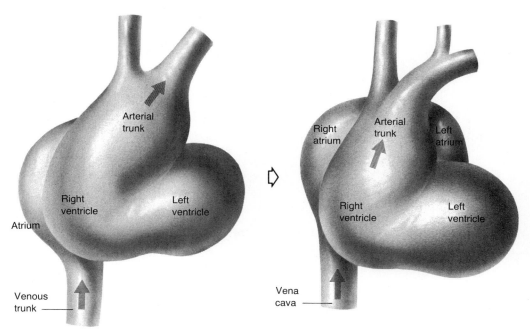

Figure 1–4. Basic architecture of the heart.

atria and the ventricles on either side. On the right, the **tricuspid valve** is formed. On the left is the **bicuspid** (more commonly called the **mitral**) valve. These funnel-shaped structures have movable inner edges that are attached by fibrous strands (the chordae tendineae) to muscular projections (the papillary muscles) arising from the floor of the ventricles.

   Another pair of valves are set at the origin of the arterial vessels. Composed of three interfacing leaflets (or cusps), these valves are referred to as the semilunar (for half-moon) valves and are designated individually as the **aortic valve** and the **pulmonary valve**.

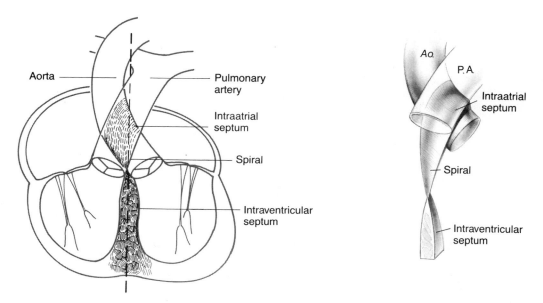

Figure 1–5. The cardiac septa: vertical partitions.

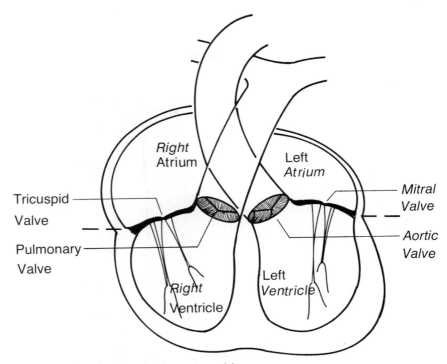

Figure 1–6. The cardiac valves: horizontal partitions.

By the end of the seventh week of life, the basic structure of the embryonic heart has developed. Next the anatomical features and functions of the mature heart that are critical to understanding the cardiac rhythms will be reviewed.

Viewed from the front, the right ventricle makes up the largest portion of the anterior surface (Fig. 1–7). Only the lateral margin of the left ventricle can be seen, its major bulk being situated posteriorly. All that is visualized of the right and the left atria are the small, thin-walled projections (the auricles) that flank the major arterial trunks: the aorta and the pulmonary artery.

In a cut-away view, the interior of the right ventricle is exposed, revealing the tricuspid valve (here partially sectioned), its outer rim affixed by a fibrous ring adjoining the right atrium (Fig. 1–8). The string-like chordae tendineae are seen, arising from the papillary muscles and attaching to the free edges of the valve. Two of the cusps of the semilunar (or pulmonary) valve are depicted at the origin of the pulmonary artery. The thick, muscular intraventricular septum is drawn perpendicular to the plane of vision; it forms the medial walls of both the right and the left ventricles.

A portion of the left ventricle can be seen in this diagram, the larger portion extending behind the intraventricular septum. Note the much thicker lateral wall of this chamber compared with that of the right ventricle. Comparable features are observed: the mitral (or bicuspid) valve lying at the junction with the left atrium and its chordae tendineae-papillary muscle apparatus. The aortic valve in the left ventricle cannot be seen in this drawing; it lies at the origin of the aorta at the same level as the pulmonary valve, and it has a similar semilunar configuration.

The pathways through which blood flows in the heart are depicted in a schematic representation in Figure 1–9. First considering the chambers on the right side, the right atrium fills with blood delivered by the superior and inferior venae cavae. During atrial contraction, this blood is ejected through the tricuspid valve into the right ventricle. Filling in somewhat less than 0.2 second, the right ventricle then contracts. This action forces open the pulmonary valve, through which blood is ejected into the pulmonary artery and from there into the lungs. At the same time, contraction of right ventricular

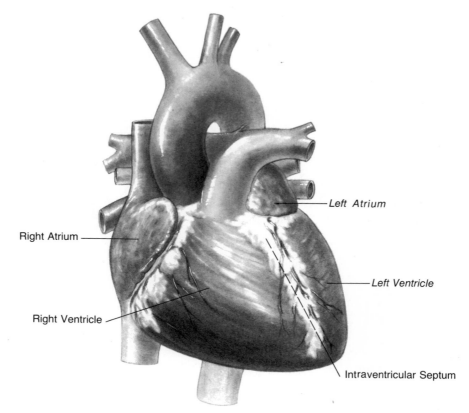

Right Atrium

Left Atrium

Left Ventricle

Right Ventricle

Intraventricular Septum

Figure 1–7. Anterior surface of the heart.

forces shuts the tricuspid valve, thus preventing backflow into the right atrium. Apposition of the tricuspid valve edges is effected by the chordae tendineae, which prevent billowing (or prolapse) of the valve back into the right atrium during ventricular systole. Increased tension on the chordae is exerted by the papillary muscles, which participate in the ventricular contraction.

A comparable series of events simultaneously occurs in the chambers of the left side (Fig. 1–10). Blood from the lungs is brought to the left atrium by the pulmonary veins. On contraction of the left atrium, this oxygenated blood is pumped into the left ventricle through the mitral valve.

Once filled, the left ventricle, by far the most powerful chamber of the heart, contracts, opening the aortic valve and ejecting blood into the aorta, thus providing the systemic arterial flow (Fig. 1–11). During contraction, the mitral valve is forced shut, the chordae tendineae restricting the backward movement of the valve edges.

Contraction (or **systole**) of the ventricles is immediately followed by relaxation (or **diastole**) during which the intraventricular pressure falls abruptly (Fig. 1–12). The relatively higher pressures within the aorta and the pulmonary artery snap shut the semilunar valves, an action exerted through the elastic properties of the walls of the aorta and the pulmonary artery. The sequence of events constituting a single heartbeat is then completed. It will begin again with filling of the atria, atrial contraction, and opening of the atrioventricular valves.

With each heartbeat, somewhat more than half the amount of blood contained in each ventricle is ejected, about 70 ml in a human adult. This ejected blood is termed the **stroke volume**. Cardiac output refers to the total volume of blood ejected over a period of time. By convention, **cardiac output** is the stroke volume multiplied by the number of ventricular contractions in 1 minute. A heart beating at a rate of 80 con-

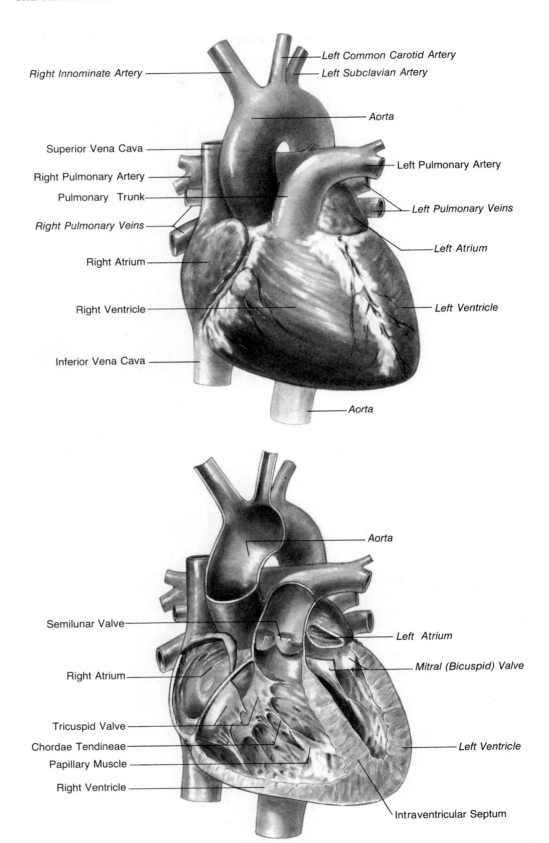

Right Innominate Artery

Left Common Carotid Artery

Left Subclavian Artery

Aorta

Superior Vena Cava

Right Pulmonary Artery

Pulmonary Trunk

Right Pulmonary Veins

Right Atrium

Right Ventricle

Inferior Vena Cava

Left Pulmonary Artery

Left Pulmonary Veins

Left Atrium

Left Ventricle

Aorta

Aorta

Semilunar Valve

Left Atrium

Mitral (Bicuspid) Valve

Right Atrium

Tricuspid Valve

Chordae Tendineae

Papillary Muscle

Right Ventricle

Left Ventricle

Intraventricular Septum

Figure 1–8. Anterior aspect of the heart, exterior and interior.

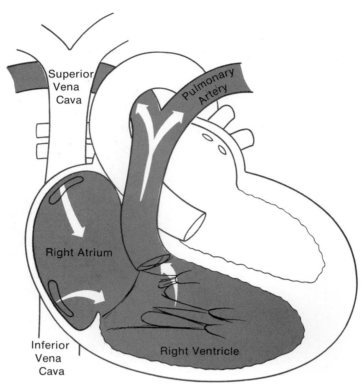

Figure 1–9. Pulmonary blood flow.

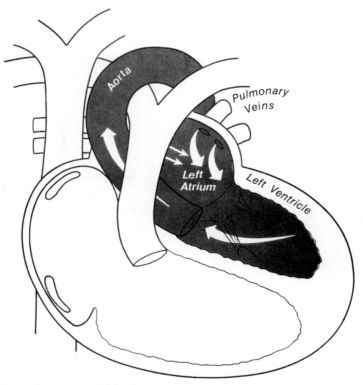

Figure 1–10. Flow of oxygenated blood.

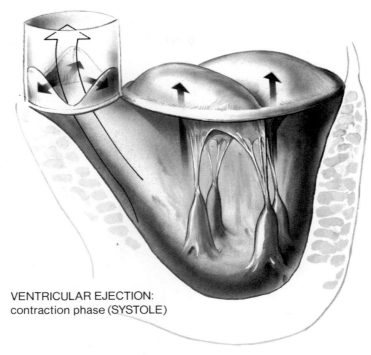

VENTRICULAR EJECTION:
contraction phase (SYSTOLE)

Figure 1–11. Mitral valve during systole.

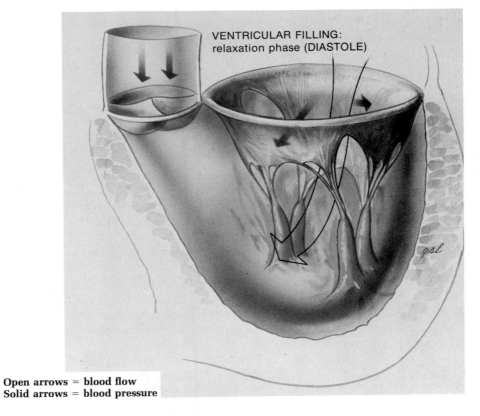

VENTRICULAR FILLING:
relaxation phase (DIASTOLE)

Open arrows = blood flow
Solid arrows = blood pressure

Figure 1–12. Mitral valve during diastole.

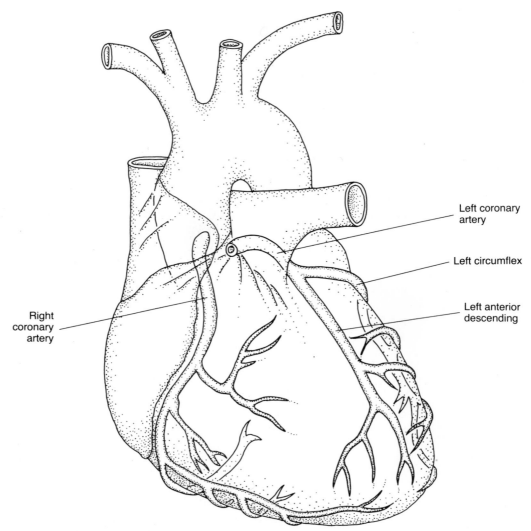

Figure 1–13. Distribution of the coronary arteries.

tractions per minute and with a stroke volume of 70 ml has a cardiac output of 5.6 liters a minute (80 × 70 ml = 5600 ml), which is within the normal range for an adult.

Blood is supplied to the heart by the **coronary arteries**, which arise from the aorta immediately distal to the aortic valve (Fig. 1–13). There are two coronary arteries, a right and a left, each about the size of a soda straw. They extend along the epicardial (outer) surface of the heart (the Latin word *corona* means "crown") and proceed toward the cardiac apex.

The right coronary artery extends along the groove between the right atrium and the right ventricle, proceeding on the right border of the heart to the apex, inferiorly. Its branches supply the right ventricle and the posterior portion of the left ventricular apex. In addition, it is distributed to the superior and the posterior regions of the intraventricular septum.

Within a few millimeters of its origin, the left coronary artery divides into two branches, (1) the anterior descending artery and (2) the circumflex artery. The anterior descending branch follows the groove between the right and the left ventricles. It supplies the anterior wall of the left ventricle as well as the anterior aspect of its apex. Branches from this artery also perfuse most of the intraventricular septum.

The circumflex artery is located posteriorly. It passes over the ring where the left atrium and the left ventricle adjoin. This branch conveys blood to the left atrium and to the posterior and the diaphragmatic walls of the left ventricle.

At the apical region of the heart, the terminal segments of the right and the left coronary arteries meet to form an anastomotic network. Although the number of connections of these two vessels is relatively small, it does increase with aging. In obstructive disease of the coronary arteries, the extent to which the heart is compromised depends in large part on the measure of development of this collateral circulation.

All along the path of the coronary arteries, small branches arise and penetrate into the myocardium (Fig. 1–14). They eventually anastomose with other end arterioles arising from arterial branches on the endocardial (inner) surface.

Atherosclerosis, the most important disease of the heart in the general population, predisposes to plaque formation (atheroma) in the proximal portion of the coronary arteries, tending to occlude the vessels (Fig. 1–15). The most dangerous site for such a lesion is in the main stem of the left coronary artery, impeding blood flow into both the anterior descending and the circumflex arteries and consequently endangering viability of the left ventricle.

Advanced obstructive disease of a coronary artery may result in permanent damage to the heart, termed **myocardial infarction**. Degrees of stenosis that permit adequate cardiac circulation at rest may become critical during exercise or other states of intensified physiological demand. The result is temporary inadequacy of cardiac blood flow (ischemia), producing the syndrome of **angina pectoris**. In addition, coronary atherosclerosis is the most common cause of **myocardial insufficiency**. Furthermore, ischemic heart disease from atherosclerosis is frequently responsible for **cardiac rhythm disturbances** by interfering with the normal formation and conduction of impulses.

The specific types of rhythm disorders produced by an obstructive lesion of a given coronary artery or its branches tend to be predictable according to the structures of the electrical pacemaker and pathway systems involved. However, the anatomy of the arterial distribution varies considerably from one individual to another, so that identifying the incriminating vessels on the basis of the type of arrhythmia produced is not highly accurate. Even so, knowledge of the relationship between the location of an

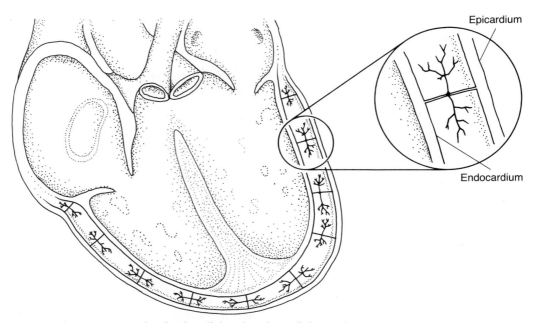

Figure 1–14. Anastomosis of epicardial and endocardial vessels.

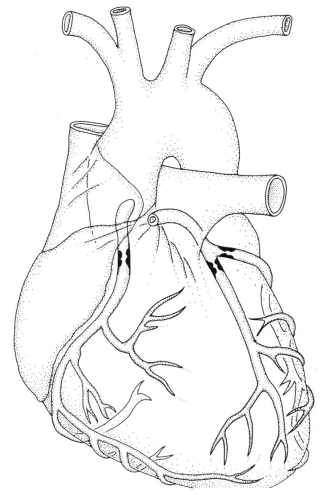

Figure 1–15. Proximal coronary artery lesion.

arterial obstruction (as may be determined by the electrocardiogram) and the most likely disturbance in rhythm to be expected is useful in clinical management.

The basic anatomy of the heart is illustrated in the schematic view in Figure 1–16. All four chambers are shown, with the atrial and ventricular septa cut in cross section. The sequences of impulse formation and impulse conduction will be discussed throughout the book, using this diagram for reference.

THE MYOCARDIUM

The heart has one function—to perform as a pump. (Actually, this long-held generalization has been modified somewhat now that atrial natriuretic polypeptide, which acts as a hormone in fluid volume regulation, has been discovered.) This mechanical function is served by the contractile fibers of the heart, which make up about 90% of the entire cardiac mass. All the other components of the heart support the pumping action:

- The valves limit blood flow to only one direction when the cardiac chambers contract.

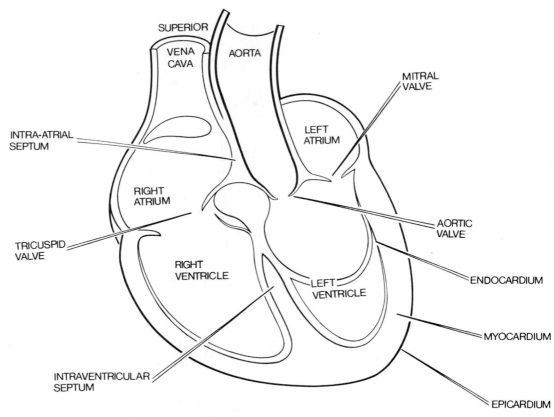

Figure 1–16. Basic anatomy of the heart.

- The pericardium facilitates the smooth movement of the heart within the mediastinum while resisting sudden cardiac dilation from severe hemodynamic stresses.
- The electrical impulse formation and conduction tissues regulate the rate of pumping and the sequence in which the cardiac chambers are activated.

Reducing this admirably integrated mechanism to its most elementary level, we focus on the sarcomere, the unit of contraction. Understanding the function of this cardiac muscle fiber provides a basis for developing a strong working knowledge of the more specialized elements that produce and transmit electrical impulses and are responsible for maintaining the rate and the rhythm of the heart.

THE SARCOMERE

Sarcomeres are cells that have the capacity to shorten or contract; they are the basic muscle fibers of the heart. When observed under the light microscope, a sarcomere appears as a rectangular structure characterized by cross-bands (Fig. 1–17). An individual sarcomere is not easy to discern because each forms an interlacing network with adjoining sarcomeres by numerous shared branches. Where sarcomeres meet end to end, the cells are separated by an intercalated disk, a modification of the cell membranes. The masses of sarcomeres are arranged in parallel so that the force of all the units on contraction is exerted in a single orientation (Fig. 1–18).

The sarcomeres, functioning in concert, compose two separate masses, or syncytia. One syncytium forms the walls of the atria; the other makes up the ventricular

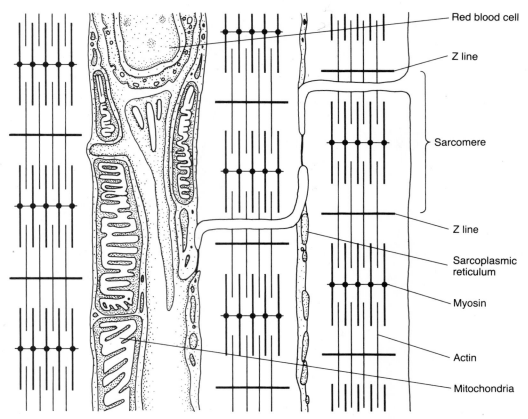

Red blood cell

Z line

Sarcomere

Z line

Sarcoplasmic reticulum

Myosin

Actin

Mitochondria

Figure 1–17. Cardiac myofibrils, demonstrating the basic unit, the sarcomere (extending from a Z line to an adjacent Z line and including interdigitating actin and myosin fibers). Portions of mitochondria interspersed between myofibrils are also shown.

walls and the intraventricular septum. These functionally independent muscle masses join at the two fibrous rings, serving as the cardiac "skeleton" to which are also attached the atrioventricular valves. Normally, the syncytia of the atria and the ventricles are electrically isolated from each other by the fibrous rings. Stimuli can pass from one to the other only by a specialized pathway, the atrioventricular node, located where the rings come together.

The cross-bands (or striations), which are so conspicuous on microscopic inspection, represent rods of fibrous protein lying side by side (Fig. 1–19). These protein rods are composed of two types of filaments, the thick filament and the thin filament. The thick filament is made up of the protein myosin, which has coiled arms projecting along its length. Each projection ends in a small, globular mass, the myosin head, containing enzymes essential for the process of contraction. The enzymes, principally adenosine triphosphatase (ATPase), interact with the companion contractile filament, actin.

Actin, a thin filament, is actually composed of two threads of the protein globulin. This pair of threads forms a cylindrical spiral. In three-dimensional geometry, the actin filaments overlap the myosin bundles in such a design as to surround each myosin filament by six actin filaments. Additional protein structures lie between the myosin and the actin fibers, and these proteins serve to regulate the interaction between the two contractile elements.

The mechanical **force of contraction** is created when electrochemical cross-bridges are established between the actin filament receptor sites and the heads of myosin. On coupling, the myosin head swivels on its coiled stem, generating a pulling tension on

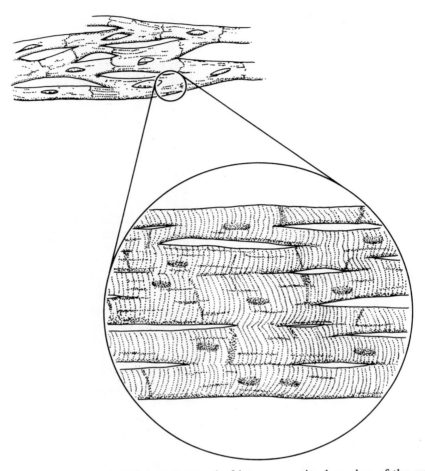

Figure 1–18. The cardiac syncytium, composed of interconnecting branches of the myofibrils. (Modified from Guyton AC: Textbook of Medical Physiology, 7th ed. Philadelphia, WB Saunders, 1986.)

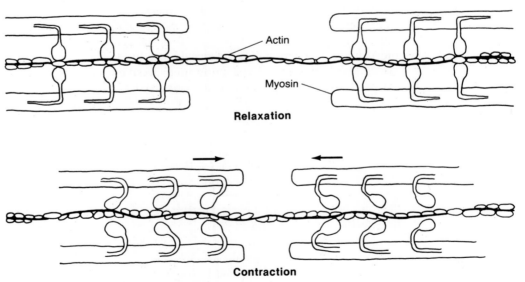

Figure 1–19. Actin-myosin relationship.

the attached actin. This tension draws the actin filament closer toward the center of the myosin bundle. Thus, the degree of overlapping is increased and the sarcomere, in effect, shortens.

The rotation of the myosin head requires **metabolic energy**, which is supplied by the high-energy phosphate bonds contained in adenosine triphosphate (ATP). These packets of stored energy are found in the sarcoplasm and are produced in the mitochondria, organelles containing the enzymatic systems for producing oxygen-consuming work. ATPase, the enzyme that catalyzes the hydrolysis of ATP (thus releasing the high-energy phosphate bonds), is stored on the heads of myosin.

The strength and velocity at which the sarcomere contracts are determined by the number of cross-bridges developed between the actin and myosin filaments. Determining factors include the quantity of calcium ions arriving at the receptors of the regulator proteins by way of the sarcoplasmic system of channels. In addition, the degree of overlapping of actin and myosin filaments before contractions has an important bearing on the number of interacting receptor sites established.

The Resting Sarcomere

In the noncontractile (or resting) state, a sarcomere is about 2.0 microns long. (One micron represents 0.001 mm.) When myosin and actin are brought into the reactive state, the sarcomere shortens to about 1.8 microns.

As is characteristic of all excitable cells, the sarcomere absorbs chemical energy from circulating nutrients and transforms this energy into an **electrical gradient** across the membrane of the cell. This gradient, known as the **transmembrane potential**, is created by the process of developing an uneven distribution of certain ions on either side of the cell membrane, an energy-consuming activity that is carried out by the cell membrane itself. The unequal concentration of ions, such as sodium and potassium, on opposing sides of the membrane causes an electrochemical pressure or tension. It is this tension, built up by the metabolic work of the cell membrane, that is suddenly released on stimulation of the sarcomere and provides the energy for developing a contraction.

Electrochemical pressure has been measured in a single cardiac muscle fiber by techniques involving glass microelectrodes inserted directly into the sarcomere (Fig. 1–20). Expressed in millivolts, changes in transmembrane potential throughout the process of contraction and relaxation have been recorded.

The changes in transmembrane potential that occur through an entire cycle of contraction and relaxation are called the **action potential**. The action potential of an individual sarcomere will be described briefly. The electrochemical events represented are similar to those involved in the specialized cells and in the cells that are responsible for cardiac pacemaker activity and impulse conduction. Consequently, the sarcomere

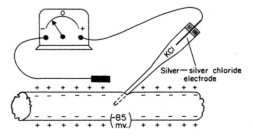

Figure 1–20. Measurement of the membrane potential of the nerve fiber using a microelectrode. (From Guyton AC: Basic Human Physiology: Normal Function and Mechanisms of Disease. WB Saunders, Philadelphia, 1977.)

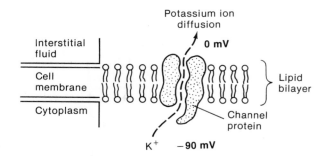

Figure 1-21. Transmembrane potential of the resting sarcomere.

can serve as a model for gaining a basic understanding of the action potential; this information will then serve as a foundation for developing a working concept of the electrophysiology of the heartbeat. Confident interpretation of the disorders of cardiac rhythm depends on sound knowledge of the causal mechanisms at a cellular level. Further, such knowledge is the basis for the rationale for modern treatment of these disorders through pharmacological and electronic interventions.

The transmembrane potential represents the electrical current at any instant developed between the extracellular and the intracellular fluid (that is, across the cell membrane). The transmembrane potential of the resting cell (diastole) is depicted in graphic terms in Figure 1-21. Here, the fully charged (or resting) sarcomere has an electrical gradient of 90 millivolts (mv), the interior of the cell being electrically **negative** in relationship to the exterior. Supposing that the cell were totally neutral (i.e., the distribution of similar ions on either side of the cell membrane were equal); then the transmembrane potential would be zero (and, of course, the cell would possess no stored energy).

The most important factor in development of the transmembrane potential is the leakage of potassium ions from inside the cell into the interstitial fluid that bathes the exterior of the cells. Because each potassium ion carries a positive charge, the interior of the cell becomes electrically negative.

In the cardiac sarcomere, potassium ions leak out of the cell until the transmembrane potential decreases to about -90 mv. At this level, the cell membrane becomes impermeable to potassium ions and further exodus ceases. The cell has then reached its fully **polarized** state and will remain so as long as the sarcomere enjoys adequate oxygen, nutrients, removal of metabolic by-products, and favorable temperature, or until it receives an external stimulus causing the release of its stored energy.

During the resting state of high electrical tension, the cell membrane also maintains a virtually impermeable barrier to sodium and calcium ions. Normally at a concentration or 140 to 150 mEq/liter in the extracellular fluid, sodium is only about 10 mEq/liter in the intracellular fluid of the sarcoplasm (Fig. 1-22). Calcium ions are normally at a concentration of approximately 5 mEq/liter (or 10 millimoles/liter) in the extracellular fluid and less than 1 mEq/liter in the intracellular.

The Activated Sarcomere

On stimulation by any force of sufficient intensity—whether electrical, mechanical, or chemical— the voltage gradient across the cell membrane undergoes an abrupt and profound change. This disturbance results in the contraction and relaxation sequence of the sarcomere.

The span during which the sarcomere discharges its stored energy and then replenishes it is separated by convention into five distinct intervals, designated Phase 0

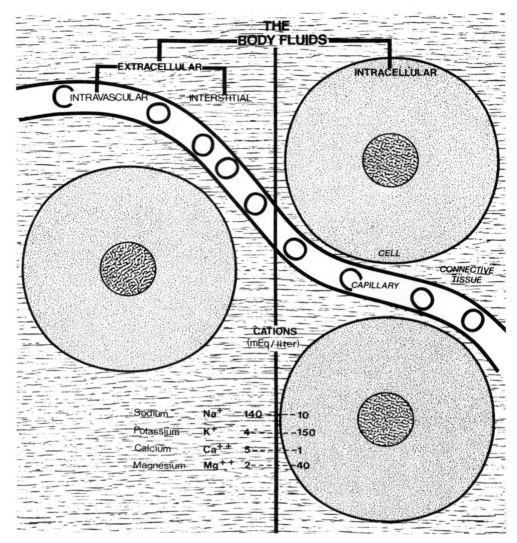

Figure 1–22. Distribution of the body fluids in tissue, with concentrations of the major cations in the extracellular and intracellular compartments.

through Phase 4 (Fig. 1–23). The explanation of action potentials begins with a description of Phase 4, representing the fully polarized state of the resting sarcomere in which a maximum negative voltage gradient is established. The steps in release and restoration of this energy will now be presented.

PHASE 0: DEPOLARIZATION

When excited by a stimulus of sufficient magnitude, the sarcomere abruptly discharges its stored energy. This sudden loss of polarity, Phase 0, is referred to as **depolarization**. It is accomplished by the following mechanism:

The wall of the cell contains "gates" that are impermeable to sodium ions when the cell is in its fully polarized, or resting, state despite great differences in sodium concentration in the extracellular and the intracellular fluid. An external stimulus alters the cell membrane in such a way as to suddenly open up these gates to sodium ions (see Fig. 1–23). With the stimulus-activated change in permeability, sodium pours into the cell. Because this influx is so rapid, the entry sites are called **fast channels**. To be effective in initiating the change in permeability, the stimulus must be of sufficient intensity to open up enough channels to cause an **all-or-none** reaction.

The surge of positively charged sodium ions into the cell obliterates the electrical gradient instantly. The transmembrane potential shifts from the electronegative charge of −90 mv to electrical neutrality. However, the sodium influx is so massive that a small electrically positive "overshoot" is created to about +10 mv at the end of the depolarizing event. (This brief period of intracellular positive transmembrane potential is known as **reverse potential**.) Represented graphically, Phase 0 is aptly named the **rapid upstroke** or **spike potential** of the action potential curve.

The spike potential expresses the release of electrical energy developed by the sarcomere. In turn, this energy initiates the interaction of myosin and actin filaments, thereby expending the energy for biological work in the form of shortening the muscle cell. In addition, the energy serves as a stimulus to adjoining sarcomeres, thus passing the electrical disturbance from cell to cell, each transference bringing about a similar discharge of energy (and subsequent contraction) until all the sarcomeres in the syncytium have been depolarized.

The description of the action potential now turns to the subsequent steps by which the depolarized sarcomere restores its electrochemical energy: the process of **repolarization**. These steps depend on the metabolic work performed by the cell membrane to shift the electrolytes against their own concentration gradient.

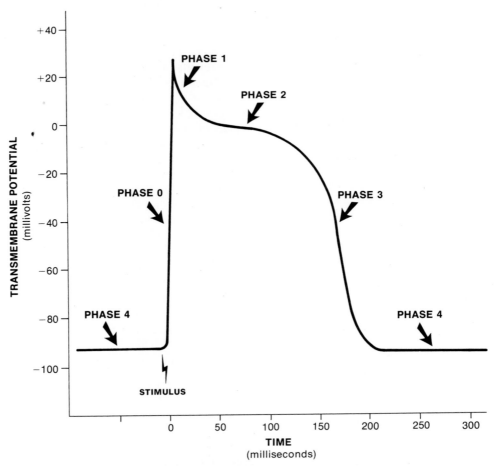

Figure 1–23. The action potential. Phases of activation of the excitable cell.

PHASE 1: EARLY REPOLARIZATION

At the peak of the rapid upstroke, the gates through which sodium moved so freely clamp shut. There follows a return in the transmembrane potential from its maximum positive charge toward zero (electrical neutrality), as is evident from the graph shown in Figure 1–23. This reduction in electropositivity, which occurs fairly rapidly, represents the beginning of restoration of cellular energy.

The movement of ions in Phase 1 probably reflects the combination of several factors, most predominantly the cessation of sodium influx. The extrusion of potassium ions from the cell also plays a role in reducing intracellular electropositivity. Further, chloride ions, possessing a negative charge, move into the cell, most likely through special chloride channels interspersed throughout the cell membrane.

PHASE 2: THE PLATEAU

As electrical neutrality is approached in Phase 1 repolarization, the slope of the action potential curve levels out somewhat abruptly (see Fig. 1–23). The plateau thus formed is the longest segment of the entire action potential and is referred to as Phase 2. This delay in repolarization is determined principally by the late entry of calcium ions into the cell.

The cell membrane contains channels that transport calcium preferentially. However, calcium ions move much more slowly through these channels than does sodium through the fast channels. Consequently, they are known as the **slow channels** for calcium. Although they open as soon as the cell is stimulated, the bulk of calcium does not cross the cell membrane until *after* the rapid upstroke and the early recovery period. With their positive electrical charges, calcium ions exert the net effect of slowing down the rate at which the cell recovers its full electronegative potential. For much of Phase 2, this in-rush of calcium ions results in a virtual standstill in the action potential curve.

Actually, relatively small amounts of calcium enter the cell through the slow channels, not in sufficient quantity to trigger the mechanism of contraction. The increase in intracellular calcium is enough, however, to release calcium ions stored in sac-like structures, the cisternae, located in the reticulum of the sarcoplasm as shown in Figure 1–17. On release, these ions migrate from the reticulum to the depths of the sarcomere along an extensive network of fluid-filled channels. The channels, by invagination, form transverse tubules that lead directly into the myofilaments.

On contact with the receptor sites of actin, calcium ions are bound immediately to the regulator proteins. This binding alters the structural relationship of actin filaments and exposes their reactor sites to the myosin heads. It can be appreciated that the infusion of calcium ions into the regions of the myofilaments, occurring during Phase 2 of the action potential, is responsible for lifting the blocking action of the modulator proteins, thus setting the stage for the formation of electrochemical cross-bridges between actin and myosin.

In addition to the entry of calcium ions into the cell, another important event occurs in Phase 2: conductance of potassium ions back into the cell. Cellular energy is required to move potassium against its own concentration gradient—that is, from the low concentration in the extracellular fluid to the high concentration within the cell. This influx of positive charges contributes to the plateau effect of the Phase 2 curve, probably through selective channels separate from those already described.

PHASE 3: LATE REPOLARIZATION

After approximately 0.3 second, the plateau is interrupted by a distinct alteration in the slope of the action potential curve (see Fig. 1–23). The transmembrane potential now moves much more rapidly toward the fully charged electronegative state of the resting cell. This acceleration of repolarization—designated Phase 3—is the result of several forces acting in concert: cessation of entrance of calcium ions, shift again toward loss of potassium ions from the intracellular fluid, and ejection of sodium ions in the sarcomere into the extracellular fluid. This latter event is accomplished against a strong concentration gradient.

Migration of these ions in repolarization is accompanied by a receding of intracellular calcium from the contractile proteins back into the sarcoplasmic cisternae, where they are stored until the next depolarization occurs. The regulator proteins once again separate actin filaments from the myosin heads, and the contractile elements regain their resting state and relax, the sarcomere returning to its former length.

Phase 3 continues until sodium ions are nearly completely extruded from inside the cell and until the calcium ions return to their prestimulation distribution both inside and outside of the cell. In addition, potassium ions continue to leak through the cell wall. The transmembrane potential falls steadily, finally leveling off at about -90 mv, Phase 4. The cell wall then becomes resistant to further changes, and the sarcomere has returned to its original resting state, thus completing the action potential.

PHASE 4: FULL POLARIZATION

With development of the maximum transmembrane potential, the cell is metabolically recovered, now poised, ready to respond to the next stimulus by releasing its stored energy (see Fig. 1–23). As long as the sarcomere is healthy, it will maintain this stable electronegative polarity until once again confronted with an external stimulus.

On beginning the study of cardiac arrhythmias, it is essential to understand that the contractile elements of the myocardium—the sarcomeres—must be triggered to discharge by an external stimulus. In this respect, sarcomeres contrast sharply with the specialized cells of the heart that generate and conduct impulses. These cells with unstable membranes have the capacity to stimulate themselves. They will be discussed in subsequent chapters, as they determine the mechanisms responsible for cardiac rate and rhythm. First, however, the principles by which the electrical activity of the heart is recorded will be explained and the electrocardiogram introduced.

2 The Electrocardiogram

ELECTROCARDIOGRAPHIC PAPER
COMPONENTS OF THE CARDIAC CYCLE
ELECTROCARDIOGRAPHIC COMPO-
  NENTS
Review
STANDARDIZATION MARKERS
DETERMINATION OF RATE
The Ruler Method
The Grid Method
The Scan Method
THE STANDARD ELECTROCARDIOGRAM
Bipolar Limb Leads
Unipolar Limb Leads
Unipolar Precordial Leads

COMPONENT ABNORMALITIES
Chamber Enlargement
ST Segment Deviation
Q Wave Changes
T Wave Changes
QRS Axis Deviation
ARTIFACTS
CARDIAC RHYTHM MONITORING
ELECTRODE PLACEMENT FOR
  MONITORING
Suggested Electrode Placement
Alternative Systems for Monitoring
Automatic Warning Systems

The action potential described in Chapter 1 refers to the individual myocardial cell. The action potentials of large numbers of cells produce a composite waveform. Because the masses of sarcomeres in the atria and in the ventricles are not stimulated simultaneously, the processes of depolarization and repolarization are spread over a period of time. Consequently, the composite action potentials of the two sets of chambers appear quite different from that obtained from an individual sarcomere. Recorded from the skin surface, this summation of myocardial action potentials creates the **electrocardiogram (ECG)**.

Electrical activity from the heart emits small currents on the body surface. In fact, skeletal muscles produce electrical disturbances on the body surface as well (which is the basis of the electromyogram). However, these skeletal muscle currents are not visible in the ECG when the subject is lying at rest. The surface currents produced by cardiac activity are extremely small, so that an electrical amplifier is necessary to generate visible complexes on a recording. The instrument devised for recording the surface electrical activity of the heart is called an **electrocardiograph** (Fig. 2–1).

The electrocardiograph transmits the emitted electrical activity to a sensing component through wires connected to electrodes that are placed on the skin. On reception, these electrical disturbances are amplified and transcribed onto recording paper by a vertically moving pen or stylus. This written image of cardiac electrical activity is typically produced by contact of the paper with a heated or inked stylus. By convention,

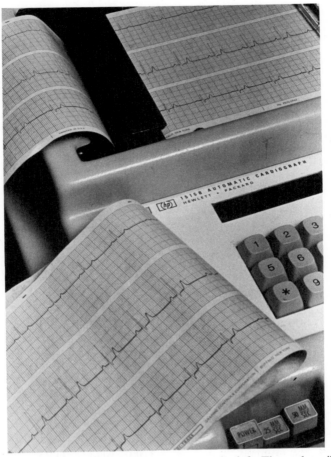

Figure 2–1. The electrocardiograph. The paper moves to the left. The stylus vibrates vertically.

an upward deflection of the stylus is designated **positive**; a downward deflection, **negative** (Fig. 2–2).

The form of the ECG represents an interaction between the vertically moving stylus and the horizontally moving paper. When no electrical activity is emitted by the heart, the stylus does not deflect and the moving paper records a straight line. Because the net effect of electrical activity is in neither a positive nor a negative direction, the straight line occurs at a zero point on the recording paper, a reference point known as the **baseline** or the **isoelectric line**.

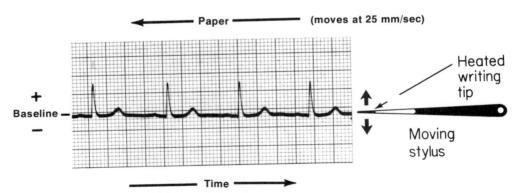

Figure 2–2. Representation of the activity of an electrocardiograph.

The ECG reflects the intensity and the direction of all electrical activity generated by the heart at any given instant in time. These events are a function of stylus oscillations. In addition, the ECG, by presenting a sequential series of instantaneous points, prints a continuous recording on which the duration of events can be determined, using a standardized rate of paper movement.

As the reader progresses in this study, he or she must keep in mind that the ECG represents a continuum of electrical disturbances emitted by the heart. In turn, these disturbances are a composite of depolarization-repolarization activity occurring in all sarcomeres at each instant. Furthermore, the ECG does *not* measure the contraction-relaxation processes themselves; the mechanical events of muscle activity are the aftermath of the electrical events recorded.

ELECTROCARDIOGRAPHIC PAPER

To facilitate measuring the electrical activity of the heart, the paper on which the ECG is recorded has standardized grid markings (Fig. 2–3). By convention, the grid lines, in both the vertical and horizontal directions, are exactly 1 mm apart. (The illustration provided here is enlarged five times to better display the details.) For more convenient inspection, every fifth line, both horizontally and vertically, is imprinted more heavily.

Because deviations of the stylus caused by electrical currents occur in the vertical plane, the magnitude of deviation is measured by the 1-mm gradations of the horizontal lines. In the electrocardiographic cycle presented in Figure 2–4, measure from the baseline to the peak of the largest upward deflection. Its magnitude is 13.5 mm in a positive direction. The millimeter value, when applied to the height of deflections, is often converted to a millivolt value (1 mm = 1 mv).

Elapsed time on the ECG is measured by the vertical grid lines. The paper moves against the stylus from a right to left position so that events on electrocardiographic paper are always read from left to right. The standard rate for passing the paper past the stylus is 25 mm per second. At this speed, the distance between vertical grid lines represents 0.04 second (see Fig. 2–4). The distance between five vertical grid lines is 0.20 second (the time elapsed from one heavy vertical line to the next). One second is represented by 25 1-mm vertical lines, or more conveniently by five heavy vertical lines.

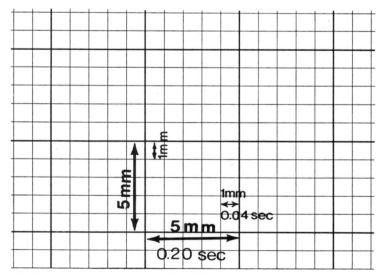

Figure 2–3. Grid dimensions of electrocardiographic paper.

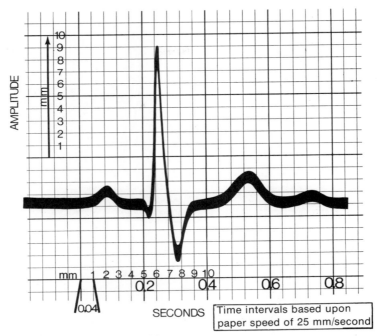

Figure 2–4. The electrocardiographic grid system.

COMPONENTS OF THE CARDIAC CYCLE

Normally, the heart is activated in a well-defined, sequential order in which atrial depolarization precedes ventricular depolarization. To illustrate the system of activation, we use a schematic view of the heart throughout the book. In Figure 2–5, all four chambers are shown with the atrial and the ventricular septa cut in cross section. Each site of impulse formation and the conduction pathways will be presented with this diagram for reference.

The process of electrical activation begins in a small nest of specialized cells situated high in the right atrium. Referred to collectively as the **sinus node** (Fig. 2–6), these cells periodically discharge an electrical impulse that then spreads through the various regions of the heart. Although other cells in the heart are also capable of emitting impulses spontaneously, the sinus node has the most frequent inherent rate of firing. Consequently, it serves as the dominant pacemaker of the heart.

Although the sinus node generates an impulse of enough intensity to transfer energy to adjacent tissues, the electrical disturbance is so small that the energy transmitted to the body surface cannot be picked up by the electrocardiograph. Thus, depolarization of the sinus node—the first step in the cardiac cycle— is electrocardiographically **silent** because it produces no movement of the stylus.

The electrical impulse emitted by the sinus node spreads to sarcomeres in the surrounding right atrium (Fig. 2–7). From there, the impulse propagates from one cell to another until the entire myocardial wall of both atria is depolarized. The general direction of the wave front created is from right to left and from the upper atria downward. As the wave of depolarization progresses, an infinite number of sequential electrical disturbances occur; they deflect the stylus and result in inscription of a continuous electrocardiographic deflection on the moving paper. The wave front causes the stylus to rise to a peak; then it falls as electrical activity in the atria gradually subsides. The figure inscribed by depolarization of the atria is designated the **P wave**.

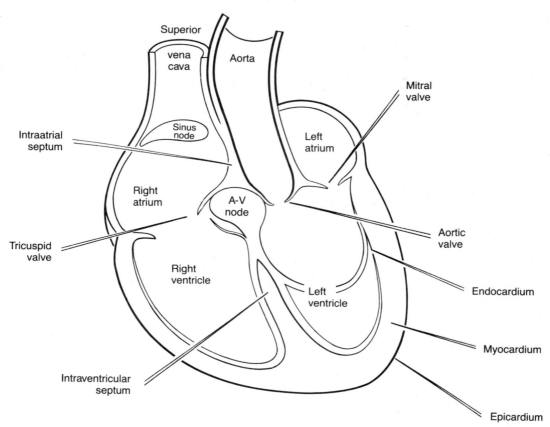

Figure 2–5. Basic anatomy of the heart.

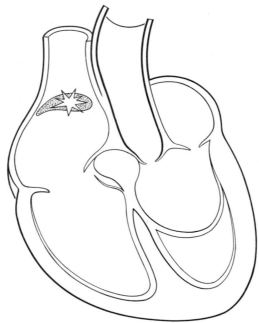

Figure 2–6. Impulse formed in the sinus node.

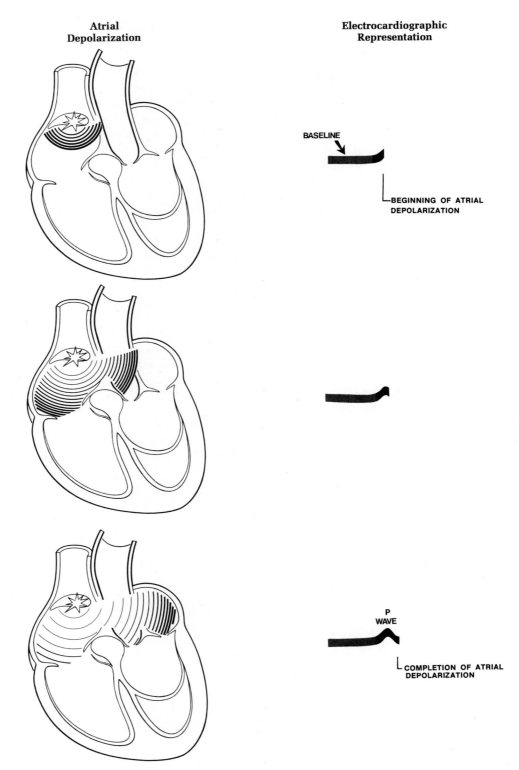

Figure 2–7. Atrial impulse conduction.

The processes of repolarization of the atria must occur to restore kinetic energy. However, the electrocardiographic deflections produced are relatively small. Because these deflections generally occur simultaneously with depolarization of the ventricles, a far greater electrical event, atrial repolarization is usually obscured on the ECG.

As impulses transmitted through the atria reach the junction between atria and ventricles, they stimulate another cluster of specialized cells located in the lower intraatrial septum (Fig. 2–8). Called the **atrioventricular** (or A-V) node, these cells form pathways for impulse conduction, serving as an electrical bridge from the atria to the ventricles. Depolarization of the A-V node is relatively slow, and only a minute amount of electrical energy is released. As a result, the segment on the ECG occurring at the time of A-V node depolarization is electrically silent, and the stylus remains at the baseline for a brief period immediately after the P wave. This duration from the beginning of atrial activation to the beginning of ventricular activation is called the **PR interval**.

Emerging from the A-V node, impulses enter the ventricles by way of a compact tract of conducting fibers, the **bundle of His**, or common bundle, which straddles the proximal portion of the intraventricular septum (Fig. 2–9). From there, impulses continue into the ventricles as the common bundle separates into a **right branch** and a **left branch**. These branches provide routes for rapid conduction of the impulses throughout the intraventricular septum and to the endocardial surface of the free ventricular walls. The terminal elements of this conduction pathway system are the **Purkinje fibers**.

Figure 2–10 illustrates the components of normal conduction from sinus node activation to Purkinje fiber response in a schematic format.

From the Purkinje fibers, impulses penetrate to the interior of the ventricular myocardium, setting off a succession of depolarizations of sarcomeres and resulting in ventricular contraction (Fig. 2–11). The depolarizing wave front progresses from endocardial to epicardial surfaces of the wall.

The sequence of activation of the ventricles can be divided into three overlapping phases. Ventricular depolarization begins in the intraventricular septum, normally proceeding from the left toward the right surface. In the second phase, the right ventricle is activated, usually resulting in a sudden change in the electrocardiographic inscription. This event is then followed by depolarization of the much larger muscle mass of the left ventricle, which then dominates the inscription. As depolarization in both ventricles subsides, the stylus returns to baseline.

The entire sequence of ventricular depolarization represented on the ECG is called the **QRS complex** (Fig. 2–12). The components of the QRS complex will be defined shortly, under Electrocardiographic Components. It is enough to mention at this point that depolarization of the ventricles involves a large muscle mass (compared with the atria) and that it occurs very rapidly. Thus, the inscription produced is generally much

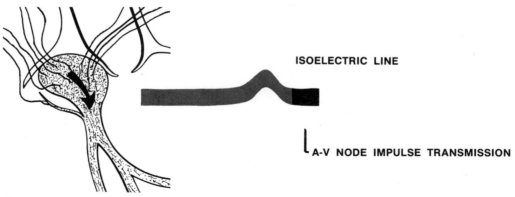

ISOELECTRIC LINE

A-V NODE IMPULSE TRANSMISSION

Figure 2–8. The atrioventricular node.

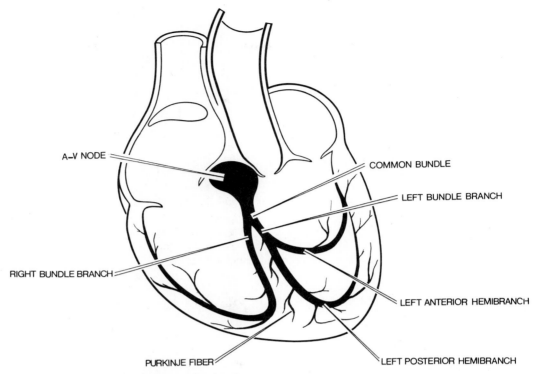

Figure 2–9. Anatomy of the conduction system.

greater in amplitude than the P wave, and it has much sharper angles. The thinner line inscribed reflects the faster-moving stylus.

Immediately after the QRS complex, a period of low electrical activity appears, an interval referred to as the **ST segment** (Fig. 2–13). This portion of the cardiac cycle is usually observed as an isoelectric line or one having a gradual sloping configuration toward the baseline.

As must occur in all excitable tissues of the neuromuscular system, the ventricles repolarize before subsequent activation can take place once again. The repolarization phase causes a prominent figure on the ECG, designated the **T wave** (Fig. 2–14). Be-

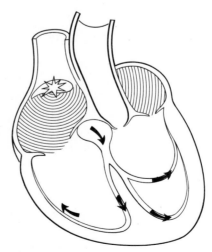

Figure 2–10. Pathways of conduction.

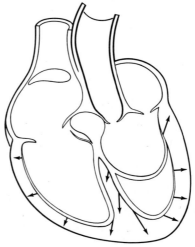

Figure 2–11. Early ventricular depolarization.

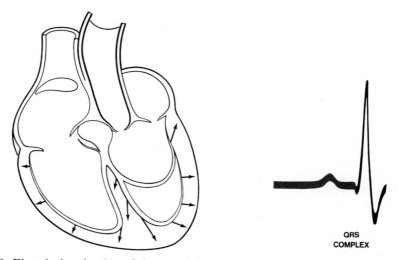

Figure 2–12. Electrical activation of the ventricles.

QRS
COMPLEX

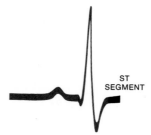

ST
SEGMENT

Figure 2–13. Period of electrical inactivity.

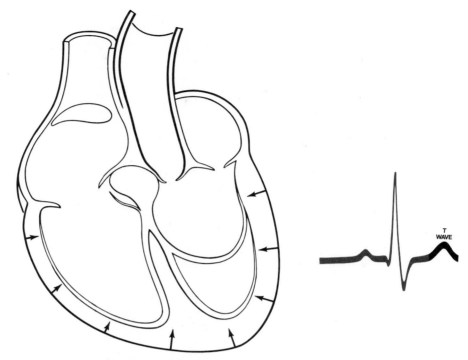

Figure 2–14. Ventricular repolarization.

cause this process is relatively slow, inscription of the T wave is considerably longer than that of the QRS complex, and the configuration is much less angular.

The major electrical forces of repolarization of the ventricles are transmitted from the epicardial to the endocardial surface. Therefore, the T wave deflection is generally in the same direction as the largest deflection of the QRS complex.

The last component of the cardiac cycle is a small, rounded deflection called a **U wave** (Fig. 2–15). The electrophysiological events responsible for this inscription are uncertain. One explanation is that the U wave represents repolarization of the Purkinje fibers themselves, occurring at a definitive time after the ventricular sarcomeres have repolarized.

Having reviewed the nomenclature ascribed to various components of the cardiac cycle, the reader may be interested in the historical basis for this chosen alphabetical sequence. At the beginning of this century, the science of electrocardiography emerged. At that time, general physiology had already developed at a rapid rate. Because so many physiological phenomena had already been described according to alphabetical designation, starting with the letter A, the acknowledged founder of electrocardiography, Willem Einthoven of Leyden, the Netherlands, appreciated the desirability of

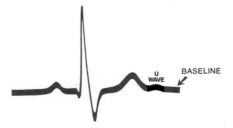

Figure 2–15. Late repolarization.

having more distinctive terminology. Thus were derived the symbols assigned to the ECG: the letters PQRST. It was Einthoven, incidentally, who introduced the string galvanometer to better observe electrophysiological actions and the photograph to record them.

ELECTROCARDIOGRAPHIC COMPONENTS

To identify components of the cardiac cycle correctly by electrocardiography, it is easiest first to locate the QRS complex. Of course, this component is not the initial event in the cardiac cycle, but its distinctive features render it a useful landmark. The QRS complex represents a brief but intensive electrical activity occurring in a large muscle mass, the ventricles. Its rapid inscription thus produced consists of a thin line with sharply angular characteristics. Practice in first recognizing the QRS complex will prove rewarding for developing an approach to interpretation, particularly when the patterns of arrhythmias become more complicated. For orientation, we begin these exercises in identification with the QRS complex.

A series of relatively simple ECGs are presented here to permit identification of various components, demonstrating the great variation in form of these components

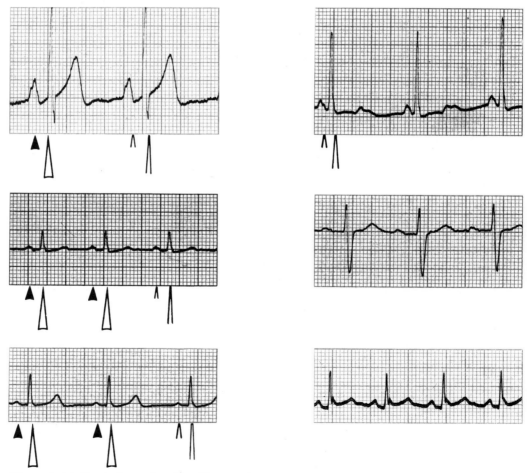

Figure 2–16. Symbols used to identify complexes.

from one tracing to another. For assisting the reader in identification, symbols for the P wave and the QRS complex are used. A short, solid arrow indicates the P wave; a tall, open arrow indicates the QRS complex (Fig. 2–16). These symbols may be hand-written (note complexes identified by hand). The beginner can adopt the symbols for annotating practice tracings. Complete the labeling of the strips in the right column.

In Figure 2–17, ECGs are presented for identifying the QRS complexes. In tracing *A*, all QRS complexes are labeled by a long, open arrow. Note that all complexes are identical in form. In tracing *B*, you should complete the labeling of the QRS complexes. Again, all complexes in the tracing are similar in configuration, but they are strikingly different from those of tracing *A*.

To review, an upward deflection on the ECG is designated **positive**; a downward deflection, **negative**. In tracing *A*, QRS complexes are wholly upward (and are thus designated positive). In tracing *B*, the QRS complexes are completely negative.

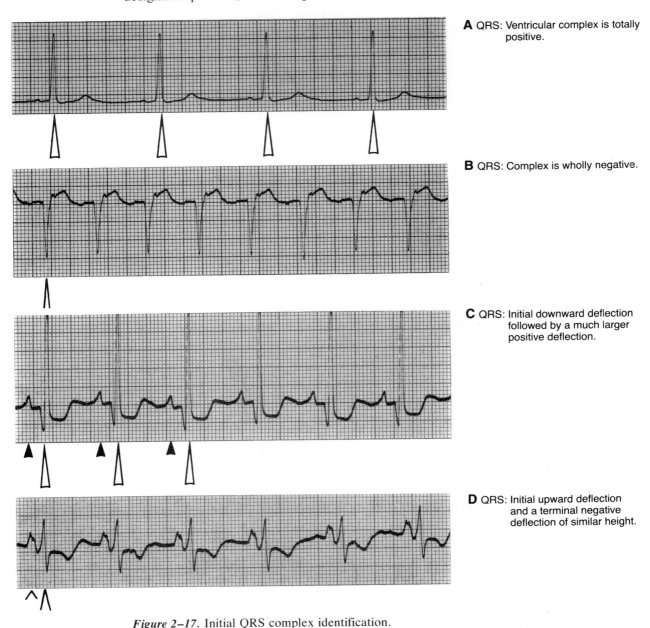

A QRS: Ventricular complex is totally positive.

B QRS: Complex is wholly negative.

C QRS: Initial downward deflection followed by a much larger positive deflection.

D QRS: Initial upward deflection and a terminal negative deflection of similar height.

Figure 2–17. Initial QRS complex identification.

Now complete the identification and marking of QRS complexes in tracings *C* and *D*. Note that in both tracings, these complexes have both upward and downward deflections. Even so, all complexes on the same tracing are identical and easy to identify because of their thin-lined and sharply pointed characteristics.

Components of the QRS complex follow standardized nomenclature. The initial deflection, if it is downward (negative), is called the **Q wave**. Q waves are designated in the tracings on the left (Fig. 2–18). Label the Q waves in the tracings on the right. Note the great differences in amplitude of these waves.

The **R wave** is the first upward component of the QRS complex. It may follow an initial downward deflection (Q wave) or may be the initial deflection of the QRS complex. Sometimes the R wave is the only figure of the complex, being a single positive deflection. Variations of R waves are presented in Figure 2–19 for identification and labeling. Large differences in amplitude of this component are obvious.

A downward deflection immediately following the R wave is called the **S wave**. Once again, variations in amplitude are evident in the examples given for identification (Fig. 2–20).

The QRS complex sometimes consists of a simple downward deflection (wholly negative). This variation is referred to as a **QS complex**. A tracing with this configuration is provided in Figure 2–21.

The QRS complex occasionally contains a second upright deflection immediately after the S wave. It is called **R prime** (written R′). Mark this component in the example given in Figure 2–22.

In the same format, a downward deflection that follows an R′ is referred to as **S prime** (S′). An example of S′ is provided in Figure 2–23 for identification.

Having established the identity of the QRS complex, next look for the P wave,

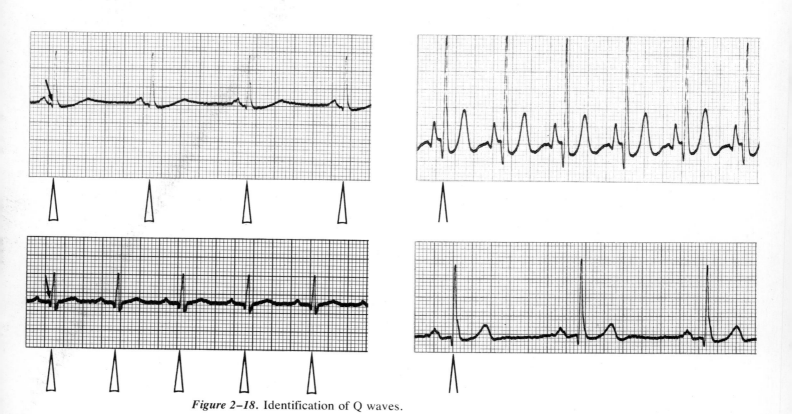

Figure 2–18. Identification of Q waves.

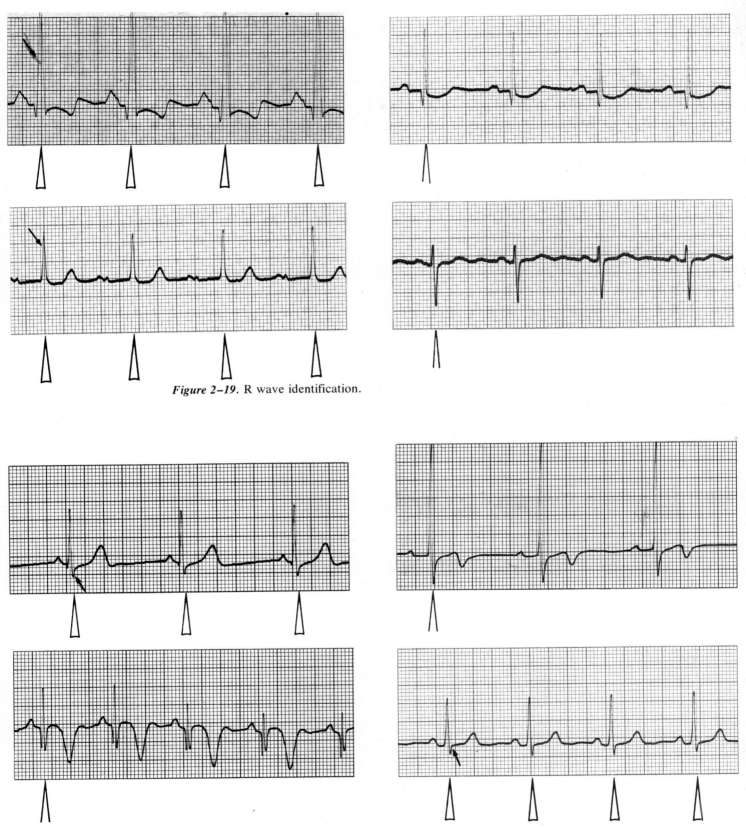

Figure 2–19. R wave identification.

Figure 2–20. Identification of S waves.

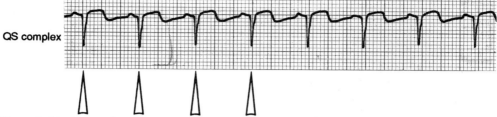

QS complex

Figure 2–21. A completely negative deflection is called a QS complex.

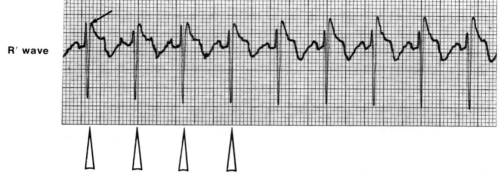

R′ wave

Figure 2–22. Ventricular complex with R′ component.

which normally precedes it (to the left). The contour of P waves is much less sharply angular than that of QRS complexes, and the line inscribed is considerably thicker. The configuration of P waves may be upright, downward, biphasic (having two directions), rounded, or bipeaked, as demonstrated in the examples in Figure 2–24. Locate the QRS complex in each tracing on the right, then the P wave inscribed immediately before, labeling the latter with a small, closed arrow.

Amplitude is an unreliable criterion for distinguishing QRS complexes from P waves, because the latter may not always be larger. Examples of this are presented in Figure 2–25. Label both P waves and QRS complexes of all cardiac cycles.

Close examination reveals that the P wave terminates at the baseline and that the inscription remains isoelectric until the onset of the QRS complex. The total duration of the P wave plus that of the isoelectric period defines an extremely important measurement in electrocardiography—the **PR interval**. The range of this interval in normal individuals is between 0.12 and 0.20 second. For practice, this range of normal is found in the tracings in Figure 2–26. Remembering that the interval between two vertical lines represents 0.04 second, the PR interval should be easy to determine.

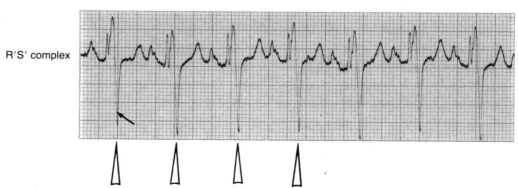

R′S′ complex

Figure 2–23. Complex with both R′ and S′ components.

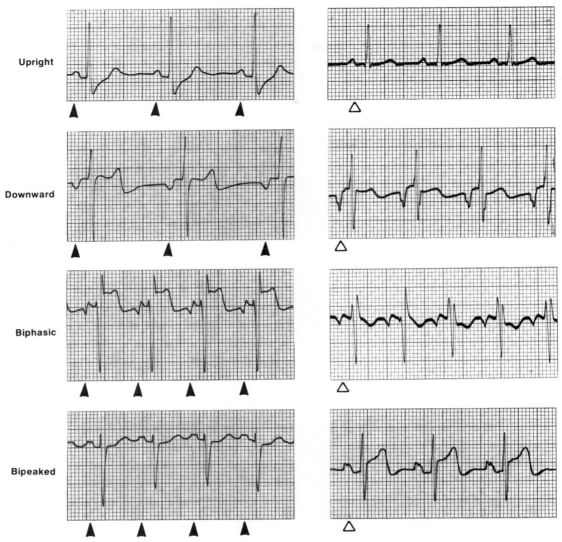

Figure 2–24. Variability of P wave configuration.

The PR interval allows for the optimal synchronization of atrial and ventricular contractions. After the P wave, the atria eject blood into the ventricles. The isoelectric silence of the A-V node conduction time permits completion of atrial contraction before activation of the ventricles. If the ventricles contracted immediately, they would contain a lesser amount of blood, and the stroke volume during ventricular systole would be decreased.

The normal QRS duration is 0.11 second or less; it is abnormal if longer than 0.12 second (Fig. 2–27). A QRS complex falling between these two definitive limits is equivocal. Of course, very careful measurements are required to make distinctions in this

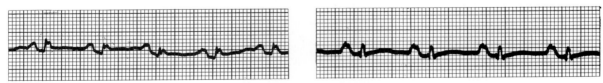

Figure 2–25. P wave amplitude exceeds the height of the QRS complex.

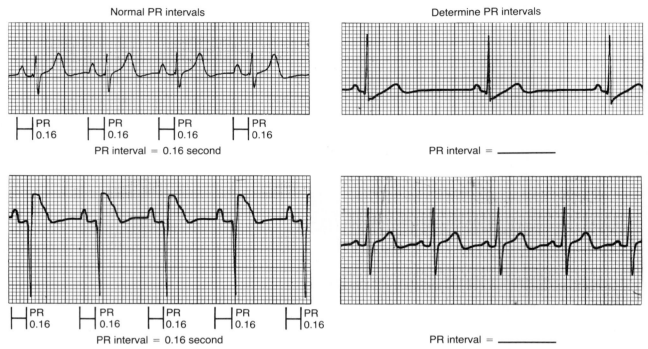

Figure 2–26. PR interval duration within normal range of 0.12 second to 0.20 second.

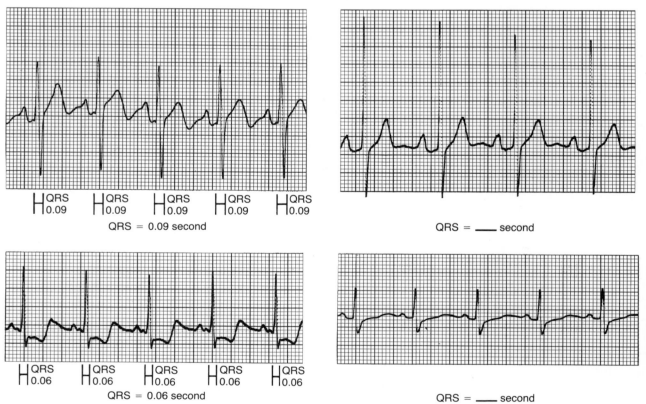

Figure 2–27. Normal duration of the QRS of less than 0.11 second. Determine the durations of the QRS complexes in the two unmeasured rhythm strips.

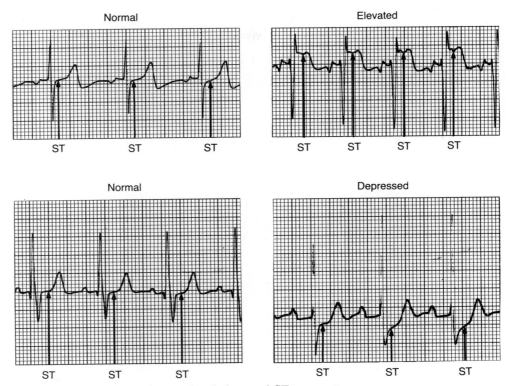

Figure 2–28. Comparison of normal and abnormal ST segments.

intermediate range. The tracings that follow provide opportunities to measure the intervals of the QRS complexes.

The terminal portion of the QRS complex leads into the isoelectric (or nearly so) line known as the **ST segment**. This period represents the relatively inactive phase of ventricular physiology, the delay following depolarization and preceding repolarization. The ST segment ends at the beginning of the T wave. This separation is sometimes quite arbitrary when there are gradually merging contours. In abnormal states, the ST segment may be displaced off the isoelectric line (either elevated or depressed) or may exhibit an upward or a downward slope. Several examples of normal and abnormal ST segments are shown for identification (Fig. 2–28).

The **T wave**, corresponding to repolarization or recovery of the ventricles after depolarization, occurs after the more or less isoelectric ST segment. The transition is usually gradual, and the contour of the T wave gently curved. T waves occur in many different forms: simple upright or downward, double peaked, rounded, acutely angular, nearly flat or extremely tall, and sometimes biphasic. A T wave always occurs after a QRS complex, even though it may be difficult to observe because of low amplitude. Examples of various forms of T waves are provided for labeling (Fig. 2–29). In each of these tracings, locate the QRS complex *first*, then the P wave that precedes it. Scan the entire tracing to ascertain that the coupling of P waves and QRS complexes is consistent throughout. Finally locate the T wave, observing its amplitude and configuration.

Because of the possible variability in the T wave appearance, identification of this cycle component may be difficult, especially in the presence of some abnormal rhythms.

The **U wave**, which follows the T wave, is always relatively small in amplitude and has gradual contours. It is often very difficult or even impossible to discern the U wave because of its inconspicuous nature. Because the U wave may become confused with either P waves or T waves, it is important to identify U waves with the highest degree

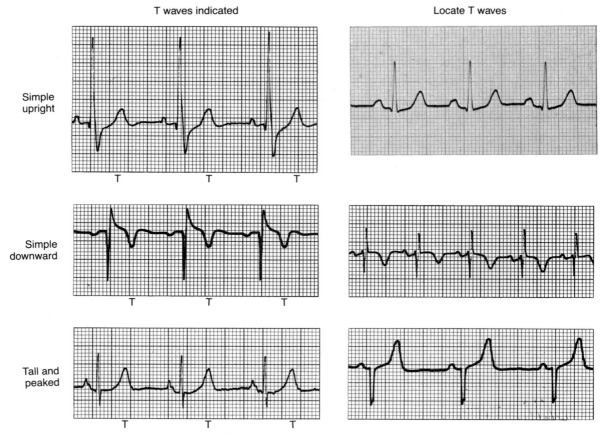

Figure 2–29. Identification of T waves.

of confidence. Ordinarily, an isoelectric line separates the T wave and U wave, but this is not always so. It may fall on the terminal slope of the preceding T wave or even on the succeeding P wave. In any case, it must be appreciated that the U wave is a component of the preceding cardiac cycle and that in irregular rhythms it falls in a consistent time relationship with the preceding T wave, not with the P wave that follows it.

A U wave is not always a component of the electrocardiographic cycle. It is most often seen in tachyarrhythmias or electrolyte abnormalities. The significance of its presence or absence is not clearly understood.

U waves are present in each of the tracings in Figure 2–30. In each, the reader should now be able to correctly label the P wave, QRS complex (and its various components), ST segment, T wave, and U wave.

A pictorial summary of the electrocardiographic components described is presented in Figure 2–31 in stylized version for clarity. Each designated feature of the represented cardiac cycle should be well understood before proceeding further.

In the ECGs in Figure 2–32 (all taken from adults), the reader should select one cardiac cycle in each tracing and label each component of that cycle. Then compare this cycle with all others in the tracing, noting shape, height (amplitude), and width (duration) of each component, and compare with the corresponding component of the adjacent cycles. Remarkable similarity can be observed throughout. With each tracing, do not forget to identify a QRS complex first; then use this component as a reference point for finding the other components of that cardiac cycle.

Figure 2–30. Correctly label the P wave, QRS complex, ST segment, T wave, and U wave on strips A and B.

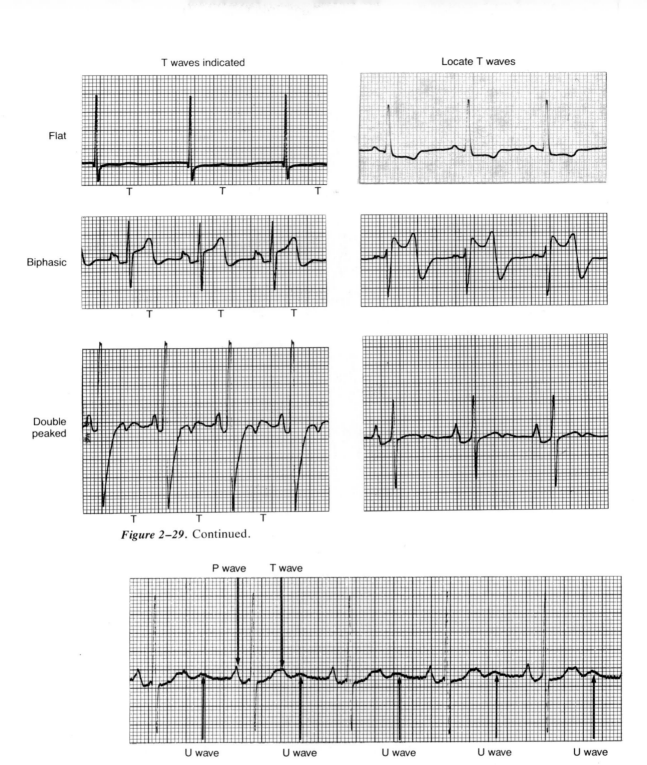

Flat

T waves indicated

Locate T waves

T   T   T

Biphasic

T   T   T

Double
peaked

T   T   T

Figure 2–29. Continued.

P wave   T wave

U wave   U wave   U wave   U wave   U wave

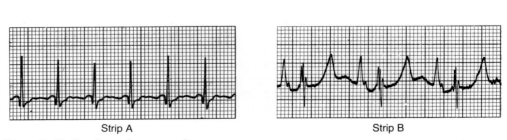

Strip A

Strip B

Figure 2–30. See legend on opposite page.

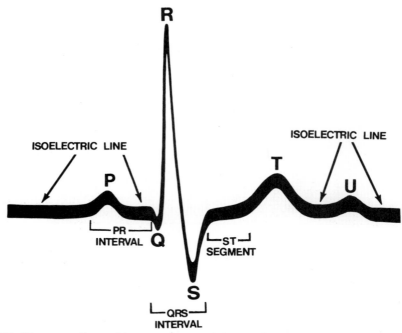

Figure 2–31. Electrocardiographic components of the cardiac cycle.

Review

The electrophysiological events that are represented by the ECG are summarized in Table 2–1. Correlating each event with the appropriate figure on the ECG in Figure 2–33 will reinforce the basic understanding of the normal cardiac cycle.

STANDARDIZATION MARKERS

The electrocardiograph amplifies electrical signals from the body surface. To ensure that the degree of amplification is the same on each recording, an adjustable reference marker is provided. A key on the instrument deflects the stylus for testing. By convention, the amount of deflection from baseline is 10 mm, and this amplitude indicates that amplification is 10 millivolts. A knob for adjusting the deflection is used to bring it to exactly 10 mm. The deflection must originate directly from the baseline; those that are superimposed on a component of the cardiac cycle must be ignored. Typical standardization markers are shown in the ECGs in Figure 2–34.

For clinical electrocardiography, the adjustment of amplitude affects all components of the ECG in their vertical dimensions. Proper standardization is imperative for interpreting the size of cardiac chambers. For example, enlargement or dilation of either atrium often results in increased amplitude of the P wave. Increased wall dimension of the ventricles is associated with an increased amplitude of the QRS complex.

If the cardiac rhythm is the only focus of interest, as in rhythm monitoring, standardization of amplitude is not critical. However, it is important in interpretation that standardization markers not be mistaken for components of the cardiac cycle. Because these markers correspond to the instant that the operator depresses the standardization key, they do not fall in any constant time relationship to the natural cardiac cycle.

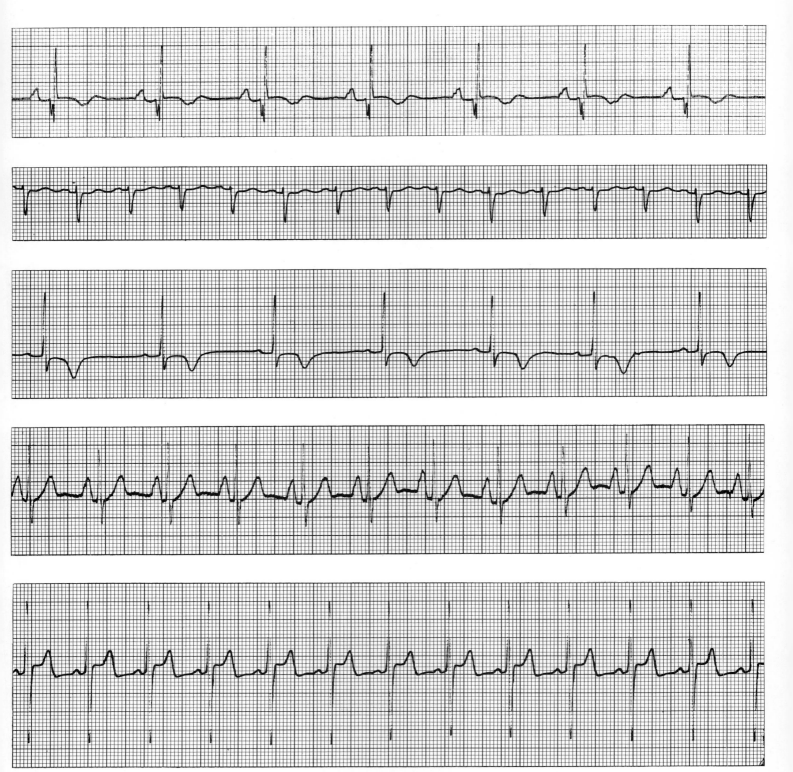

Figure 2–32. Sample rhythm strips for practice in labeling.

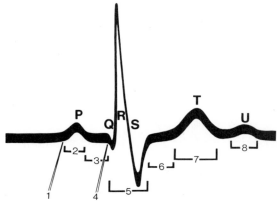

Figure 2–33. Sequential electrical events of the cardiac cycle.

Table 2–1. ELECTROPHYSIOLOGICAL EVENTS
REPRESENTED BY THE ELECTROCARDIOGRAM

Sequential Electrical Events of the Cardiac Cycle	Electrocardiographic Representation
1. Impulse from the sinus node	Not visible
2. Depolarization of the atria	P wave
3. Depolarization of the A-V node	Isoelectric
4. Repolarization of the atria	Usually obscured by the QRS complex
5. Depolarization of the ventricles	QRS complex
a. intraventricular septum	a. initial portion
b. right and left ventricles	b. central and terminal portions
6. Quiescent state of the ventricles immediately after depolarization	ST segment: isoelectric
7. Repolarization of the ventricles	T wave
8. Afterpotentials following repolarization of the ventricles	U wave

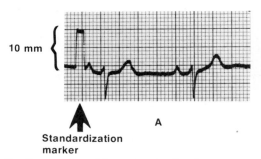

Figure 2–34. Typical deflection produced by a standardization system.

For practice, indicate the standardization marker(s) in each of the tracings in Figure 2–35. Which of these ECGs is properly standardized?

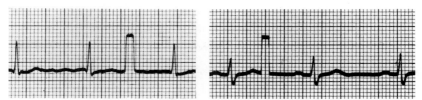

Figure 2–35. Identification of standardization artifacts.

DETERMINATION OF RATE

The rate of cardiac cycles can be determined from the ECG using several techniques. All methods presuppose that the recording was made at a standardized speed of paper movement. For clinical electrocardiography, this standard is generally accepted as 25 mm per second, the speed of all tracings presented in this book.

The Ruler Method

Considering convenience and accuracy, cardiac rate is best determined with a **rate ruler**. Such a ruler is provided on the first page inside the front cover; it can be removed and cut flush to the edges. The ruler is also useful for measuring duration of cardiac events in seconds.

THE ONE-BEAT RULER

Using the one-beat edge of the rate ruler (Fig. 2–36), place the reference arrow on a distinct point of one cardiac cycle. A point of the most prominent deflection of the QRS axis is usually most convenient, although any point can be used if the corresponding point is used in subsequent cycles. Find the identical point on the following cycle (to the right). The rate in cycles per minute is indicated at this location on the scale. In the example in Figure 2–37, the rate is 53 cycles per minute.

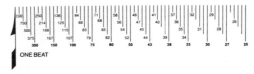

Figure 2–36. The one-beat ruler.

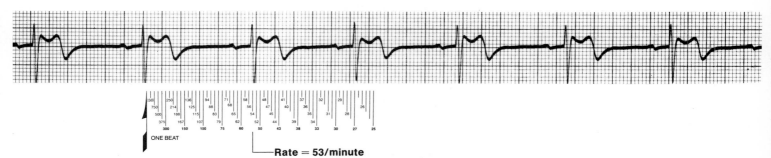

Figure 2–37. Determining the heart rate using the one-beat ruler method.

The one-beat ruler provides easy and fairly accurate measurements, particularly at slow, regular rates. It must be understood that only the interval between two consecutive beats is used to represent the rate for an entire minute. Accuracy of this extrapolation is less true the more irregularly the beats fall. To improve accuracy in highly irregular rhythms, several intervals should be sampled and an average made.

The one-beat ruler is especially handy for abnormally slow rhythms. It can be used for rhythms as slow as 25 cycles per minute. Determine the rate in the example of an extremely slow rate shown in Figure 2–38. The average rate in beats per minute is in the high 50s.

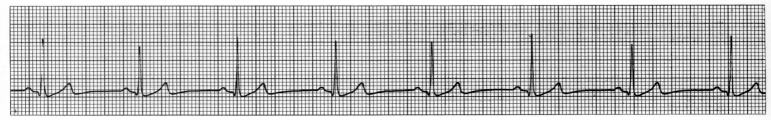

Figure 2–38. Rate determination with the one-beat ruler.

THE THREE-BEAT RULER

The three-beat ruler (Fig. 2–39) employs the same basic principles as the one-beat except that it samples across three cardiac cycles. In effect, it averages the intervals between consecutive beats so that the 1-minute extrapolation is more accurate.

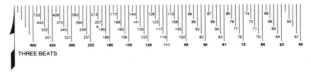

Figure 2–39. The three-beat ruler.

To use the three-beat ruler, line up the reference arrow of the ruler with a well-defined point on a cardiac cycle and count the subsequent three cycles. Read off the rate, expressed for 1 minute, on the corresponding point of the third cycle. In the example in Figure 2–40, the rate is 85 cycles per minute.

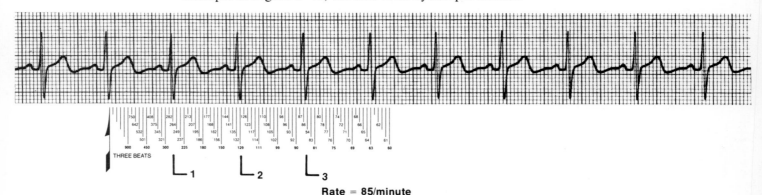

Rate = 85/minute

Figure 2–40. The three-beat ruler being used to determine rate.

Because the gradations are more gradual than on the one-beat ruler, this ruler is more accurate at rapid rates. Note that as the rate gets faster, the interval between a given rate difference becomes shorter (e.g., the actual distance between rate markings

80 and 90 is much less than between 60 and 70). This spacing follows a logarithmic scale. Determine rates in the tracings in Figure 2–41. The rate range in the top strip is 88 to 96 beats per minute; the bottom strip rate is between 150 and 160 beats per minute.

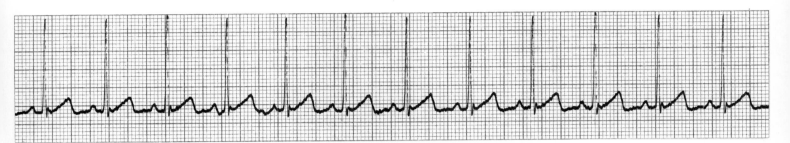

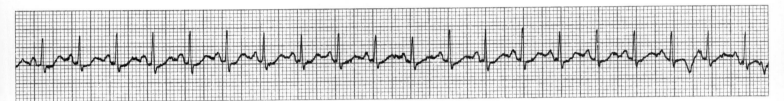

Figure 2–41. Determine rate using the three-beat ruler.

The Grid Method

Another useful method for rapidly and fairly accurately determining heart rate involves estimating the interval between two consecutive beats by the 0.2-second markers (heavy vertical lines) on the grid. In the example in Figure 2–42, identical points of the designated QRS complexes fall precisely on adjacent heavy vertical lines. Thus, cardiac cycles occur 0.2 second apart. This duration is divided into 60 to give the number of cycles in 1 minute (60.0 seconds ÷ 0.20 second = 300 beats per minute).

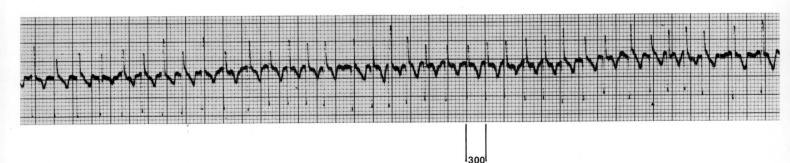

Figure 2–42. Cardiac cycles occur on heavy grid marks.

Seldom does a human heart beat as rapidly as 300 beats per minute, but this tracing is included as a demonstration of grid measuring. Actually, the tracing was obtained on a fox terrier being evaluated for a heart murmur, subsequently found to be an intraventricular septal defect.

Similarly, beats occurring at 0.4-second intervals (two heavy grid lines apart) denote a rate of 150 per minute.

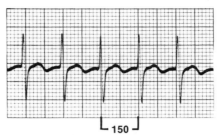

When the cardiac cycle repeats itself three heavy grid lines apart, the interval is then 0.6 second. In 1 minute, 100 such cycles occur (60 seconds ÷ 0.6 second = 100 per minute).

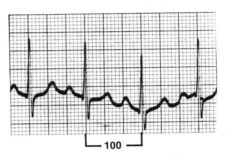

Corresponding points of adjacent cardiac cycles that are exactly 0.8 second (or 20 mm) apart indicate a rate of 75 per minute. This represents an interval of four heavy grid lines.

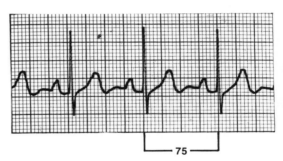

When adjacent beats are 1.0 second or five heavy grid lines apart, the rate is 60 per minute. This interval is 25 mm.

Because the normal heart rate of a resting adult is between 60 and 100 beats per minute, the three and five heavy grid line intervals serve as handy reference points for quickly determining if the cardiac rate is within normal limits.

Table 2–2 summarizes cardiac rate estimation by the grid method. Memorizing the range of normal will prove highly worthwhile in clinical work.

As with the ruler techniques, the grid method is based on equidistant cycles throughout the minute represented by adjacent beats. For exceptionally irregular rhythms, comparing several intervals is essential.

Difficulty may be encountered when no sharply defined portion of a cycle component lies precisely on a heavy grid line. In such cases, it is helpful to use calipers

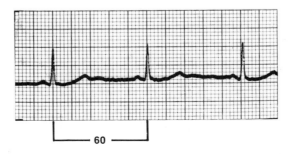

Table 2–2. THE GRID METHOD

Number of Large Squares	Interval Between Beats	Rate Per Minute	
1	0.2 sec	300	
2	0.4 sec	150	
3	0.6 sec	100 ⎫	
4	0.8 sec	75 ⎬ normal sinus rhythm	
5	1.0 sec	60 ⎭	
6	1.2 sec	50	
7	1.4 sec	43	
8	1.6 sec	37	
9	1.8 sec	33	
10	2.0 sec	30	

(mechanical dividers) (Fig. 2–43). The points of the calipers are placed on corresponding portions of adjacent beats, then moved (being careful not to alter the instrument's splay) to place one point on a heavy grid line. The second point is placed to the right along a horizontal plane, and the estimation of rate made where this point falls.

A straight edge of a piece of paper can easily substitute for calipers. Place the edge just above the tracing and mark the corresponding portions of adjacent cycles (Fig. 2–44, *top*). Then place the left marker on a heavy grid line and estimate the rate at the right marker as demonstrated in Figure 2–44, *bottom*.

Owing to the logarithmic nature of these intervals, the interpreter must take into account their peculiarities. For example, if the right marker falls exactly halfway be-

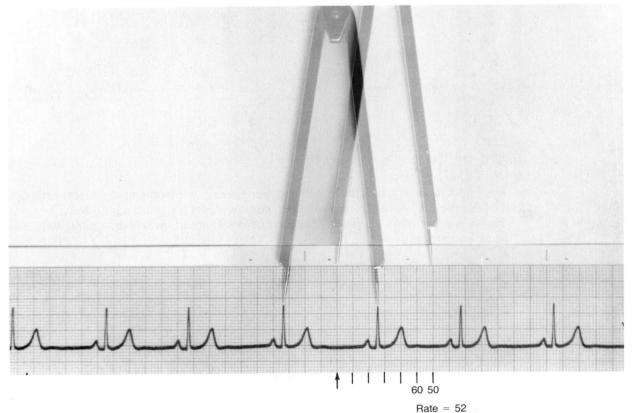

60 50

Rate = 52

Figure 2–43. Using calipers in application of the grid method for rate determination.

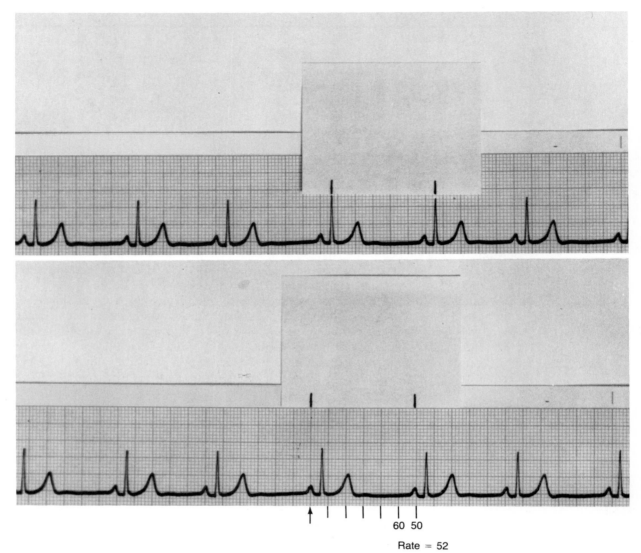

Figure 2–44. Paper edge used to facilitate grid technique.

tween 60 and 70, the rate is not 65 beats per minute. It is somewhat slower, estimated at 64 per minute. Actually, such precise measurements are seldom required in ordinary clinical interpretations, although they are of great importance when dealing with electronic pacemaker rhythms.

The Scan Method

To be strictly accurate for rate, all cardiac cycles occurring in 1 minute must be counted. This method is cumbersome, time-consuming, and wasteful of paper. An acceptable compromise, most suitable for very irregular rhythms, is available, using the markers found on the edge of most standard electrocardiographic paper. These markers are ordinarily placed at 3-second intervals (less often, 1-second intervals). Using 6-second intervals, during which all beats are counted, is highly satisfactory for ease and practicality.

There are 10 6-second intervals in 1 minute. Therefore, counting all cardiac cycles that fall between two adjacent 3-second markings will represent the rate for one-tenth

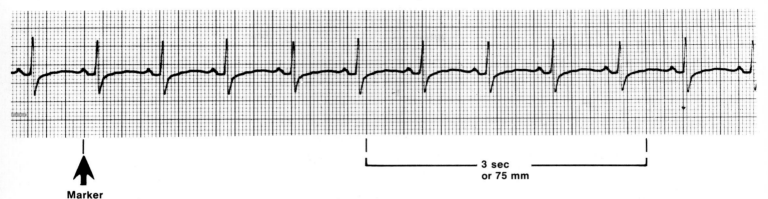

Marker

Figure 2–45. Determining rate using ECG paper interval markers.

of a minute. Simply multiplying this rate by 10 provides the rate for 1 minute. Count the number of cycles in 6 seconds in the tracing in Figure 2–45.

Calculations
Number of beats in 6 seconds	9
Number of 6-second intervals in 1 minute	<u>10</u>
Beats per minute (9 times 10)	90

The scan method is most useful for rhythms exhibiting extreme irregularity. However, it is also helpful when the rate is so extremely slow that it is beyond the scale of a rate ruler. Accuracy, on the other hand, is greater at rapid rates. Determine rates using the scan method in the tracings in Figure 2–46, representing rates of great variability. The average rates are 40, 130, and 70 beats per minute, respectively, from top to bottom.

THE STANDARD ELECTROCARDIOGRAM

Recordings made from electrical signals emitted from the body surface vary in configuration according to the sites at which the electrodes are placed. The standard ECG employs consistent electrode sites. In addition, a system has been devised in which signals from surface current are "summarized" by several electrodes, which then serve as a single electrode. Each combination of electrodes used for a recording is known as a **lead**. There are 12 such leads in the standard ECG.

The single-lead ECG is comparable to a single photograph taken of a three-dimensional object. The standard (12-lead) ECG resembles a series of photographs taken from different vantage points. Of course, the subject does not change, but the perspective varies with each lead. The electrocardiographer uses this information to reconstruct a stereoscopic view of the sequence of electrical activation of the heart.

In the most simple form of electrocardiographic recording, three electrodes are required. Two of these electrodes sense the electrical activity at different sites on the body (Fig. 2–47). Any difference in activity results in a flow of current between the electrodes, and this energy in turn moves the stylus. The third electrode, known as the **ground** lead, serves to eliminate electrical activity from extraneous sources.

There are two types of electrode combinations in the 12-lead ECG: bipolar and unipolar. The **bipolar** form is simply the two-electrode combination in which the electrical signal received by the electrocardiograph represents the difference in potential between the two electrodes. Ordinarily, the electrodes are placed on the extremities.

The **unipolar** system also senses the electrical potential between two poles. How-

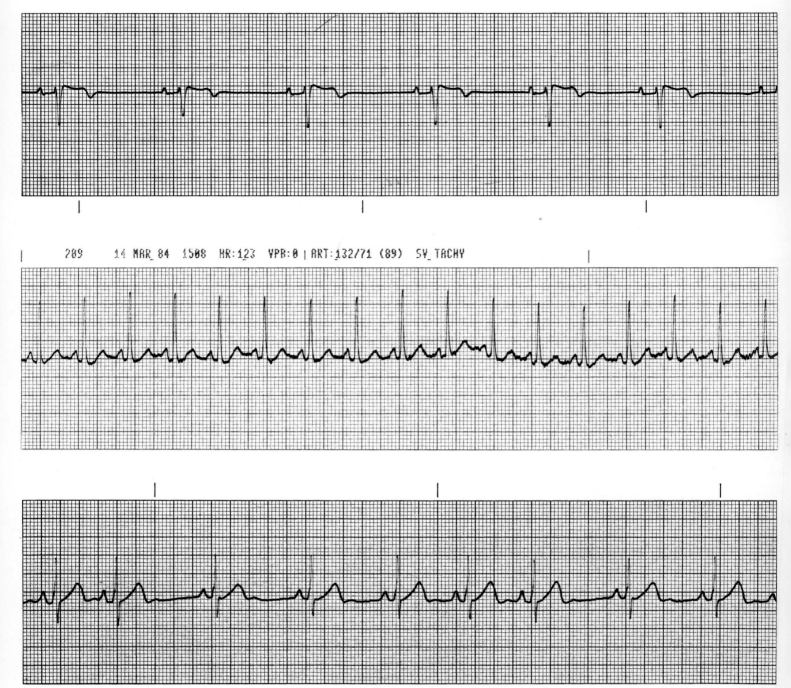

Figure 2–46. Determine the rate using the scan method.

ever, one of the poles is composed of the sum of potentials from three extremity electrodes. These potentials when combined almost completely cancel each other out so that the composite potential is virtually zero. It is therefore referred to as the **indifferent** electrode. The second pole consists of a single electrode, or **exploring** electrode. Thus, the unipolar leads record potentials between a single site and a zero point. The lead may be confined to the extremities, or the exploring electrode may be placed directly

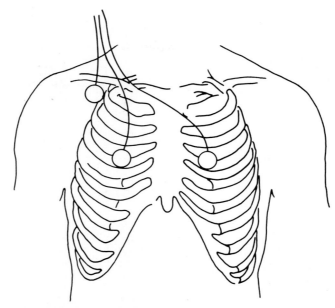

Figure 2–47. Placement of the three-electrode lead system on the thorax.

on the chest at various points. In the latter situation, the arrangement is referred to as a **precordial** lead.

In the standard ECG, the electrode attached to the right leg (color coded green and designated RL) is always a nonrecording ground lead. In all of the electrode systems, it serves to minimize interference from static electricity and other external currents.

Although cardiac rhythms usually can be interpreted from a single lead of the standard ECG, it is useful to have a basic understanding of the various leads. In addition, long-term rhythm monitoring generally requires some improvisation from the standard placement to display the optimally visualized waveforms. Therefore, a brief description of the leads from the standard ECG is provided here. The leads represented were taken from a 48-year-old man who was in excellent health and jogged daily (Fig. 2–48).

Bipolar Limb Leads

Leads I, II, and III make up the three sets of the bipolar limb leads of the standard ECG. Lead I "reads" across the chest horizontally from the right arm (RA) to the left arm (LA). Lead II records potentials diagonally across the chest, more or less along the longitudinal axis of the heart, from the right arm to the left leg (LL). Lead III senses vertically between the left arm and the left leg. Thus, the electrical activity of the heart is recorded in the frontal plane of two dimensions from three electrical sightings.

In the bipolar limb lead system (also called the triaxial system), the RA electrode is always the electrically negative pole. The LL electrode is always the electrically positive pole. The LA is positive in lead I and negative in lead III.

The electrocardiographic representation of cardiac events on the different bipolar limb leads is shown in a composite sketch (Fig. 2–49). The ECG was recorded on the same 48-year-old man with normal cardiac function. For convenience, the limb leads are transposed to the chest in a triangular form with the LL electrode in the center. For practical purposes, this transposition produces negligible change.

Remember that the processes of depolarization generally proceed from the base

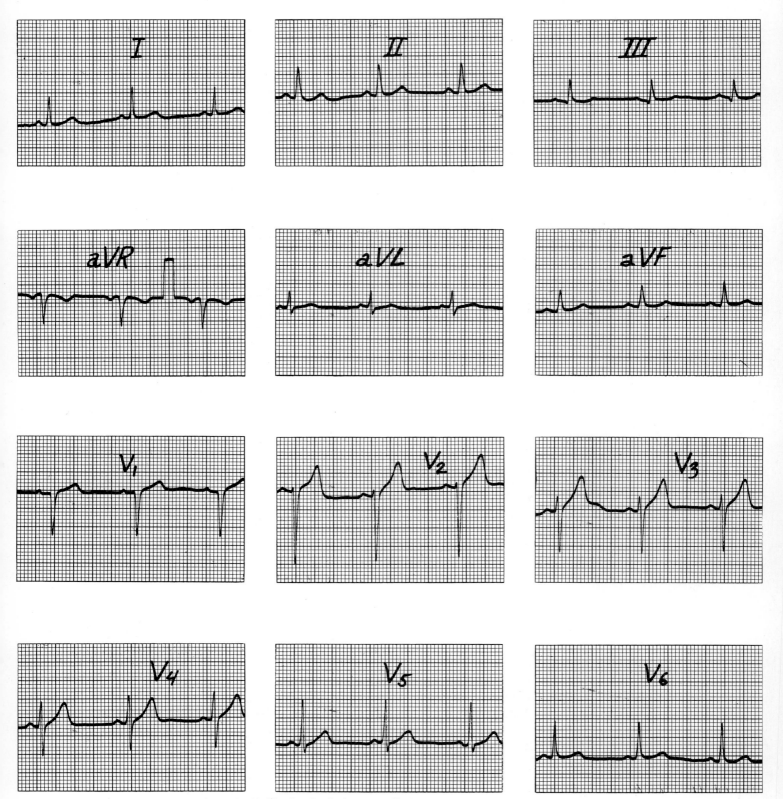

Figure 2–48. Twelve-lead electrocardiogram.

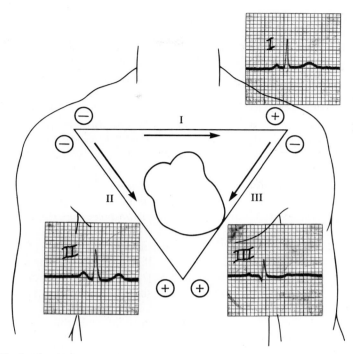

Figure 2–49. Bipolar leads.

of the heart (in the right atrium) toward the apex. Also, the deflection is upward (positive) when the depolarization wave moves toward the positive electrode of the recording set. The more directly pointed toward the positive electrode the electrical current, the greater will be the amplitude of the deflection.

LEAD I. The P wave (atrial depolarization) is wholly upright as the wave front proceeds from the right atrium toward the positive electrode (LA). A small Q wave (left-to-right septal depolarization) is followed by a tall R deflection (predominantly left ventricular depolarization) as the electrical front passes toward the LA electrode. The S deflection is small, representing the terminal depolarization forces, moving through the right ventricle toward the negative electrode. The T wave is upright, indicating that the ventricular repolarization is principally in a right-to-left direction.

LEAD II. The configuration of components of the cardiac cycle in lead II is generally similar to that of lead I because the positive electrode remains to the left of the negative electrode. The P wave, small Q, tall R, and small S deflection are usually little different in these two leads. The T wave varies inappreciably. Minor differences in the direction of depolarization and repolarization do result in some advantages in either lead for rhythm monitoring, as will be explained later.

LEAD III. The positive electrode is located at the apical aspect of the heart. The resultant P wave is usually of lower amplitude than in leads I and II, and it is more likely to be biphasic. The Q wave is usually deeper and the R deflection less prominent.

It can be appreciated that the position of the heart and the relative dominance of the individual chambers affect the direction and the magnitude of the various inscriptions. Indeed, these variations are of great importance for interpreting the position and chamber dimensions on the ECG.

In Figure 2–49, compare the waveform recorded from the three bipolar limb leads, noting each component for direction and amplitude. Sketch mentally or literally the predominant directions of the wave fronts in each phase of the cardiac cycle, identifying the represented component on the ECG, until the correlations become familiar.

Unipolar Limb Leads

Whereas the bipolar limb leads just described project changes in electrical potentials sensed across the chest, the unipolar limb leads reflect predominantly local potentials. In this system, an electrode placed on the right arm, left arm, or left leg provides the positive pole. The other pole is actually a composite of sensing electrodes on each of the extremities. A summation of their electrical potentials is virtually negligible because they tend to cancel each other out throughout the cardiac cycle. This zero point is located in the middle of the chest and is therefore referred to as the **central terminal**.

The three unipolar limb leads are termed aVR, aVL, and aVF. The letters *R*, *L*, and *F* refer to the limb lead that acts as the **positive electrode**. *V* represents a **unipolar lead**. The letter *a* stands for **augmented**, referring to the increased electrical potential achieved by internal separation of the signal between the exploring electrode and the central terminal. This modification increases the amplitude of waveforms by about 1½ times.

The unipolar limb lead tracings in Figure 2–50 are from the same standard ECG of the healthy man used to illustrate the bipolar leads reviewed in Figure 2–49. The drawing places the limb electrodes on the thorax and the LL electrode midline, and the central terminal is equidistant between positive electrodes.

Again, study each of the represented leads in relationship to the components of the cardiac cycle. Note that in lead aVR the P wave, the major portion of the QRS complex, and the T wave are negative (in a downward deflection). This configuration results from the wave fronts of atrial depolarization, the preponderance of ventricular depolarization and ventricular repolarization proceeding away from the positive pole (RA electrode). The small R deflection is caused by the relatively small depolarizing

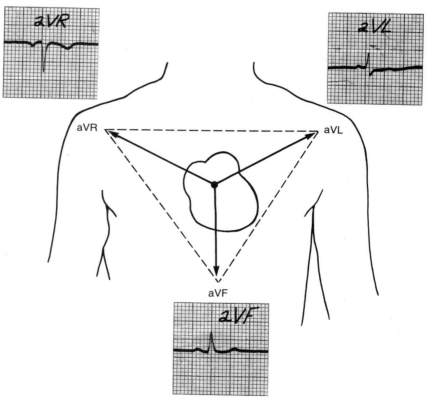

Figure 2–50. Unipolar limb leads.

activity occurring in the intraventricular septum, proceeding briefly toward the right arm. Similarly, visualize the inscriptions of the other two augmented leads.

Unipolar Precordial Leads

Instead of the positive electrodes being placed on the limbs, they are placed on six designated sites on the anterior chest in the unipolar precordial lead system. The central terminal arrangement for the negative (or zero point) electrode remains in effect. This system provides a vantage point of predominant local electrical activity close to the anterior and left lateral surfaces of the heart, which is projected in a sagittal plane (as opposed to a frontal plane in the limb leads).

Electrode location for the positive electrodes of the precordial leads are depicted (Fig. 2–51). These **V leads** are designated by number starting at the right lower sternal border. In Figure 2–51A, the placement on the anterior chest wall is depicted. B represents a sagittal section of the thorax with cardiac cycles (from the subject identified in the two preceding figures) appropriately placed near the represented electrode. Here, the atrial depolarization wave proceeds away from the positive electrode of lead V_1 and toward that of lead V_6 (downward and upward P wave, respectively). Intraventricular septal depolarization moves toward lead V_1 (small R) and away from lead V_6 (small Q). The predominant ventricular depolarization occurs away from lead V_1 and toward lead V_6 (large S and large R, respectively). A transition of QRS between predominantly negative and predominantly positive is seen in lead V_4, in which the upward and downward deflections are of nearly equal magnitude.

The electrode arrangements of the standard ECG are summarized in Table 2–3. Selection of the various leads on the electrocardiograph automatically determines the unipolar or bipolar sensing.

All 12 leads of the standard ECG are present, obtained from a healthy 28-year-old woman (Fig. 2–52).

At this stage, the reader should be able to correlate the events observed in each lead with the major electrophysiological events occurring. Keep in mind the location of the positive electrode in each lead. Note the direction, amplitude, and duration of the various components of a single cardiac cycle in relationship to specific electrical events:

Atrial depolarization	(P wave)
Septal depolarization	(Q deflection)
Early ventricular depolarization	(R deflection)
Late ventricular depolarization	(S deflection)
Ventricular repolarization	(T wave)

Some variations in configuration of these components are observed when comparing the ECGs of this patient and the one previously studied. These differences relate to individuality in the direction, magnitude, and velocity of the wave fronts that govern the electrocardiographic response. The reader will appreciate, even from this limited study, that the standard ECG provides information on the size of cardiac chamber thickness (waveform amplitude), the rate of electrical impulse conduction through the chambers (interval durations), and the spatial orientation of superimposed electrical events (vectors).

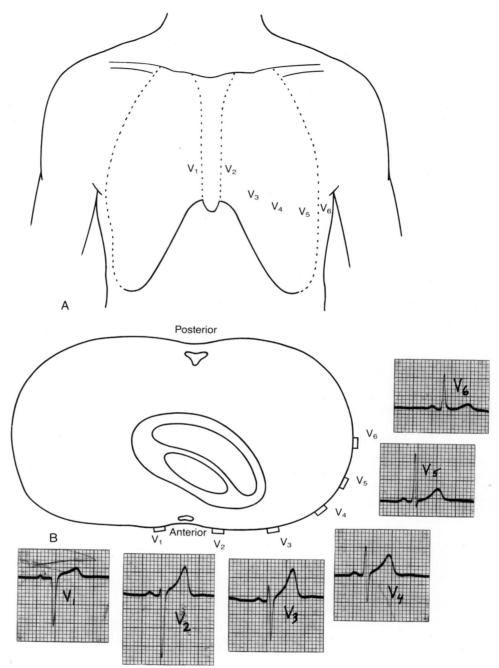

Figure 2–51. Precordial leads.

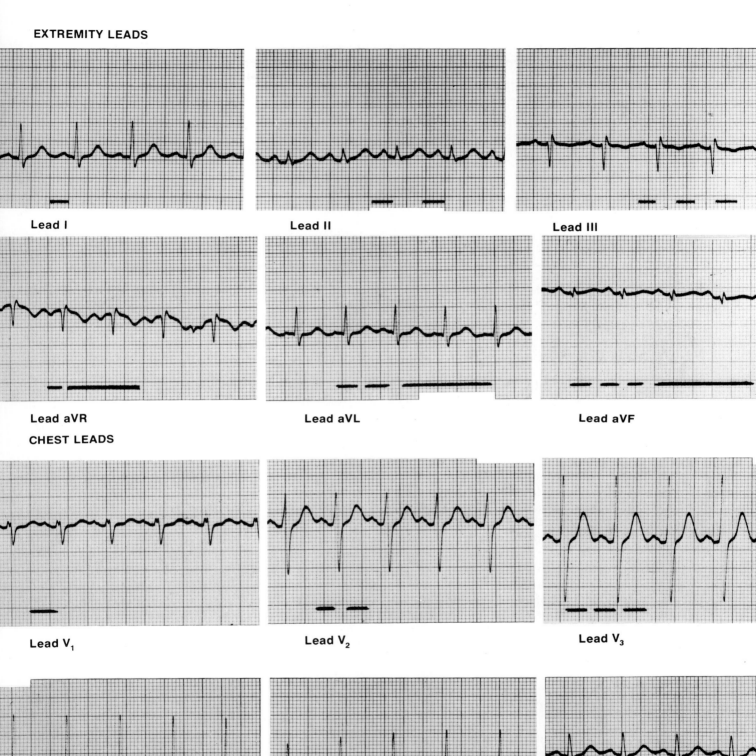

Lead I   Lead II   Lead III

Lead aVR   Lead aVL   Lead aVF

CHEST LEADS

Lead V₁   Lead V₂   Lead V₃

Lead V₄   Lead V₅   Lead V₆

Figure 2–52. Example of the standard electrocardiogram.

Table 2–3. STANDARD ELECTROCARDIOGRAM LEADS

		Leads	Positive Electrode		Negative Electrode
Bipolar	1.	I	Left arm	and	Right arm
	2.	II	Left leg	and	Right arm
	3.	III	Left leg	and	Left arm
Unipolar	4.	aVR	Right arm		
	5.	aVL	Left arm		Central terminal*
	6.	aVF	Left leg		
Precordial	7.	V_1	Right of sternum in 4th intercostal space (4th ICS)		
	8.	V_2	Left of sternum in 4th ICS		
	9.	V_3	Midway between V_2 and V_4		Central terminal*
	10.	V_4	Midclavicular line in 5th ICS		
	11.	V_5	Midway between V_4 and V_6		
	12.	V_6	Lateral chest in 5th ICS		

* The *central terminal* is a combination of electrode potentials, producing a summation effect. This serves as the single negative or *indifferent* electrode. The specific combination of electrodes for each lead is automatically determined in the lead selector switch.

COMPONENT ABNORMALITIES

Because the electrical activity of the heart is affected by a great many factors, it is not surprising that the ECG—a graphic expression of depolarization and repolarization—may give an indication of disturbances in any of these factors. The patterns of the ECG may be altered by insufficient blood flow (ischemia), inflammatory conditions of the myocardium (myocarditis) or surrounding membrane (pericarditis), major disturbances of electrolyte balance (e.g., hyper- and hypokalemia), metabolic disorders (e.g., myxedema), drug action (e.g., with digitalis), and cardiac contusion (the steering-wheel injury being the most common cause). Any abnormality that results in cardiac chamber enlargement (either hypertrophy or dilation) produces characteristic electrocardiographic changes. These conditions may include systemic hypertension (left ventricular hypertrophy), mitral valve stenosis (left atrial enlargement), chronic obstructive airway disease (right ventricular hypertrophy), and tricuspid insufficiency (right atrial enlargement), to mention only a few possibilities.

As an introduction to these abnormal patterns found on the ECG, a few of the most common conditions in which classic features of the represented condition are demonstrated and described will be presented. These exercises should give the reader some concept of general electrocardiographic interpretation. It must be understood, however, that these examples are not directly pertinent to the cardiac arrhythmias and that further definitive explanations are beyond the scope of this book.

Chamber Enlargement

Atrial enlargement is reflected in the morphology and the amplitude of the P waves. When only one of the atria is enlarged, characteristic features are commonly present on the ECG. In the two examples provided here, enlargement of the right and the left atria is clearly demonstrated (Fig. 2–53).

Ventricular enlargement is expressed by increased amplitude of the QRS complex and to some degree ST segment deviation and changes in T wave amplitude. The left ventricle undergoes compensatory hypertrophy in response to aortic stenosis, systemic hypertension, and athletic conditioning. Left ventricular enlargement is suggested when the combined amplitudes of the S deflection in lead V_1 and the R deflection in lead V_5

A   B

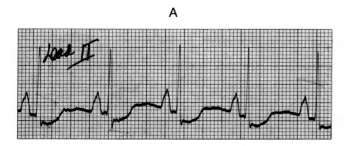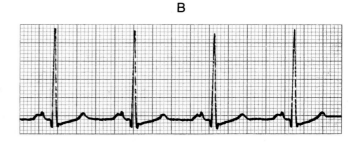

Right atrial enlargement   Left atrial enlargement

Figure 2–53. Examples of right and left atrial enlargement. The contour and amplitude of the P wave may reveal enlargement (hypertrophy or dilation) of the atria. (*A*) The tall, peaked P waves have an amplitude greater than 3 mm. The tracing is from a patient with severe pulmonary emphysema with high pulmonary arterial pressure. The resultant enlargement of the right atrium produces this typical "P pulmonale" pattern. (*B*) P waves are broad and bipeaked, reflecting prolonged depolarization in a large left atrium. The "P mitrale" pattern is from a 24-year-old woman who was found to have mitral valve stenosis.

is greater than 35 mm. (The strict amplitude criteria required for this determination bear out the importance of ascertaining that the amplitude standardization marker on the electrocardiograph has been tested and adjusted, if necessary, to exactly 10 mm, as described earlier in this chapter in the section entitled Standardization Markers.)

In the example of left ventricular enlargement presented in Figure 2–54, the subject is a 20-year-old cross-country runner with no medical problems. In this instance, the sum of S in V_1 ($= 4.5$ mm) and R in V_5 ($= 37$ mm) is 41.5 mm, thus fulfilling the criteria. The exceptionally tall R deflection in lead V_5 is attributed to increased thickness of the wall of the left ventricle, a condition developed through athletic training of the endurance type. Incidentally, additional features of changes typical of vigorous physical training can be observed in this resting tracing: (1) the slow heart rate (48 beats per minute); (2) the elevated takeoff of the ST segment in lead V_5 at its junction with the QRS complex (the J point); and (3) the tall and peaked T wave in lead V_5.

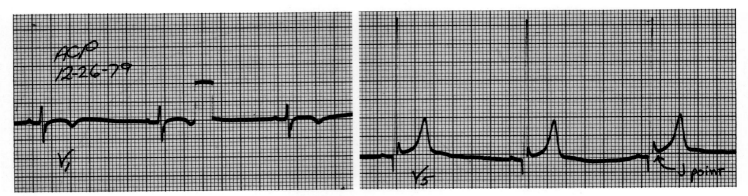

Figure 2–54. Ventricular enlargement.

ST Segment Deviation

Inflammation, ischemia, and metabolic changes in the myocardium displace the ST segment from the isoelectric line. The patterns of deviation provide critical clues in the diagnosis of acute and chronic heart disease.

Disturbances of repolarization in the ventricles tend to shift the ST segment from the baseline. This characteristic deviation in myocardial ischemia constitutes the definitive diagnostic criterion for the positive (abnormal) exercise stress test. For comparison, a normal response to exercise is presented first.

NORMAL EXERCISE STRESS TEST

Figure 2–55 demonstrates a normal maximum exercise stress test using Kattus' protocol in a 65-year-old man who maintains a moderate level of regular athletic exercise.

The heart rate is at the maximum anticipated level for the patient's age. In all

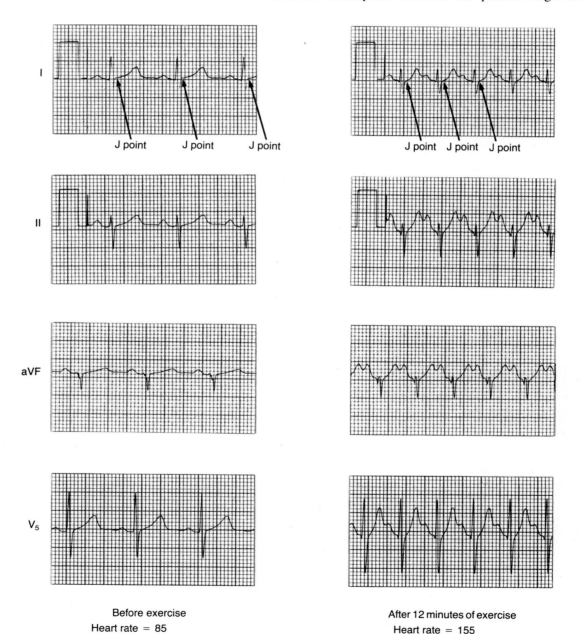

Before exercise

Heart rate = 85
Blood pressure = 105/75

After 12 minutes of exercise

Heart rate = 155
Blood pressure = 170/60

Figure 2–55. Select leads of a normal stress test electrocardiogram showing complexes before and after exercise.

leads, the J point of the ST segment is at the isoelectric line (using for reference the horizontal line after the P wave and before the QRS complex). The ST segment itself is upward sloping (except in aVR) in its entirety.

Locate the standardization marker in the series of tracings shown in Figure 2–55. It is included to emphasize the importance of checking this reference point whenever amplitude criteria are required.

ABNORMAL EXERCISE STRESS TEST

Individual complexes of representative leads are shown in Figure 2–56 to demonstrate development of an ischemic pattern.

In lead V_5, the ST segment depression becomes progressively deeper. As maximum exercise is approached, the contour becomes gradually flattened and horizontal to 3.5 mm in reference to the isoelectric line. This is a markedly positive study. The patient, a 46-year-old bank executive, was found on angiography to have major obstructive disease in the main stem of the left coronary artery.

As a rule, ST segments are depressed in leads in which the positive electrode is toward the area of acute ischemia. For example, ST segments are lower than the isoelectric line in lead V_5 in anterolateral wall ischemia; they are lower in lead aVF with ischemia of the inferior walls of the ventricles.

Twenty-five minutes after an elderly man experienced the onset of retrosternal chest pain at home, the Emergency Medical Technologist transmitted the tracing shown in Figure 2–57A.

Using the isoelectric segment between the end of the T wave and the beginning of a P wave as a reference (arrow), marked ST segment elevation is observed. This finding is often present at the onset of myocardial infarction, a sign designating the **hyperacute** phase.

Fifteen minutes later, on arrival at the hospital, the ST segment was markedly depressed in reference to the isoelectric line (Fig. 2–57B).

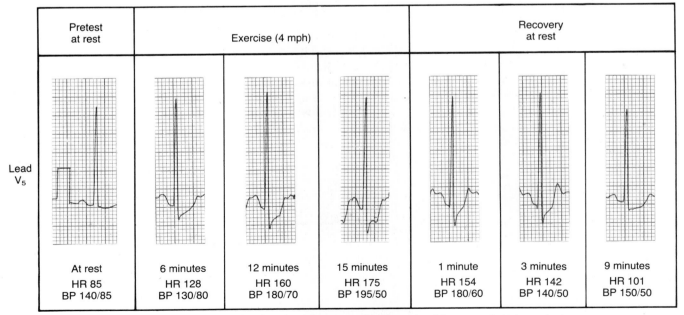

Pretest at rest	Exercise (4 mph)			Recovery at rest		
At rest	6 minutes	12 minutes	15 minutes	1 minute	3 minutes	9 minutes
HR 85	HR 128	HR 160	HR 175	HR 154	HR 142	HR 101
BP 140/85	BP 130/80	BP 180/70	BP 195/50	BP 180/60	BP 140/50	BP 150/50

Figure 2–56. ST segment changes reflecting a positive exercise stress test.

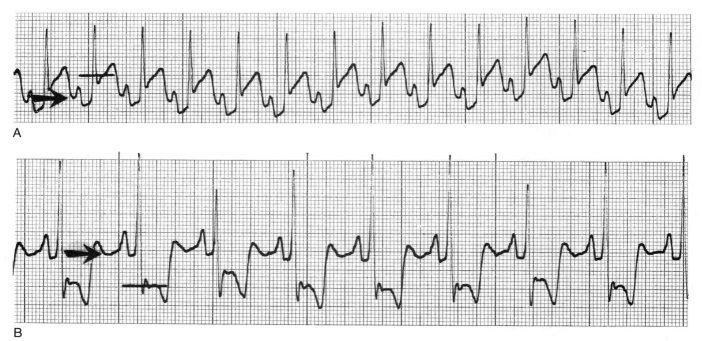

Figure 2–57. Changes in the ST segment reflect typical alterations seen in inferior wall ischemia.

Later development of abnormal Q waves in leads II, III, and aVF signified the evolution of an inferior myocardial infarction.

Similarly, ST segments are often elevated in acute ischemia when the cause is a spasm of a coronary artery, a condition known as Prinzmetal's (or variant) angina. Elevation of ST segments in nearly all leads is commonly present in acute pericarditis, reflecting the irritation on the adjoining epicardium over a widespread area. In addition, persistent elevation of ST segments over a region of the heart may reflect ventricular aneurysm.

Figure 2–58 demonstrates the ST segment changes that occur during an episode of acute myocardial ischemia. In lead V_3, the ST segment lies on nearly the same horizontal plane as the baseline (labeled BL). The ST segment is observed to rise gradually as it moves toward the T wave. This recording was obtained during a routine office checkup on a 71-year-old man with angiographically documented coronary artery disease. As the patient was leaving the office, he suddenly felt chest pressure in the midsternal area. On repeated ECG, the same lead reveals marked deviations in the level of ST segments. The onset of ST is now about 5 mm below the baseline reference point. In addition, the ST segment descends briefly before rising sharply to merge into

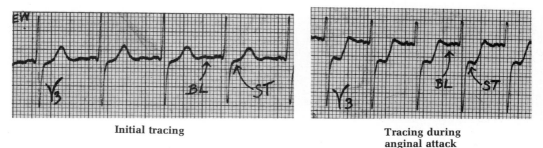

Initial tracing   **Tracing during anginal attack**

Figure 2–58. ST segment change.

the T wave. The symptom and the electrocardiographic abnormalities subsided within 2 minutes after the patient took sublingual nitroglycerin.

Q Wave Changes

Normally, the intraventricular septum depolarizes in less than 0.03 second. In leads having a Q wave, it is inscribed within this period. In myocardial injury, the affected area of muscle loses its capacity to generate action potentials, an event most characteristically recognized on the ECG by alteration of the initial portion of the QRS complex. Depolarization of viable myocardium during this period distorts the early QRS complex, often resulting in an abnormally long Q wave in leads normally exhibiting a Q wave, and may even produce a Q wave *de novo* in leads in which there was no Q wave before infarction.

Although an abnormal Q wave may regress in duration and amplitude as the heart recovers from infarction (or even disappear altogether), it usually persists as a permanent electrocardiographic "scar." The pattern of leads in which such abnormal Q waves appear helps to locate the area of myocardial damage. For example, a Q wave (absence of a small R) in leads V_1 and V_2 indicates anterior wall infarction. A Q wave of 0.04 second or longer in leads II, III, and aVF is evidence of an inferior wall infarction. An abnormal Q wave in leads V_5 and V_6 suggests a lesion in the anterior-lateral wall. These and other patterns of infarction localization may be envisioned, appreciating that the initial forces of ventricular depolarization proceed away from the direction of the injury, thus producing an initial negative deflection (Q wave) in leads in which the positive electrode is in the vicinity of the infarct.

The 12-lead ECG shown in Figure 2–59A was recorded on a 75-year-old man who presented with chest pain and nausea. Typical QRS complex changes of classic inferior wall infarction are most evident in the bipolar and unipolar limb leads, especially leads II, III, and aVF. Specifically note the deep Q waves in leads III and aVF, which exceed 0.04 second. (Compare with the normal 12-lead ECG shown in Figure 2–48.)

In Figure 2–59B, the pattern of anteroseptal myocardial infarction is evident, recorded from a 68-year-old man with retrosternal chest discomfort. The changes in the precordial leads of the standard ECG, which are most revealing, are described.

Normally, the R deflection increases progressively as the chest electrode is moved toward the left from the V_1 to the V_6 position (see Fig. 2–48). In the tracing in Figure 2–59B, no R deflection is observed in lead V_1, and there is a small R in lead V_2. In lead V_3, instead of having a larger positive deflection, R is absent and ventricular depolarization produces a QS complex. Farther leftward, a small R is present in V_4, and this deflection gains amplitude proceeding to leads V_5 and V_6; however, it remains abnormally reduced in these leads. These patterns indicate that the anterior free wall and septal regions do not generate appreciable electrical activity while the remaining portion of the myocardium depolarizes predominantly in a posterior lateral direction. Associated with the acute ischemic event are the ST segment elevation in leads V_3, V_4, and V_5 and T wave inversion in leads V_3 through V_6.

T Wave Changes

The T wave is an extremely sensitive indication of physiological and pathological changes in repolarization activity within the ventricles. Transient fluctuations in amplitude are observed in innumerable and diverse situations: during exercise or acute emotional stress, when drinking cold liquids (related to the proximity of the esophagus and the posterior left ventricular wall), and with digitalis effect, pericarditis, myocarditis, myocardial ischemia, ventricular hypertrophy and aneurysm, and electrolyte dis-

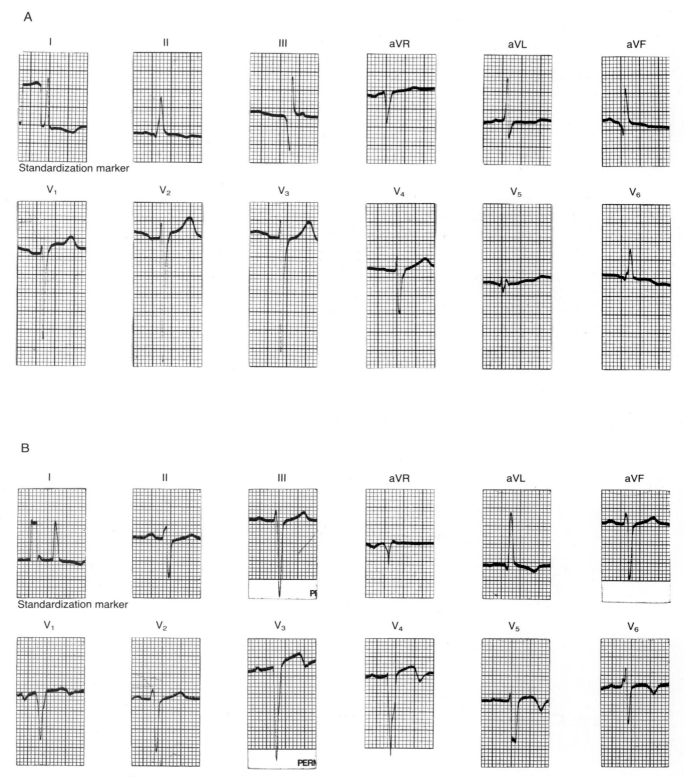

Figure 2–59. (*A*) Inferior myocardial infarction. (*B*) Anteroseptal myocardial infarction.

turbances. These changes in T wave amplitude may be of such magnitude that an alteration in polarity actually occurs (e.g., from an upward to a downward inscription).

The ECG shown in Figure 2–60 on the left side (from lead V_1) was taken on a periodic examination for management of angina pectoris. Five days later, the patient incurred an anterior myocardial infarction. At this time, the tracing on the right (also lead V_1) exhibits a reversal of polarity of the T wave. Note, in addition, the elevation of ST segments above baseline, sometimes observed within the first few hours of the onset of myocardial infarction.

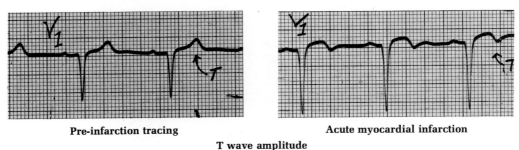

Pre-infarction tracing   **Acute myocardial infarction**

T wave amplitude

Figure 2–60. Change in T wave configuration during the infarction process.

T wave amplitude and contour may be profoundly altered in disorders of electrolyte balance. Severe hyperkalemia may distort the ECG in a characteristic way. Most typical is an increase in amplitude of the T wave with a sharply angled peak (or "tenting"). In addition, P waves and U waves tend to become reduced in amplitude. In the extreme, hyperkalemia widens the QRS complex and fatal dissolution of ventricular depolarization may ensue. Figure 2–61A exhibits these abnormalities in a 14-year-old boy who sustained acute renal failure after a bicycle accident. His serum creatinine at the time of hospital entrance was 8.3 mg/dl, and potassium was 7.8 mEq/liter.

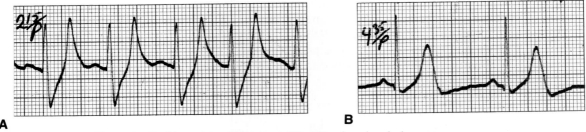

A   **B**

Figure 2–61. Alteration of T wave with potassium level changes.

Sodium bicarbonate was given by intravenous infusion as an emergency measure, and peritoneal dialysis was started. Within a relatively short period, the striking T wave amplitude and tenting were reduced, the P waves became more prominent, and most importantly the QRS complexes were narrowed to within normal limits (Fig. 2–61B).

U waves have little diagnostic significance. However, they are sometimes unusually tall when marked hypokalemia is present.

QRS Axis Deviation

An electrocardiographer uses the direction of the combined electrical forces occurring during ventricular depolarization to assess the relative preponderance of the ventricles. These combined forces, the summation of *all* electrical activity, are represented in a single event, averaging both direction and magnitude, and are referred to as a **vector**. In respect to ventricular depolarization, this vector is known as the QRS **axis**. Shifts in the direction of the axis are caused by enlargement of either ventricle or by alterations in the depolarizing wave front, such as in conduction pathway defects.

Vectors in electrocardiography are expressed in degrees of the compass (Figure 2–62). In the frontal plane, the zero point coincides with the location of the positive electrode of lead I (3 o'clock position). The negative electrode of this lead is at 180° (9 o'clock). Thus is defined a horizontal line on which the hexaxial system of reference is devised. When a vector direction points below this line, it is given a positive value from 0° to 180°. When directed above, it is designated negative, from 0° to 180°.

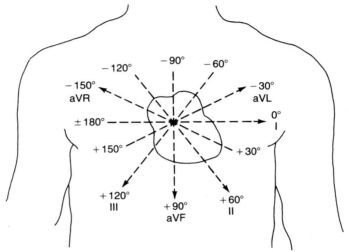

Figure 2–62. Hexaxial system.

Infants, having a relatively powerful right ventricle, normally have a QRS axis directed downward and somewhat to the right to about +120°. Reviewing the electrode positions of each of the standard limb leads, the reader can anticipate the general appearance of an infant's QRS complex. As shown in Figure 2–63, the averaged forces of ventricular depolarization produce a tall R deflection in lead aVF (positive electrode at +90°) and a deep S deflection in lead aVL (negative electrode at +150°). The mean

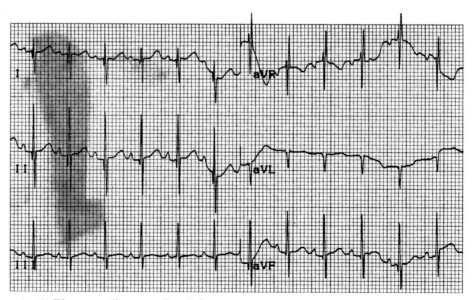

Figure 2–63. Electrocardiogram of an infant.

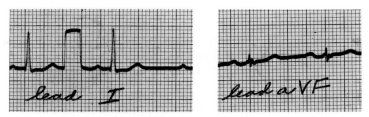

QRS axis = 0°
(leftward, horizontal axis)

Figure 2–64. Electrocardiogram with a horizontal axis.

QRS electrical axis is also pointed forward (toward the right ventricle), producing a prominent R deflection in lead V_1 and a small R deep S deflection in lead V_6 (not shown).

As individuals age, left ventricular activity gradually becomes dominant in mass and contractile force. Thus, the QRS axis shifts leftward. In a normal adult, the QRS axis lies between $+120°$ and $-30°$.

When the QRS axis is located precisely at 0°, the QRS complex in lead I is taller than in any other lead (pointing directly toward the positive electrode) as shown in Figure 2–64. At the same time, the QRS axis is perpendicular to the vertical orientation of lead aVF; it lies halfway between the positive and the negative electrodes. The resultant inscription is half above baseline and half below. All other leads reflect transitional configurations between leads I and aVF.

A contrasting pattern is found when the QRS axis is exactly vertical (pointing at $+90°$). A tall R deflection appears in lead aVF (its positive electrode coincides with $+90°$), while lead I exhibits approximately equal R and S deflections (the vector is oriented between the positive and negative electrodes) (Fig. 2–65).

A counterclockwise rotation of the QRS axis beyond $-30°$ is abnormal and is designated left axis deviation (LAD). This condition may be caused by enlargement (either hypertrophy or dilation) of the left ventricle, by delayed impulse conduction through the left ventricle, or by loss of right ventricular mass. Systemic hypertension, aortic stenosis, diffuse ischemic disease of the left ventricle, conduction block of the left anterior fascicle, and right ventricular infarction all are typically associated with LAD. Because the perpendicular point between the positive and negative electrodes of lead II is at $-30°$, this lead is most helpful in defining LAD. LAD is present when the S deflection is more prominent than the R deflection (predominantly a negative vector direction) in lead II.

Right axis deviation (RAD) is defined as a QRS axis beyond $+120°$. Here, lead aVR is the critical determinant because $+120°$ lies halfway between the positive and the negative electrodes. In RAD, the QRS complex in lead aVR is predominantly upward or positive. (It is normally downward.) RAD may be the result of obstructive airway disease, pulmonary valve stenosis, or impulse conduction disturbances of the left posterior fascicle.

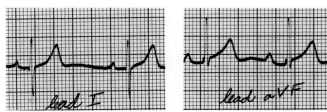

QRS axis = 90°
(vertical axis)

Figure 2–65. Vertical axis on the electrocardiogram.

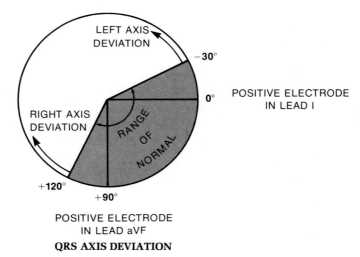

QRS AXIS DEVIATION

Figure 2–66. QRS axis deviation ranges.

For ease in envisioning the landmarks of QRS axis deviation, Figure 2–66 depicts the limits of normal in relationship to the critical lead determinants.

Of course, readers cannot expect to be proficient in general electrocardiographic interpretation on the basis of these several examples. Yet even when concentrating on the patterns of arrhythmias, reference is frequently made to the concepts presented. As already stated, the introductory information with illustrations offered here is meant to provide useful acquaintance with the standard ECG.

ARTIFACTS

Many factors may interfere with proper recording of an ECG. These can often be identified by characteristic features known as **artifacts**. An interpreter must always be alert to the possibility of artifacts, which may mimic genuine rhythm disturbances or may obscure others. The telltale signs of frequently encountered artifacts are presented for familiarization.

In the lefthand tracing in Figure 2–67, representing lead I, a clear baseline is present. At the end of this tracing, however, the RL (ground) electrode has disconnected

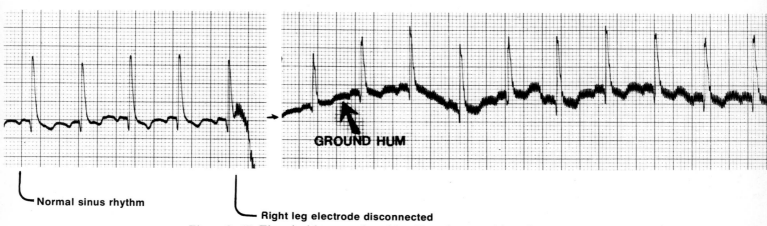

Figure 2–67. Electrical hum produced by 60-cycle ground interference.

and the inscription immediately becomes irregular and wanders off the paper. Within a few seconds, the stylus has returned to a recording position, as observed in the righthand tracing. A broad, jagged baseline is now evident as the stylus oscillated rapidly as a result of extraneous electrical currents no longer eliminated by the ground lead, an artifact referred to as **ground hum**. This pattern is typical of **60-cycle electrical interference** from ordinary power sources. Despite this difficulty, the components of each cardiac cycle can still be identified, but not so clearly.

Movement of the patient commonly results in wandering of the baseline. During the recording of Figure 2–68, the patient raised her right arm, on which was taped the RA electrode. The inscription responds by a sudden shift from the established baseline. Note also a mild degree of 60-cycle electrical interference from improper grounding, in this instance from a hypothermia unit.

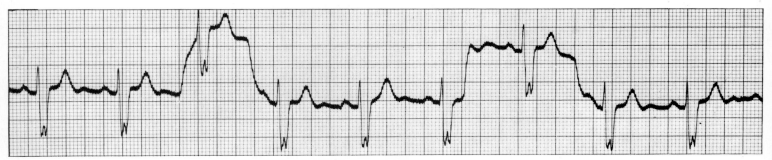

Figure 2–68. Baseline drifting from patient movement.

The patient whose ECG is shown in Figure 2–69 had a rapid, fairly regular tremor associated with Parkinson's disease. The movement is responsible for the small baseline oscillations recorded (which are slower than those found in ground hum). An ECG taken during sleep (when tremulousness is minimal) reveals normal sinus rhythm with clearly discerned P waves and sharp baseline.

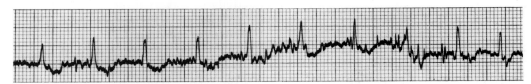

Figure 2–69. Artifact from muscle tremor.

The inability to obtain clear rhythm strips can also result from interference by equipment in the environment. In Figure 2–70, the pumping action of an intravenous controller creates periodic small deflections of the baseline. The cause of these deflections was positively identified when the controller was turned off, and only normal cycle complexes are seen on the rhythm.

The importance of good electrode contact is demonstrated in Figure 2–71. The LA electrode was loosely attached, and insufficient electrical transmission gel was used. On correcting these deficiencies, a satisfactory recording is obtained.

For monitoring of the cardiac rhythm, excellent and sustained electrical contact is essential. The skin-electrode interface must be prepared with special diligence to assure a stable, artifact-free tracing over a long period of surveillance. The well type of electrode, which holds an appreciable amount of gel, is preferred to the plate electrode.

To minimize resistance to small electrical currents between the skin and the electrode, the operator should prepare the skin by rubbing briskly with gauze and bland solvent such as alcohol or acetone. This technique removes surface oils and the most

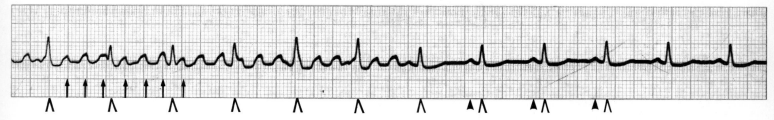

Figure 2–70. Artifact created by an intravenous infusion flow rate controller. Note baseline deviations in the beginning of the strip. These ceased when the controller was discontinued.

superficial layer of cornified epidermis, both of which impede electrical flow. Shaving may be necessary for satisfactory electrode adherence.

Cardiac rhythms are sometimes grossly misinterpreted because of patient movement artifact, particularly from those movements that are repeated and even rhythmical. Examples of such confusion artifacts are hiccups, coughing, nodding, and tapping the foot. In Figure 2–72, the artifact is the result of movement from brushing the teeth. Of course, this activity does not affect the cardiac rhythm, and QRS complexes can be discerned throughout (although with difficulty).

CARDIAC RHYTHM MONITORING

Application of the electronic **oscilloscope** at the bedside has enabled clinicians to observe and record the cardiac rhythm continuously during an extended time. Patients at high risk of developing physiologically compromising or lethal arrhythmias can thus be constantly assessed. Furthermore, the information gained from the uninterrupted observation of cardiac rhythm activity in acutely ill patients has greatly improved our understanding of the natural evolution of arrhythmias.

The oscilloscope is a cathode-ray tube that receives electrical potentials from electrodes in the same manner as the electrocardiograph (Fig. 2–73). It differs from the electrocardiograph in that an electron "gun" in the stem of the tube fires electrons toward the screen end of the tube. The beam of electrons emitted by the gun is focused to a point falling on the screen. A visual image is formed at this point by excitation of fluorescent material in the screen, causing it to glow.

The electron gun reflects changes in incoming electrical activity by projecting vertical oscillations on the tube screen. The amplitude of these inscriptions is regulated by an adjustable amplifier. The factor of time is projected by a sweep circuit that proceeds horizontally from left to right. (The electrocardiographic write-out differs in that the paper rather than the writer moves horizontally.) Inspection of the focused beam on the screen is rendered easier by momentary fixation from the fluorescence.

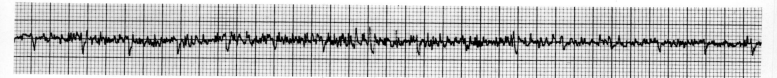

Figure 2–71. Continuous electrical interference from faulty lead attachment.

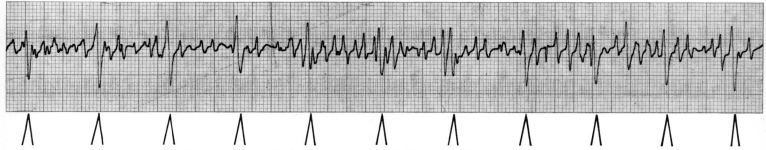

Figure 2–72. Artifact created by brushing the teeth. The electrical activity caused by the muscle contractions interferes with clear visualization of the cardiac complexes.

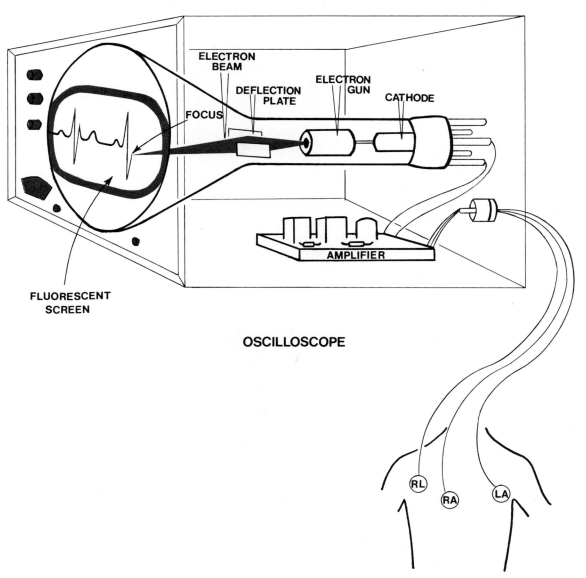

Figure 2–73. Adaptation of the cathode-ray oscilloscope to electrocardiographic monitoring.

ELECTRODE PLACEMENT FOR MONITORING

For continuous surveillance of the cardiac rhythm during a long period, it is highly desirable that the patient be relatively unencumbered by electrodes and wires and that a clearly discernible rhythm pattern, to which automatic alarm sensors are sensitive, be obtained. Many variations from the procedure used in standard electrocardiography have been devised to achieve these ends.

The ideal monitoring pattern for cardiac rhythms should embody the following features:

1. The baseline is stable. The limb electrodes are transferred to the chest, thus freeing the extremities and at the same time minimizing distortions of the rhythm pattern due to the patient's movements. If significant baseline wandering due to the movement of respiration occurs, improvement is usually obtained by attaching the electrodes closer to the sternum.

2. P waves and QRS complexes are clearly discernible to facilitate rapid and precise identification of the rhythm.

3. One complex of each cardiac cycle is outstanding in amplitude. Instruments that have heart rate alarm systems incorporated into them determine rate by detecting deflections of specific amplitude. Thus, if one complex is distinctly larger, the electronic sensor will receive one—and only one—signal for each heartbeat.

4. Electrical interference from outside sources is negligible. Monitoring instruments and nearby electrical equipment (including the bed itself) must be thoroughly grounded. When interference cannot be controlled by carefully eliminating potential causes at the bedside, failure of the three-pronged outlet plug should be suspect. Of course, the RL electrode (the ground plate) must be placed on the skin with the same careful preparation as with the recording electrodes.

5. Chest electrodes are placed far enough apart to allow application of the defibrillation paddles, should this form of treatment be required in an emergency.

6. Electrodes are securely affixed to the skin. Shaving of trunk hair is often required before scrubbing with an organic solvent. For patients who sweat appreciably, application of an antiperspirant spray to the electrode area improves adherence.

Most monitoring systems require the use of only three electrodes (in contrast to five for the standard ECG). Two of the electrodes measure the electrical current between the points of attachment, and one is used for electrical grounding. This system provides only one electrocardiographic picture, but, with a few exceptions, it is convenient and entirely suitable for cardiac rhythm interpretation. It must be remembered, however, that moving electrodes from their prescribed positions on the extremities (for the standard ECG) to the chest also changes the forms and amplitudes of the various complexes. Therefore, the special electrode arrangements for monitoring the cardiac rhythm should *not* be used to detect patterns of chamber hypertrophy, myocardial ischemia and infarction, or metabolic disturbance, all of which ordinarily require using at least several leads of the conventional 12-lead ECG. In rhythm monitoring, interpretation of complex arrhythmias and conduction defects can often be facilitated by the supplemental use of strips taken from the standard ECG.

Those specialty care units that adhere to a single electrode placement system for all patients sacrifice the advantages of individualized pattern characteristics for simplicity. Rather, a systematic technique for obtaining the most advantageous rhythm monitoring tracing can be easily learned and should be used.

Suggested Electrode Placement

Of the many arrangements devised for lead selection and placement of electrodes, the one recommended here has the advantage of simplicity while providing for flexible adaptation to individual patients (Fig. 2–74). (No single prescribed placement arrangement will invariably furnish an ideal monitoring pattern on all patients!)

STEPS

1. Select lead I on the cardiac oscilloscope monitor.
2. Attach the RL electrode securely to a convenient place on the right upper anterior chest or to the lateral chest wall on either side. This electrode is the electrical ground. It is *not* a recording electrode, and therefore its position is not critical.
3. Attach the RA electrode securely to the right of the sternum, about midway along its length.
4. The LA electrode is now applied over the left chest. In most instances, a satisfactory rhythm tracing can be obtained with the LA electrode in this position. However, there is great variation in patterns among individuals, and several positions for this electrode should be tried before finally attaching it to the chest. If disposable adhesive electrodes are used, it is cost-effective to expend one for determining optimal LA electrode placement. Once this position is established, a fresh electrode is then securely attached. (Because moving an adhesive electrode from place to place causes loss of stickiness, the testing electrode should be replaced. Considering the importance of obtaining a good monitoring lead, this procedure does not seem wasteful.)

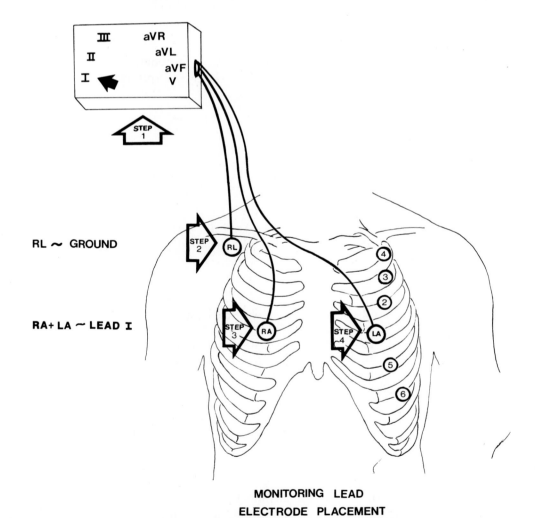

**MONITORING LEAD
ELECTRODE PLACEMENT**

Figure 2–74. Steps for placement of electrodes on the chest to obtain the ideal monitoring lead.

The best position for the LA electrode is determined by placing it upward and downward on the left precordium. The electrocardiographic pattern is observed for each position and the best one chosen according to the criteria already described. The value of having a clearly readable tracing cannot be overemphasized, and the few minutes required to explore several positions for the electrode is well worth the effort.

Alternative Systems for Monitoring

Alternative systems for electrode placement and lead choice are commonly used; two will be described here. These systems also produce excellent patterns for rhythm monitoring in most patients. Whatever system is adopted, however, it is important that all persons responsible for preparing the patient for monitoring follow that system.

One method, if the fixed approach is chosen, consists of attaching the RA (negative) electrode to the right upper parasternal area (Fig. 2–75). The LL (positive) electrode is placed near the apex of the heart. The RL (ground lead) electrode can be attached to the left upper chest. Lead II is dialed on the monitor, and in fact this arrangement gives a pattern closely comparable to lead II on the standard ECG. In most patients, it provides an upright P wave of relatively large amplitude (the normal atrial depolarization wave front proceeds toward the positive pole of this bipolar system). The amplitude of the R deflection is generally high in adults (although the wide variations in QRS vector render this parameter less dependable).

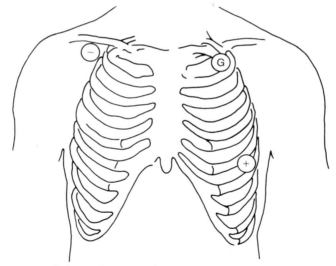

Figure 2–75. Placement of electrodes when using lead II for monitoring.

An additional monitoring technique finds wide use and is referred to as the MCL$_1$ system. It is based on the unipolar leads and is a modification of the precordial arrangement. The "exploring" electrode (LA) is placed at the V$_1$ area, where a distinct P wave can often (but certainly not always) be found. The RA electrode is placed on the left shoulder, and the ground (RL) electrode is positioned on the right shoulder (Fig. 2–76). This system allows repositioning of the exploring electrode over the chest until a satisfactory monitoring pattern is observed.

The pattern obtained in the MCL$_1$ system at V$_1$ may be a downward inscribed P wave. In an adult, the predominant QRS deflection is also downward. This situation may require that the alarm setting be adjusted to the negative deflection, as will be described next. An advantage of the MCL$_1$ method is the distinctive configurations of the bundle branch conduction abnormalities.

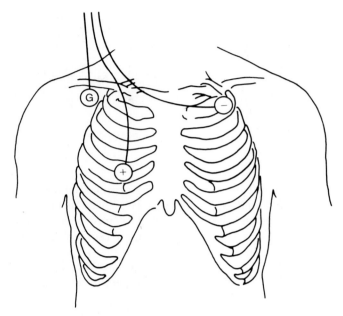

Figure 2–76. MCL₁ lead electrode placement.

Automatic Warning Systems

A **visual** and/or **auditory** alarm signal is incorporated into most cardiac rhythm monitoring oscilloscopes. These alarms are activated by heart rates that occur more rapidly or more slowly than a preset limit. The instrument senses any vertical oscillation beyond a predetermined amplitude, and its sensitivity is adjusted so that one, and only one, deflection of each cardiac cycle falls within the sensitivity range. Thus, each heartbeat should produce one signal to the alarm system. Because the system cannot distinguish signals from various components of the cardiac cycle (e.g., P wave from T wave), painstaking effort must be taken to assure that the electrocardiographic pattern selected contains a solitary outstanding vertical deflection.

A positive deflection on the oscilloscope can be detected with the sensor mechanism. A single, tall, upright QRS component (R spike) is the most suitable element of the cardiac cycle to fall within the sensitivity range of the instrument. All other components should be well below this amplitude. If the sensitivity is set too low, some or all of the cardiac cycles will not be counted, and a slower than true heart rate will be registered. If the sensitivity is too high, more than one component of each cycle may provide a detected signal, and a greater than true rate will be counted. False counting in either direction, when sufficiently great, activates the alarm. Proper selection of the cardiac cycle pattern and setting of tolerable rate limits will minimize miscounting by the instrument and help avoid excessively frequent false alarms.

Some oscilloscopic instruments have a switch that reverses polarity, creating a vertical inversion, in effect a mirror image of the cardiac pattern (Fig. 2–77). This device is useful when the QRS complex has a deep, downward spike and the clinician chooses to monitor with a predominantly upright deflection. The situation just described is most applicable to monitoring with the MCL₁ lead system. An additional technique that can be used to enhance the ability of the equipment to identify the ECG signal when the patient has a predominantly negative complex is to reverse the positive and negative monitoring electrodes so that the complex becomes predominantly upright.

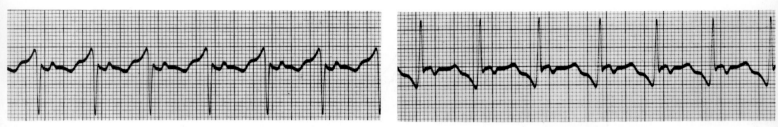

Figure 2–77. First position of suggested cardiac monitoring lead. Same electrode position, reversed polarity.

Whenever the monitoring arrangement is modified from the usual method, a notation should be made at the oscilloscope to denote the alteration.

In attempting to establish the electrode positions for obtaining an ideal monitoring pattern, observe the following characteristics in the three examples in Figure 2–78:

1. Distinct P wave.
2. Single, tall, upright spike in QRS complex.
3. P and T waves of small amplitude relative to amplitude of upright spike of QRS complex.

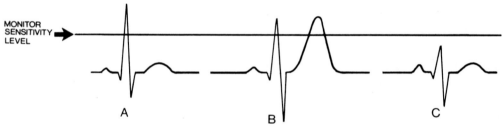

Figure 2–78. Monitoring lead patterns.

The ideal pattern for monitoring is cycle A.

Cycle A: Clearly identifiable complexes with relative sizes permitting sensing of only the tall QRS complex.

Cycle B: Height of T wave is equal to QRS (thus both will be sensed by the monitor).

Cycle C: All complexes are too short to activate the sensing mechanism of the monitor.

Table 2–4. LEAD SUITABILITY

	A Ideal	B T Wave Too High	C R Spike Too Low
	R well above sensitivity level	Double rate will be indicated	No signal will be sensed
	No interference likely from relatively small P and T waves	Tachycardia by alarm warning system	Bradycardia by alarm warning system
Corrective maneuvers		Reposition **left arm** electrode or reverse polarity of instrument	Increase **gain** on instrument

Table 2–4 summarizes lead suitability for each of the three preceding electrocardiographic cycles. Reference is made to the sensitivity level, and it should be clear that "A" is the only acceptable situation.

Which of the following practice strips are good monitoring leads? Suggest changes when indicated. (All numbered ECGs require answers, which may be found in a special section at the end of the book.)

The pulse rate limits can be set so that a considerable margin is left to allow for extraneous signals such as the patient's movements. As a rule, the upper limit can be set about 30 beats per minute above the average heart rate of the individual. The lower limit may be routinely set at 50 per minute. However, if the average heart rate is close to this, the limit should be set slower than 50, perhaps 10 beats per minute below the average rate. These limits usually permit instant indications of significant changes in rate without producing an excessive number of false alarms.

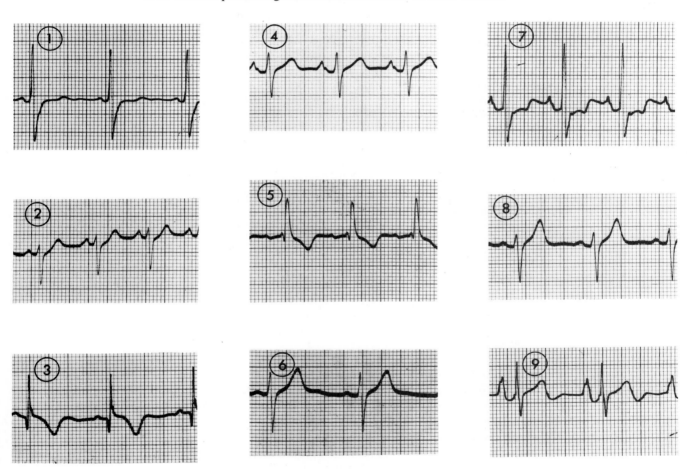

3 The Sinus Node

IMPULSE FORMATION
Action Potential
Normal Sinus Rhythm
AUTONOMIC NERVOUS SYSTEM
Structure
Physiology
Regulatory Mechanisms
SINUS NODE: IMPULSE FORMATION
Excitation
Sinus Tachycardia
SINUS NODE: IMPULSE FORMATION
Depression
Sinus Bradycardia

Sinus Pause
Sinus Arrest
The Vasovagal Reflex
Carotid Hypersensitivity
DYNAMIC RHYTHM PROFILE
SINUS NODE DYSFUNCTION
Etiologies of Sinus Node Dysfunction
Characteristics of Sinus Node Dysfunction
SINUS NODE: IMPULSE CONDUCTION
Depression
Sinoatrial Block
PREPARATION OF A CARDIAC RHYTHM
   NOTEBOOK

IMPULSE FORMATION

The muscular elements of the heart require a dependable pacemaker to set the rate at which they contract. Furthermore, such a pacemaker must be exquisitely sensitive to regulating the rate of cardiac contraction in response to the continual—often drastic—changes in physical and metabolic demand. Because the heart rate is a basic determinant of cardiac output (together with stroke volume), the critical role of the pacemaker in adjusting the rate can be readily appreciated.

The responsibility of the cardiac pacemaker is assumed by a small cluster of cells lying in the wall of the right atrium near the entrance of the superior vena cava (Fig. 3–1). Known collectively as the **sinus node** (or sinoatrial node), the cells rhythmically emit small electrical impulses that propagate directly to the contractile elements or reach these elements by way of other cells specialized for impulse conduction. Thus, the electrical activity of the sinus node, minuscule as it is, normally provides a recurring impulse that dictates the rate at which the heart beats. The pacemaker, in turn, depends on a system capable of conducting each impulse to all the sarcomeres of the heart to ensure that the sarcomeres contract in proper synchrony.

Scattered throughout the fibers and dense collagen matrix that make up the sinus node are nests of small cells. Referred to as **P** (for pacemaker) cells, they differ sharply

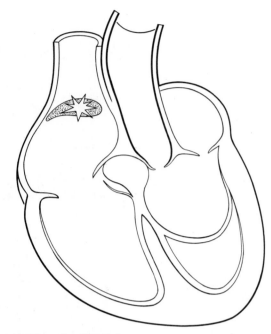

Figure 3–1. The sinus node: impulse formation.

from the ordinary sarcomeres that make up the working muscular component of the heart.

Although derived embryologically from the sarcomeral stem cell, the P cells have lost the function of contractility and have acquired that of impulse formation. They have rudimentary myofibrils with few cross-striations, and they are relatively sparse in mitochondria. Furthermore, the sarcoplasmic reticulum, in which calcium ions are stored during electrical diastole, is poorly developed. Although the contractile sarcomeres interdigitate extensively, there are few intercellular connections between the P cells, and these connections have limited access to the surrounding atrial tissue.

Impulses generated by the P cells are not conveyed directly to the atrial mass or to the principal conducting system. Instead, these impulses are transmitted to intermediary cells that surround the sinus node. Designated **T** (for transitional) cells, these intermediate cells are more elongated than P cells, and they contain more highly developed myofibrils. In addition, mitochondria are more abundant. In these respects, the T cells are shorter and less well endowed with myofibrils and mitochondria than are the sarcomeres. Therefore, the T cells can be considered transitional anatomically as well as functionally between those cells that only produce impulses and those that only contract.

The sparse interconnections between the P cells and the T cells probably account for the relatively slow rate of conduction for impulses emerging from the sinus node to the surrounding atria. In addition, the abundant neural fibers of the autonomic nervous system that terminate in this area correlate with the high degree of sensitivity to autonomic stimulation of the sinus node mechanism for impulse formation. The complex interconnection may also explain in part the susceptibility of the sinus node perimeter to degenerative disease.

In most individuals, blood to the sinus node is supplied by a branch of the right coronary artery (Fig. 3–2). However, about a third of the population have this branch to the sinus node originating from the left circumflex artery.

The sinus node artery does not terminate in the sinus node but rather pierces it at its center, proceeding on to supply portions of the intraatrial septum and the free

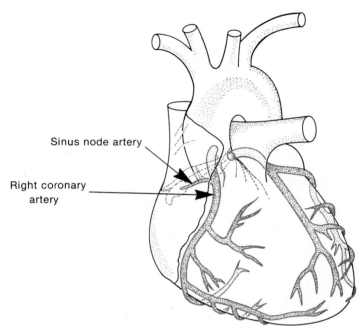

Figure 3–2. Coronary artery distribution to the sinus node.

wall of the right atrium. In microscopic cross section, the sinus node artery appears very large relative to the size of the sinus node itself. This unique arrangement may have an important physiological implication as a rate-controlling servomechanism.

Mechanical stretch of the P cells produces an acceleration in the rate at which they emit impulses. Such stretching may be exerted by a reduction in the caliber of the central artery of the sinus node. Indeed, the dense network of collagen material surrounding this artery is richly supplied with neural endings and probably enhances this interrelationship. When the artery constricts (as in hypovolemic shock), a pulling tension is exerted on the surrounding tissue, thus stretching the P cells and resulting in a physiologically appropriate acceleration in the rate of impulse formation.

Distention of the central artery of the sinus node, in contrast, relaxes the P cell tension, causing the rate of impulse emission to slow. Distention may be produced by vasodilating drugs or by overloading the intravascular capacitance. (This deceleration response, however, may be overridden by other autonomic adjustments.)

Action Potential

The action potential of the sinus node deserves careful study because it is a valuable key to understanding the special properties of this pacemaker, its normal adaptations to physiological stresses, and the various pharmacological agents and diseases that affect the heart.

For reference, it will be recalled that the resting sarcomere (Phase 4) maintains a transmembrane potential of about -90 millivolts (mv) and that this steady state persists under favorable metabolic support until caused to fire (or depolarize) by a stimulus impinging on it.

One important difference between the action potential of the typical sarcomere and that of the sinus node is that the latter generates a transmembrane potential of only about -60 mv. In even sharper contrast, the transmembrane potential of sinus node cells is *not* maintained in a steady state pending stimulation. In fact, once the maximum transmembrane potential is achieved, a gradual decay in electrical potential occurs spontaneously. This decrease in voltage gradient across the P cell membrane is known as **spontaneous diastolic depolarization**.

DEPOLARIZATION

Cell membranes of the sinus node depend on the slow channels for depolarization. Consequently, entry of calcium ions rather than sodium is the dominant electrolyte transfer on stimulation of the P cells. This distinction is reflected in the slope of Phase 0 of the action potential curve.

     PHASE 0: RAPID DEPOLARIZATION. When the falling transmembrane potential in the sinus node reaches a critical level of about −40 mv, the rate of depolarization suddenly increases (Fig. 3–3). This acceleration is reflected in the abrupt change in the slope of the action potential curve, identifying the beginning of Phase 0. The loss of intracellular electrical negativity proceeds until the state of neutrality is reached, the end of Phase 0.

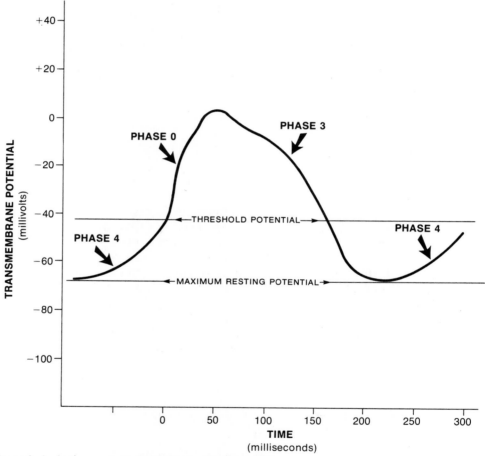

Figure 3–3. Action potential of cells in the sinus node.

Thus, we have observed slow, spontaneous depolarization (Phase 4), then more rapid depolarization (Phase 0), both occurring *without* the influence of an external stimulus. In effect, the gradual loss of transmembrane potential in the "resting" cell proceeds to a definable point at which the changing gradient itself acts as a stimulus to initiate fast depolarization. This description introduces the concept of **automaticity:** the property by which an excitable cell has the capacity to discharge energy by self-stimulation.

EARLY REPOLARIZATION

Distinct Phase 1 and Phase 2 repolarization described for the sarcomere is virtually absent in the action potential of the sinus node cells. This absence is explained in the paragraphs that follow.

PHASE 1. There is no rapid influx of sodium in the P cells. Consequently, little or no overshoot is developed for the electrochemical forces at the termination of Phase 0.

PHASE 2. In the absence of an appreciable sodium influx, there is no interplay between fast channel repolarization and slow channel repolarization as is characteristic of the contractile sarcomere. Instead, repolarization of automatic cells is limited almost entirely to the dynamics of Phase 3.

PHASE 3: REPOLARIZATION. Immediately after the point of transmembrane electrical neutrality produced by Phase 0 depolarization, cations are transported across the cell membranes in energy-absorbing processes. Potassium ions are pumped into the cell from the extracellular fluid while sodium and calcium ions are removed from the intracellular fluid. These events continue until the potential once again approaches -60 mv. At this gradient, reversal of cations occurs, leading to another cycle of firing.

PHASE 4: SPONTANEOUS DEPOLARIZATION. The P cells do not maintain their maximum diastolic potential but, once achieved, immediately begin to lose potassium from the intracellular fluid. Thus is initiated a gradual loss of membrane potential, which will culminate in another action potential, as described in the beginning of this section.

Normal Sinus Rhythm

Up to this point, we have given attention to the individual heartbeat: its electrophysiological basis, identification of its components by electrocardiographic representation, and the mechanics of determining the measuring intervals and rates of beating. Now, attention will advance to consideration of the dynamics of rhythmic beating characteristic of the diseaseless state, a condition referred to as **normal sinus rhythm**.

The rhythmicity of sinus node impulses in a young fetus is strikingly erratic. As a fetus develops, the degree of irregular beating diminishes although the rhythm remains noticeably variable (Fig. 3–4). Neonates commonly exhibit some irregularity of the heartbeat (sometimes markedly so), but with maturation the sinus node gradually steadies. Even so, the rhythm does not become perfectly regular but varies somewhat in a pattern that coincides with the phases of respiration. This characteristic of slight speeding during inspiration and slight slowing during exhalation persists throughout life.

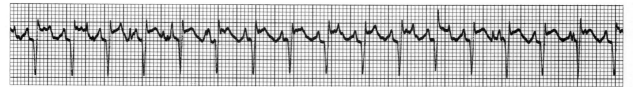

Figure 3–4. Sinus rhythm in a 1-day-old infant. The extremely rapid rate (160 beats per minute) is typical of neonates.

The electrocardiogram (ECG) shown in Figure 3–5 was obtained from a recumbent person without any evidence of cardiac disease or systemic illness. First, scan the entire tracing, noting that all cycles are similar in form to one another in respect to individual components: P waves, QRS complexes, and T waves. In addition, the interval between successive cycles appears to be similar, suggesting a regular rhythm. However,

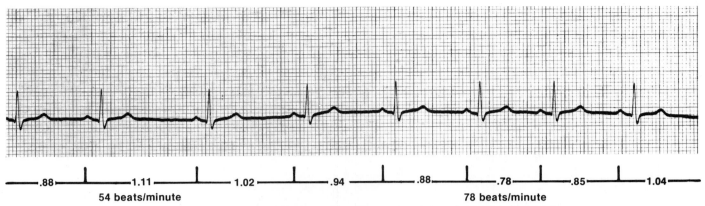

.88 — 1.11 — 1.02 — .94 — .88 — .78 — .85 — 1.04

54 beats/minute   **78 beats/minute**

Figure 3–5. Normal rhythm demonstrating periodicity of the normal heartbeat.

measurement of the time interval (or rate) between beats reveals that a slight variation is present. (Use the one-beat ruler to determine the rates from cycle to cycle, which have been labeled in time intervals for you.) A pattern with alternating periods of slight acceleration and slowing is revealed. These variations in rate (slowest = 54; fastest = 78) represent the physiological rhythmicity of the normal heartbeat.

The rhythmic changes just pointed out are explained on the basis of hemodynamic reflexes occurring in the heart. When the lungs expand with inspiration, their blood volume increases. This small redistribution decreases the volume of blood in the right cardiac chambers, resulting in some reduction in pressure on their walls. The sinus node is exquisitely sensitive to such changes and responds by increasing its rate of firing. The mechanism here is an acceleration in the rate of spontaneous depolarization (Phase 4).

During exhalation, the process is reversed. Blood in the right atrium and right ventricle increases in volume, owing to a reduction in the volume capacitance of the pulmonary circulatory bed. The resultant rise in intraatrial pressure is associated with some deceleration of sinus node firing.

Thus is described one feature of normal sinus rhythm: the phasic variations in rate associated with respiration. The degree of variation may be barely perceptible or may, in some individuals, be extremely prominent. In any case, the point is made that the heart does *not* beat with metronome-like periodicity but in a slightly irregular but recurring pattern. (The term *regular* is reserved for those rhythms that do not vary in rate from cycle to cycle, rhythms that are abnormal and will be presented later on.)

Figure 3–6 represents an exaggeration of the **normal phasic rate changes** and is

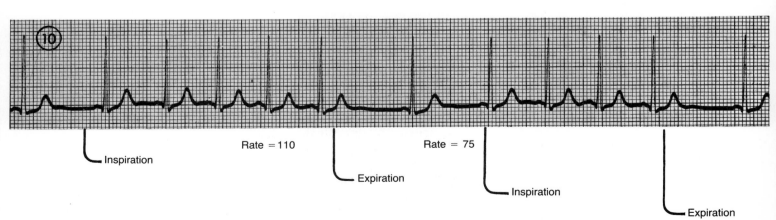

Inspiration   Rate = 110   Expiration   Rate = 75   Inspiration   Expiration

Figure 3–6. Sinus rhythm variations associated with quiet respirations.

presented to demonstrate the phenomenon clearly. Confirm the rates during inspiration and expiration.

In Figure 3–7, compare the shortest and the longest PP intervals. This tracing illustrates the marked moment-to-moment changes in heart rate that may occur in normal individuals.

The following tracings illustrate normal sinus rhythm. In each tracing, label all components of one cycle. Also, determine the interval between cycles; it may be expressed as rate, using the one-beat ruler.

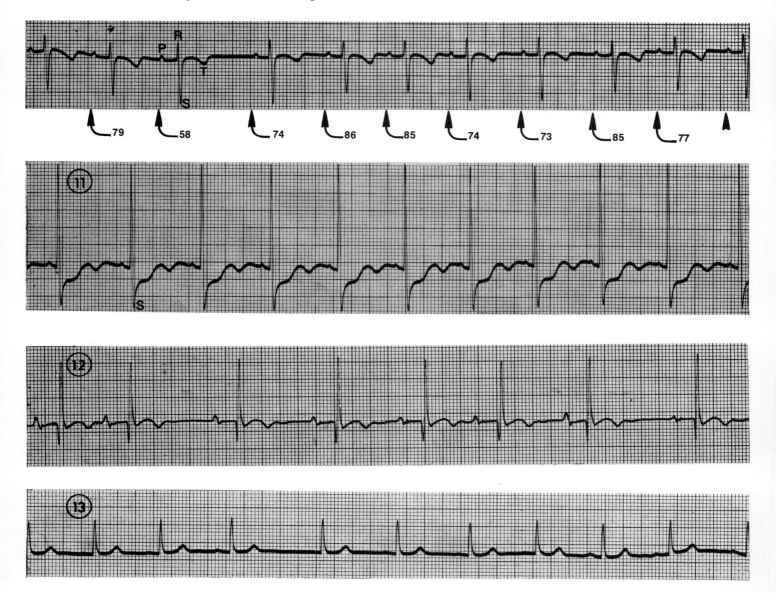

Components can sometimes be difficult to recognize. In rhythm strip 13, some complexes have P waves with extremely low amplitude, but they can be positively identified on close inspection.

An additional characteristic of normal sinus rhythm is a firing rate between 60 and 100 beats per minute. This limit is entirely arbitrary because normal individuals may have rates that either exceed or are slower than the range given. One important factor in determining normal rate is age.

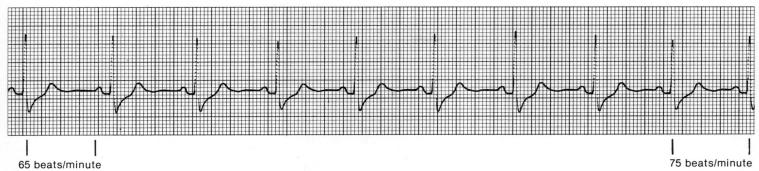

65 beats/minute   75 beats/minute

Figure 3–7. Normal sinus rhythm.

Normally, the heart rate of a fetus varies from 120 to 160 beats per minute. A neonate when sleeping may have a heart rate as slow as 70, but during activity it may rise to 180 per minute. The average heart rate in a week-old baby at rest is about 140 per minute and at 1 year about 120 per minute. Average rate slows further by the age of 6 years, to less than 100 per minute at rest and to about 80 per minute in adolescence. The resting heart rate of adults is determined by a host of factors: size, physical conditioning, concurrent physiological or pathological conditions, and environmental factors such as temperature. Substantial alterations are superimposed by physical activity, posture, emotional stress, and digestive function.

Thus, normal sinus rhythm can be defined according to the following three criteria:
1. Each heartbeat results from an impulse generated in the sinus node.
2. A slight rhythmic variation occurs in association with the phases of respiration.
3. The rate is between 60 and 100 beats per minute.

SINUS ARRHYTHMIA

Some individuals have an exaggerated natural slowing and speeding of the heartbeat associated with respiration, a condition referred to as **sinus arrhythmia** (Fig. 3–8). It is most common in adolescents and young adults but may occur in any age group.

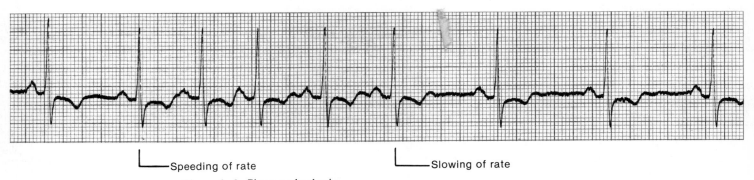

Speeding of rate   Slowing of rate

Figure 3–8. Sinus arrhythmia.

Examples of this form of periodicity are demonstrated in the tracings in Fig. 3–9). As can be seen in the two examples, this slowing-speeding pattern can be striking in some persons. In the examples, the slowest and most rapid cycles are expressed as beats per minute.

In almost all instances, sinus arrhythmia is a benign condition as it is merely an accentuation of a normal phenomenon. Athletic conditioning, in fact, is often associated with this irregularity. It is only of significance clinically when the intervals of the slowest

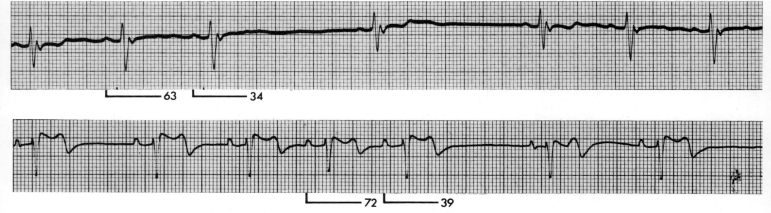

Figure 3–9. Note the variance in cycle-to-cycle intervals.

beats are so marked that normal cardiac output is impaired, a rare event. Pronounced irregularity may also result in awareness of the heartbeat, a symptom known as palpitations.

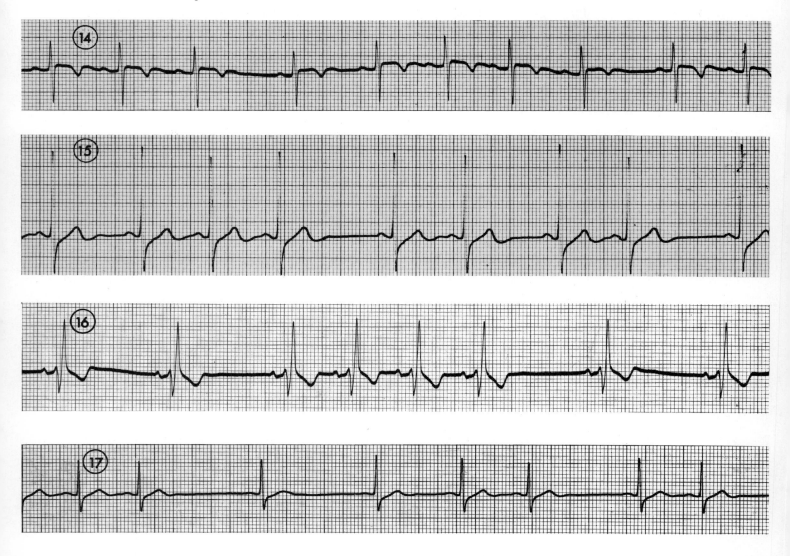

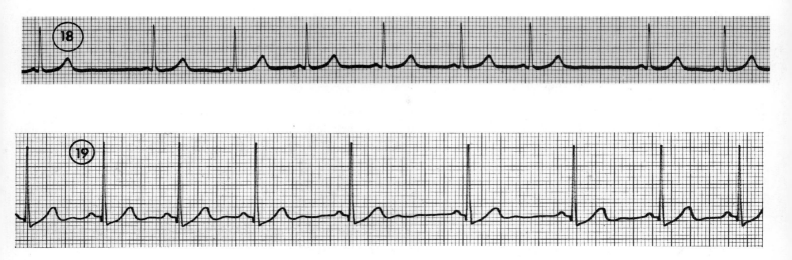

In test strips 14 to 19, examples of sinus arrhythmia, mark off each cardiac cycle and determine the fastest and slowest rates, using the one-beat ruler.

To further demonstrate the natural dynamics of sinus node rhythmicity, a simple physiological manuever is analyzed.

Deep, forced breath holding intensifies the phasic variations in rate of the sinus node pacemaker. This physiological response depends on reflexes that involve pressure-volume sensory receptors in the heart, blood vessels, and autonomic nervous system and on chemical factors of the blood. Reflex slowing is demonstrated in strips taken from a healthy 40-year-old man during prolonged breath holding in deep inspiration.

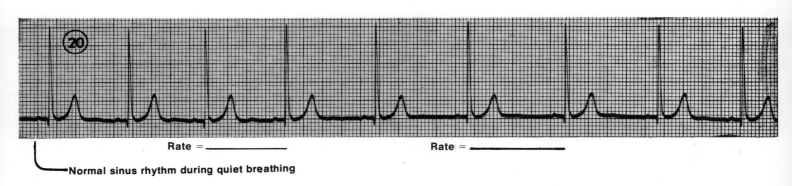

Rate = _____   Rate = _____

Normal sinus rhythm during quiet breathing

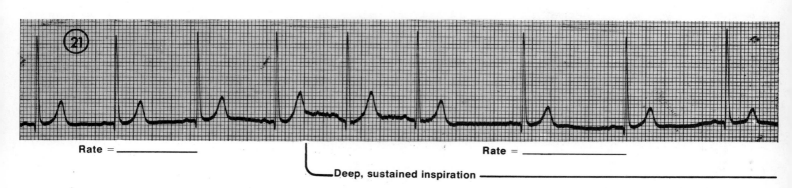

Rate = _____   Rate = _____

Deep, sustained inspiration

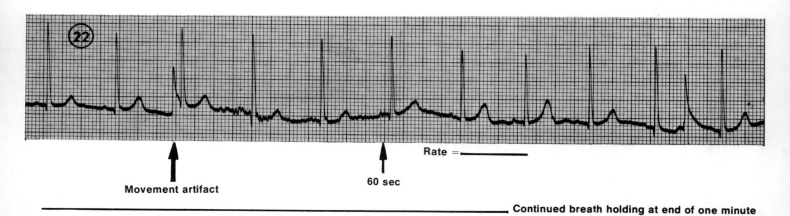

Movement artifact

60 sec

Rate =_____

_____ Continued breath holding at end of one minute

The first few beats are often accelerated on deep inspiration, from sudden expansion of total lung capacity. This expansion results in an increased blood volume in the lungs, a decreased blood volume in the right heart chambers, and the reflex production of a more rapid sinus beat. After this initial response, neural control becomes dominant, causing significant slowing of impulse formation. When breath holding is prolonged, the carbon dioxide level in the blood eventually rises, causing gradual speeding of the rate.

Review the preceding examples from Figure 3–4 to Figure 3–9 to determine the rhythmic variation in cycle-to-cycle intervals that typify sinus rhythms.

SINUS IRREGULARITY

Marked variations in sinus node pacing in which there is no phasic association with respiratory dynamics are occasionally encountered (Fig. 3–10). Such erratic rhythms reflect an instability in the processes of automaticity in the sinus node. They are often an indication of an abnormal condition, most commonly infant prematurity, digitalis toxicity, and degenerative disease of the sinus node itself. Sometimes, however, sinus irregularity is found without any detectable cardiac disorder. The condition, incidentally, is often referred to as **nonrespiratory sinus arrhythmia**.

Several ECGs demonstrating sinus irregularity are presented. Carefully inspect each P wave to ascertain that there is no variation in contour or amplitude despite the striking changes in rate. Measure out the rate of the fastest and the slowest intervals (using the one-beat ruler) to appreciate the degree in rate variations. Note that there is no pattern of alternating speeding and slowing that could be associated with respiration.

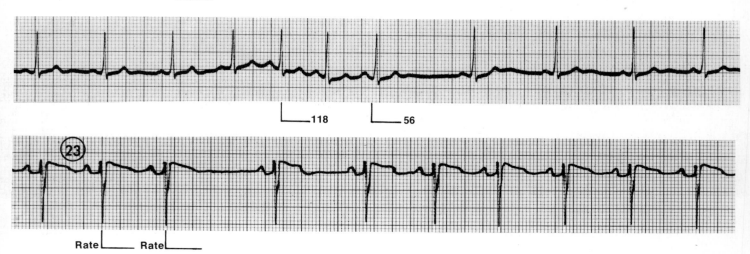

118   56

Rate____ Rate____

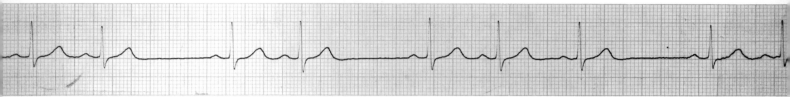

Figure 3–10. Sinus irregularity.

These variations in rate of impulse formation are determined in part by a complex neural mechanism known as the **autonomic nervous system**. This network affects smooth muscle and glands throughout the body, continually adjusting the involuntary functions of organs to the physiological demands of the organism. In the heart, the autonomic nervous system serves a prominent role in regulating the rate as well as the velocity of impulse conduction and the strength of contractions.

Autonomic control is divided into two highly integrated functional entities, the **sympathetic** and **parasympathetic** nervous systems. This subject is introduced at this point to provide a basic understanding of cardiac dynamics that can then be developed throughout the text. Its importance in the genesis of cardiac arrhythmias and in their clinical management cannot be overemphasized.

AUTONOMIC NERVOUS SYSTEM

The heart rate is continually adjusted by a complex and sensitive regulatory mechanism responding to extracardiac stimuli. Body position, physical activity, respiration, temperature, blood volume, peripheral vascular tone, and emotional reactions all modify the frequency of impulse formation. Thus, the pulse is modulated to the demands of cardiac output. This finely tuned mechanism is also affected by many drugs and may be deranged by various diseases.

A major influence on reflex cardiac activity is exerted by the **autonomic nervous system**, composed of two counterbalancing forces: the sympathetic and the parasympathetic divisions (Table 3–1 and Fig. 3–11). The opposing effects of the two divisions maintain a delicate balance, which can be tipped in favor of one or the other by any of innumerable physiological and pathological factors.

Table 3–1. DIVISIONS OF THE AUTONOMIC NERVOUS SYSTEM INNERVATING THE HEART

| | The Autonomic Nervous System | | |
	Sympathetic	*Parasympathetic*	
Peripheral nerves	Cardiac plexus	Vagus nerve	
Types of fibers	Effector	Effector	Sensory
Source	Cerebral cortex Thalamus Hypothalamus Spinal cord	Brain stem nuclei	Aortic root and arch Carotid sinus
Distribution	Sinus node Atria A-V node Ventricles	Sinus node Atria A-V node	Brain stem nuclei

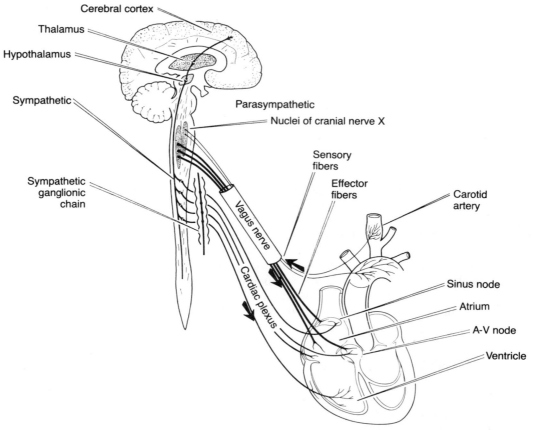

Figure 3–11. Composite diagram of the autonomic nervous system divisions innervating the heart.

Structure of the Autonomic Nervous System

STRUCTURE OF THE SYMPATHETIC NERVOUS SYSTEM

This complex network originates in cells of the brain stem. Its neurons to the heart course downward in the spinal cord, and branches emerge from the upper thoracic region to form the cardiac plexus. These branches have terminal branches in both the sinus and the atrioventricular (A-V) nodes and in the muscle of the atria and ventricles.

The brain stem nuclei that govern heart rate receive neural impulses from the cerebral cortex. Thus, stimuli from cognitive senses are intimately involved in the regulatory action of the sympathetic nervous system on sinus node function.

STRUCTURE OF THE PARASYMPATHETIC NERVOUS SYSTEM

This system includes the cranial nerves, of which the tenth is distributed to the heart. The nuclear center of this nerve is in the brain stem, and the effector fibers make up the **vagus nerve**, terminating at the sinus and A-V nodes. These fibers are also distributed to atrial musculature but not, to any appreciable extent, to ventricular tissue.

The vagus nerve also contains sensory neurons that convey impulses from vascular structures near the heart to the central nervous system. These neurons arise from the arch of the aorta and the internal carotid arteries and terminate in the tenth cranial nerve nucleus. Changes in pressure and chemistry within these vessels are transmitted to the nuclear center by these sensory fibers and may evoke reflexes by the effector fibers of the vagus nerve, known as the vasovagal reflexes.

A chemical substance known as a **neurohumoral transmitter** is stored in the nerve endings of the sympathetic and parasympathetic nervous systems. Impulses coursing through the autonomic nerves cause release of this substance, which in turn initiates a response of effector cells in the immediate vicinity. The difference between a sympathetic and parasympathetic response depends on the chemical nature of the transmitter substance.

Physiology of the Autonomic Nervous System

PHYSIOLOGY OF THE SYMPATHETIC NERVOUS SYSTEM

The neurohumoral transmitter at sympathetic nerve endings is **norepinephrine** (or noradrenaline). When this agent is discharged from terminal sympathetic nerve branches, responsive effector cells are stimulated, resulting in a sympathetic action. In the heart, sympathetic stimulation tends to *excite* the rate of impulse formation in automatic tissue. In addition, the velocity of cardiac impulse propagation in the conductile fibers is accelerated, and the force of contractile fibers is increased.

Another source of sympathetic neuronal stimulation is the adrenal gland. The adrenal gland synthesizes and stores norepinephrine and epinephrine (adrenaline). When stimulated, the gland secretes these hormones into the bloodstream, which carries them to the various receptor organs. Their direct action on the heart, through a hormonal mechanism, is similar to that of neurally transmitted norepinephrine.

These endogenous agents are referred to as sympathetic or adrenergic agents, and the effects elicited by them are called sympathetic or adrenergic responses. These terms are applied interchangeably regardless of the origin (neural or adrenal) of the stimulating transmitter. The sympathetic nervous system affects the heart by excitation of automaticity, conductivity, and contractility.

In electrophysiological terms, the adrenergic agents act by accelerating the rate of diastolic depolarization of automatic cells. In effect, these agents increase the slope of the Phase 4 segment of the action potential (Fig. 3–12). The mechanism is not completely understood but is thought to involve the more rapid entry of calcium ions into the resting cells. This action on the automatic cells of the heart has been designated one of the β (beta) effects (the other beta effect being an increase in the contractile force of the myofibril).

Enhanced adrenergic effect on the heart may be caused by exertion, standing, emotional stress, and reduction in blood volume. It is mediated through release of norepinephrine from neuronal terminals of sympathetic cardiac fibers. The frequency of impulses generated by centers in the brain and coursing through the sympathetic neurons determines the intensity of norepinephrine release. Thus, the tone of sympathetic activity is controlled by the central nervous system by impulse-generating cells that are responsive to chemical and pressure changes in the blood.

Strong adrenergic stimulation can also be effected by discharge of norepinephrine and epinephrine from the adrenal medulla. The usual cause of this hormonally mediated reaction is hypoglycemia or sudden emotional disturbances, as from fright or anger.

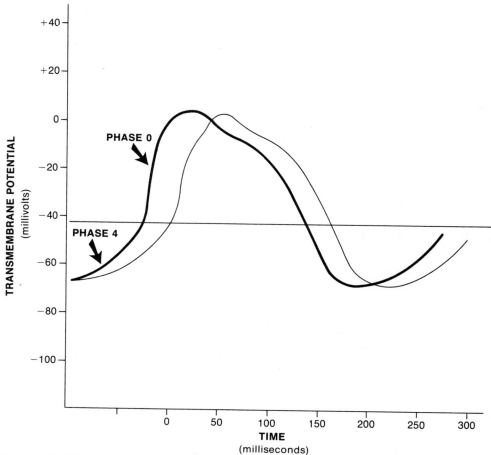

Figure 3–12. Effect of beta-adrenergic stimulation on the action potential. The slope of diastolic depolarization is steeper (heavy line) than that of the unaffected action potential (light line).

PHYSIOLOGY OF THE PARASYMPATHETIC NERVOUS SYSTEM

Stimulation of parasympathetic fibers causes release of **acetylcholine** at the system's nerve endings. The vagus nerve, subserving parasympathetic function to the heart, has a general inhibitory influence on the rate of cardiac impulse formation and on the velocity of conduction. The force of myocardial contractility is not altered substantially by vagal stimulation. Acetylcholine and its analogues are known as cholinergic agents, and the effects of vagal stimulation are known as cholinergic responses, which tend to *depress* automaticity and conductility within the heart.

The principal clinical use of cholinergic agents is for stimulation of smooth muscle of the hollow viscus. For example, bethanechol (Urecholine) has a limited application in the management of urinary retention and gastrointestinal atony. Patients on this or similarly acting drugs are often found to have an unusually slow heartbeat because of the enhanced vagal tone.

Figure 3–13 illustrates the relationship between adrenergic and cholinergic stimulation of myocardial fibers.

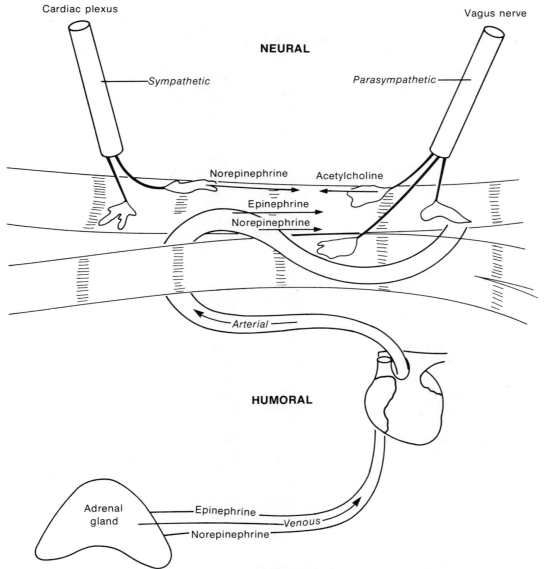

Figure 3–13. Adrenergic and cholinergic stimulants.

Regulatory Mechanisms of the Autonomic Nervous System

The sympathetic and parasympathetic nervous systems maintain a delicate balance of opposing forces—excitation and depression—on the electrical sequences of cardiac activity. A great number of variables may affect the stability of this regulatory mechanism, by either stimulating or inhibiting either system, causing a shift in the relative influence in favor of one or the other.

This dynamic equilibrium of the autonomic nervous system is analogous to a car moving at a steady speed, with continuous pressure (**tone**) applied to both the accelerator (**sympathetic**) and brake (**parasympathetic**) pedals. The driver may go faster by increasing the accelerator pressure (**adrenergic stimuli**) or slower by pushing harder on the brake (**cholinergic stimuli**) (Fig. 3–14).

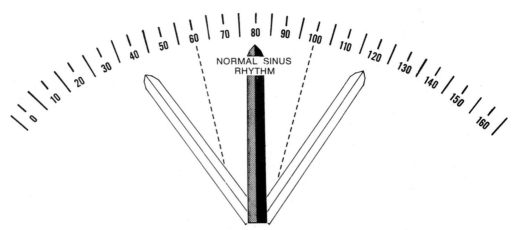

Figure 3–14. Balance of sympathetic and parasympathetic forces.

The driver can also change the rate of motion by letting up on either controlling pedal. Decreased pressure on the accelerator leaves a predominating braking influence, and the car slows **(adrenergic inhibition)**. If, during the steady state, braking action is reduced and accelerator tone held constant, the car's velocity increases **(cholinergic inhibition)**.

We shall now apply these principles of autonomic nervous system control in the study of normal sinus rhythm and the variations of sinus impulse formation.

The endogenous neurotransmitter substances norepinephrine and epinephrine belong to a general class of agents known as the **catecholamines** (in reference to their common carbon-ring nucleus structure). A number of these agents with adrenergic activity are used clinically and are derived from exogenous sources, including chemical synthesis. The catecholamines more commonly used are norepinephrine (Levophed), epinephrine (Adrenalin), isoproterenol (Isuprel), dopamine (Intropin), metaraminol (Aramine), phenylpropanolamine (in many preparations for the common cold), and phenylephrine (Neo-Synephrine). All have a similar effect on the heart, although the potency of each differs markedly. In contrast, each is characterized by individual actions on vasomotor tone and on other organ systems under control of the sympathetic nervous system.

SINUS NODE: IMPULSE FORMATION

Excitation

In this text, excitation denotes intensification of activity in automatic or conductive tissues. Excitation of these tissues produces an increase or acceleration of pacemaker rate or conduction velocity. Factors that cause changes in this direction in impulse formation and conduction are referred to as excitatory or stimulatory. Such factors may be of a physiological, pharmacological, or pathological nature.

These factors will now be explored in relationship to excitation of impulse formation in the sinus node. The result is sinus tachycardia (ST), depicted in Figure 3–15.

Sinus Tachycardia

When the sinus node is driven or excited to discharge at rates over 100 per minute, the term **sinus tachycardia** is applied.

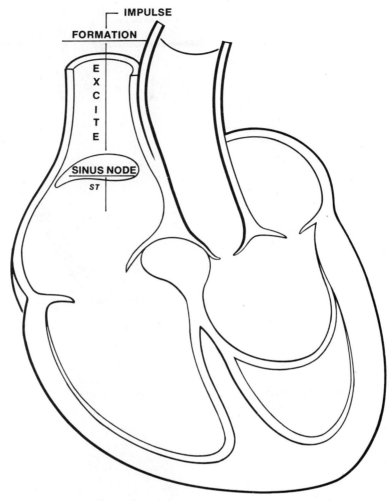

Figure 3–15. Sinus tachycardia.

As the sinus rate speeds (see rhythm strips 24 and 25), the P wave of a cycle appears closer to the T wave of the previous beat, and at very rapid rates it becomes harder to distinguish. (This emphasizes the importance of selecting a clear, discernible waveform on monitored patients.)

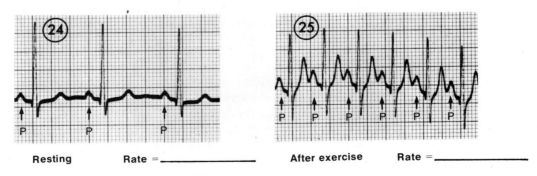

Referring to our driving analogy, the accelerator is pressed harder by adrenergic stimuli, and the sinus node responds by increasing its rate of impulse formation (Fig. 3–16).

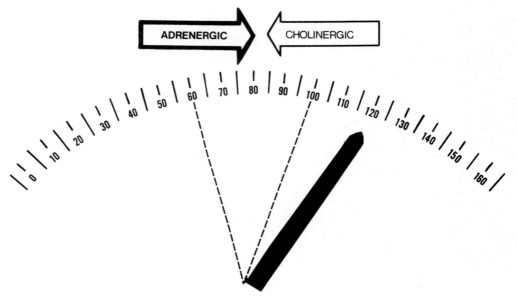

Figure 3–16. Sympathetic tone increases, producing speeding of rate.

Figure 3–17 illustrates the acceleration of sinus rate in response to climbing stairs. Determine rates for the series.

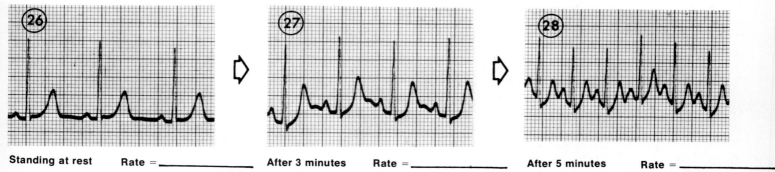

Standing at rest   Rate = _____   **After 3 minutes**   Rate = _____   **After 5 minutes**   Rate = _____

Figure 3–17. Physiological response to exercise.

A portion of an ECG obtained during an exercise stress test is provided to demonstrate the natural acceleration of heart rate during various degrees of physical exertion. Although two or three leads are ordinarily used for recording during exercise testing, the issue at point is shown here with only one lead, lead V_5. In this study, a 21-year-old female laboratory technician underwent exercise testing to evaluate recurring palpitations. No evidence of a cardiovascular disorder had been discovered on initial physical examination and resting ECG. The exercise stress test was performed on a treadmill according to the Bruce protocol, a method of adding increments of work at 3-minute intervals by progressively increasing both the speed and the incline of walking. Three minutes is chosen routinely for each increment in work level because it generally matches the time required for the body to adjust to added exertion and to reach a new steady state at a higher level.

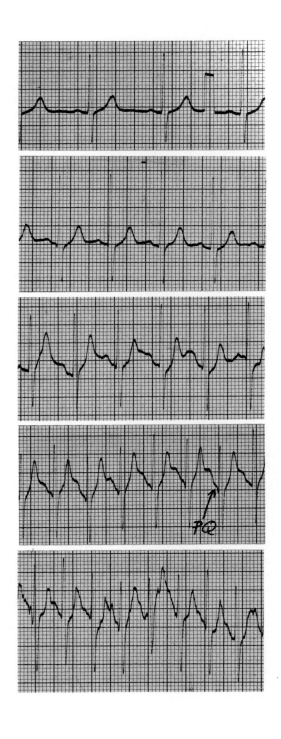

Standing
Rate = 76
   Blood pressure = 126/70

Stage 1
1.7 mph at 10% grade for 3 minutes
Rate = 110
   Blood pressure = 136/72

Stage 2
2.5 mph at 12% grade for 3 minutes
Rate = 130
   Blood pressure = 150/70

Stage 3
3.4 mph at 14% grade for 3 minutes
Rate = 172
   Blood pressure = 182/66

Stage 4
4.2 mph at 16% grade for 2-1/2 minutes
Rate = 200
   Blood pressure = 200/66

The test was stopped somewhat prematurely in Stage 4 because of marked, generalized fatigue. The subject recovered promptly with a cool-down work load of 1.7

mph at 0% grade for several minutes. Note the following features of the exercise response:

1. The heart rate increases with each added work load. Here, the highest rate was 200 beats per minute; it represents the maximal heart rate, because it was achieved through exertion to the point of exhaustion. The maximal heart rate for a healthy individual can be predicted with considerable accuracy according to age. A rule of thumb for this prediction is to subtract the subject's age from 220. In this example, the maximum heart rate is as anticipated.

2. As the heart rate quickens, the cardiac cycles appear closer together on the ECG, thus shortening the baseline intervals between a T wave and the subsequent P wave. At very rapid rates, this baseline is eventually eliminated. In Stage 3, the P wave is seen to fall on the down slope of the T from the previous cardiac cycle. When this occurs in sinus tachycardia, the reference point for the isoelectric line becomes the PQ segment, that brief interval between the end of the P wave and the beginning of the QRS complex.

3. Movement of the subject at vigorous exercise causes some wandering of the recording, as shown in Stage 4. Where adjacent QRS complexes are fairly level, the J point portion of the ST segment is observed in relationship to the level of the previous PQ segment. In this example, the ST segment is found to be neither depressed nor elevated, and the finding represents a normal (or nonischemic) response in a maximal stress test. Deviation of the ST segment is an indication of exercise-induced ischemia of the myocardium.

4. The systolic blood pressure rises progressively with each increment of work load, thus paralleling the heart rate response. This, too, is a normal response to exercise, and in stress testing, systolic pressure is an important parameter in assessing hemodynamic integrity. Also normal for isotonic exercise (the kind of exercise performed by relatively low level but repeated exertions, as on treadmill walking) is a nearly constant diastolic blood pressure, as witnessed here.

The subject did not experience palpitations during the stress test despite the marked tachycardia. Thus, the cause for her episodes of palpitations remains unexplained. On the other hand, the cardiovascular system was assessed at extreme physiological demand, and no disturbance in heart rhythm or evidence of organic disease was revealed. This information is helpful in reassuring individuals with such symptoms that prove elusive to definitive diagnosis.

Sinus tachycardia is a natural response to certain physiological and pathological factors and is not actually an arrhythmia. It may be induced by conditions affecting the myocardium (ventricular failure, myocarditis) or by a diversity of extracardiac disorders. Clinicians must alway keep in mind that sinus tachycardia is the result of an underlying process, whether physiological or pathological. The rhythm should never be considered as a primary disorder by itself. Although the cause may be entirely innocuous, it may also be the most outstanding (and occasionally the only) clue to a serious organ disturbance.

Sinus tachycardia may occur from increased metabolic demand (fever, hyperthyroidism) and elevated circulatory flow (heat exposure, anemia, arteriovenous communications). Shock, congestive heart failure, acute myocardial infarction, and pulmonary embolism accelerate the heart rate, tending to compensate for diminished blood flow. Hypoxia and hypercapnia are physiochemical conditions leading to sinus tachycardia. Sinus impulse formation is stimulated by sympathetic nervous system forces (emotional excitation, pain reflexes, adrenal gland responses, and adrenergic drugs) and by suppression of parasympathetic nervous system tone (cholinergic inhibitor drugs). Smoking may cause sinus tachycardia through the action of nicotine on sympathetic excitation.

The following tracings (29 and 30) were obtained from a 21-year-old woman who had viral gastroenteritis and a temperature of 100.8° and experienced lightheadedness on standing. Notice the changes in rate and blood pressure that follow the change from a recumbent to a sitting position. The acute viral illness, with fever and the prolonged bed rest, contributes to this symptomatic postural response.

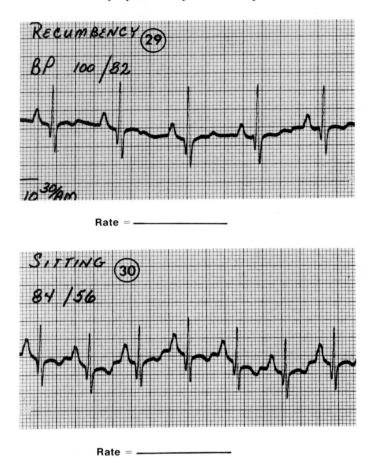

Rate = _____

Rate = _____

An increase in heart rate may also follow subcutaneous administration of epinephrine for bronchial asthma, as can be seen in Figure 3–18.

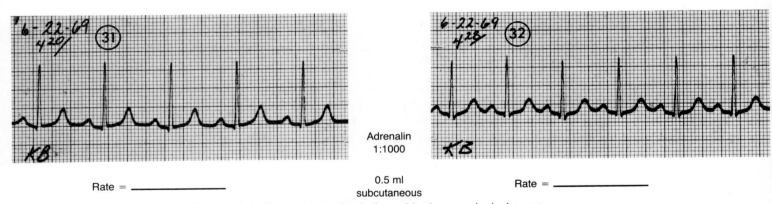

Adrenalin
1:1000

0.5 ml
subcutaneous

Rate = _____   Rate = _____

Figure 3–18. Sympathetic stimulation with pharmacological agent.

Sinus tachycardia may also result from a decrease of neurogenic tone (releasing brake pressure), which normally inhibits sinus node activity (Fig. 3–19). For example, atropine, the prototype of a number of anticholinergic agents that have parasympathetic inhibiting action, blocks the release of acetylcholine. In the vagus nerve, this action renders the normal sympathetic tone unopposed, thus creating a wholly dominant adrenergic effect. It should be noted that many mixed proprietary drugs contain derivatives of atropine, especially the sedatives, analgesics, and medications used to treat the common cold and gastrointestinal disturbances. Agents that cause cardioexcitation through inhibition of parasympathetic tone are termed **vagolytic**.

Example: Atropine

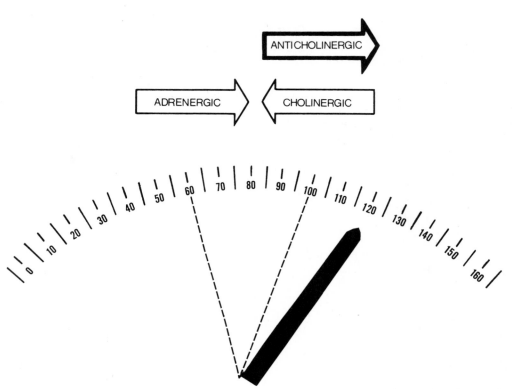

Figure 3–19. Inhibition of parasympathetic tone, producing speeding of rate. Sympathetic forces now dominate.

Thus, atropine inhibits the steady stimulation of the vagus nerve by its anticholinergic effect. The normally present braking action of vagal tone is released, and the sinus rate speeds up.

Figure 3–20 demonstrates the effect of the cholinergic inhibiting agent atropine, occurring within 5 minutes after its administration by intravenous injection.

Conversely, increased vagal tone, by reflexes from external pressure applied over the carotid artery, produces an abrupt slowing in the sinus rate (Fig. 3–21).

Digitalis is used primarily to treat myocardial insufficiency because of its salutary effect on the contractile force of the myocardial fiber. In addition, digitalis affects the heart by increasing parasympathetic activity to the atrial and A-V nodal structures. Clinicians can use this property of digitalis for accentuating vagal tone to advantage in certain arrhythmias. In Figure 3–22, the tracings were obtained from a 65-year-old man with congestive heart failure before and after institution of digitalis therapy.

As can be seen, sinus rate slows. Clinically, pulmonary congestion improved, presumably from both more effective myocardial contractility and the slower rate with enhanced vagal tone.

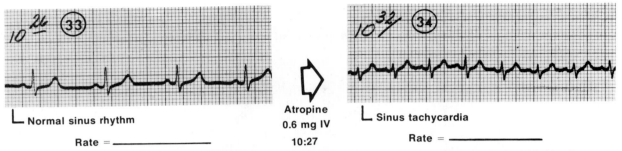

Normal sinus rhythm

Rate = _____

Atropine
0.6 mg IV
10:27

Sinus tachycardia

Rate = _____

Figure 3–20. Excitation of sinus node impulse formation by pharmacological block of parasympathetic control.

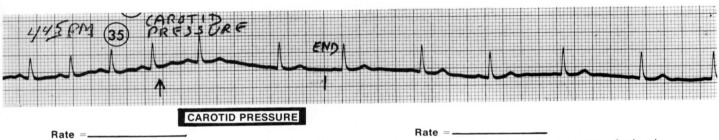

CAROTID PRESSURE

Rate = _____   Rate = _____

Figure 3–21. Transition from sinus tachycardia to normal sinus rhythm by parasympathetic stimulation.

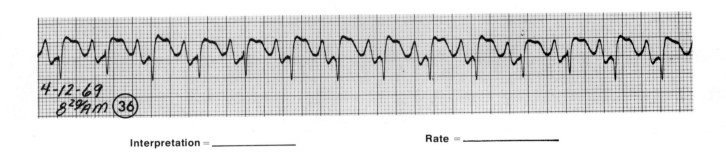

Interpretation = _____   Rate = _____

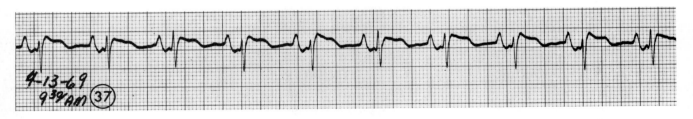

Interpretation = _____   Rate = _____

Figure 3–22. Before and after digitalis therapy.

EXAMPLES OF SINUS TACHYCARDIA

In test strips 38 to 43, label representative P, QRS, and T. Calculate rate by all three methods.

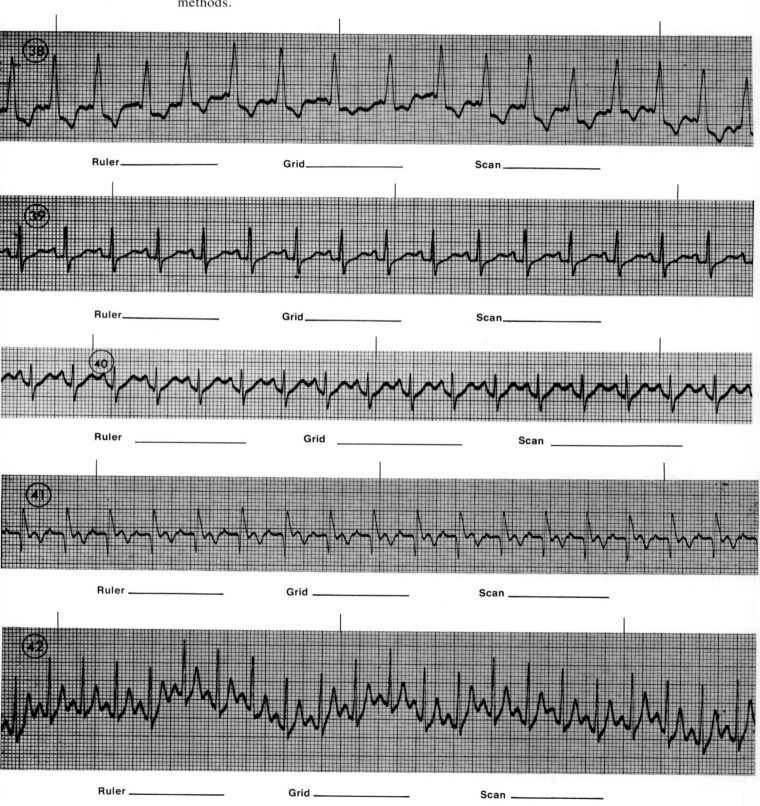

Ruler_____ Grid_____ Scan_____

Ruler_____ Grid_____ Scan_____

Ruler_____ Grid_____ Scan_____

Ruler_____ Grid_____ Scan_____

Ruler_____ Grid_____ Scan_____

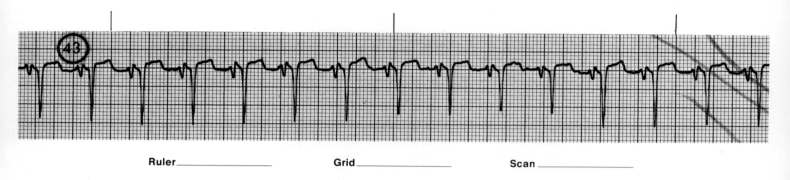

Ruler_____ Grid_____ Scan _____

SINUS NODE: IMPULSE FORMATION

Depression

Depression is considered here as the converse of excitation. Factors that depress impulse-forming or conducting tissues cause slowing of pacemaker rate or conduction velocity. Inhibition of these determinants may be produced by physiological, pharmacological, or pathological factors. Such depression of impulse formation in the sinus node results in abnormal slowing of sinus pacing, as depicted in Figure 3-23. (Bold type is used to emphasize the particular site and disturbance being discussed. Arrhythmias previously presented in the text are maintained in the schema in light type to illustrate the relationships.)

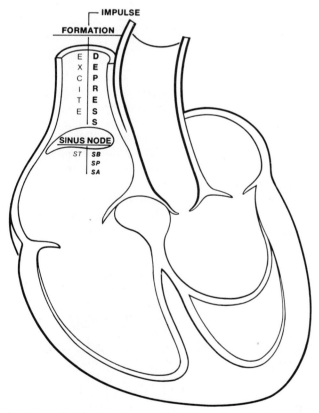

Figure 3–23. Impulse formation in the sinus node. SB = sinus bradycardia; SP = sinus pause; SA = sinus arrest.

Sinus Bradycardia

A sinus node pacemaker rate less than 60 per minute is termed **sinus bradycardia**.

Normal individuals with a strong degree of parasympathetic tone often have sinus bradycardia. This rhythm is most commonly found in young adults, especially those conditioned by vigorous athletics. Test strip 44 is an example of sinus bradycardia recorded from a 37-year-old dance exercise instructor. She was considered to have *physiological* bradycardia (rather than *pathological*) as a result of a high level of physical training, and in the absence of a history of any cardiovascular disorder or symptoms or physical findings suggesting such. (Note the fine oscillations throughout the record, reflecting an artifact from inadequate electrical grounding.)

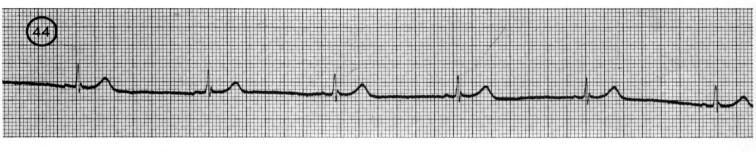

Ruler _____   Grid _____   Scan _____

Sinus bradycardia may also occur when the metabolic rate is reduced, as during sleep, and in myxedematous or hypothermic states. Increased intracranial pressure may cause an abnormally slow pulse. Sudden appearance of sinus bradycardia in a patient with cerebral edema or subdural hematoma is an important clinical observation, because it is evidently the result of stimulation of the parasympathetic center by excessive intracerebral pressure. Sinus bradycardia is sometimes present in acute myocardial infarction (especially of the inferior wall) as a result of interruption of blood supply to the sinus node.

Test strip 45 is a tracing obtained from an elderly nursing home patient with abdominal distention. The diagnosis of severe hypothyroidism was made after hospital admission.

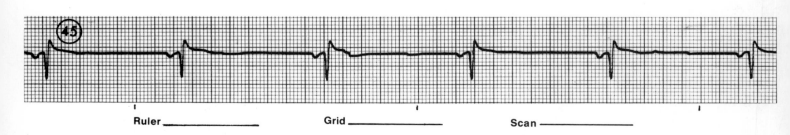

Ruler _____   Grid _____   Scan _____

EXAMPLES OF SINUS BRADYCARDIA

For test strips 46 to 50, identify components and determine rate.

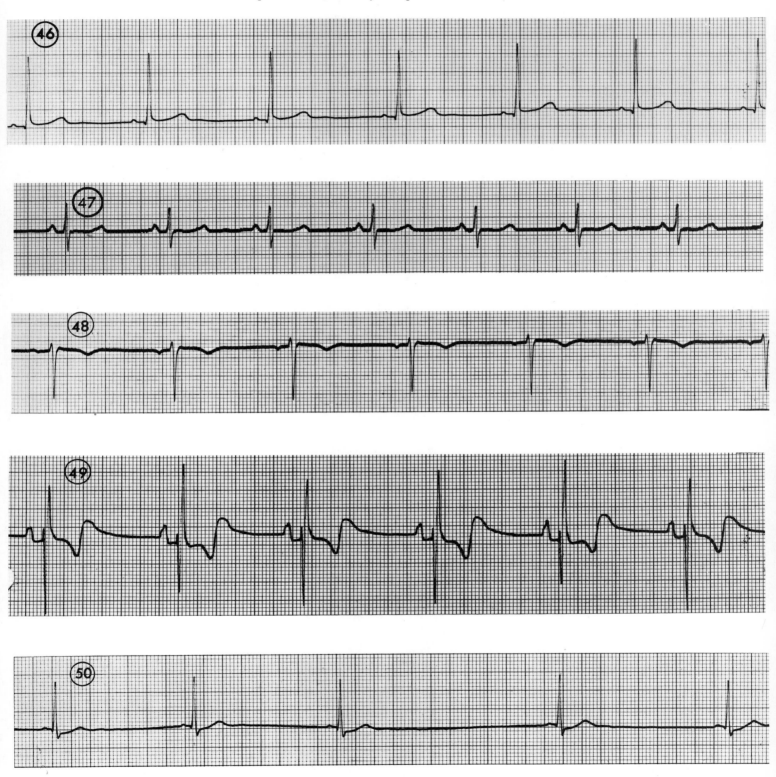

Rate: for shortest interval = _____   for longest interval = _____

Figure 3–24 illustrates an extremely slow rate, falling beyond the one-beat ruler scale (less than 25 beats per minute). An accurate rate can be obtained by determining the distance between beats. There are 90 mm between the first and second cardiac cycles. Because each millimeter represents 0.04 second, the interval represents 3.6 seconds (90 × 0.04). Divide the seconds in 1 minute (60) by the interval seconds (3.6) to obtain the rate in minutes: 60 ÷ 3.6 = 17 beats per minute.

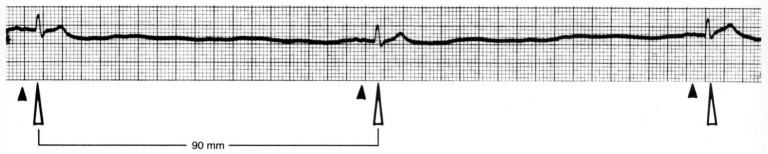

90 mm

Figure 3–24. Example of severe pathological depression of sinus node impulse formation. This tracing was recorded in a patient brought to the emergency room with terminal carbon dioxide poisoning.

Depressed rhythms of sinus node impulse formation may be produced by the following:

1. **Decreasing sympathetic tone:** Reserpine depletes stored adrenergic substances in sympathetic nerve endings. Propranolol (Inderal) inhibits the neurotransmission of norepinephrine by blocking the receptor sites at which the catacholamine acts. Accordingly, propranolol is designated a beta-blocking agent. Slowing of the pulse rate is produced by both agents (Fig. 3–25). Loss of cardiac sympathetic tone also results from complete cervical sympathectomy, leaving the vagus nerve intact and essentially unopposed.

Example: Propranolol

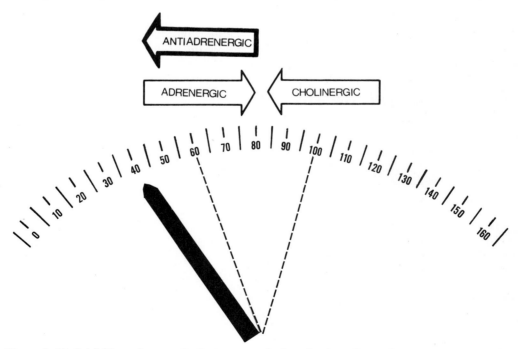

Figure 3–25. Inhibition of sympathetic tone, producing slowing of rate. Parasympathetic forces now dominate.

Clonidine (Catapres) and methyldopa (Aldomet), used in the treatment of hypertension, reduce sympathetic tone by inhibiting adrenergic activity in the central nervous system.

2. **Increasing parasympathetic tone:** Vagal stimulation characteristically leads to reflex slowing of sinus node impulses by increasing cholinergic tone (Fig. 3–26). This may be produced by manual pressure over a carotid artery or by vomiting, forced voiding, and straining at stool (forms of the Valsalva maneuver). Other mechanisms that enhance cardiac parasympathetic tone include pressure on the eyeballs, coughing, immersion of the face in cold water, pulling on the tongue, and nose blowing. In fact, these techniques are used to overcome certain forms of excessively rapid heartbeat.

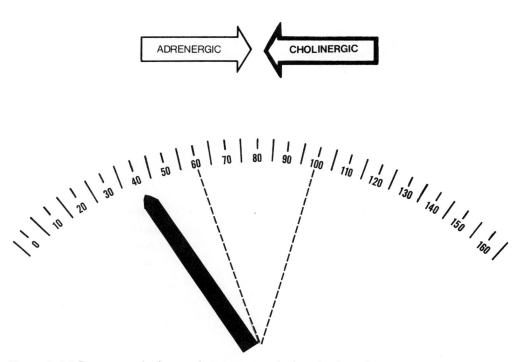

Figure 3–26. Parasympathetic tone increases, producing slowing of rate.

Carotid pressure is a convenient way of increasing vagal tone and slowing the heart rate, and much can be learned of an individual's cardiac autonomic nervous system with this maneuver (Fig. 3–27). Certain precautions are required, however. The pressure should be light and of brief duration; the patient must be recumbent; and cardiac activity must be continuously monitored. Known carotid artery or cerebrovascular disease is a relative contraindication for its use. It is imperative to be prepared for any resultant arrhythmias that may require immediate therapy.

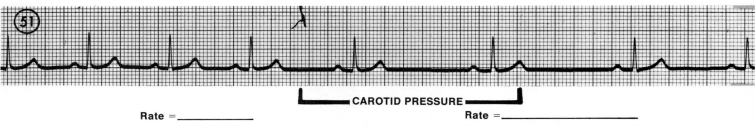

Rate = _____   Rate = _____

Figure 3–27. Sinus rate slowing with carotid stimulation for 2.0 seconds. Note that the bradycardia persists after release of the pressure.

Slowing of the sinus rate typically occurs with deep inspiration, as demonstrated in Figure 3–28. Note that there is actually an *increase* in heart rate for the first few beats on inspiration, a phenomenon related to the dynamics of pulmonary blood volume as described earlier in this chapter.

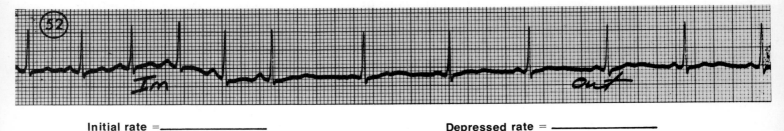

Initial rate = _____   Depressed rate = _____

Figure 3–28. Sinus slowing during full inspiration.

In Figure 3–29, what is the change in rate produced by carotid pressure?

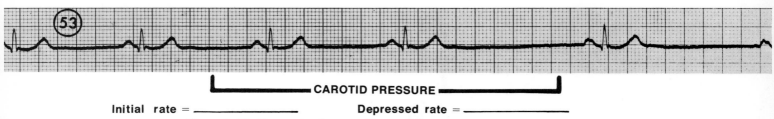

Initial rate = _____   Depressed rate = _____

Figure 3–29. Sinus rate change with carotid pressure.

Sinus tachycardia shows pronounced but gradual slowing of rate in response to carotid pressure (Fig. 3–30). This characteristic helps differentiate sinus tachycardia from rhythms that arise from impulse-forming tissue outside of the sinus node. Note also the gradual resumption of rate after release of carotid stimulation.

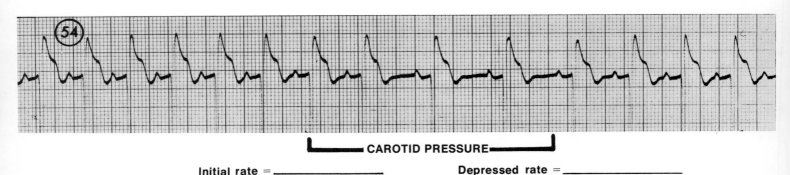

Initial rate = _____   Depressed rate = _____

Figure 3–30. Slowing of sinus tachycardia.

3. **Calcium channel blockers:** The sinus node is heavily dependent on the influx of calcium ions during depolarization. Drugs that interfere with passage of calcium through the cell membrane "gates" (Fig. 3–31) may adversely affect sinus activity, particularly in individuals who have sinus node dysfunction.

The calcium channel blocking agents have various degrees of effect on sinoatrial and A-V nodal activity and on arterial vasodilation and myocardial contraction, all of which require calcium ions for impulse formation and conduction and for the actin-myosin interaction. Of drugs in this group, verapamil (Calan, Isoptin) is most likely to

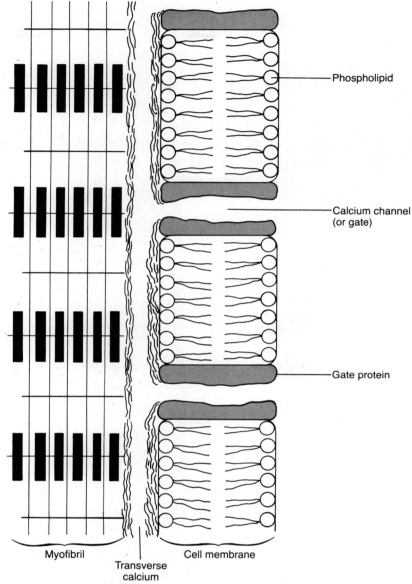

Phospholipid

Calcium channel
(or gate)

Gate protein

Myofibril

Transverse
calcium

Cell membrane

Figure 3–31. Calcium channels that penetrate the cell membrane and form transverse channels along the myofibrils are shown. The calcium channel blocking drugs inhibit the passage of calcium ions through the membrane.

depress the sinus node. In descending order of effect, diltiazem (Cardizem) and nifedipine (Adalat, Procardia) tend to inhibit sinus node function. Nicardipine (Cardene) has negligible effect.

Sinus Pause

A momentary cessation of sinus impulse formation followed by spontaneous resumption of cadence is referred to as sinus pause (see strip 55). Such events may be found in normal persons with a high degree of vagal tone or they may result from digitalis effect or from disease within the sinus node, most commonly fibrodegenerative disease, and acute myocardial infarction.

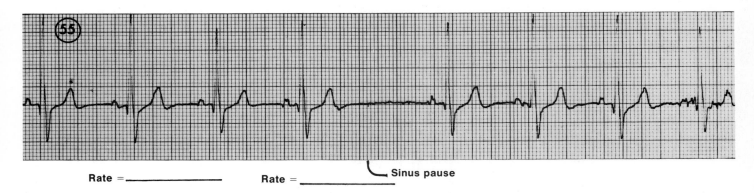

Rate = _____   Rate = _____ ⌐ Sinus pause

Test strip 56 was recorded while a patient in the Coronary Care Unit (CCU) was straining on a bedpan. Such effort represents a form of Valsalva maneuver.

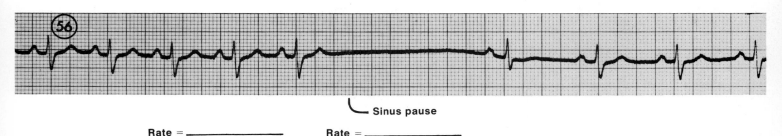

⌐ Sinus pause

Rate = _____   Rate = _____

Special forms of sinus pauses are described further under Sinus Node Dysfunction and Sinoatrial Block in this chapter.

EXAMPLES OF SINUS PAUSE

In strips 57 to 59, compare the basic with the delayed rate.

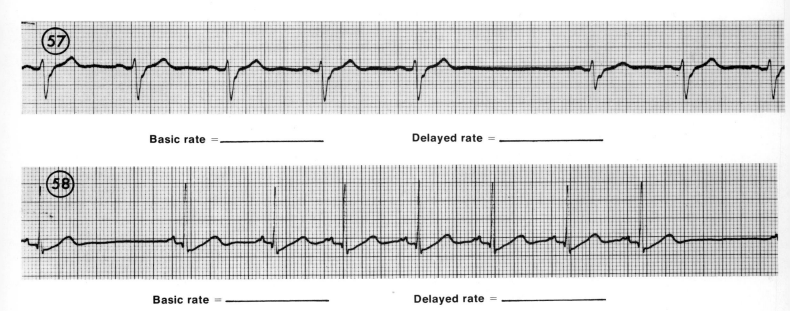

Basic rate = _____   Delayed rate = _____

Basic rate = _____   Delayed rate = _____

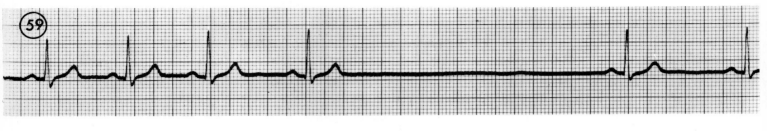

Basic rate = _____   Delayed rate = _____

Sinus Arrest

A prolonged failure (more than 3 seconds) of sinus node automaticity is referred to as **sinus arrest**. In the case of severely delayed or even permanent cessation, an alternative or secondary impulse-forming tissue outside the sinus node maintains the heartbeat. (This mechanism will be discussed in Chapter 4.)

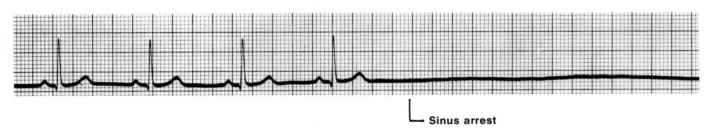

Sinus arrest

The series of tracings that follow demonstrates sinus arrest and the resumption of sinus node activity after mechanical stimulation. A 68-year-old man incurred a sudden brief period of syncope of uncertain cause. He was admitted to the CCU, where he was found to have sinus bradycardia. Continuous tracings obtained a few hours after admission revealed sudden failure of sinus impulse formation. (**Horizontal arrows at the end of one tracing and the beginning of another indicate that the recordings are continuous. This system of notation will be used throughout this book.**)

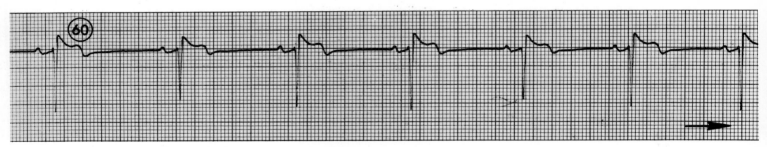

Sinus bradycardia: Rate = _____

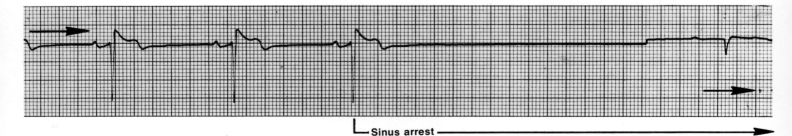

Sinus arrest

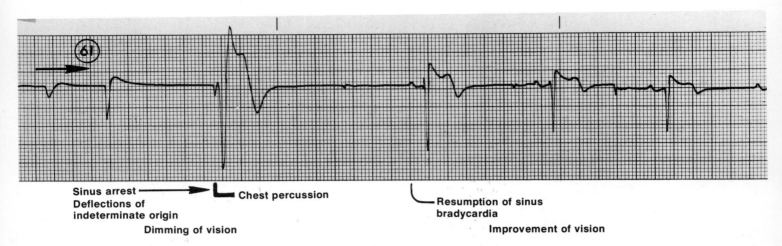

Sinus arrest ———➤ **Chest percussion**
Deflections of
indeterminate origin   **Resumption of sinus**
                                            bradycardia
        Dimming of vision
                                        Improvement of vision

Determine the entire duration of asystole (cessation of ventricular activity) (__ seconds). A sharp thump over the sternum (precordial thump) with the fist induces a cardiac response. Note that the mechanically stimulated ventricular complex has a greater duration than the spontaneous complexes, indicating a slow rate of impulse conduction in the ventricles.

Treatment of sinus bradycardia may be accomplished with agents that increase sympathetic tone (e.g., isoproterenol) or inhibit parasympathetic impulses (e.g., atropine). These drugs may also be given for control of vasovagal hyperactivity and for emergency treatment of severe sinus pauses or sinus arrest.

The following clinical sequence begins with a tracing showing severe sinus bradycardia in a 48-year-old man during endotracheal intubation for anesthesia, a strong vagal stimulation. Treatment with the vagolytic agent atropine was started.

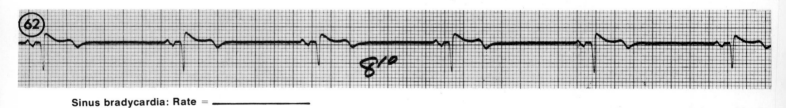

Sinus bradycardia: Rate = _____

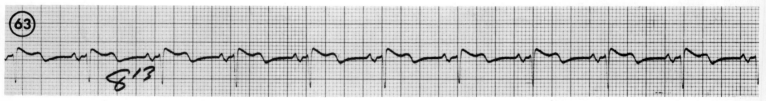

Normal sinus rhythm   Rate = _____

The Vasovagal Reflex

Normally, a modest slowing of heart rate occurs on stimulation of pressure-sensitive neural endings (or baroreceptors) located in the arch of the aorta and at the bifurcation of the carotid artery in the neck. The reflex bradycardia is mediated by afferent impulses conveyed from these arteries by the glossopharyngeal nerve to cardiac and vasomotor control centers in the brain stem. By a classic feedback system, stimulation of these sensory neurons intensifies the brain stem center activity, resulting in an increase in tone of the efferent vagus nerve. This enhanced vagal tone causes inhibition of impulse formation in the sinus node, as explained earlier under Physiology of the Parasympathetic Nervous System. The response in its entirety is referred to as the vasovagal reflex, denoting the circuit from vascular origin to central nervous system to vagal fibers to sinus node.

The vasovagal reflex can be elicited by pressure or light massage in the area of the carotid pulsation.

A vasovagal response is represented in Figure 3–32. The patient is a 66-year-old artist who complained of occasional episodes of lightheadedness with sweating and weakness when standing suddenly from a crouched position and on turning the neck to extreme degrees. The physical examination and ECG were unremarkable except for left axis deviation. With very light pressure applied to the right carotid artery, his lightheadedness (but not the other symptoms) was reproduced and this continuous ECG recorded.

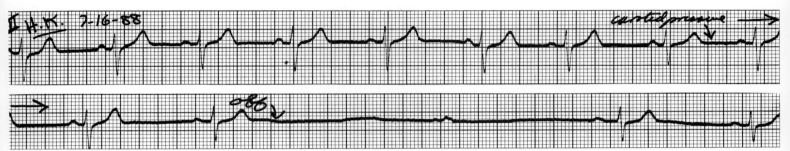

Figure 3–32. Vasovagal response.

Normal sinus rhythm is interrupted on vagal stimulation by sinus slowing followed by a period of ventricular inactivity for 4.3 seconds (the interval between QRS complexes flanking the pause). Very mild graying of vision was experienced near the end of this period. Note that one atrial waveform that occurs is not conducted to the ventricles. Sinus bradycardia supervened for a half minute thereafter, with complete clearing of symptoms. Severe cardiac slowing was the presumed cause of his spontaneous symptoms, and a decision was made to prevent further such episodes with an electronic pacemaker.

An interesting form of the vasovagal reflex occurs in fainting from intense emotional experiences. Evidently, these reactions (e.g., to the sight of blood or to threatening situations) set into motion a strong adrenergic response. A secondary stimulation of the parasympathetic nervous system occurs, probably from the sudden rise in blood pressure affecting the baroreceptors in blood vessels. The result is a profound systemic vasodilation together with a severe bradycardic reaction. Adequate cerebral circulation cannot be maintained, and lightheadedness or frank syncope supervenes momentarily.

Carotid Hypersensitivity

In some individuals, slowing of the sinus rate with stimulation of the carotid artery baroreceptors is exaggerated, occasionally extremely so. Such a response, referred to as carotid hypersensitivity, occasionally results in extremely slow rates. It is most commonly encountered in patients with coronary artery disease, but there are many other associated underlying conditions. It is occasionally found in persons without any detectable incriminating disease, including healthy youths in excellent physical condition.

Carotid hypersensitivity is demonstrated in Figure 3–33, obtained from a 60-year-old woman who complained of repeated episodes of lightheadedness, most likely to occur when carrying heavy grocery bags. With right carotid pressure applied with the

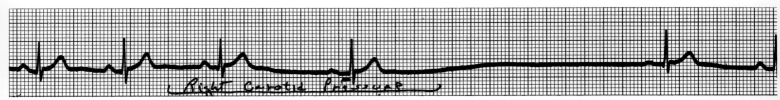

Figure 3–33. Severe sinus slowing after carotid stimulation.

patient in the recumbent position, she did not experience symptoms during this period of prolonged cardiac standstill of 3.20 seconds. Normal sinus rhythm was resumed with release of carotid pressure.

The hyperreactive carotid stimulation-sinus node response represents an abnormality of neural control of the sinus node. It is not a result of intrinsic disease of the sinus node, although carotid hypersensitivity is commonly found in patients with sinus node dysfunction.

Actually, few patients with demonstrated carotid hypersensitivity have symptoms from it. Bradycardia-induced syncopal attacks may result from tight neckwear, shaving the neck, or hyperextension or extreme rotation of the neck. Increased vagal tone from the Valsalva maneuver on straining may precipitate episodes of severe bradycardia. Administration of a combination of cardiodepressor drugs such as propranolol and quinidine to individuals with a tendency toward carotid hypersensitivity can result in symptomatic bradycardia through this mechanism.

In hypersensitive patients, special care must be exercised to avoid excessive carotid artery stimulation, even during simple tasks of shaving and washing. This precaution is extended to those with recent myocardial infarction, who seem especially predisposed to carotid hypersensitivity during the acute phase.

DYNAMIC RHYTHM PROFILE

At this point, it is interesting and helpful for the reader, working with a partner, to record and interpret his or her own ECG under various conditions. By this exercise, the beginning electrocardiographer can observe the physiological variations of the heartbeat. The electrode placement may be that described for cardiac monitoring of a patient in a CCU. Locate a single lead that has well-visualized components and is relatively free from movement artifact.

Procedure:
I. Attach right arm and left arm electrodes.
   A. Select lead I on the machine.
   B. Record. Add the right leg electrode and record again; then compare.*
II. Obtain a rhythm strip during the following conditions (modifications may be indicated for individuals with cardiac or pulmonary disorders or with various physical disabilities):
   A. Supine, normal breathing.
   B. Deep inspiration—hold for at least 30 seconds.
   C. Full, forced exhalation.
   D. Valsalva maneuver (strong expiratory force against a closed nose and mouth to make the ears "pop").
   E. Standing:
      1. Immediately.
      2. After 1 minute.

---

* Some electrocardiographic machines will not operate unless the right leg ground lead is attached.

    F. Exercise:
        1. Immediately after exercise (running in place, deep knee bends, climbing steps, sit-ups, performed to the point of mild fatigue).
        2. One minute after exercise.
    G. Sitting—after rest and return of rate to baseline heart rate.
    H. Carotid pressure (only under supervision of a physician). Adverse reactions may occur in hypersensitive persons.
  III. Inspect each portion of the dynamic profile and correlate changes in rate with activity or maneuver. Also note any unusual beat forms or prominent irregularity of rhythm and set aside for later interpretation.
  IV. Cut the ECG at convenient and uniform lengths and select representative sections. This series can be mounted in the same format as the example dynamic cardiac rhythm profile that follows. Write in the heart rate where major changes occur.

The series of rhythm strips presented here was taken from a 20-year-old nursing student. Lead I was used, and the electrodes RA, LA, and RL were attached to the chest wall as described for the special monitoring lead.

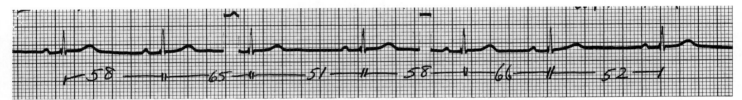

The above tracing, taken during recumbency, reveals prominent sinus irregularity, the rate changes varying with the phases of respiration. The predominantly slow rate is probably related to athletic conditioning gained from regular jogging.

In the tracing below, the heart rate suddenly quickens on taking a deep breath because of hemodynamic changes related to expansion of pulmonary blood volume and temporary alterations in cardiac filling. Shortly thereafter, however, increased vagal tone from deep breath holding dominates, and the sinus rate slows.

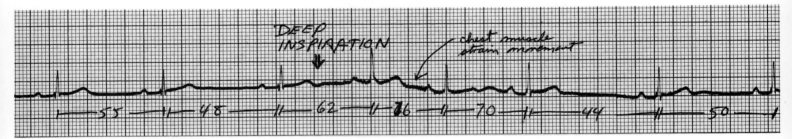

The effects of strong vagal tone, induced by the Valsalva maneuver, are demonstrated in the next rhythm strip. The sudden development of marked sinus bradycardia is observed. Considerable baseline artifact is present owing to muscular contractions required for the maneuver.

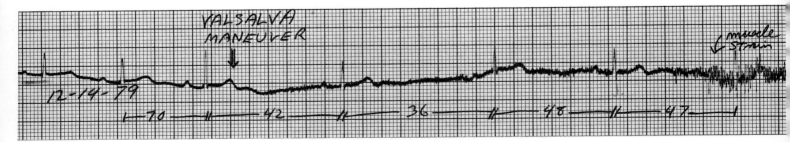

A slight acceleration in sinus rate occurs on standing, as is seen on the following tracing. The faster resting rate is one of the mechanisms by which the general circulatory function is preserved in the face of the increased cardiac demand imposed by the upright position.

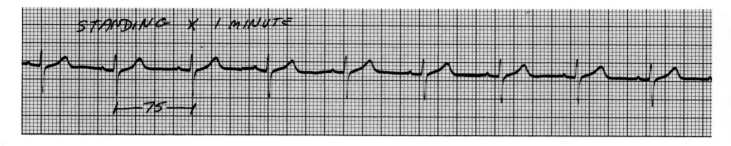

With relatively mild exercise, specifically, running in place for 1 minute, the heart rate increases moderately, as demonstrated in the tracing below.

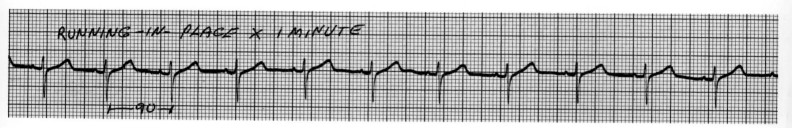

After more vigorous exercise, the sinus rate is accelerated even further, as demonstrated in the next tracing. Such changes are critical features of the normal supportive responses to the stress of physical exertion.

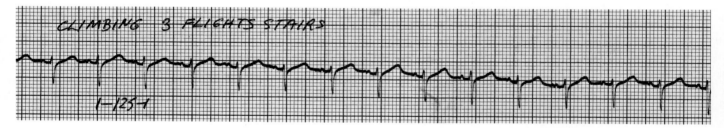

Compare your dynamic rhythm profile with those of others. You are likely to find considerable and even marked variation in responses, even among entirely normal individuals. Factors that play a role in this variability include resting sympathetic and parasympathetic tone, peripheral vascular reactivity to positional changes, body build, physical conditioning, psychological state, and smoking habits.

SINUS NODE DYSFUNCTION

Alterations in automaticity of the sinus node have been described as they occur in association with influences of the autonomic nervous system. We have observed the effects of stimulation of the parasympathetic nerves to the sinus node region and of inhibition of sympathetic tone. In addition, the sinus node is susceptible to intrinsic disorders (severe sinus bradycardia, sinus pauses, sinus arrest) that disturb its normal rhythmicity. Such conditions are known as sinus node dysfunction.

Two mechanisms may be responsible for intrinsic disease of the sinus node:

1. Injury to the P cells, resulting in disturbed capability for producing impulses.

2. Injury to T cells, limiting the transmission of impulses from the sinus node to the surrounding atrial cells.

Etiologies of Sinus Node Dysfunction

Sinus node dysfunction is now being recognized as a very frequent cause of symptomatic bradycardia and erratic cardiac rhythms, particularly in elderly patients. A large number of underlying diseases may be causally related to sinus node dysfunction, summarized in the following list:

- Degenerative disease. A progressive fibrosis (a sclerodegenerative process) that is directly related to aging is probably the predominant cause of sinus node destruction. This condition appears to be independent of ischemic heart disease, which is also more prevalent in the aging population.
- Ischemic coronary arterial disease. The cause may be chronic arterial stenosis, spasm, or thrombus resulting in acute myocardial infarction.
- Inflammatory disease. Myocarditis, collagen vascular disease (as systemic lupus erythematosus).
- Infiltrative disease. Amyloidosis, hemochromatosis, metastatic carcinoma, muscular dystrophy.
- Metabolic disorders. Hypothyroidism, hyperthyroidism, hypercarbia, hypokalemia, hypothermia.
- Drug toxicity. Certain drugs at cardiotoxic levels may induce sinus node dysfunction even in persons with no intrinsic disease of the sinus node. In those with an underlying condition affecting the sinus node, such drugs, even at ordinary pharmacological levels, may induce or seriously aggravate sinus node dysfunction. Digitalis, quinidine, lidocaine, and atropine are the most commonly incriminated agents.
- Sleep apnea. Severe bradycardia associated with sinus node failure has been documented in many individuals who develop respiratory depression during sleep.

Characteristics of Sinus Node Dysfunction

Sinus node dysfunction may become manifest by one or several distinctive features:

1. Sinus bradycardia. Usually in the range of 40 to 55 beats per minute in a resting individual, this rhythm occurs without association with athletic conditioning, metabolic disorder, or cardiodepressor drugs.

2. The sinus pacemaker does not accelerate as expected in response to increased physical work (chronotropic incompetence). Exertional tolerance is reduced as a result of rate-related limitation in cardiac output. Failure of an appropriate rise in heart rate during exercise is particularly troublesome for individuals who also have impaired myocardial contractility or cardiac valve disease.

3. Another sign of sinus node disease (and a frequently overlooked sign) is the *absence* of sinus tachycardia in patients who would be expected to have a rapid heart rate. For example, a patient with congestive heart failure, pneumonia, fever, or severe

anemia may have a second condition affecting impulse formation. The tracing in Figure 3–34 was obtained from a 58-year-old woman with severe hypotension, shortly after she received an injection of chlorpromazine for severe nausea. Subsequently, the diagnosis of primary amyloidosis was made; it had been previously unsuspected.

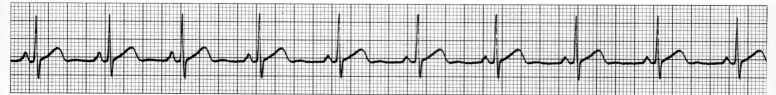

Figure 3–34. Sinus rhythm unresponsive to stimulation to increase rate.

In another example, abnormal sinus node function was observed in a 61-year-old man admitted to the hospital for suspected myocardial infarction. Fine inspiratory rales were present at both lung bases, and jugular veins were moderately distended at 15° from recumbency, suggesting both left and right myocardial insufficiency. The admission tracing obtained on the monitoring lead is shown (Fig. 3–35).

The most striking feature of this ECG is the extremely deep T waves together with moderate depression of ST segments, commonly found during the early phase of acute myocardial infarction. The presence of sinus bradycardia is wholly inappropriate in congestive heart failure, when the usual compensatory response is an acceleration of heart rate. This association suggests that the sinus node itself is involved in the ischemic injury.

4. The physiological slowing and speeding of sinus rate in response to respiratory dynamics is blunted or absent altogether.

5. Episodic sinus arrest. Sinus pauses and sinus arrest are common findings in this syndrome. Sinus arrest can last for several seconds or minutes; sinus standstill may eventually become permanent.

6. Lack of the characteristic acceleration of sinus rate from drugs. Testing for this response is usually performed with isoproterenol (an adrenergic agent) or atropine (an inhibitor of parasympathetic tone).

7. Frequent association with other forms of cardiac abnormalities affecting impulse-forming and impulse-conducting tissues outside of the sinus node. Such diffuse involvement often results in failure of the normal "escape" or "rescue" pacemakers of the atria or ventricles to function when the sinus node ceases pacemaker activity. Various forms of conduction defects may be found in the A-V node and in the His-Purkinje system.

8. Tachycardias may interrupt the usual slow sinus rhythm in sinus node dysfunction. These paroxysms of tachycardia result from activated pacemakers that lie outside of the sinus node, called ectopic pacemakers. This susceptibility to tachycardias is incurred by the coexistence of a slow heart rate and defects in impulse conduction that are scattered throughout the atria. The mechanism involves reentrant circuits, which will be explained in Chapter 4. As may be anticipated, the bradycardia-tachycardia syndrome is manifest in the more advanced stages of sinus node dysfunction.

9. Prolonged sinus arrest (or sinoatrial block) typically occurs on termination of a tachycardia. Indeed, the expression **sick sinus syndrome** was introduced in a report in 1967 describing the long period of sinus standstill commonly observed immediately after electric shock treatment of rapid atrial rhythms. Although the example from this report that is presented here (Fig. 3–36) is complex, bradycardia with an absence of an effective sinus rhythm is recorded immediately after cardioversion.

Popular use, incidentally, has resulted in the term **sick sinus** being applied to all forms of sinus node dysfunction. We chose to adhere to the latter term, which is more consistent with traditional medical terminology.

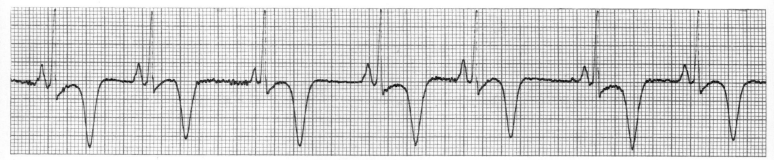

Figure 3–35. The inability of the sinus node to compensate by increasing the rate of impulse formation is demonstrated in this strip of sinus bradycardia in a patient in congestive heart failure.

In Figure 3–37, a tachycardia of atrial origin is present initially. Suddenly the tachycardia ends; an extraordinarily long pause of 3.4 seconds occurs before a sinus beat appears. During this period, the patient in the CCU complained of transient palpitations followed by giddiness.

Several hours later, severe and irregular sinus bradycardia was observed (Fig. 3–38), another sign of a severely disturbed sinus pacemaker.

Because sinus node dysfunction has the propensity for prolonged sinus inactivity following an episode of tachycardia, symptoms of lightheadedness or syncope immediately after an episode of rapid palpitations are highly suggestive of sinus node dysfunction. The disorder in these patients is generally accompanied by concurrent disease in subsidiary pacemakers and in the major conduction pathways. Indeed, prolonged cardiac standstill subsequent to a paroxysm of tachycardia is probably the most common cause of serious symptoms associated with sinus node dysfunction.

Symptom-related manifestations of sinus node dysfunction are usually intermittent, and evidence of the syndrome may not be present on random electrocardiography. A clinician who suspects that sinus node dysfunction is the basis for symptoms can enlist special studies to provide a definitive diagnosis. Those available are long-term recording of the cardiac rhythm, even during full activity, and intracardiac electronic pacing techniques.

Ambulatory rhythm recording is obtained using a cassette taping device. Periods of 24 hours are usually recorded. During this time, patients can be physically active, and the time of experienced symptoms is marked on magnetic tape. The taped information is subsequently descrambled electronically, and a clinician may observe the cardiac rhythm for the entire period, either at rapid speed for surveying or at real time in the ordinary electrocardiographic form. In a small portion of a 24-hour record in

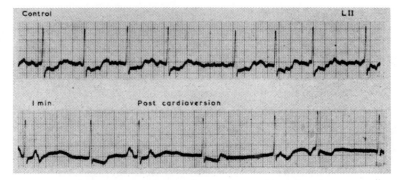

Figure 3–36. Sinus arrest following cardioversion. (From Lown B: Electrical reversion of cardiac arrhythmias. Br Heart J 29:469, 1967.)

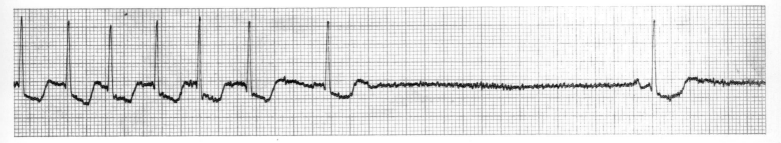

Figure 3–37. Tachycardia-bradycardia rhythm.

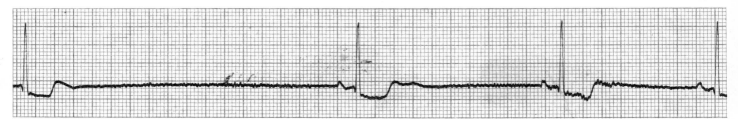

Figure 3–38. Severe bradycardia in the same patient as in Figure 3–37.

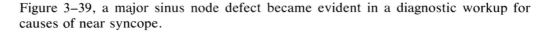

Figure 3–39, a major sinus node defect became evident in a diagnostic workup for causes of near syncope.

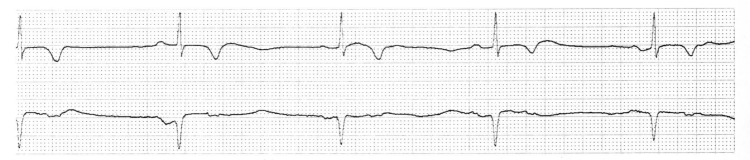

Figure 3–39. Rhythm strip showing severe depression of sinus node impulse formation (rate = 37 per minute) obtained with 24-hour ambulatory monitoring equipment.

The second method of establishing (or excluding) the diagnosis of sinus node dysfunction requires introduction of an electrode wire by peripheral vein into the right atrium. An external electronic pacemaker then stimulates the heart by emitting impulses at a rate faster than the natural heart rate. An indication of sinus node dysfunction is the phenomenon of delayed reappearance of a sinus rhythm following sudden cessation of the electronically paced tachycardia. This duration is called the **sinus node recovery time**.

More than half of the permanent electronic pacemakers implanted in the United States are for treatment of sinus node dysfunction. The objective is to ensure that the heart rate does not slow beyond a preset rate. In many patients, episodic tachycardias no longer occur when the heart beats faster under electronic control. In those who continue to have tachycardias, cardiodepressor drugs may be used safely. (Such drugs are contraindicated in this syndrome without the protection of an electronic pacemaker.)

SINUS NODE: IMPULSE CONDUCTION

Depression

To review sinus node electrophysiology, an impulse is generated within P cells in the center of the node. The impulse is then transmitted to T cells at the periphery of the sinus node, from which it propagates to the myocardial cells of the surrounding atrium. This orderly transmission may be affected by diseases, drug effects, or neural conditions that delay the emergence of the impulse from the sinus node or prevent it altogether. Such disorders may be called **T cell dysfunction** and are included in the general category of sinus node dysfunction. The distinguishing feature from those forms described earlier is the failure of impulse conduction rather than impulse formation within the sinus node. Called **sinoatrial block**, the condition is represented under Depression: Impulse Conduction in Figure 3–40.

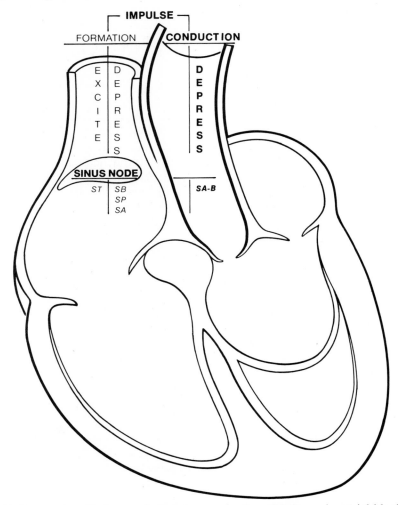

Figure 3–40. Depression of sinus node impulse conduction. SA-B = sinoatrial block.

Sinoatrial Block

Sinoatrial block–the failure of an impulse already generated to emerge from the sinus node—cannot be determined directly by electrocardiography. This limitation is the result of the extremely small electrical disturbance of the impulse. Instead, the presence of sinoatrial block (also termed sinus exit block) must be determined by inference, and this distinction depends on the timing of the interrupted sinus rhythm (Fig. 3–41).

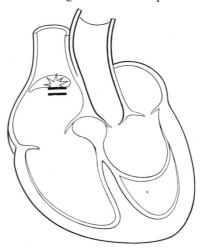

Figure 3–41. Double bars show blocking of impulses emanating from the sinus node.

In appearance on the ECG, sinoatrial block resembles a sinus pause, produced by an abrupt slowing of sinus impulse formation. The distinguishing feature, however, is that the intrinsic rhythm of the sinus node is not interrupted. The P wave following the pause picks up in time with the established cadence of the sinus node. This results in a pause that is precisely twice the duration of the preceding cardiac cycles. In other words, the duration of the sinus pause from P wave to P wave is double the PP interval of the usual beats. This phenomenon is depicted in Figure 3–42.

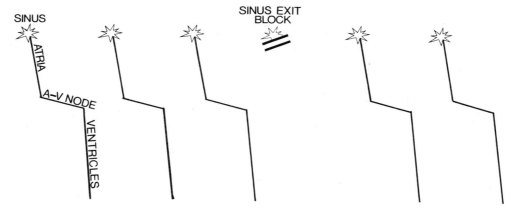

Figure 3–42. The stars represent sinus impulse formation and the lines the course and time of impulse conduction. Impulse blockage is depicted in the fourth cardiac cycle, in which the sinus impulse does not penetrate into the atria. Note that there is no change in the cadence of the sinus beat.

In this diagram, note that the interval between the two beats that flank the delay is precisely twice the interval between the normally timed beat. In commonly applied terminology, the PP interval spanning the delay is two times the PP interval of the normal rhythm.

In Figure 3–43, normal sinus rhythm appears initially. After the third beat, a delay occurs. This event appears to be a sinus pause (failure of sinus node impulse formation). However, when P waves are measured out with calipers, it can be demonstrated that

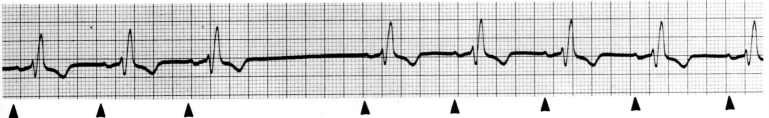

Figure 3–43. Example of sinoatrial block.

subsequent P waves appear without any change of cadence. This is not likely to happen in sinus pause. More probably, the sinus node discharges an impulse on time during the apparent missed beat, but it does not exit from the sinus node to stimulate an atrial response. The basic rhythmicity of the sinus node is not disturbed.

The differences in pause duration between these two forms of sinus node dysfunction—(1) a defect in impulse generation versus (2) a defect in impulse conduction—are explained at the cellular level:

- P cell dysfunction. In this condition, action potentials in the pacemaker cells are generated with an erratic timing. A pause thus resulting has a random duration.
- T cell dysfunction. Sinoatrial block is ascribed to failure of transitional cells at the sinus node perimeter, and it does not disturb the intrinsic rhythmicity of action potentials generated in the pacemaker cells. Consequently, the exit block causes merely a single missed beat. The duration of the pause is equal to the duration of two cardiac cycles at the usual rate. Indeed, it is the temporal relationship of pause duration to normal cycle length that allows an electrocardiographer to infer that sinoatrial block has occurred.

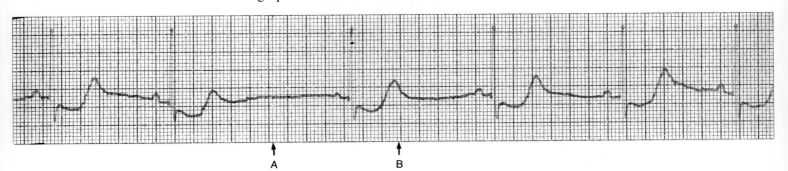

Figure 3–44. Sinus pause (see text for explanation of arrows A and B).

Compare these relationships of timing with that of the strip in Figure 3–44. Here the PP interval of the pause is not twice the naturally occurring PP interval. One assumes that the depolarization sequence of the pacemaker cells is fired erratically. A blocked (or "concealed") sinus impulse would be expected to occur 32 mm (or 1.28 seconds) after the preceding P wave (arrow at A) and the subsequent P wave (arrow at B) to appear at 32 mm after that presumed point. In fact, the cycle after the pause appears only 16.5 mm after the expected P wave. This implies a sinus cadence change rather than failure of transmission of a single sinus impulse.

Causes of sinoatrial block are similar to those listed for causes of impulse formation depression in the sinus node. They include degenerative fibrosis, myocardial ischemia, inflammatory and infiltrative conditions, and drug toxicity. In fact, many patients with advanced sinus node dysfunction are thought to have a progressive disease that begins in the pacemaker cells, resulting in bradycardia, and eventually involves the transitional cells, producing sinoatrial block.

The preeminent cause of sinoatrial block is ischemic coronary arterial disease. In addition, there is a strong propensity for patients with sinoatrial block to develop disorders of impulse conduction in the atrial mass and in the A-V node. These patients commonly have symptomatic bradycardia and the bradycardia-tachycardia syndrome. Consequently, the detection of sinoatrial block has important implications in patient management.

Excessive vagal tone may sometimes produce sinoatrial block, even in healthy persons. Indeed, superb athletic conditioning attained through endurance exercise is a predisposing factor. Usually, however, sinoatrial block induced by vagal stimulation is found in individuals with sinus node disease. Closed glottis straining and pressure over the carotid artery may induce episodes of lightheadedness or syncope. In these instances, a series of blocked sinus beats (often in conjunction with blocked impulses in the A-V node) results in profound bradycardia.

Persons with sinoatrial block are also susceptible to untoward action of various drugs. By its vagotonic effect, digitalis may precipitate symptomatic sinoatrial block. Drugs that inhibit adrenergic tone or depress cell activity directly (such as quinidine) can produce similar adversity. Sinoatrial block may also be responsive to pharmacological intervention, as demonstrated in the following example.

A 67-year-old woman was admitted to the CCU shortly after an episode of mid-anterior chest discomfort (sensation of heaviness) associated with weakness and a giddy feeling. Sinoatrial block interrupting normal sinus rhythm was discovered on admission, as illustrated in the next strip, and this condition was treated with a parasympathetic blocking agent.

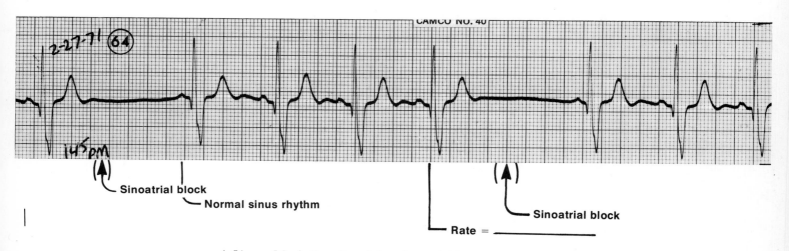

1:51 PM: Mark the site of the sinoatrial block.

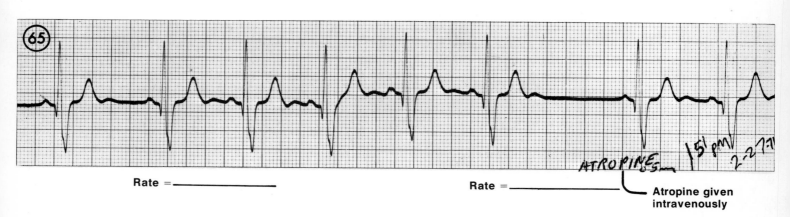

2:00 PM: Nine minutes after the administration of atropine, the sinus rate has increased, and sinoatrial block is no longer present.

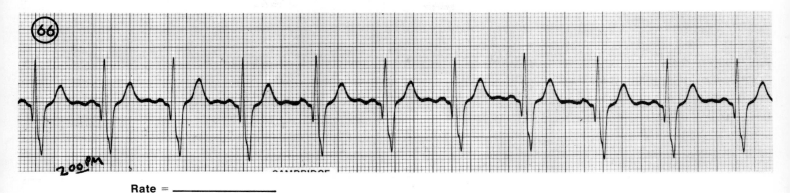

Rate = _____

The pharmacological suppression of parasympathetic activity resulted in acceleration of **impulse formation** (sinus rate increased) and **impulse conduction** (sinoatrial block abolished).

Permanent sinoatrial block cannot be distinguished from sinus arrest (failure of impulse formation). In both conditions, continued cardiac activity depends on the development of pacemakers outside of the sinus node in the atria, the A-V junctional tissues or the ventricles, or an external electronic source.

It can be appreciated that sinoatrial block may occur with successive sinus impulses. The result is again a pause, but the duration is longer than that associated with a single sinus exit block. In these instances, the PP interval at the pause is three, four, or more times the PP interval of normally conducted beats. These higher degrees of block are more serious because the associated bradycardia is more severe.

LADDERGRAMS

At this point in the text, a schematic representing a cardiac rhythm is introduced. This method is particularly useful for analyzing complex arrhythmias, and the learner may find it helpful to apply this process as rhythms are reviewed. Referred to as a **laddergram**, a diagram of each cardiac cycle is constructed to depict each impulse formed and the route and time interval of conduction throughout the heart. A laddergram for normal sinus rhythm is presented to familiarize readers with its basic form (Fig. 3–45). Additional laddergrams will be provided for the various arrhythmias.

At the left of the diagram, the areas of the conduction system are shown. The stars represent the site (or sites) of impulse formation. The lines depict the course of conduction, with the slant of the line indicating the duration (time interval) for the conduction. Interruption of conduction is illustrated by two heavy lines crossing the line of conduction and the absence of the conduction line below the block.

The electrical activity of each beat is expressed in a laddergram by using a sloping line for each zone of conduction: the atria, the A-V node, and the ventricles. The line begins at the point at which the cardiac cycle is initiated (i.e., the pacemaker). Note that in Figure 3–45 the line starts at the onset of the P wave and proceeds downward and to the right to the end of the P wave. At the A-V node, the line changes its slope, falling less precipitously, thus expressing the slower conduction velocity through this pathway. As the impulse enters the ventricles to form the QRS complex, the line drops off more sharply, representing the more rapid conduction velocity through the Purkinje fibers. Further examples of the laddergram will be presented along with the various arrhythmias.

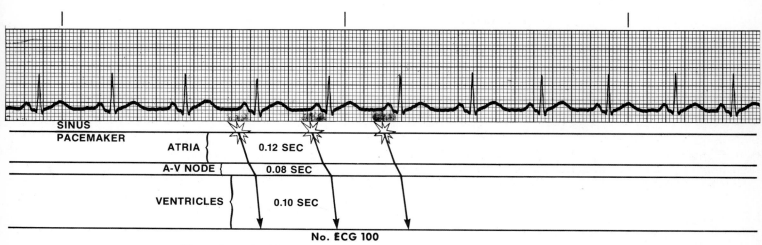

Figure 3–45. Laddergram for normal sinus rhythm.

PREPARATION OF A CARDIAC RHYTHM NOTEBOOK

A valuable collection of examples of arrhythmias can be assembled from routine ECGs and monitoring tracings in hospitals of any size. These may be taken from clippings not selected for the permanent record. Almost all the examples used in this text are discarded portions of recordings taken in community hospitals.

A well-developed notebook may serve as a log or as a ready bank of arrhythmias for review and teaching. In addition, selecting appropriate tracings will increase rhythm scanning acuity and encourage careful interpretation, labeling, and display.

Examples in the notebook should be arranged by some orderly system. The format of this book or some other system may be followed. Each tracing should be clearly labeled with the name (or initials) of the patient and the date for reference. Record pertinent drugs and activity. Interpretations may be written under each tracing or included on a separate answer sheet.

Tracings in this book have been cut at 20 cm (or 8 seconds) and mounted on regular-sized typing paper. Longer strips, if preferred, can be placed along the long axis of the paper, or a larger notebook size may be used. Changing rhythm patterns are highly desirable for teaching purposes. These interesting tracings can usually be cut and mounted as serial tracings, indicating continuity with bold arrows. A glue pencil is handy for mounting; rub the adhesive on the mounting paper rather than directly on the ECG to avoid causing marks. Acetate folders are advantageous for protecting the tracing from slipping and from inadvertent marking such as with caliper points. Notebook tab dividers provide easy reference to rhythm categories. A section containing arrhythmias of all types makes an excellent file for review and for teaching.

Symbols can be placed on the ECG with any convenient marker, such as a ballpoint or fine-tipped felt pen.

4 The Atria

IMPULSE FORMATION
Atrial Escape Complex
Atrial Escape Rhythm
Wandering Atrial Pacemaker
ATRIA: IMPULSE FORMATION
Excitation
Atrial Premature Complex
Blocked Atrial Premature Complexes
The Refractory Period
Multifocal Atrial Premature Complexes

Atrial Tachycardia
Electrocardioversion
Atrial Tachycardia with Atrioventricular
   Block
ATRIAL FLUTTER
Treatment of Atrial Flutter
ATRIAL FIBRILLATION
Treatment of Atrial Fibrillation
SELF-EVALUATION: STAGE 1

IMPULSE FORMATION

Cells scattered throughout the atrial wall, like those of the sinus node, possess the property of automaticity. In effect, the cells undergo spontaneous Phase 4 depolarization. However, the action potential of atrial pacemaker cells differs strikingly from that of the sinus node cells and in some aspects more resembles the action potential of the myofibrils, described earlier.

Automatic cells in the atria have a greater resting transmembrane potential than do sinus node cells. In addition, they have a slower rate of decline during Phase 4 depolarization (Fig. 4–1). These important characteristics endow the atrial cells with a slower inherent rate of automatic firing, simply because it takes longer for these cells to reach the point of self-stimulation. In normal sinus rhythm, the impulses from the sinus node propagate through the atria, stimulating sarcomeres and automatic atrial cells before the latter have a chance to form their own impulses. In this way, the more rapidly firing sinus node dominates the atrial beat.

Phase 0 depolarization of atrial automatic cells is much more abrupt than in cells of the sinus node. The upstroke, in fact, much more closely approximates that of the myofibrils. The phases of repolarization are also similar to those of the myofibril, assuming a more distinct identity than in the P cells while taking longer to attain full repolarization.

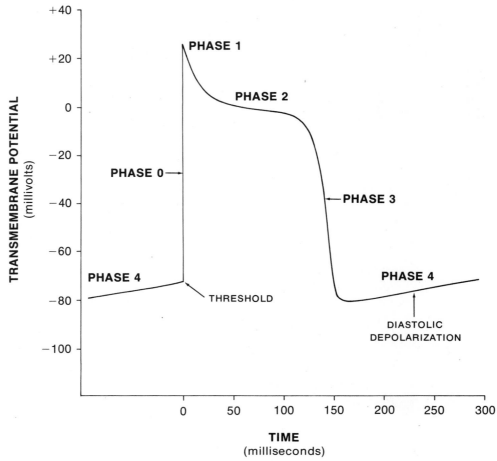

Figure 4–1. Action potential of the automatic atrial cell.

Atrial Escape Complex

From the preceding description of comparative action potentials, it can be readily appreciated that if sinus firing became ineffective (either because of failure of sinus impulse formation or because of sinus exit block), the automatic cells of the atria would be free to develop their own spontaneous firing. This eventuality is exactly the expected response when the sinus node function is interrupted by disease, drugs, or extreme vagotonic reflexes. Thus, an impulse originates from an ordinarily latent pacemaker site in the atria. Such a beat is referred to as an **escape beat**.

In an atrial escape beat, the impulse arises in the atrium and disperses throughout it, including to the sinus node. As in normal conduction originating in the sinus node, the impulse travels to the ventricles via the atrioventricular (A-V) node (Fig. 4–2). Such impulses may arise from either the right or the left atrium.

Depolarization from an ectopic atrial focus proceeds in a different direction than does that of a depolarizing wave front originating in the sinus node. This results in an electrocardiographic change, represented by a variation in P wave contour. The PR interval may also be altered. The impulse, after penetrating the A-V node, continues along normal conduction pathways, so that the QRS complex and T wave of the beat are similar to those of sinus beats.

Note below the delay in the rate of sinus beats (in this case induced by carotid pressure). During this slowing, a beat that has an altered P wave configuration appears.

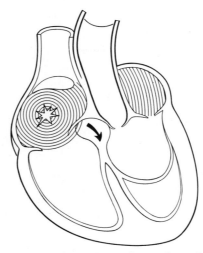

Figure 4–2. Schematic view of atrial impulse formation and conduction.

The associated QRS complex and T waveforms are identical to those of the sinus beats. This cardiac cycle is an atrial escape beat.

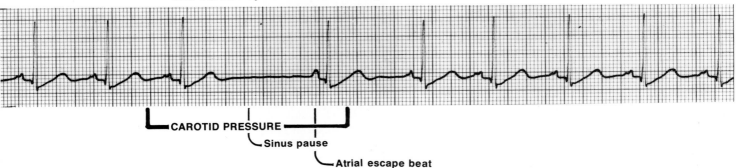

CAROTID PRESSURE

Sinus pause

Atrial escape beat

Atrial Escape Rhythm

Successive atrial escape beats that result from sustained suppression of sinus impulse formation to below a certain rate establish an **atrial escape rhythm**. Again, this phenomenon is a normal physiological event that protects the heart from standstill in the presence of prolonged failure of impulse formation or conduction in the sinus node.

In test strip 67, progressive slowing of the sinus pacemaker leads to a sustained rhythm in which P waves have an altered configuration. QRS complexes and T waves remain unchanged. These are atrial escape beats that maintain a nearly constant rate. In the example given here, sinus slowing was a spontaneous event in a patient with documented sinus node dysfunction but with no associated symptoms.

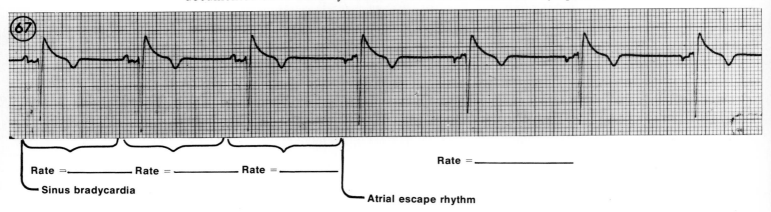

Rate = _____   Rate = _____   Rate = _____

Rate = _____

Sinus bradycardia

Atrial escape rhythm

After the slowing of the sinus rate with vagal stimulation in Figure 4–3, a rhythm supersedes in which the P wave form and PR interval are altered. Presumably, a pacemaker in the atria is activated on suppression of the sinus node, and the atria are now depolarized in a different sequence. This tracing demonstrates a sustained escape rhythm from an atrial focus. Note that the escape rhythm rate is *slower* than that of the sinus rhythm.

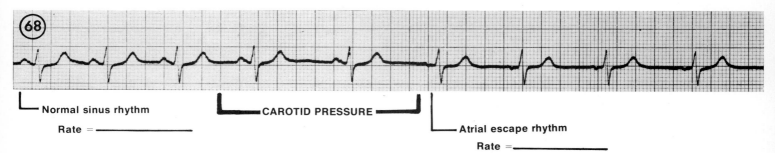

Figure 4–3. Atrial escape rhythm induced by vagotonic maneuver.

The rate of spontaneous diastolic depolarization of those cells in the atria that have the capacity for automaticity is such that the inherent rate of an atrial escape rhythm is set at about 50 beats per minute. Thus, one would expect that sustained atrial pacing of the heart would appear whenever the sinus rate fell below 50 beats a minute. In actuality, those factors that slow the sinus rate (e.g., high vagal tone, drugs, sclerosing fibrosis) are often operative on atrial pacemaker cells as well. This shared suppressing influence explains the common condition of sinus bradycardia, well below this inherent rate without evidence of automaticity in atrial pacemakers.

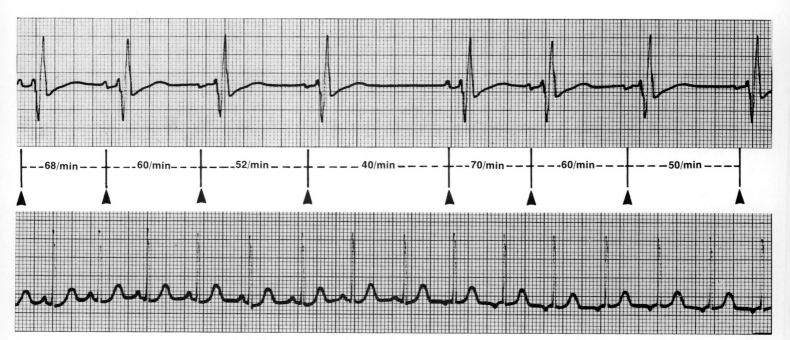

Figure 4–4. Two examples of wandering atrial pacemakers. Note variable cycle rate and P wave configuration with similarity of QRS complexes and T waves.

Wandering Atrial Pacemaker

Another variation in atrial rhythms is the shifting of impulse formation from focus to focus within the atrial tissue, virtually with every beat. Sinus beats may be interspersed throughout, P waves are of many forms, PR intervals vary, and the cadence tends to be somewhat irregular. Ventricular complexes are without alteration. This rhythm is called a **wandering atrial pacemaker** (Fig. 4–4). Wandering atrial pacemaker should not be confused with sinus irregularity. In the latter, atrial depolarization originates from the sinus node and occurs in a uniform sequence; consequently, all P waves look alike.

A wandering pacemaker may be associated with ischemic disease involving the sinus node, or it may occur as a manifestation of an inflammatory state (e.g., acute rheumatic fever). Digitalis, probably by enhancing vagal tone, may cause the arrhythmia. Often, however, a wandering atrial pacemaker may be found without any other sign of cardiac disease.

ATRIA: IMPULSE FORMATION

Excitation

The rate of diastolic depolarization of automatic fibers in the atria may be accelerated by certain forms of physical, pathological, and pharmacological stimuli. When this rate of Phase 4 depolarization exceeds that of automatic cells in the sinus node, an impulse will be generated in the atria before a normal sinus impulse can be emitted. The result is an impulse formed in the atria themselves; this impulse can then propagate throughout the atria and may travel into the ventricles by way of the A-V node. Thus, this ectopic (meaning "out of place") impulse acts as a pacemaker of the heart for one beat.

Characteristic of the atrial impulse formed by accelerated depolarization is the appearance of the resultant beat *earlier* than that which might be expected in a sinus rhythm. In this way, the excited automatic focus produces a *premature* beat. Quite obviously, this timing occurs in sharp contradiction to that of the escape atrial beat, which follows a *delay* in the sinus rhythm.

Atrial premature beats may occur as isolated events that interrupt normal sinus beating, or they may appear in succession, thus establishing a rapid rhythm of atrial origin. The various forms of these atrial tachyarrhythmias will be described individually (Fig. 4–5).

Atrial Premature Complex

A single beat that arises in the atria from early excitation of an automatic focus is called an **atrial premature complex** (APC). The pattern of normal sinus rhythm is interrupted by a beat having the following features:

1. It appears early in the cardiac cycle.
2. The P wave is altered in shape (similar to atrial escape beats).
3. The QRS complex and the T wave are similar to those of beats of sinus node origin (the events of ventricular depolarization and repolarization proceed in the ordinary sequence).
4. The pacing cadence of the sinus node is altered.

These features are demonstrated in pictorial form for easy identification (Fig. 4–6). Using calipers, set the normal sinus rate and observe how this cadence is altered in the sinus beat that follows the premature beat.

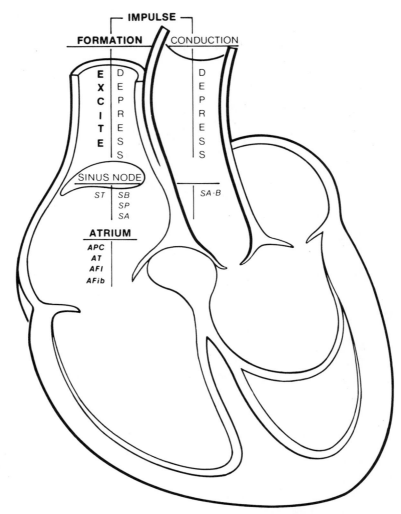

Figure 4–5. Atrial impulse formation: excitation. APC = atrial premature complex; AT = atrial tachycardia; AFl = atrial flutter; AFib = atrial fibrillation.

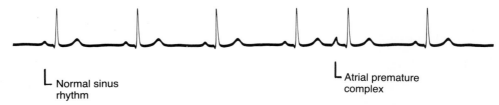

Figure 4–6. Comparison of normal sinus rhythm and atrial premature complex.

LADDERGRAM OF ATRIAL PREMATURE COMPLEX

The dynamics of an APC can be better understood by representation on the laddergram (Fig. 4–7). Depicted are changes in the origin of the atrial impulse and in the direction of the wave front propagation. Note the previously mentioned characteristics of the resultant atrial beat: prematurity, P wave contour change, and the similarity of the QRS and T waveforms to those of sinus beats.

The antegrade (forward) direction of the atrial wave front is represented by the

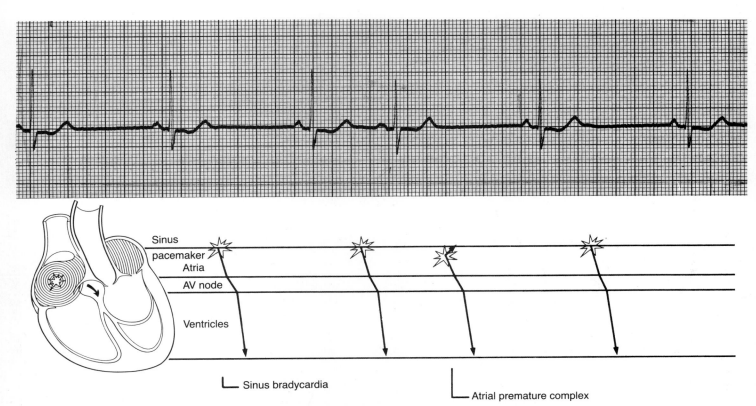

Figure 4–7. Laddergram of an atrial premature complex.

downward pointing arrow, passing through the atrial mass, then into the A-V node and to the ventricles by the usual conducting system. Also shown, by the upward pointing arrow, is the retrograde (backward) direction to part of the atria, depolarizing this portion in a reverse sequence (and accounting for the alteration in P wave contour). Note that reverse atrial depolarization is completed before the antegrade impulse reaches the ventricles so that the P wave is transcribed on the electrocardiogram (ECG) before the QRS complex occurs.

As the retrograde wave front reaches the high right atrium, it may penetrate the sinus node itself. Thus, the sinus node is caused to depolarize prematurely. The early firing prevents completion of the natural sinus action potential in development, and the cadence of the sinus node is disturbed momentarily. Consequently, the sinus pacemaker is reset by the atrial premature beat.

IDENTIFYING ATRIAL PREMATURE COMPLEXES

The interval between the ectopic P wave and the P wave of the subsequent sinus beat usually measures approximately the same as the interval between two sinus beats (Fig. 4–8). This similarity demonstrates that the time required for the sinus node to recover from an external stimulus and to fire again spontaneously is about the same time required between normal beats.

Sometimes, however, the duration of the atrial to sinus interval (P′P) is considerably greater than that between sinus beats (PP). This phenomenon is found in the ECG in Figure 4–9. Inspect the components of the APC on this tracing. The P wave generated by the atrial impulse varies in form from that of the sinus-initiated beats; however, the QRS complex remains unchanged.

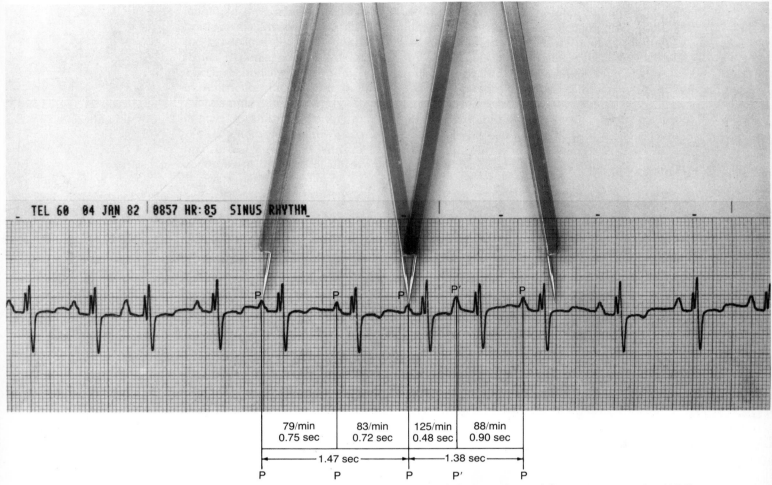

79/min 0.75 sec	83/min 0.72 sec	125/min 0.48 sec	88/min 0.90 sec
P	P	P P'	P

Figure 4–8. Calipers are used to demonstrate the influence of an atrial premature complex (APC) on sinus cycling. The calipers placed at the fifth and seventh sinus beats (P) show normal cycling for three beats. The calipers (without altering the relationship of the points) are then repositioned to span three cycles including the APC (P') at beat eight. (Note the change in the T wave, indicating superimposition of the P wave.) The P of the sinus beat following the APC has occurred earlier than if the sinus node had been routinely firing, indicating a change in sinus cadence. Subsequent sinus beats occur at expected intervals. The rates and intervals for sinus P to sinus P (P-P), sinus P to the P of the APC (P-P') and the APC P to the subsequent sinus P (P'-P) are also identified.

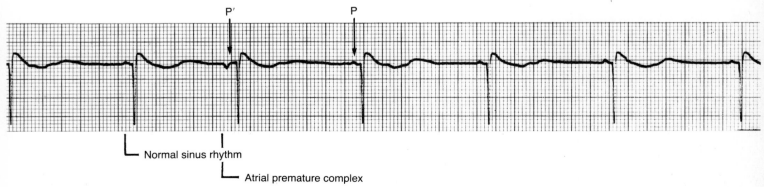

Normal sinus rhythm

Atrial premature complex

Figure 4–9. Note the interruption of the sinus rhythm by an early beat having an altered P wave.

In this tracing, the interval between the APC and the subsequent sinus beat (use calipers and measure from P′ wave to P wave) is slightly longer than the interval between sinus beats that follow. This minor delay may reflect either (1) the additional time required for the retrograde atrial impulse to travel to the sinus node or (2) "fatigue" of the sinus node from the premature stimulation resulting in slower repolarization, and consequently some delay in forming the next impulse.

TERMINOLOGY

The cardiac cycle recorded on the ECG represents electrical events only. The long-used term **contraction** indicates that a mechanical event has occurred as well, and this relationship is not always true. (Depolarization can occur without muscular action resulting.) Consequently, the terms **beat** and **complex** have gradually replaced contraction in general usage. They do not imply an associated myocardial action, although one does infer from them a sense of related events. Both terms are used interchangeably in this book. More precise, perhaps, is the word **depolarization**, although this nomenclature is less commonly used.

In the next three ECGs, identify APCs. Observe prematurity, alteration in the P waveform, and the interval following the APC. Is this interval equal to or longer than that between sinus beats?

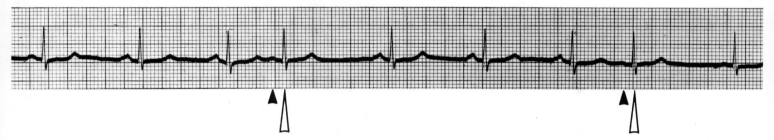

Basic rhythm: normal sinus rhythm. Rate = 60 to 65 per minute. Ectopic beat(s) = two APCs.

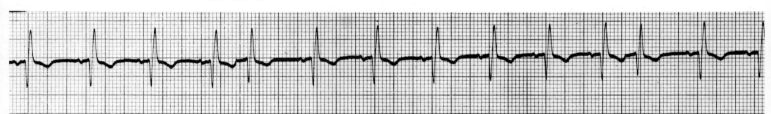

Basic rhythm: normal sinus rhythm. Rate = 92 per minute. Ectopic beat(s) = two APCs.

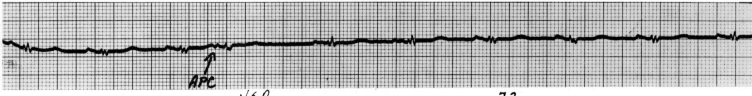

Basic rhythm = _N S R_   Rate = _72_

Ectopic beats = _1 APC_

The frequency of APCs is extremely variable. The examples below are arranged in order of increasing frequency. Identify and label each APC.

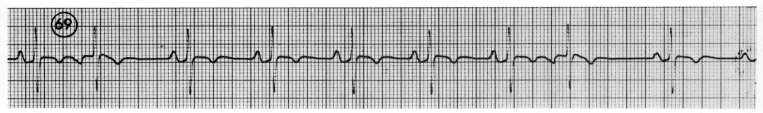

Basic rhythm = _NSR_   **Rate =** _____

Ectopic beats = _2 APCs_

APCs may appear so early that they occur before ventricular repolarization of the previous beat has been completed. The P wave of the premature beat is thereby superimposed on the T wave of the preceding beat. This combination of simultaneous events is usually not difficult to identify when other normal components are compared. In test tracing 70, the first APC (beat 4) exhibits a clearly discernible P wave. In the last beat of the tracing, the APC occurs so early in the cycle that the P wave is observed only as a small deflection of the downward slope of the previous T wave. Similar early APCs are demonstrated below.

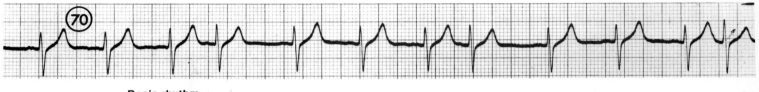

Basic rhythm = _____   **Rate =** _____

Ectopic beats = _____

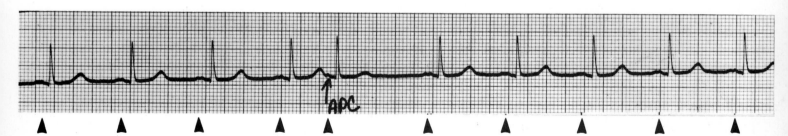

Basic rhythm = _NSR_   **Rate =** _72_

Ectopic beats = _1 APC_

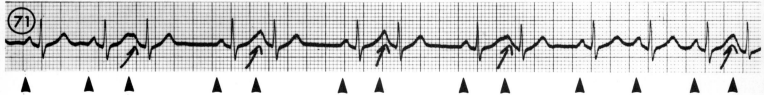

Basic rhythm = _NSR_   **Rate =** _____

Ectopic beats = _5 APCS_

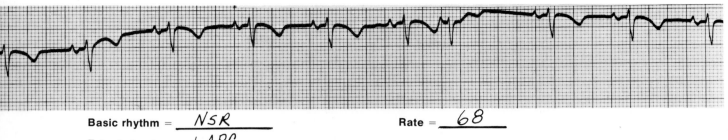

Basic rhythm = ___*NSR*___   Rate = ___*68*___

Ectopic beats = ___*1 APC*___

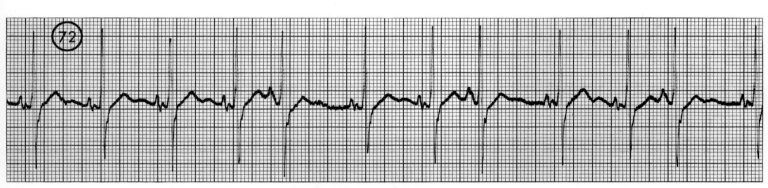

Basic rhythm = _____   Rate = _____

Ectopic beats = _____

An APC becomes less distinct when its P wave falls near the peak of the T wave. The combined components can sometimes be recognized only by the increased amplitude of the T wave preceding a premature QRS. For each of the following examples, determine basic rhythm and rate, locate the APC, and note the following:

1. The degree of prematurity by comparing the rates of normal and premature beats.

2. The contours of normal P, QRS, and T components compared with those of premature beats.

Label the cardiac cycles; estimate rate per minute for sinus and atrial beats.

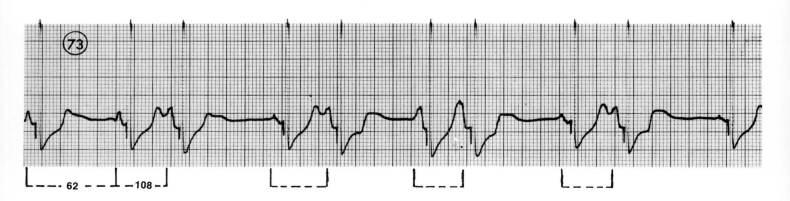

Note in tracing 74 that two consecutive APCs occur.

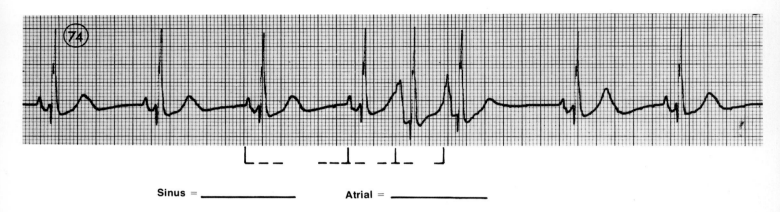

Sinus = _____   Atrial = _____

Locate all P waves of atrial premature beats and designate with arrows in test tracings 75 and 76.

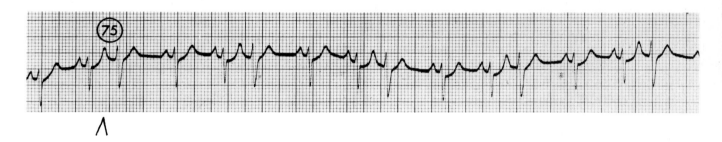

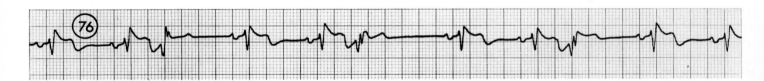

In Figure 4–10, two APCs occur in succession. The P wave of the first of the paired APCs is superimposed on the T wave of the previous beat, causing the latter to appear taller and more peaked. The second APC occurs relatively earlier in the next cycle and can be identified before the T wave of the previous beat. It does not produce a T wave any taller than those of sinus beats.

APCs may assume a constant pattern in relation to normal beats. If every second

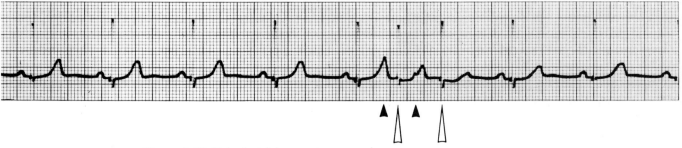

Figure 4–10. Paired atrial premature complexes.

beat is an APC, the term **atrial bigeminy** is applied. By definition, atrial bigeminy has one sinus beat alternating with an atrial beat (i.e., sinus:atrial = 1:1).

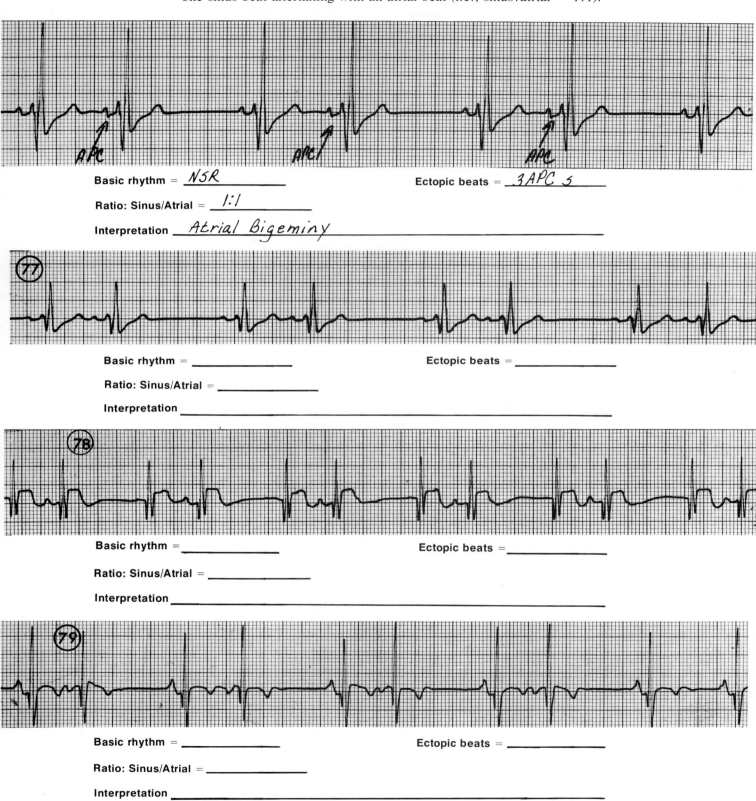

Basic rhythm = *NSR*

Ectopic beats = *3 APC s*

Ratio: Sinus/Atrial = *1:1*

Interpretation *Atrial Bigeminy*

Basic rhythm = _____

Ectopic beats = _____

Ratio: Sinus/Atrial = _____

Interpretation _____

Basic rhythm = _____

Ectopic beats = _____

Ratio: Sinus/Atrial = _____

Interpretation _____

Basic rhythm = _____

Ectopic beats = _____

Ratio: Sinus/Atrial = _____

Interpretation _____

Test strips 80 and 81 represent *compound* arrhythmias (i.e., they have more than one disturbance in rhythm). Note the sinus bradycardia (depression of impulse formation: sinus node) and APCs (excitation of impulse formation: atria).

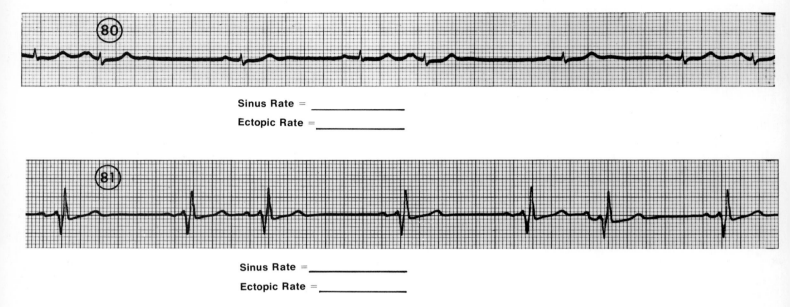

Sinus Rate = _____

Ectopic Rate = _____

Sinus Rate = _____

Ectopic Rate = _____

Blocked Atrial Premature Complexes

An APC may take place so soon after the previous beat that ventricular repolarization is not sufficiently complete, and the A-V node or the ventricles cannot respond to the new stimulus. In other words, the premature impulse from the atria arrives at the A-V node or the ventricles at a time when they are refractory to depolarizing excitation. The nonconducted impulse is dissipated within the conduction pathways, and ventricular conduction does not follow. Such an ectopic beat is described as **blocked** or **dropped**. It can be identified by the appearance of an early P wave of abnormal configuration that is not followed by a QRS complex.

With blocked APCs (Fig. 4–11), the normal sinus rhythm is interrupted by frequent APCs that are not conducted to stimulate the ventricles. Note that the APCs prolong the interval between QRS complexes. Clinically, a blocked APC is one of the causes of delays or pauses in heart sounds and pulse rhythmicity. Yet the interval between the APC and the subsequent P wave is about the same as that between consecutive P waves. In effect, the blocked APC resets the timing mechanism of the sinus node, which then begins a new action potential.

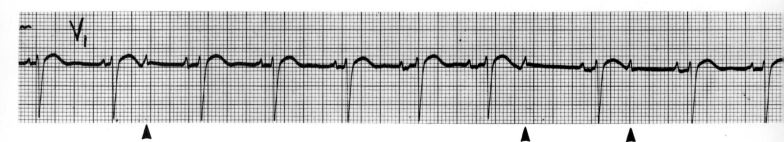

Figure 4–11. Examples of blocked atrial premature complexes.

APCs sometimes fall on the T wave of the previous beat. In Figure 4–12, they can then be identified by the change in contour of the T wave (to a biphasic form) coupled with a subsequent pause in the sinus rate.

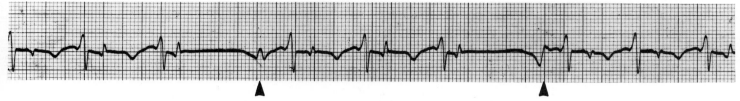

Figure 4–12. Blocked APCs. Note the biphasic T wave.

The distortions of T waves are caused by superimposition of ectopic atrial depolarization occurring at the time of ventricular repolarization as seen in Figure 4–13.

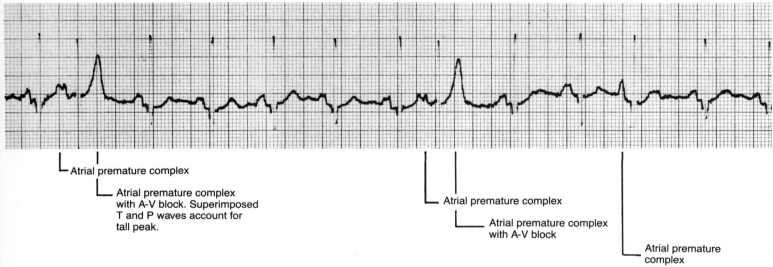

└ Atrial premature complex

    └ Atrial premature complex with A-V block. Superimposed T and P waves account for tall peak.

└ Atrial premature complex

    └ Atrial premature complex with A-V block

        └ Atrial premature complex

Figure 4–13. Conducted and nonconducted atrial premature complexes.

The APC is identified in the first of the next four strips. Locate the blocked APCs in the remaining three examples.

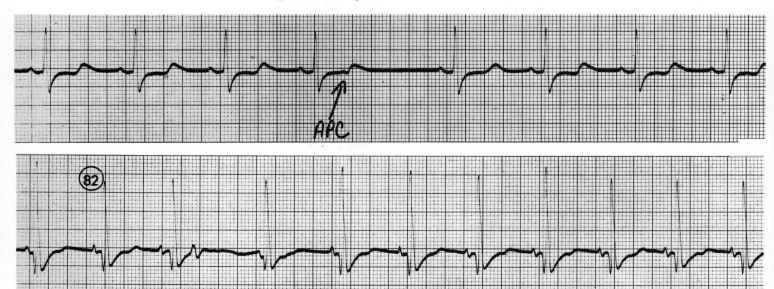

APC

82

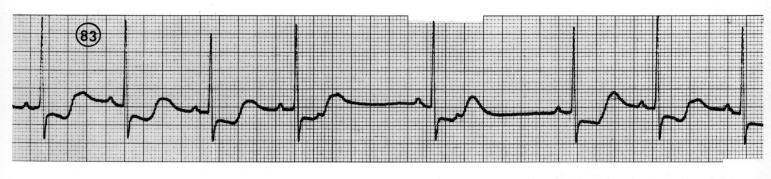

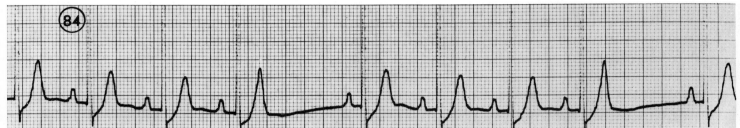

Note in test tracing 84 that the T wave preceding each pause is taller and more peaked than other T waves. An APC has presumably occurred precisely at the time of the T wave's highest amplitude, causing it to be increased further in amplitude and changing its contour somewhat. The APC happened so early in the normal cardiac cycle that the conduction mechanism had not recovered enough to carry this new impulse. The atrial and sinus nodes are depolarized, but further development of the beat is blocked (interpretation: blocked APCs). Note that considerable delay in sinus rhythmicity is imposed by the premature beats.

Identify the blocked APCs in test strip 85.

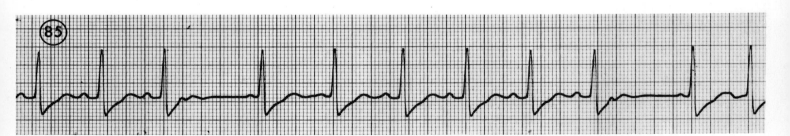

A dropped APC is an example of an electrical event within the cardiac cycle that is affected by the time relationship to the previous beat. This phenomenon introduces an important concept in understanding arrhythmias—the refractory period.

The Refractory Period

Because depolarization represents the release of stored energy, the phenomenon cannot occur when the cell has been depleted of energy. Thus, a stimulus, however great, cannot provoke a response after depolarization until the cell has had time to restore its electrical charge. This refractoriness to stimulation is known as the **absolute** refractory period. It is a phenomenon occurring in all excitable cells, automatic or otherwise.

As the process of repolarization proceeds, the cell gradually restores enough electrical energy to respond to a new stimulus. However, until the electrical charge has been fully restored, the intensity of stimulus required to induce depolarization is greater than that required when the cell is in its resting state. This period, occurring during the later stage of repolarization, is referred to as the **relative** refractory period. It is a stage in which the threshold for excitation is higher than that of the fully repolarized cell.

Figure 4–14 depicts a normal action potential upon which are superimposed two stimuli during repolarization. One stimulus occurs during the absolute refractory period, the other in the relative refractory period.

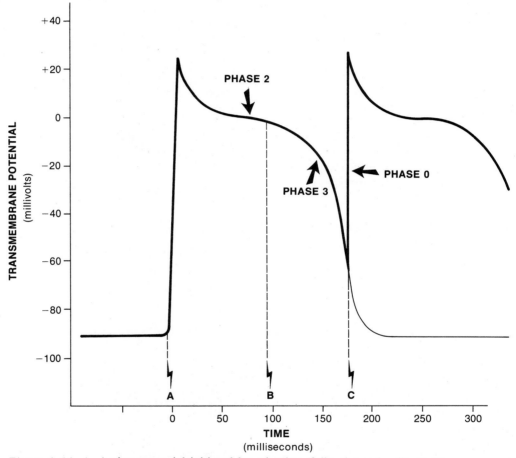

Figure 4–14. *A*, Action potential initiated by stimulus (fully charged cell). *B*, No response to stimulus, regardless of intensity (absolute refractory period). *C*, Action potential initiated but increased stimulus intensity necessary (relative refractory period).

The cell that is excited during the relative refractory period not only requires greater stimulatory force, but the upstroke of its action potential (Phase 0) is slowed. These phenomena will be seen to have critical significance in the genesis of problems of both impulse formation and conduction and in contractile responses of the myofibril.

The blocked APC is an example of the refractory period phenomenon occurring in the A-V conduction system. The premature atrial impulse obviously propagates throughout the atria (because a P wave is developed), demonstrating that the atrial mass has sufficiently recovered from the previous depolarization to respond to a new stimulus at the time of the APC. On the other hand, no ventricular response is forthcoming. The atrial impulse wave front evidently strikes the conduction pathways lead-

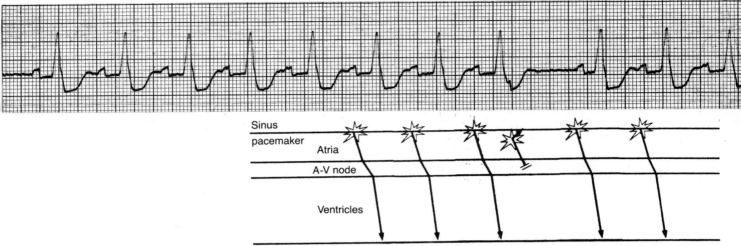

Figure 4–15. Blocked atrial premature beat using a laddergram to demonstrate absence of conduction.

ing to the ventricles during the refractory period of those tissues. Consequently, they are incapable of transmitting the atrial impulse, so that ventricular stimulation does not occur (Fig. 4–15). Refractoriness of conductile fibers is described in detail in subsequent chapters.

Multifocal Atrial Premature Complexes

Premature beats may arise from multiple atrial pacemaker sites. The resultant wave front from each originating focus propagates in a somewhat different sequence of depolarization. The effect is to produce P waves of somewhat differing contour from beat to beat. This rhythm disorder, known as multifocal atrial premature beats, is shown in Figure 4–16.

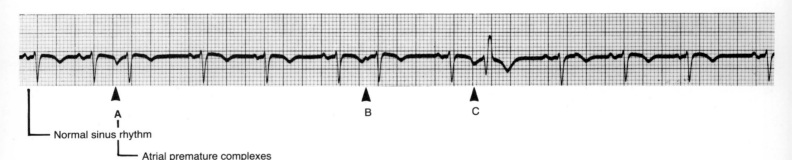

Figure 4–16. Multifocal atrial premature complexes.

Compare atrial beats A, B, and C. Note the strong dissimilarity of the associated P waves. The impulses initiating each of these beats are presumed to originate in various locations in the atrial wall, causing the wave front to radiate in somewhat differing directions. Also note an incidental finding: the change in QRS morphology and duration associated with the P wave at C. This phenomenon will be discussed in Chapter 8.

Clinically, it is important to distinguish multifocal APCs from wandering atrial rhythms. The latter represent shifting sites of impulse formation within the atria occurring when impulse formation in the sinus node falls below a critical rate or when it fails altogether, the atrial automatic impulses acting as an escape rhythm. In contrast, multifocal APCs are the result of changing sites from atrial pacemakers that have been excited to rapid firing. This increased automaticity may be an expression of drug toxicity (most notably from digitalis) or from a metabolic disturbance (such as hypoxia or acidosis).

Atrial Tachycardia

Three or more APCs occurring consecutively establish, by definition, atrial tachycardia. This form of tachyarrhythmia may persist for only a few seconds or may be sustained for hours or even days.

In the ECG shown in Figure 4–17, a typical APC appears at A, interrupting the sinus rhythm. At B, another APC that has like features of abnormal P wave morphology and normal QRS complex and T wave occurs. After this beat, however, there is a succession of similar beats, producing a very rapid rate. This tachycardia suddenly stops at C, and the sinus rhythm is resumed. The short burst of rapid beating, evidently arising from an atrial focus, is called **atrial tachycardia**.

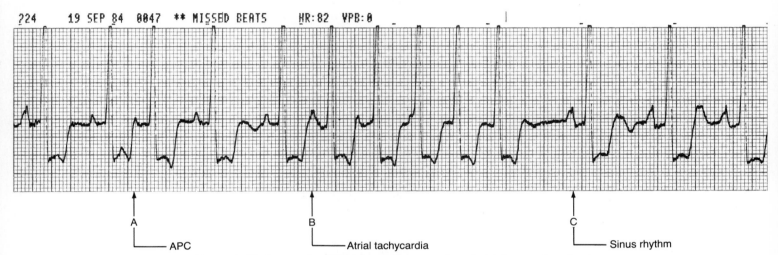

Figure 4–17. Onset of atrial tachycardia—a series of atrial premature beats.

There are two basic mechanisms that produce atrial tachycardia. These mechanisms have important implications in cardiology as they reflect fundamental differences in etiology, interpretation by electrocardiography, and approach to therapy. The two forms are as follows:

1. **Enhanced automaticity.** Excitation of an atrial focus is produced by physiological disturbances that accelerate the rate of spontaneous depolarization and result in rapid firing.

2. **Impulse reentry.** Premature stimulation of the atria is caused by a delayed impulse from a depolarizing wave front in a localized zone that returns to normal atria and evokes a second depolarizing response.

It can be appreciated from these definitions that atrial tachycardia can be produced by either accentuation of automatic impulse formation or by depression of impulse conduction. These mechanisms, which are admittedly complex, will be described individually as they apply to the sequence of topics.

MECHANISMS OF ATRIAL TACHYCARDIA

ENHANCED AUTOMATICITY. As mentioned at the beginning of this chapter, cells having the capability of forming impulses are distributed throughout the atria. These fibers, which have the inherent property of spontaneous diastolic depolarization (giving them the potential for automatic firing), may be excited by a multitude of disturbances. Such factors exert an excitatory effect by (1) decreasing the maximum transmembrane potential (thereby moving it closer to the threshold point for spontaneous discharge) or (2) increasing the rate of Phase 4 spontaneous diastolic depolarization (Fig. 4–18). In either case, the result is a more rapid approach to the threshold point at which the Phase 0 spike potential is triggered.

As already described, the natural decay rate of the transmembrane potential normally reaches threshold in the sinus node before it occurs in automatic cells within the atria. When a physiological disturbance brings the atrial cells to this trigger point *before* that in the sinus node, an impulse is generated in the atria. This impulse then propagates to the remaining atrial tissue as a radiating wave front and eventually descends through the A-V node to enter and stimulate the ventricles. In this way, the ectopic impulse controls a cardiac cycle.

Thus far, we have described a mechanism for production of an APC in which excitation of automatic cells is responsible. When the accelerated rate of spontaneous diastolic depolarization is sustained, by whatever incriminating factor, continued rapid beating supersedes sinus node control of the heart. In effect, atrial tachycardia results.

It is important to understand that the excited atrial fibers, firing rapidly, dominate the heartbeat. The pacemaker cells of the sinus node that are set to periodic activation at a slower rate are therefore continuously suppressed by the atrial pacemaker. The "fault" essentially lies in the abnormal atrial cells, not in the sinus node.

Characteristics. The characteristics of atrial tachycardia that suggest that enhanced automaticity is responsible are as follows:

1. The heart rate is generally in the range of 120 to 160 beats per minute. However, the rate may be as slow as 100 or as rapid as 240 beats per minute.

2. P wave morphology differs from that associated with sinus rhythm (as with APCs). P waves inscribed during atrial tachycardia sometimes vary in contour from beat to beat (similar to the findings described for multifocal APCs), indicating numerous areas of enhanced automaticity. In other forms, P waves in the tachycardia are identical, and it is inferred that there is a single focus of origin.

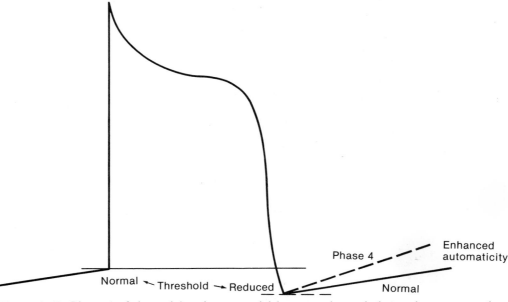

Figure 4–18. Phase 4 of the atrial action potential has an enhanced slope when compared to normal.

3. The rhythm may be slightly irregular; occasionally it is conspicuously erratic. This rhythm does not, however, exhibit the phasic variations associated with respiration that are normally found in sinus rhythms.

4. The onset of tachycardia usually exhibits a gradual acceleration for several beats (the so-called warm-up) until the maximum rate is established.

5. P wave morphology gradually changes over several beats at the onset of the tachycardia, from that of the sinus node to that of the established ectopic pacemaker. This transition coincides with the gradual acceleration of the initiating rhythm.

6. The offset (termination) of the tachycardia tends to occur by gradual slowing, the transition to a sinus pacemaker being characterized by progressive deceleration of atrial firing until the sinus node takes over control of the heartbeat.

7. Parasympathetic stimulation (as imposed by vagotonic maneuvers) usually produces little or no change in the rate of the ectopic atrial pacemaker.

Features of enhanced automaticity are found in the example of atrial tachycardia shown in Figure 4–19.

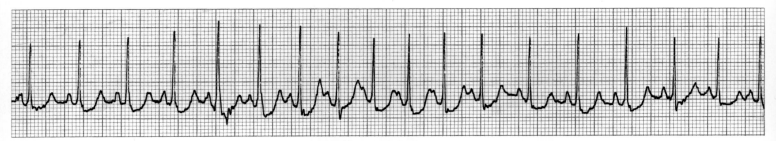

Figure 4–19. Atrial tachycardia exhibiting characteristics of tachycardia resulting from enhanced automaticity.

Clinically, atrial tachycardia produced by enhanced automaticity has serious implications. It is most often observed in the setting of intrinsic heart disease with superimposed abnormalities of a diverse nature. The principal causes of such ectopic atrial beating are as follows:

1. **Myocardial.** Ischemia, infarction, cardiomyopathy, and blunt trauma (contusion).

2. **Metabolic.** Endogenous catecholamine surge (from pain, emotional excitement, and sudden strenuous physical activity), hypoxia, acidosis, and alkalosis.

3. **Electrolyte.** Hypokalemia, hypercalcemia, hypocalcemia and, hypomagnesemia.

4. **Pharmacological.** Digitalis toxicity (the most common drug-induced form), adrenergic agents (such as norepinephrine or dopamine), and alcohol. Patients with underlying myocardial disease are often highly sensitive to the arrhythmia-provoking properties of these chemicals.

Treatment of atrial tachycardia caused by enhanced automaticity often proves difficult unless the underlying causative disturbance can be alleviated. Indeed, a diligent search must be conducted to identify such conditions, most notable of which are systemic hypoxia, myocardial ischemia, insufficiency, and inflammation or drug toxicity.

Atrial tachycardia of this class is generally resistant to suppression by pharmacological agents. As a rule, those that prove most useful are drugs that directly slow Phase 4 (spontaneous depolarization) such as the calcium channel blockers (e.g., verapamil) or drugs that blunt adrenergic tone to the hyperexcitable myofibrils, especially the beta-adrenergic blockers (such as propanolol).

A brief paroxysm of atrial tachycardia is shown in Figure 4–20. The patient was being treated with digoxin and furosemide for congestive heart failure. The digoxin blood level at the time of this recording was 3.4 ng/ml, and serum potassium was 2.8 mEq/liter. Note that the rate of the tachycardia varies slightly from beat to beat. Also, the tachycardia does *not* terminate with an accelerated beat. These circumstances suggest that the tachycardia is an automatic rhythm (due to digitalis toxicity) rather than to a reentrant mechanism.

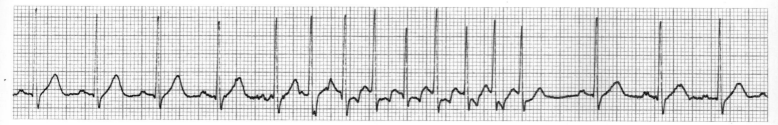

Figure 4–20. Short episode of atrial tachycardia due to digitalis toxicity.

REENTRANCE. The second form of atrial tachycardia results from reexcitation by a portion of the advancing wave front that turns back on itself, forming an electrical loop and producing an additional heartbeat. Rather than being a result of an impulse arising *de novo* (as does the ectopic beat from excited automatic fibers), the beat is the consequence of abnormal wave front propagation. In other words, the factor responsible for reentrant arrhythmias involves impulse *conduction*, not impulse formation.

Admittedly complicated, the reentrant mechanism has in recent years assumed a critically important role in the electrocardiographic interpretation of arrhythmias and in clinical management. Indeed, it is now realized that the large majority of tachyarrhythmias have reentrance as the underlying mechanism. This subject will be covered in detail in this and subsequent chapters, as applicable.

A brief review of a few points of normal physiology may be helpful. The myocardium consists of cell fibers (or sarcomeres), of which about 90% have the property of excitability, responding to stimulation by contracting and by conveying the exciting impulse to adjacent cell fibers. They do not have the property of automaticity (i.e., of producing impulses spontaneously). These individual myofibrils, making up the muscular wall of the heart, transmit a wave front fairly rapidly (compared with the very slow transmission characteristic of the sinus node and A-V node). The homogeneity of inherent conduction velocity in these fibers also ensures a fairly uniform propagation of a depolarizing wave front. Furthermore, the time required for repolarization (refractory period) of these fibers is relatively long.

These two properties of atrial myofibrils—rapid conduction velocity and long refractory period—have important implications because they ensure that the normal impulse emitted from the sinus node passes through the atria. Exiting by way of the A-V node, the impulse is not reflected back into the atria because these fibers are in their refractory state at the time of entry into the A-V node.

The foundation for the reentry concept of arrhythmias was proposed early in this century, based on observations on neurotransmission in the jellyfish and later in the hearts of turtles and mammals. Reentrant mechanisms were postulated in 1923 as the cause of atrial tachycardia. During the following decades, further insight into this theory was furnished through astute inferences in clinical electrocardiography by the outstanding pioneers in this field. With the introduction of electrophysiological techniques in the 1970s, study of intimate electrical pathways was possible in the hearts of both animals and humans from recordings taken within their chambers. The intricacies of impulse formation and conduction are now revealed with electrophysiological studies.

Myofibrils lying side by side may not have precisely the same action potential dynamics. When differences in electrophysiological properties are exaggerated, the stage is set for nonhomogeneous conduction and repolarization. If the dissimilarity is severe enough, the wave front may pass a zone of depressed tissue, enter the zone more distally, and continue in reverse direction; on exiting the zone, the impulse encounters tissue that has already recovered sufficiently from the original wave front to respond. In this way, a secondary wave front—and a new heartbeat—is generated.

The phenomenon of reentry will be explained using a series of diagrams. The principles will apply to all forms of reentrant beating, whether confined to the atria or to the ventricles or whether a circuitous reentrant pathway involves both atrial and ventricular chambers.

A wave front first passes through relatively homogenous tissue in the ordinary manner. Ahead lies a zone of tissue that is physiologically depressed (represented by the stippled area in Figure 4–21) and from an electrophysiological perspective is functionally isolated. Here the advancing wave front is slowed or blocked altogether.

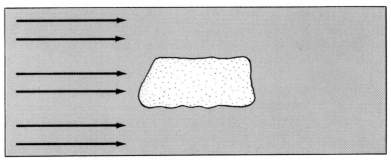

Figure 4–21. Reentry phenomenon—initial phase.

Meanwhile, the wave front flanking the island continues to propagate around the depressed zone without impairment. All the tissue that surrounds the island is soon depolarized, and the normal wave front continues (Fig. 4–22).

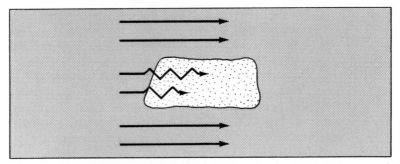

Figure 4–22. Reentry phenomenon—impulse propagating slowly through the area of depression.

Excitable cells at the more distal portion of the depressed zone may be capable of responding to the passing wave front, thus allowing an impulse to enter the zone (Fig. 4–23).

Should the fibers within the zone be responsive to this entering impulse, undergo depolarization, and then transmit this disturbance to proximal fibers, the impulse will pass along in a retrograde direction (reverse that of normal). This impulse eventually arrives at the area where the initial antegrade block was encountered (Fig. 4–24).

If the normal tissue in this area has restored its excitability after its depolarization by the time the exiting retrograde impulse reaches it, a new action potential is stimulated. Thus, another wave front is initiated, this time from a reverberating impulse,

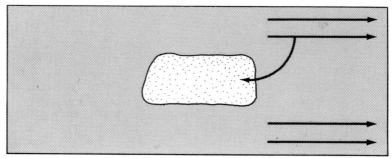

Figure 4–23. Reentry phenomenon—reentry of impulse into the area of depression.

and the wave front propagates radially (Fig. 4–25). In the atria, it courses proximally and may eventually enter the sinus node. Traveling distally, the wave front may enter the A-V node and intraventricular conduction system, initiating ventricular depolarization.

From this description, it can be appreciated that a fortuitous set of circumstances favors development of reentrant beats. These factors include the following:

1. Relatively rapid conduction of the wave front around the island of depressed tissue.

2. Aborted conduction of an antegrade impulse in the island.

3. Intact function of the depressed zone to pass an impulse in a retrograde direction. (The combination of numbers 2 and 3 is called unidirectional block.)

4. Relatively rapid repolarization of tissue (e.g., a short refractory period) at the site of exit of the retrograde impulse. (Normally, protection against reentrant beating is preserved by the long refractory period of muscle fibers.)

In other words, a normally or rapidly conducted impulse bypassing a depressed zone and/or a rapid recovery of tissue surrounding the depressed zone allows time for a retrograde impulse to exit from the zone into responsive tissue. The result is production of a second cardiac cycle from the original impulse. This reverberant or echo impulse is expressed as an APC.

The exit-reentrant impulse sometimes enters the depressed zone and emerges to again form a cardiac cycle (Fig. 4–26). When this repetitive cycling is sustained, the mechanism for an atrial tachycardia is established. This activity may recur for a few beats or may continue for prolonged periods.

Eventually, however, the action potentials of the involved fibers in the circuit lose their responsiveness to the rapidly incoming stimuli, a phenomenon referred to as detrimental conduction. The circuiting impulse consequently becomes interrupted and the tachycardia stops abruptly. The term **paroxysmal**, as applied to this reentrant arrhythmia, refers to its characteristic sudden onset and sudden cessation (Fig. 4–27).

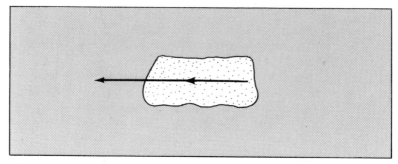

Figure 4–24. Reentry phenomenon—impulse arriving at site of initial antegrade block.

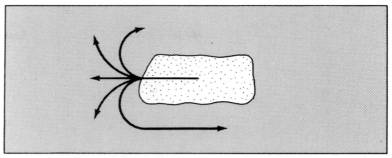

Figure 4–25. Reentry phenomenon—initiation of conduction from a reverberating impulse.

The distinction between tachycardias of reentrant origin and of enhanced automaticity has important implications in management and prognosis. Detection of an automatic tachyarrhythmia alerts a clinician to underlying causative cardiac pathology or systemic disease such as severe hypoxia. A reentrant tachyarrhythmia, on the other hand, represents a functional dissimilarity in adjacent fibers that is not necessarily associated with heart disease. Indeed, a tachycardia of this type is considered a benign condition even if it produces symptoms ranging from palpitations to weakness, lightheadedness, and even fainting.

Characteristics. The features of reentrant arrhythmias that are most helpful in differentiating them from the automatic arrhythmias are as follows:

1. **Sudden onset.** Beginning with a premature beat, the reentrant tachycardia appears at a sustained rapid rate. The warm-up period observed from enhanced automaticity is not present. The reentrant tachycardia also can be deliberately induced with a properly timed and placed electrical impulse.

2. **Rate regularity.** The interval from beat to beat is usually constant. This metronome-like periodicity helps differentiate the tachycardia from that due to enhanced automaticity, which is typically somewhat irregular in timing. A slight phasic pattern of rate can generally be detected in sinus tachycardia, differentiating excitable sinus rhythms from those initiated in the atria.

3. **Responsiveness to parasympathetic stimulation.** By altering either conduction velocity or the refractory period in one segment of the reentrant loop, vagal stimulation may interrupt the tachycardia. Automatic mechanisms are resistant to vagotonic maneuvers.

4. **Responsiveness to electric shock.** A properly timed external electrical impulse simultaneously depolarizes myofibrils in both the reentrant loop and in the surrounding tissue. The stimulus is usually effective in terminating the tachycardia. In tachycardias caused by enhanced automaticity, electric shock is seldom effective.

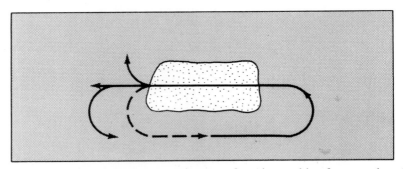

Figure 4–26. Reentry phenomenon—reentering waveform is capable of repeated cycling.

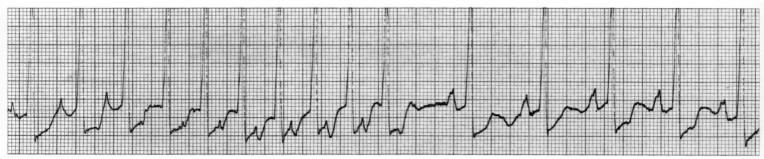

Figure 4–27. Paroxysmal reentrant arrhythmia.

5. **Responsiveness to pharmacological intervention.** Tachyarrhythmias of reentrant type tend to be highly responsive to certain drugs. Digitalis and the calcium channel blocking agents (most notably verapamil) prolong the refractory period; quinidine accelerates impulse conduction. Both actions counter the completion of a full loop circuit, thereby ending the continuous reentrant impulse.

6. **Sudden termination.** When the reverberating impulse can no longer complete its cycle in the reentrant circuit, the tachycardia for which it is responsible stops instantly.

A final distinction has a clinical basis. Persons with reentrant tachycardias involving the atria often have no other form of heart disease, and systemic causal factors cannot be found. They may occur at any age. In fact, a substantial portion of subjects with reentrant tachycardias (even those that produce severe symptoms) are young, vigorous, healthy adults. Certainly, these tachyarrhythmias are incurred in persons with myocardial or valvular heart disease or with serious metabolic disorders, but the incidence is far different from that associated with tachycardias from enhanced automaticity, in which such underlying conditions are anticipated.

An example of paroxysmal atrial tachycardia is shown in Figure 4–28. Note that normal sinus rhythm is precipitously interrupted by a rapidly beating rhythm. Identify the following features:

- Abrupt onset.
- Rapid rate of 136 per minute that is *precisely* regular (compare RR intervals, using calipers).
- Change in configuration of P waves, now superimposed on the downward slope of the preceding T waves.
- Similarity of QRS complexes in morphology and in duration between sinus and tachycardia beats. (Ventricular depolarization remains unchanged.)
- The paroxysmal tachycardia ends suddenly to be replaced by the sinus rhythm. (The last beat of the tachycardia is noted to occur at a slightly slower rate than

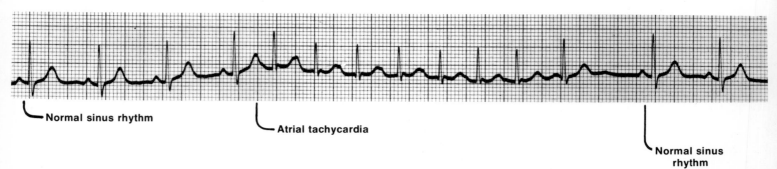

Normal sinus rhythm

Atrial tachycardia

Normal sinus rhythm

Figure 4–28. Paroxysmal atrial tachycardia.

its predecessors. In automatic tachycardias, the gradual slowdown to cessation usually involves several consecutive beats.)

The paroxysmal tachycardia that follows (Fig. 4–29) is preceded by an APC. This initial excitable beat exhibits altered ventricular conduction, a condition referred to as aberration, which will be explained in detail later. In the remaining beats of the tachycardia, QRS complexes more closely resemble those of the sinus beats. This association is common in reentrant tachycardias, signaling that the reentrant impulse circuit that occurs a single time may also course repeatedly through the loop. Indeed, reentrant paroxysmal atrial tachycardia may be considered to begin with a premature beat.

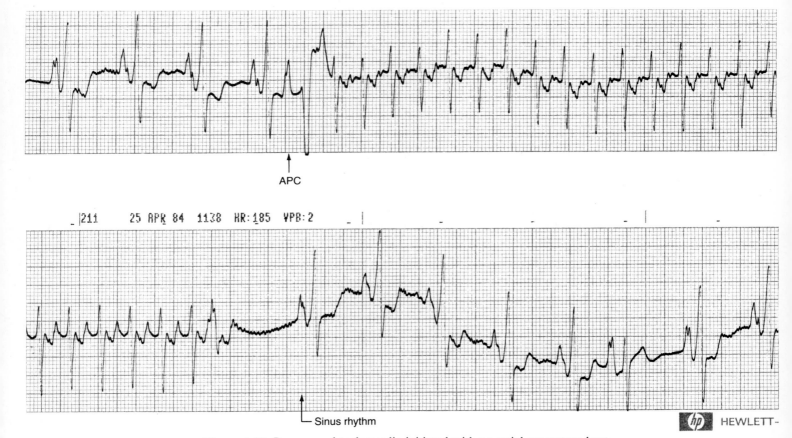

Figure 4–29. Paroxysmal tachycardia initiated with an atrial premature beat.

During the recording of this tachycardia, which lasted 10 seconds, the patient was aware only of palpitations. When paroxysms are more prolonged, when the heart rate is more rapid, or when there are concurrent conditions that already compromise the circulatory system, subjects may experience weakness, anxiety, breathlessness, lightheadedness, and even syncope. These clinical expressions of diminished cardiac output are, in part, the result of ventricular contractions occurring so rapidly that diastolic filling is insufficient. The onset of sustained tachycardias is commonly associated with the most intense symptoms because activation of peripheral vascular reflexes to compensate for the reduction in cardiac output requires a few seconds.

Persons who complain of the precipitous onset of such symptoms that abate as suddenly are suspect of having some form of reentrant atrial tachycardia. Attacks may be induced by adrenergic stimulation. Common examples are emotional outbursts, physical stress of heavy lifting, coffee or alcohol ingestion, and vasoconstricting nose drops. Often, however, no triggering factor can be identified.

Test tracing 86 represents atrial tachycardia.

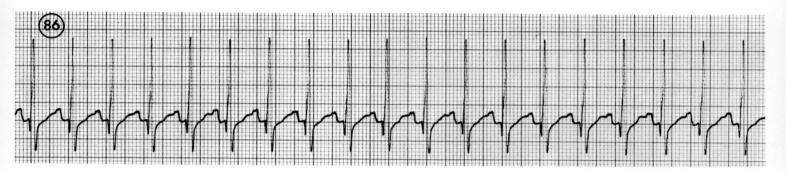

Determine: Rate = _____
Regular or irregular rhythm: _____

(Use calipers and measure several intervals between cardiac cycles. The peak of the QRS complex is a convenient place for reference.)

Also note in tracing 86 that T waves and P waves have merged, owing to the rapidity of the rate. Yet, the P wave consistently falls precisely on the same portion of the T wave in every cycle observed, and the intervals between the P wave peaks and the beginning of the QRS complexes are consistently identical. These features are found in rhythms of constant rate and are typical of reentrant atrial tachycardias.

An example of the abrupt termination of a tachycardia is demonstrated in test tracing 87. Here, the rate slows suddenly from _____ to _____ per minute. We will examine specific details of this tracing to reach an interpretation of the arrhythmia.

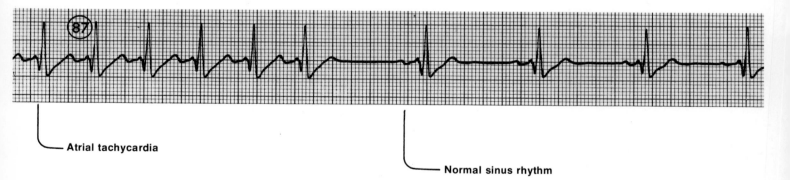

Atrial tachycardia

Normal sinus rhythm

Observe that P waves cannot be identified with certainty during the tachycardia; during the slow rhythm they are clearly evident. Their contours during the slow period are of the pattern of which pacemaker? Now compare the terminal slopes of T waves in both rhythms. Note that the inscription is slightly uneven in the rapid rhythm but is smooth in the slow rhythm. Thus, one can assume that a P wave fell during the trailing portion of the T wave when the rate was rapid, but it was of insufficient amplitude to produce a sharp deflection. Its imprint is only discernible when compared with the same region recorded later when the P wave has moved away as a result of the slower rate. Such details allow us to presume that a P wave (atrial depolarization) was present at the time of final T wave inscription (ventricular repolarization) and that the tachycardia is of atrial origin.

One may tend to mistake the low amplitude but broad positive deflection at the beginning of the QRS complex (2.5 mm) for the P wave at the rapid rate. However, this error becomes apparent on comparing the same region during the slow rhythm. Here, even in the presence of the P wave, the deflection persists unaltered, and the QRS complex remains unchanged in configuration in its entirety. On this evidence, one can conclude with confidence that the inscription in question represents an R deflection.

The last beat of the tachycardia (located 71 mm from the left border) occurs slightly earlier (= _____ beats per minute) than expected in comparison with the previous rate (= _____ beats per minute). Because of this premature beat, the refractory period of fibers somewhere in a reentrant circuit was longer than required for continuation of a reverberating impulse, and thus it could not proceed. With the reentrant beat blocked, the tachycardia ceases. On its termination, the rhythm is replaced by _____ .

We have defined this arrhythmia as a tachycardia having an atrial origin (or at least, the atria are involved in the impulse initiation) and having an abrupt termination characteristic of reentrant tachycardias. The slightly premature beat that terminates the tachycardia is also typical of this form of arrhythmia. The prompt resumption of a sinus rhythm suggests that the sinus node itself is not faulty but that its pacemaker role had simply been usurped by the more rapid ectopic pacemaker.

The sensitivity of reentrant tachyarrhythmias to parasympathetic stimulation provides an important mechanism for identifying these arrhythmias in addition to treating them. Test tracing 88 demonstrates the effect of parasympathetic stimulation induced by a vagotonic maneuver.

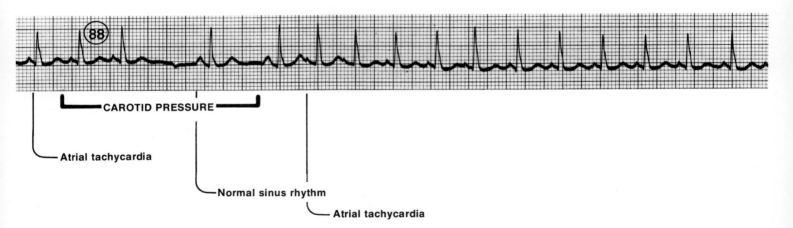

CAROTID PRESSURE

Atrial tachycardia

Normal sinus rhythm

Atrial tachycardia

At the beginning of the strip, a tachycardia is observed having sharply peaked P waves and narrow QRS complexes, all of which are identical. The rate is _____ beats per minute, and the rhythm is _____ (regular or irregular). Carotid pressure is applied. There is an immediate cessation of the tachycardia, and after a brief pause normal sinus rhythm supervenes. Here, the P waves have a more rounded peak and the PR interval is slightly longer; the QRS complexes remain unchanged in configuration. This sinus rhythm has a rate of _____ and is _____ (regular or irregular).

When carotid pressure is withdrawn, the tachycardia recurs immediately and persists. Note that there is no warm-up acceleration at its onset. Also notice that P waves of the renewed tachycardia are similar to those present previously. In this instance, we have observed the temporary suppression of a reentrant tachycardia through neurogenic disruption of the reentrant loop.

To demonstrate the difference in parasympathetic stimulation between reentrant tachycardias and sinus tachycardias, the tracing in Figure 4–30 is presented. It shows the effect of vagal stimulation on sinus tachycardia.

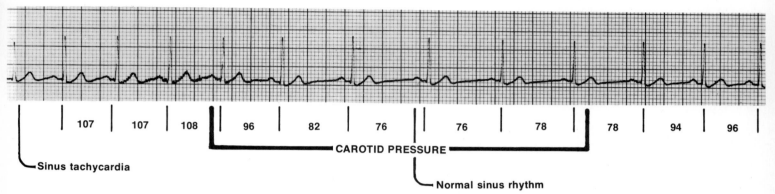

Figure 4–30. Slowing of sinus tachycardia with vagal stimulation.

Note that the rapid rate slows gradually under the influence of carotid pressure, and the rate remains slow as long as the stimulation is applied. On its release, however, the rate accelerates gradually, approaching that measured originally. In addition, P waves recorded during both the tachycardia and the normal rate are similar in contour, affirming the same pacemaker origin (i.e., the sinus node). Whatever the cause of sinus tachycardia, it persists independently of parasympathetic forces, which only modify the rate. In the instance recorded here, the patient merely had anxiety on having an ECG performed.

Because of the responsiveness of reentrant atrial tachycardias to parasympathetic stimulation, persons subject to recurring symptoms from paroxysmal atrial tachycardias often learn self-induced techniques that abort the attacks through augmented vagal tone. Yawning, gagging (the Valsalva maneuver), deep breath holding, and rubbing the neck in the carotid bulb area are such modalities. Placing the face in ice water evokes a powerful parasympathetic reflex. Clinicians commonly choose to try carotid massage as the first step in suppressing these tachycardias. An example of the successful application of this procedure is seen in Figure 4–31.

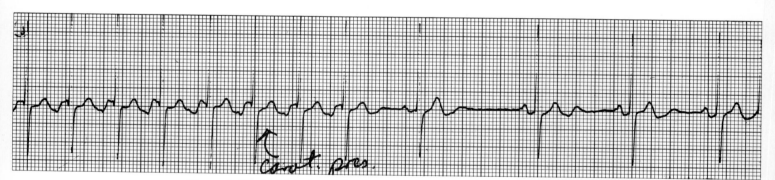

Figure 4–31. Atrial tachycardia response to augmented vagal tone.

Within 1 to 2 seconds after carotid pressure was applied, the atrial rhythm terminated. Note that prompt slowing of the atrial rate occurs just before conversion to the sinus rhythm.

The technique of carotid pressure must be applied with care, and perhaps never used on patients with compromised cervicocerebral circulation nor on those with carotid arterial bruits. Atrial tachycardia can sometimes be terminated simply by exerting light or moderate pressure on the carotid bulb. More resistant tachycardias may require a gentle but firm rotary motion, never exceeding 4 or 5 seconds, and always one side at a time. Further, the clinician performing the maneuver must be fully prepared to manage immediately any untoward eventuality, be it severe A-V block, cardiac standstill, or other complication. Given these restraints, however, carotid pressure has proved an extremely effective and safe technique for the treatment of these tachyarrhythmias.

Treatment of reentrant tachycardias with drugs may be used instead to interrupt the reverberating circuit. For example, some antiarrhythmic agents have a preferential action on certain portions of the action potential by

1. Increasing conduction velocity of normal tissue or by
2. Prolonging the refractory period of normal tissue.

In both situations, the objective is to promote arrival of the retrograde, reentrant impulse at a time when the tissue is *not* responsive, thus interrupting the repetitive circuiting.

DRUG THERAPY. Drugs used to convert atrial tachycardia to normal sinus rhythm and to maintain freedom from recurrent attacks fall into several classes. They are outlined below but described more fully in Chapter 10.

1. **Tranquilizers and sedatives.** These agents decrease sympathetic tone emanating from the central nervous system and are especially effective in patients with anxiety-induced attacks. Examples are phenobarbital, promazines (such as Thorazine), and diazepam (Valium).

2. **Adrenergic antagonists.** Direct inhibition of norepinephrine release at sympathetic nerve endings in the myocardium may be achieved with reserpine and guanethidine (Ismelin). More commonly used agents in this class are the beta-adrenergic blockers: atenolol, nadolol, metoprolol, pindolol, propranolol, esmolol, and timolol. These drugs inhibit the uptake of released norepinephrine at the receptor sites of myofibrils.

3. **Cholinergic stimulators.** Drugs that enhance parasympathetic tone in the heart are commonly used to terminate reentrant atrial tachycardias or to maintain their suppression in susceptible persons. Edrophonium (Tensilon) is the drug of choice in this class for treating an acute attack, whereas digitalis is a staple for chronic suppression of the tachyarrhythmias.

4. **Cellular suppressors.** Independent of the autonomic nervous system, agents in this class directly alter the action potential of myofibrils by slowing impulse conduction and prolonging the refractory period. By preferential action on reentrant loops, drugs such as quinidine and procainamide are often successful in interrupting the reverberating impulse. The extremely short-acting adenosine, a newly released drug, is effective for treatment of reentrant tachycardias.

5. **Calcium channel blockers.** This newest class of antiarrhythmic drugs suppresses reentrant atrial tachycardias by inhibiting the movement of calcium ions into the actin-myosin complex, thereby slowing depolarization. Their effectiveness and relative safety have rapidly led to wide use of these agents, which include verapamil and diltiazem.

Conversion of paroxysmal atrial tachycardia to a sinus rhythm by drug treatment is demonstrated in test tracings 89 and 90. This sequence is taken from a 38-year-old telephone operator who complained of a pounding in her chest lasting 12 hours. In excellent health, this woman had experienced several similar episodes during the previous 2 years, but each attack had lasted only a few minutes and each subsided spontaneously and abruptly. As the hours passed, additional symptoms of progressive weakness and a generalized soreness of the chest were felt. Librium and digoxin were administered 2 hours before the tracing shown here was recorded. Carotid pressure and the Valsalva maneuver were also tried repeatedly, to no avail.

6:20 PM:

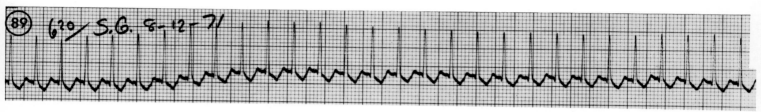

Rate = _____

Note the metronome-like regularity of the rhythm (check, using calipers). The P waves appear to merge with T waves. The segments between T wave peak and alleged P waves are consistently uniform in contour throughout. The QRS complexes are narrow (less than 0.12 second) and are identical in form.

6:21 PM: Edrophonium chloride (Tensilon) was administered by slow intravenous injection. Even before the ordinary dose of 10 mg was given, a sudden change in rhythm occurred.

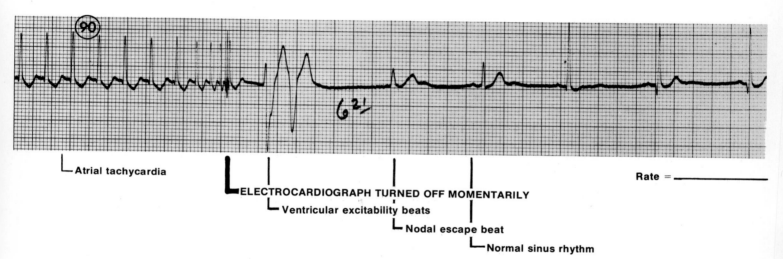

└ Atrial tachycardia

└ ELECTROCARDIOGRAPH TURNED OFF MOMENTARILY

└ Ventricular excitability beats

└ Nodal escape beat

└ Normal sinus rhythm

Rate = _____

Note that the rhythm pattern at the beginning of the tracing reveals a continuation of the previous tracing without any change in rate or pattern.

The seemingly accelerated rate and compressed deflections that immediately precede the rhythm change are in part artifactual, caused by slow movement of paper past the stylus, in turn caused by tension on the paper when the machine is first turned off.

On restarting the electrocardiograph, it appears that the very end of the tachycardia was recorded, T wave at 56 mm and the P wave at 58 mm, and that this P wave transmission was blocked at the A-V node because a QRS complex does not follow at the expected interval. Instead, the P wave is followed after a long interval by two QRS complexes having wide duration and deformed configuration. These are evidently beats from an ectopic origin, probably located in the ventricles. (Periods of enhanced automaticity often accompany strong autonomic reflexes, and such ectopic beats are common at the time of drug-induced rhythm transition.)

A beat without a preceding P wave but with narrow QRS of small amplitude follows the ectopic beats after a delay of _____ second. This beat evidently originates near the A-V node and is of the escape mechanism, to be described in Chapter 5 under the Atrioventricular Node.

The ensuing rhythm is recognized as _____ with a rate of _____ per minute.

QRS complexes become increased in amplitude, and the once downward T wave becomes upright.

With cessation of the tachycardia, the patient's symptoms disappeared immediately. Nausea, perspiration of the extremities, and abdominal discomfort occurred briefly thereafter, the side effects of Tensilon.

Tensilon achieves its effect by prolonging the action of acetylcholine through inhibiting its natural enzyme for degradation, anticholinesterase. Therefore, this drug serves to intensify activity of the parasympathetic nervous system.

A calcium channel blocking drug, verapamil, was chosen to treat a 4-year-old boy with a history of recurrent episodes of weakness, listlessness, pallor, and sweating, associated with a rapid pulse rate. On this occasion of several hours (his longest episode and his first without spontaneous remission), he was examined in the emergency department. Blood pressure was measured 90/60, and peripheral pulses were extremely weak. The initial ECG (Fig. 4–32A) revealed extreme tachycardia of nearly absolute regularity, uniformly shaped and tall peaked P waves, constant PR interval, and normal QRS complexes.

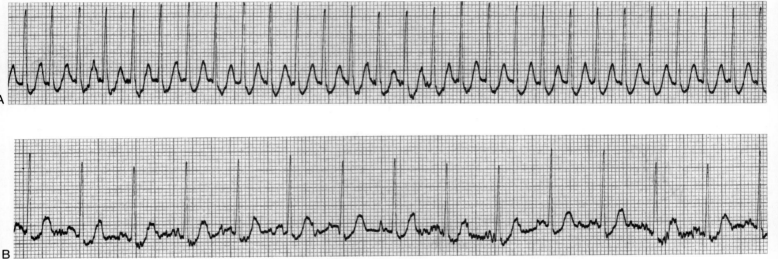

Figure 4–32. A, Initial rhythm strip of atrial tachycardia in a child. B, Normal sinus rhythm following administration of verapamil to treat atrial tachycardia.

After establishing a secure intravenous infusion, 35 mg (or 0.2 mg/kg) of verapamil was injected over 3 minutes. Two or 3 minutes later, the patient's blood pressure had fallen to 70/40 and symptoms and heart rate were unchanged. However, the pulses slowed dramatically a few minutes thereafter, and with the slowing, symptoms subsided promptly and the blood pressure rose to 104/60. The tracing in Figure 4–32B was made at that time.

Despite the baseline artifact (from the child's agitated movement), it is evident that sinus rhythm has replaced atrial tachycardia. The period of transient hypotension occurring shortly after the verapamil injection was probably related to its peripheral vasodilating action. Later, restoration of a relatively slow rhythm resulted in a sudden improvement in cardiac performance and an increase in blood pressure.

Figure 4–33 demonstrates the use of carotid pressure to convert atrial tachycardia of 2 hours duration. At first, this maneuver was unsuccessful, as was the subsequent intravenous administration of verapamil. However, 20 minutes after the drug injection, termination of the tachycardia was achieved when carotid pressure was repeated.

The general characteristics of reentrant tachycardia and premature beats that involve the atria have been presented. Actually, there are four types of such tachyar-

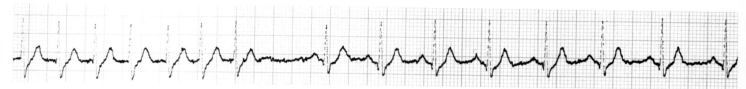

Figure 4–33. Transition of atrial tachycardia to sinus rhythm after administration of verapamil and application of carotid pressure.

rhythmias, two of which have reentrant pathways that are confined to the atria and two that have pathways that include the A-V node or the ventricles through bypass fiber tracks.

Certain features of these various reentrant tachyarrhythmias help to differentiate them. It must be acknowledged, however, that the distinguishing points are often subtle or obscure so that the four types cannot be identified with certainty from the surface ECG in many instances. Electrophysiological studies to elucidate the precise mechanism of these arrhythmias may be required. Because of this difficulty in classifying them according to extent of the reentrant loop, all forms of reentrant premature beats and tachycardias that include the atria in the loop are commonly referred to as *supraventricular*, meaning "above the ventricles." Thus, as the various mechanisms for these tachyarrhythmias have been defined by intracardiac electrophysiological investigations, the term *supraventricular* has come to be more inclusive than *atrial*.

Two forms of supraventricular tachyarrhythmias will be described directly: sinus nodal and intraatrial, these types having reentrant pathways wholly within the atria. The other two forms, having a portion of the reentrant pathways in the A-V node or in the ventricles, will be presented in Chapter 5.

SINUS NODAL REENTRY

The reentrant loop may be confined entirely within the sinus node itself owing to prominent differences of conduction velocity of internodal fibers. In other instances, the reentrant loop courses between the sinus node and adjoining atria, established through anomalous perinodal fibers.

The rate of sinus nodal reentrant tachycardias tends to be slower than those found in other supraventricular tachycardias, averaging about 120 beats per minute but sometimes as slow as 90 per minute. The P waves tend toward similarity in contour with those inscribed during normal sinus rhythm. Most often, this arrhythmia occurs in young and healthy persons, particularly those with high-grade vagal tone, such as athletes. It is also common in elderly people with sinus node dysfunction. Sinus nodal reentrant tachycardia sometimes emerges in response to drugs that enhance vagal tone (such as digitalis), those that decrease adrenergic tone (beta-adrenergic blockers), or those that alter the actin-myosin interaction (calcium channel blockers).

Furthermore, the arrhythmia is typically responsive to vagal stimulation, resulting in slowing of the rate with or without eventual termination of the tachycardia.

Figure 4–34 demonstrates the onset of a sinus tachycardia. This recording was taken while the patient was completely inactive and calm.

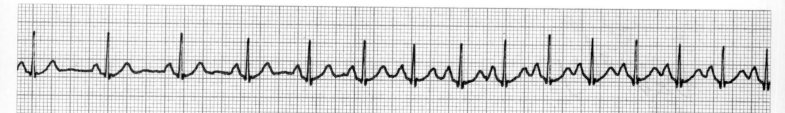

Figure 4–34. Onset of sinus tachycardia.

The following features should be noted:

Sinus rhythm with normal rate of 78 per minute at the beginning.

Sudden increase in heart rate.

After a few beats, at the more rapid rate, the rhythm becomes absolutely regular at 130 per minute.

P waves of the slow and the rapid rates are virtually identical.

The tachycardia is relatively slow.

In the absence of an apparent cause of the accelerated heart rate, it is presumed to be a nonphysiological tachycardia (i.e., a change in rhythm not in response to a functional demand). Further, it is assumed that the new pacemaker originates within (or very near to) the sinus node, because there is no appreciable alteration in the shape of the P waves. The precise regularity of the faster rate suggests a reentrant mechanism. All together, these considerations indicate a sinus node reentry tachycardia.

The relatively slow rate and the normal configuration of P waves may render sinus node reentrant tachycardia difficult to distinguish from normal sinus tachycardia. Patients are often totally unaware of the tachycardia, and the condition is found incidentally.

Ordinarily, sinus node reentrant tachycardia is asymptomatic or nearly so, and no treatment is indicated. A clinician is obligated, nevertheless, to look for an underlying abnormality, most especially sinus node dysfunction. When indicated, therapy may be effective with the same drugs sometimes associated with its cause, such as digoxin, propranolol, and verapamil. This seeming paradox is related to their relative actions on conduction velocity and refractory period of fibers within the reentrant circuit.

Of the supraventricular tachycardias encountered clinically, it is estimated that about 5% are the sinus node reentrant type.

INTRAATRIAL REENTRY

In intraatrial reentry, the entire reentrant loop lies in one or both atria, but it does *not* incorporate the sinus node. The circuit may be encompassed within the area of one cubic centimeter. These "microentry" loops can be located in any region of either atrium. In contrast, one segment of the loop may comprise a long pathway, such as Bachman's bundle, a tract of muscle fibers having preferential conduction capacity relative to adjacent fibers. This tract is more susceptible to impulse velocity-refractory period dissociation, which makes it more vulnerable to reentrant wave fronts. Bachman's bundle extends from the anterior interatrial junction to the posterior wall of the left atrium.

Reentrant tachycardias of the intraatrial type exhibit P waves that are altered in contour or in polarity (compared with sinus generated P waves) depending on the location of the reentrant loop and the direction of radial transmission from it (Fig. 4–35). The average rate of intraatrial reentrant tachycardias is somewhat faster than that

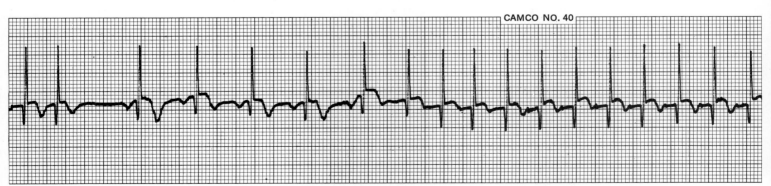

Figure 4–35. Note the altered configuration of the P wave indicating abnormal direction of conduction through the intraatrial pathway.

of sinus node reentry. Another distinction is that the intraatrial type is generally resistant to vagotonic reflexes.

It is important to distinguish intraatrial reentrant tachycardia from automatic atrial tachycardia, with which it is easily confused. A most useful differentiating point is the sudden onset and offset of the former compared with the gradual warm-up and cool-down observed with the latter. Uniformity of rate and P wave configuration is typical of the former; slight variations in rate and in morphology of P waves from beat to beat are commonly present in the latter.

Electrocardioversion

More than two decades of experience with electric shock treatment of tachycardias has firmly established this modality as a therapeutic technique. Applied directly to the chest surface at the precordium, an electrical stimulus is highly effective in instantaneously converting reentrant tachycardias to normal sinus rhythm. Further, the technique has proved relatively safe because it is performed under direct observation by the clinician.

Electric shock therapy is administered with an electronically regulated electric power source (commonly called a **defibrillator**) and two broad electrodes placed on the chest. One electrode (or **paddle**) is placed over the right atrium (midsternal area); the second electrode is placed near the cardiac apex (left lateral chest or left posterior chest base).

Instruments for electrocardioversion vary widely in design, but each instrument operates according to the same principles. The standard defibrillator discharges electrical energy in the form of direct current within a small fraction of a second. The amount of electrical energy is measured as power (or watts) applied over time (in this instance, seconds). Hence, the unit of energy used is referred to as **watt/seconds**. This unit is also known as a **joule**, named after James Prescott Joule, an English physicist of the 19th century.

Electric shock therapy for reentrant tachycardias depends on the following action. It simultaneously depolarizes all fibers that can respond to the stimulus at that instant (when the fibers are at resting membrane potential or in their relative refractory period). After depolarization, all responding fibers (myofibrils and those specialized for impulse formation and conduction) begin repolarization uniformly. When effective, the shock interrupts the reverberating impulse of the reentrant loop and allows the normally dominant pacemaker to resume its natural role.

Electric shock delivered to the heart during the hypersensitive portion of ventricular repolarization is hazardous (as explained later). Consequently, the defibrillator must be timed to fire during another portion of the ventricular cycle. The instrument is therefore preset to discharge during ventricular depolarization. This timing is assured by setting the discharge control switch to synchronize, thus assuring that discharge will automatically occur in synchrony with the QRS spike. Instrument sensitivity must also be adjusted so that it detects one and only one deflection of each cardiac cycle. The procedure for selecting the ideal monitoring lead can be followed as described in Chapter 2. To check the synchronizing accuracy of the machine, activate the synchronizing control switch and observe the oscilloscope and a rhythm strip for indication of sensing of the QRS complex.

The strips in Figures 4–36 and 4–37 illustrate the importance of the synchronizing feature. The initial strip (Fig. 4–36) was run when the machine was not programmed to fire in synchrony with the QRS. In this demonstration strip, note that discharge (as identified by the arrow in the upper border and the interruption in the normal cardiac complex trace) occurred during the recovery phase, the T wave, of the cycle.

The second strip (Fig. 4–37) was obtained after the machine was programmed to

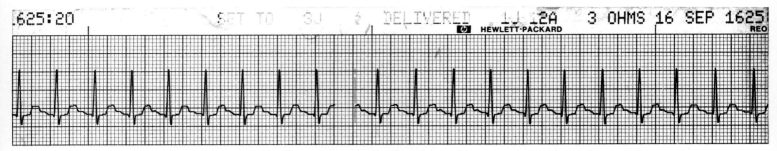

Figure 4–36. Cardioversion test strip when the machine was not programmed for synchronization. The discharge occurs during the repolarization phase (T wave).

fire in synchrony with the patient's QRS spike. Small markers at the upper edge of the strip indicate the synchronized timing. Even with the irregularity in cycling noted in the middle of the strip (under SEP), the spike appears in synchrony. The discharge in this instance occurs in conjunction with the QRS complex four cycles later.

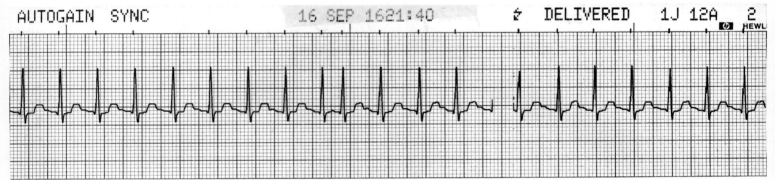

Figure 4–37. Cardioversion test strip with the machine in the synchronized mode and thus fired at the onset of the QRS complex.

Figure 4–38 illustrates a synchronized test shock in supraventricular tachycardia. The recording was obtained with the testing device in place.

The tracing begins with supraventricular tachycardia of a complex nature owing to a variable conduction defect in the A-V node. The legend denotes the moment of activation of the discharge button. The actual firing is delayed automatically until the peak of the R deflection. The shock itself obliterates the recording for 1.65 seconds before the pattern resumes. Of course, the arrhythmia is unaltered because the discharge is *not* delivered to the patient during the test procedure but the energy is expended within the testing device.

Figure 4–39 illustrates nonsynchronized test shock, an alternative method of activating the electric shock, in which discharge occurs immediately on pressing the discharge button. It is *not* timed with any event in the cardiac cycle and is used to treat arrhythmias with no definite QRS complexes. (It will be described in detail later.) The test is performed using the same electrocardiographic display as in the previous example. For this mode of delivery, the control switch is set on direct activation, which is usually designated **defibrillation**.

In Figure 4–39 note that the activator button depression and the electric shock occur simultaneously and have no relationship to the QRS complex or to any other electrical signal from the patient. The discharge is therefore not synchronous with ventricular depolarization. A transient period of electrical blackout again appears. The rhythm, as expected, is unchanged by this test shock.

Because electrical shock is an unpleasant experience at best, some form of anesthesia or sedation is administered before shocking a conscious patient. A commonly

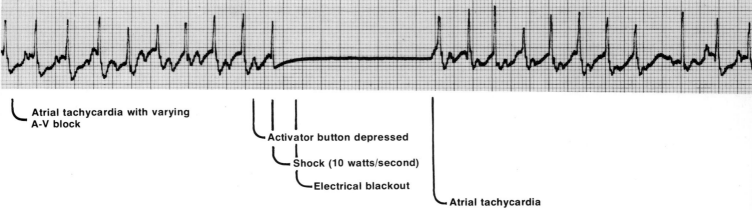

Figure 4–38. The sequence of synchronized test shock in atrial tachycardia.

used agent for electrocardioversion is diazepam (Valium), administered by titration with intermittent intravenous injections. Ordinarily, a desirable level of relaxation and analgesia can be achieved without interference with physiological defenses. In addition, patients characteristically have a peculiar amnesia for the event under diazepam effect. Testifying to the fact that a high degree of emotional tension is a factor in some patients with paroxysmal tachycardias, relief of anxiety with diazepam administration in preparation for electrocardioversion is occasionally followed by spontaneous remission of the tachycardia.

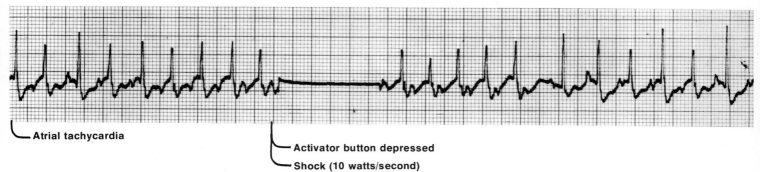

Figure 4–39. The sequence of nonsynchronized test shock.

Whether or not the shock is successful depends on a number of variables. Failure of electrocardioversion will occur when it does not interupt the reverberant impulse. An excitable focus (or foci) may continue to function automatically. The integrity of the normal impulse-formation/impulse-conducting systems may be compromised.

There is a high incidence of cardiac arrhythmias immediately after electric shock. They include severe sinus bradycardia and ectopic beats and tachycardias of either atrial or ventricular origin. These events are usually transient, however, and are soon dominated or replaced by a more stable rhythm. These arrhythmias following shock occasionally require immediate treatment, however. Obviously, electrocardioversion must be employed only with full anticipation of any rhythm complication and only when the means for their management are available.

Atrial Tachycardia with Atrioventricular Block

As the atrial rate becomes faster, the transmission capacity of the A-V node is eventually exceeded. In other words, the interval at which atrial impulses assault the A-V

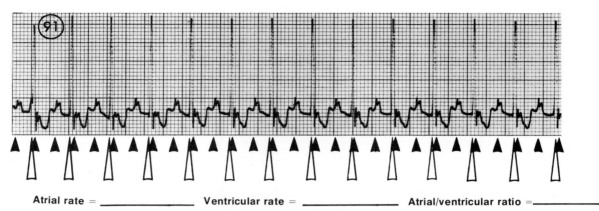

Atrial rate = _____   Ventricular rate = _____   Atrial/ventricular ratio =_____

Figure 4–40. Atrial tachycardia with 2:1 A-V block.

node is shorter than the refractory period for that tissue. This critical limit is usually about 180 transmissions per minute in most adults. Beyond this, some atrial impulses are not transmitted, much as APCs may be blocked. A physiological A-V node conduction defect results, most typically a rhythm in which every second atrial beat is not conducted (Fig. 4–40).

P waves, having highly distinctive morphology, are observed just before each QRS complex. The rate of these obvious P waves is _____ beats per minute. Note that each cardiac cycle has a constant PR interval of _____ mm (or _____ second). Also note that a deflection at the end of the QRS complex resembles these P waves. Using calipers, now measure the interval between corresponding points on the obvious P wave and on the deflection in question. (The second peak of each is handy.) You will find that this point of the latter is precisely midway between corresponding points of the flanking P waves. Thus, by configuration and by regularity of beating, we can identify the unknown inscription as a P wave, as well, but one that is blocked (is not followed by a QRS complex).

On determining the atrial rate again (to include both conducted and blocked beats), it is found to be _____ per minute with an A-V ratio of _____ : _____ . This rate, of course, is exactly twice that of the ventricular rate. The proper terminology for the rhythm is atrial tachycardia with 2:1 block.

Locate the conducted and blocked atrial complexes in test tracings 92, 93, and 94. Are they precisely equidistant? Is the PR interval of conducted beats constant? Compare the atrial and the ventricular rates.

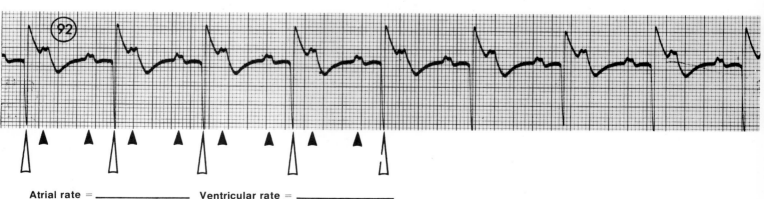

Atrial rate = _____   Ventricular rate = _____

Atrial/ventricular ratio = _____

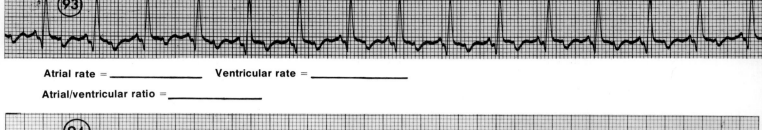

Atrial rate = _____   Ventricular rate = _____

Atrial/ventricular ratio = _____

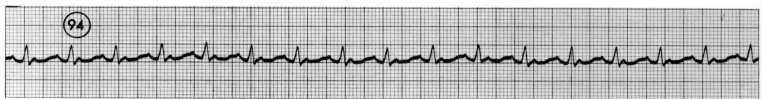

The presence of intermittent A-V block and its severity depend on the rate of the atrial rhythm and on the conductance capacity of the A-V node. In the tracing in Figure 4–41, one of the variables changes and the degree of A-V block is altered.

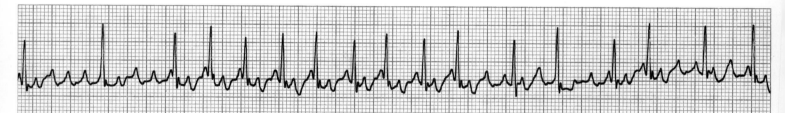

Figure 4–41. Alteration in the degree of block is seen in this example of atrial tachycardia.

At the beginning of the strip, few of the atrial beats are conducted. Then, the ability of the A-V node to accept impulses is increased and a QRS follows every other P wave. The end of the strip again shows a decrease in the capacity for conduction through the A-V node.

Inspection of the tracing in Figure 4–42 reveals a tachycardia without identifiable P waves. P waves may be superimposed on the T waves, and the slight notching on their peaks suggests that this is so. The rate is 178 beats per minute, and the rhythm has clock-like periodicity. Although the interpretation of atrial tachycardia must be considered, it cannot be made with surety.

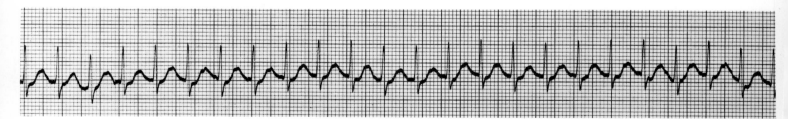

Figure 4–42. Atrial tachycardia.

To clarify the diagnosis, a parasympathetic maneuver is performed. The object is to slow the pacemaker rate and/or to cause a degree of A-V block that will expose atrial activity (Fig. 4–43).

Carotid artery stimulation is applied. There is an immediate response by slowing of the ventricular rate. Each QRS complex is now preceded by a distinct, if complex,

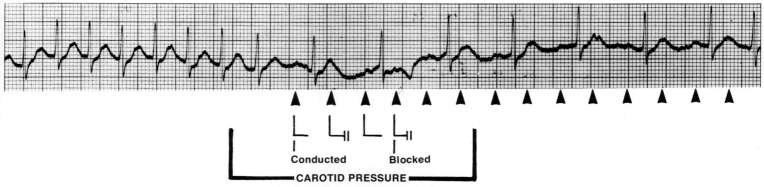

Figure 4–43. Application of carotid pressure.

P wave. Furthermore, there are blocked P waves identifiable by similarity to and equidistance from conducted P waves. Thus is established the diagnosis of atrial tachycardia with 2:1 A-V block.

Having recognized this pattern, the interpreter can go back to the earlier portion of the tracing and appreciate the presence of atrial tachycardia with 1:1 conduction of atrial beats. Note that vagal stimulation has decreased the atrial rate to 172 beats per minute (and of course the ventricular to one-half that, or 86 beats per minute).

We have demonstrated the value of a simple technique that alters autonomic tone and permits more accurate interpretation of difficult tachycardias. As already shown, such maneuvers are often successful in arresting the tachycardia. Certainly, a transition from tachycardia to normal rhythm, whether spontaneous or induced, should be studied with great care for it often uncovers very interesting dynamics of rhythm control. In addition, analyzing this period affords excellent practice for interpretation. Transitions in rhythms, in fact, are strongly featured throughout this book.

In the tracing in Figure 4–44, carotid stimulation again reveals atrial tachycardia with block as the basic rhythm. In this transition, the rhythm change is particularly interesting.

The vagotonic stimulation at first induces A-V block, but this time there are three atrial beats before the QRS complex (two blocked ones and then one conducted beat). Referred to as 3:1 A-V block, this pattern persists for two cycles, is superseded by two cycles of 2:1 A-V block, and then there is resumption of the original tachycardia with 1:1 A-V conduction. Determine the atrial rate and the fastest and slowest ventricular rates in strip 95 (Fig. 4–44).

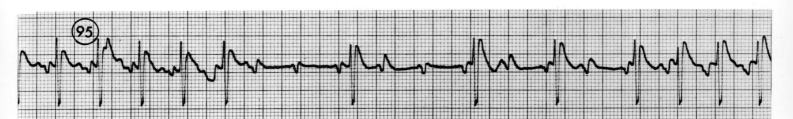

Figure 4–44. Increased degree of block in atrial tachycardia produced with vagal stimulation.

To analyze both of the preceding tracings (Figs. 4–43 and 4–44) even further, we find that the P waves are not of the smooth configuration typical of sinus rhythms. With carotid pressure, there is no gradual slowing of rate but rather an abrupt intermittent block of impulses in the A-V node. These facts, plus the very rapid atrial rates, weigh against the possibility of sinus tachycardia. Abnormal P wave morphology also precludes the diagnosis of sinus node reentrant tachycardia. Both sinus reentrant tachycardias as well as atrial reentrant tachycardias, which exhibit abnormal P wave form, are usually terminated by carotid pressure. Thus, one may suspect that the tachycardias presented are of automatic atrial origin. This tachycardia typically responds to vagal stimulation by transient increases in A-V block and not by conversion to sinus rhythm.

In strip 96, every other atrial depolarization is conducted. Measure both atrial and ventricular rates.

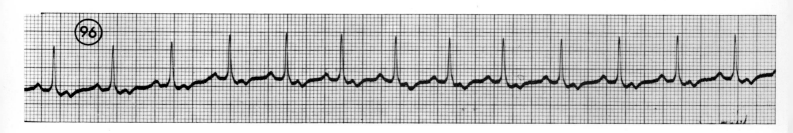

Digitalis has a special propensity for producing both excitation of impulse formation in the atria and depression of impulse conduction in the A-V node. This dual action is caused by enhanced automaticity of atrial fibers (resulting in tachycardia) and increased vagal tone in the A-V node (resulting in A-V block). Commonly, 2:1 A-V block is an expression of digitalis toxicity. The following series presents an illustrative example.

A 58-year-old woman was admitted to the hospital after 2 days of rapid palpitations and dyspnea on mild exertion. Her maintenance dose of digitalis had been increased 3 weeks before because of nocturnal dyspnea due to rheumatic valvular disease (mitral regurgitation). There were no physical signs of congestive heart failure on admission, and serum electrolyte values were within normal limits. The admission ECG is presented (test strip 97). Determine the atrial and ventricular rates.

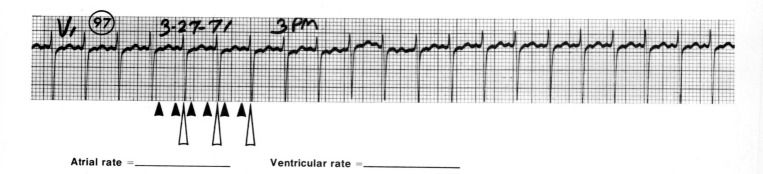

Atrial rate = _____   Ventricular rate = _____

The diagnosis of atrial tachycardia with 2:1 A-V block can be appreciated after careful measurement of intervals between P waves. The cause of the dysrhythmia was strongly suspected to be a form of digitalis toxicity, and this drug was withheld.

On the following day, atrial tachycardia persisted. However, the atrial rate slowed somewhat and the severity of A-V block decreased. Observe that after a pause in the ventricular rate, the PR intervals become progressively longer; then a blocked atrial beat occurs. The pattern then repeats itself. This is a complex form of intermittent A-V block that will be described later (under Wenckebach Phenomenon in Chapter 5).

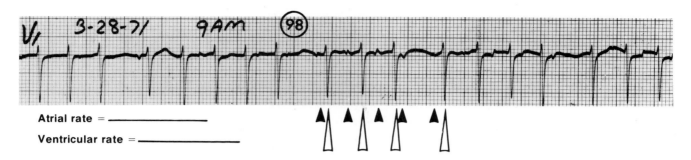

Atrial rate = _____

Ventricular rate = _____

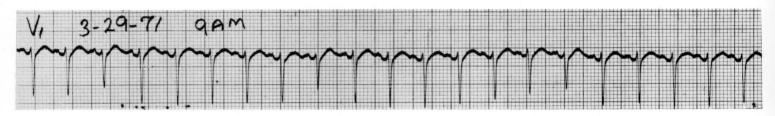

One day later, the atrial rate slowed further, and A-V block was no longer present. Atrial tachycardia with a rate of 160 per minute and 1:1 A-V conduction was the diagnosis.

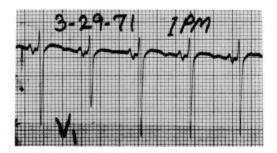

Several hours after the previous tracing, a sinus rhythm was found to have replaced atrial tachycardia. There is now no evidence of digitalis toxicity.

The biphasic P wave, incidentally, is commonly observed in lead V_1 in normal sinus rhythm.

The importance of attentive search in rhythm interpretation is exemplified in the tracing in Figure 4–45. Look carefully before arriving at a diagnosis.

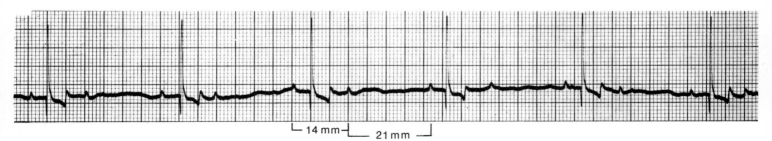

Figure 4–45. Note the difference in intervals between the conducted and the blocked P waves signifying early activation of the atria by premature beats.

One may immediately expect that 2:1 A-V block is present. In this case, the sinus or atrial beating would occur at a regular rate. Using calipers, note that the interval from the conducted P wave to the blocked P wave is considerably shorter than that between the blocked and the conducted P waves. In effect, the blocked P wave is premature. Its similarity to the sinus initiated and conducted P waves suggests that the origin is at or within the sinus node and is of the reentrant type. The constant interval between the sinus beat and the premature beat also favors a reentrant mechanism. The biphasic character of the T waves should pose no confusion when the rhythmicity is plotted out. The pattern of one normal cycle alternating with a premature beat is known as a **bigeminy**. The diagnosis, then, is sinus bradycardia with blocked bigeminal atrial (or supraventricular) premature beats. The distinction made here is of much clinical importance because blocked APCs are generally benign whereas a sinus rhythm with 2:1 A-V block has serious implications, as will be pointed out in the discussion of A-V nodal dysfunctions.

A-V block in supraventricular tachycardia may be of sufficient intensity to prohibit every other beat from penetrating the A-V node. In a few tracings of predominantly 2:1 A-V block already studied, transient periods of higher degrees of block were observed. In some tachycardias, the dominant rhythm may present with only every third, fourth, or even lesser ratio being transmitted to the ventricles.

ATRIAL FLUTTER

Atrial flutter is a tachycardia in which the atrial rate is extremely rapid, typically about 300 beats per minute, and usually within the range of 250 to 350 per minute. It may occur as paroxysms, as in reentrant tachycardias already described, in persons with no other evidence of cardiac disease. More frequently, however, it is a persistent abnormality associated with conditions causing atrial enlargement, such as valvular stenosis and chronic pulmonary disease. Degenerative disorders of the atrial wall are probably the preeminent cause.

A characteristic form of P waves presents itself, at least in some leads, as a saw-toothed pattern. Designated **F waves**, they represent a bidirectional waveform in which atrial depolarization occurs so rapidly that it appears to be virtually continuous, one wave leading directly into another without a well-defined isoelectric interval between. Figure 4–46 depicts the change in waveform commonly observed with increasing atrial rates in which the diphasic nature develops. In this illustration, atrial activity without ventricular responses is depicted for purposes of clarification.

For many decades, explanations for the mechanism for atrial flutter have had vigorous proponents representing divergent views. Some hold that a loop of anomalous conducting fibers, perhaps located around the inflow regions of the superior and inferior vena cavae in the right atrium, provide a vulnerable circuit for rapid reentrant activity. Others maintain that atrial flutter is the result of a single focus of rapid impulse emissions somewhere in the atria, most likely the most distal wall of either atrium. Thus, atrial flutter is postulated as a phenomenon of a reentrant mechanism or of enhanced automaticity. Either is probably applicable to individual cases.

Whether automatic or reentrant, atrial flutter can be thought of as a supraventricular tachycardia in which the atrial rate is extremely rapid. The rate almost always exceeds the capacity of the A-V node to transmit each wave front into the ventricles so that intermittent A-V block is a characteristic feature. Selected examples from a 12-lead ECG exhibiting the typical pattern of atrial flutter are presented in Figure 4–47.

Variations in amplitude and waveform contours of atrial complexes are noted from lead to lead. For example, in lead V_1, they are highly distinctive, but in the lateral precordial lead V_4 they are barely discernible. The broad Q wave in leads I and aVL and the small R wave in the lateral precordial leads are identifying markers of anterior lateral myocardial infarction.

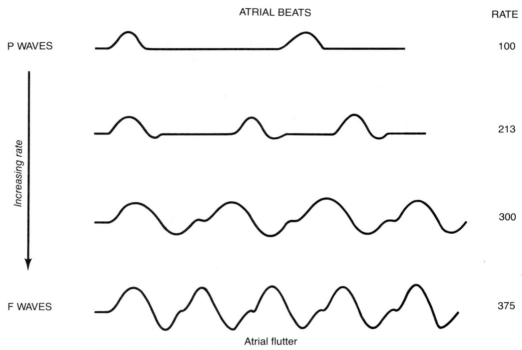

Figure 4–46. Atrial flutter. (Ventricular activity is not shown.)

Recordings from three leads of the standard ECG are presented in Figure 4–48 to demonstrate the variability of F waves.

The diagnosis of atrial flutter may be easily missed in lead V_4; F waves are distinct only in portions of lead II. In lead V_1, they are highly conspicuous. This arrhythmia developed in a patient with an acute anteroseptal myocardial infarction, accounting for the small R deflection in lead V_4.

As with atrial tachycardia, flutter can occur in paroxysms. The onset of atrial flutter and its spontaneous remission is observed for only four cardiac cycles in Figure 4–49. Slowing of the flutter rate occurs just before conversion to sinus rhythm.

If impulses from each atrial beat were transmitted in atrial flutter through the A-V node, the ventricles would be driven at a rate too fast for effective filling and pumping. In fact, such 1:1 A-V conduction is rarely encountered clinically. An untreated patient presenting initially with atrial flutter usually has a 2:1 A-V block. Even so, the ventricular rate response is quite rapid, enough to produce symptoms of palpitations if not exertional dyspnea or other manifestations of impaired cardiac performance. The tracing in Figure 4–50 was taken from a man who had experienced the sensation of a flutter in the chest at night for several days. He had previously demonstrated frequent APCs on routine ECGs but otherwise appeared healthy.

Figure 4–51 comprises representative leads from a standard ECG. Give particular attention to the marked dissimilarity of P waves in each lead. In lead I, they are practically indistinguishable. Lead III displays P waves that appear to form a continuous undulation. They are highly distinctive in lead V_1, with an apparent isoelectric separation. The atrial rate, ventricular rate, and A-V ratio have been determined.

The example of atrial flutter in Figure 4–51 demonstrates a constant ratio of atrial and ventricular beats (e.g., 4:1). In addition, the conduction time between an F wave and the subsequent QRS complex (FR interval) is also constant. Given lead I only, the diagnosis might be overlooked. These various appearances of atrial flutter demonstrate the advantage of using multiple leads in more complex arrhythmia interpretation.

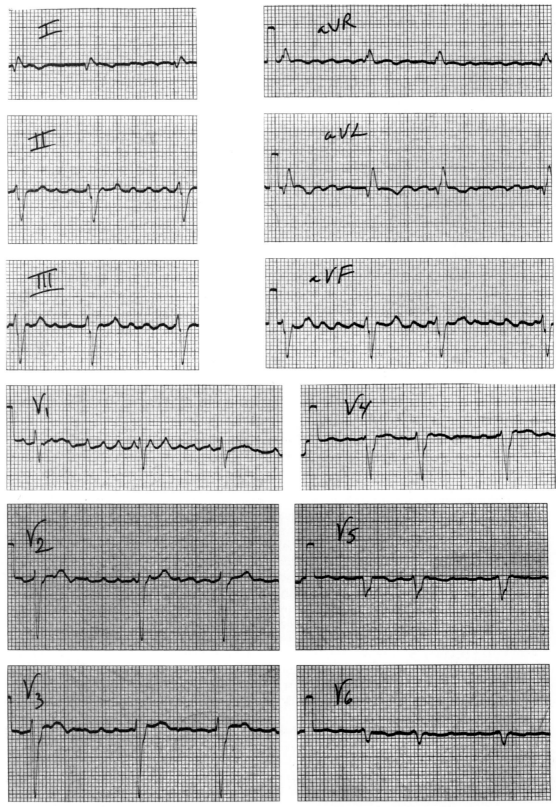

Figure 4–47. Typical pattern of atrial flutter as seen in a standard 12-lead electrocardiogram.

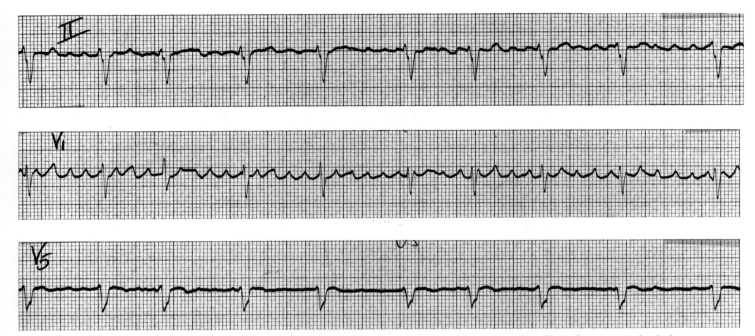

Figure 4–48. Variability of F waves can be observed in these select leads from a standard electrocardiogram.

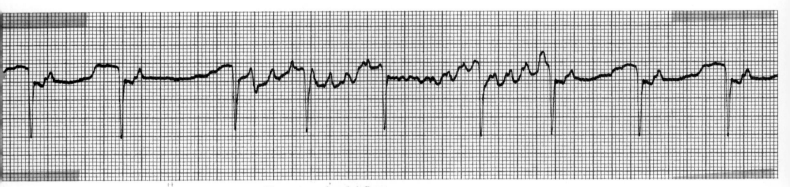

Figure 4–49. Short run of atrial flutter.

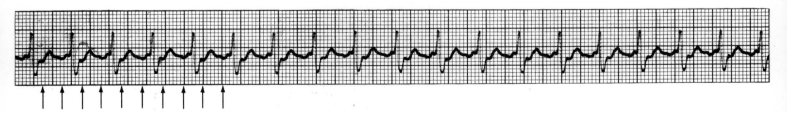

Figure 4–50. Note in this example that every other flutter wave is blocked.

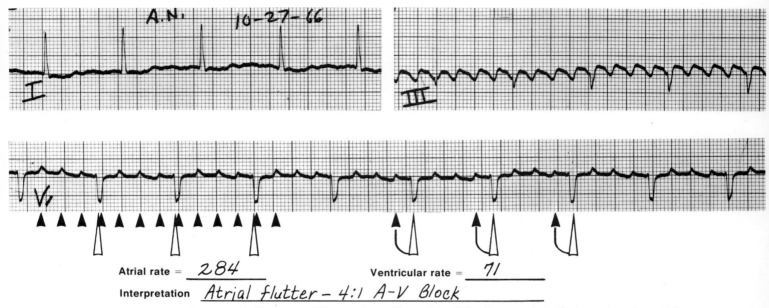

Atrial rate = *284*   Ventricular rate = *71*

Interpretation *Atrial flutter – 4:1 A-V Block*

Figure 4–51. Note the difference in configuration of the flutter waves in these three leads taken from the same patient.

These patterns of 2:1 and 4:1 A-V block are the most common forms of atrial flutter with fixed A-V conduction. That of sustained 1:1 A-V conduction, with its extremely rapid ventricular rate, constitutes a medical emergency. However, 1:1 A-V conduction can occur transiently in persons with fairly stable 2:1 or 4:1 A-V block, as demonstrated in the tracing in Figure 4–52.

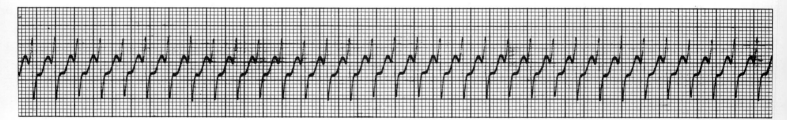

Figure 4–52. Transient episodes of 1:1 conduction in atrial flutter.

This 28-year-old patient had experienced short periods of dizziness, blurred vision, and nausea for several years. This episode was recorded by obstetrical nurses when the patient experienced palpitations and lightheadedness in the labor room. Her blood pressure was 90/60 during the rhythm, which lasted 3 minutes and terminated spontaneously.

Such temporary increases in conduction may result from adrenergic stimulation, as occurs with exercise or strong emotional reactions. Drugs, notably atropine-like agents, may precipitate 1:1 A-V conduction in atrial flutter owing to their parasympathetic blocking action. Quinidine and procainamide have anticholinergic properties and consequently can produce more severe tachycardia (even though they *also* possess a suppressant action on reentrant and ectopic pacemaker activity that is responsible for the tachycardia).

A-V block may be more intense than a ratio of 4:1, and sometimes it is severe, causing marked bradycardia. Coexisting disease within the A-V node itself is commonly responsible. Drug effect is another cause. Excessive A-V block may result from antisympathetic agents, such as the beta-adrenergic blockers (e.g., propanolol). It may be produced by agents having a vagotonic action, most notably digitalis. Vagal stimulating maneuvers can induce extreme A-V block in atrial flutter, as shown in the test tracing 99.

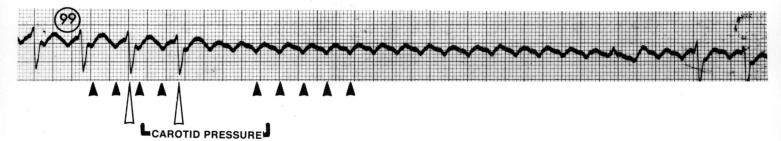

Inspection of the early portion of tracing 99 reveals typical atrial flutter with 2:1 A-V block. The F waves measure out precisely at a rate of 240 beats per minute, and the downward deflection of the blocked F wave is too close to the QRS complex to be confused with the T wave. To plan an approach to treatment according to the responsiveness to vagal stimulation, gentle carotid pressure was performed. This parasympathetic stimulation, although mild and of short duration (less than 1.5 seconds), resulted in prolonged ventricular inactivity lasting _____ seconds.

Variable A-V conduction in atrial flutter occurs when incomplete recovery and variation in transmission occur in the A-V node because of the extremely rapid atrial firing rate. This results in changes in FR intervals and contours.

In the following series of tracings, recorded from the same patient, examples of variability in the A-V ratio or the FR interval or both will be present.

1. The atrial flutter with variable A-V conduction shows changes in both the number of atrial beats that precede each ventricular beat and the interval between the F wave and the QRS complex.

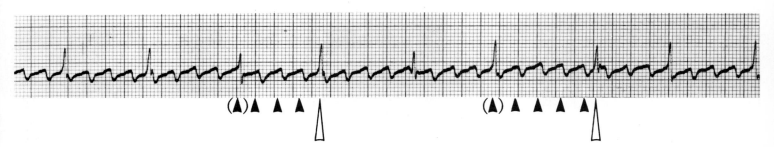

Solid arrows indicate F waves and are placed within parentheses where the F waves are obscured by the QRS complexes. Those cardiac cycles so labeled have variable A-V block.

2. When the patient takes a deep breath and holds it, physiological A-V block is markedly increased, owing to respiratory stimulation of parasympathetic control. A variable A-V numerical relationship and variable FR intervals are still present.

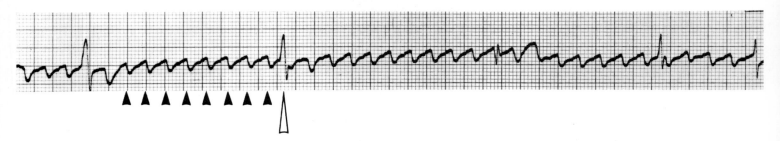

At times the atrial rate is as much as 10 times faster than the ventricular rate, and at other times only 4 times faster. Remember to include the F waves that occur simultaneously with (and may be obscured by) the QRS complexes. Note that QRS complexes vary in both contour and duration. This variation is probably the result of superimposed F waves, which have a slight change in timing relationship with the QRS complexes from beat to beat.

3. An increase in A-V conduction frequency was produced by light exercise, adrenergic stimulation the accountable factor. Even though no acceleration of atrial rate occurs, the ventricular rate has increased. Determine the A-V ratio. Are FR intervals constant?

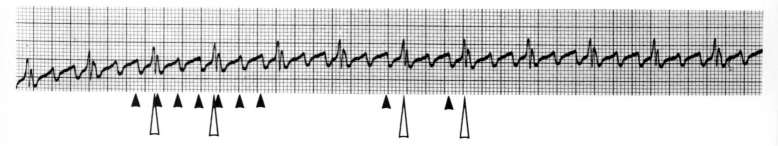

Every third atrial beat is conducted to the ventricles. Therefore, the A-V ratio is 3:1. The FR interval is constant throughout. For reasons that are not well understood, atrial flutter with an A-V ratio of 3:1 is distinctly unusual. One explanation is that the first blocked atrial beat may interfere with A-V transmission of the atrial beat that immediately follows, although this phenomenon (a form of concealed conduction) cannot be determined from the surface ECG.

The following tracings are examples of atrial flutter. In each, you are requested to analyze the strip carefully, determining atrial and ventricular rates, A-V ratios, and FR intervals when appropriate.

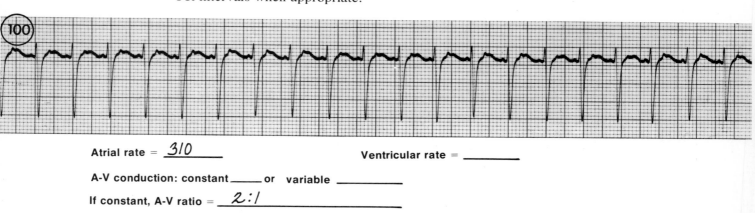

Atrial rate = _310_   Ventricular rate = _____

A-V conduction: constant_____ or variable _____

If constant, A-V ratio = _2:1_____

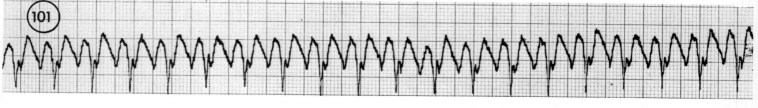

Atrial rate = _____   Ventricular rate = _145_

A-V conduction: constant _✓_ or variable _____

If constant, A-V ratio = _____

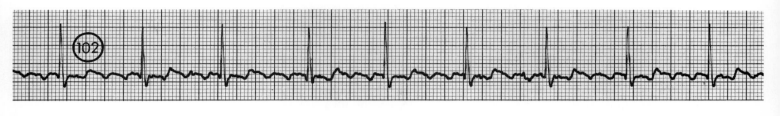

Atrial rate = _____   Ventricular rate = _____

A-V conduction: constant _____ or variable _____

If constant, A-V ratio = _____

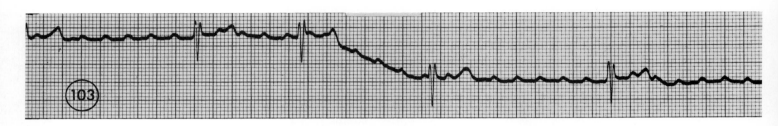

Atrial rate = _____   Ventricular rate = _____

A-V conduction: constant _____ or variable _____

If constant, A-V ratio = _____

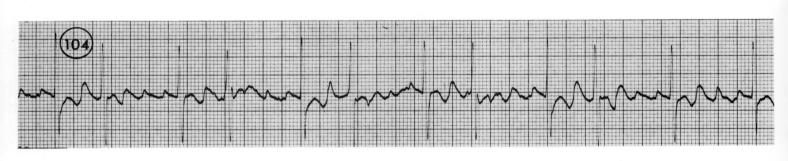

Atrial rate = _____   Ventricular rate = _____

A-V conduction: constant _____ or variable _____

If constant, A-V ratio = _____

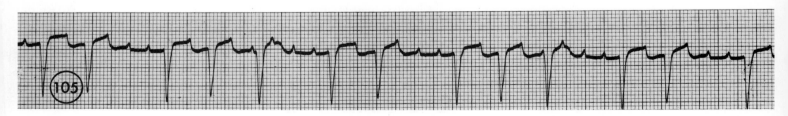

Atrial rate = _____   Ventricular rate = _____

A-V conduction: constant _____ or variable _____

If constant, A-V ratio = _____

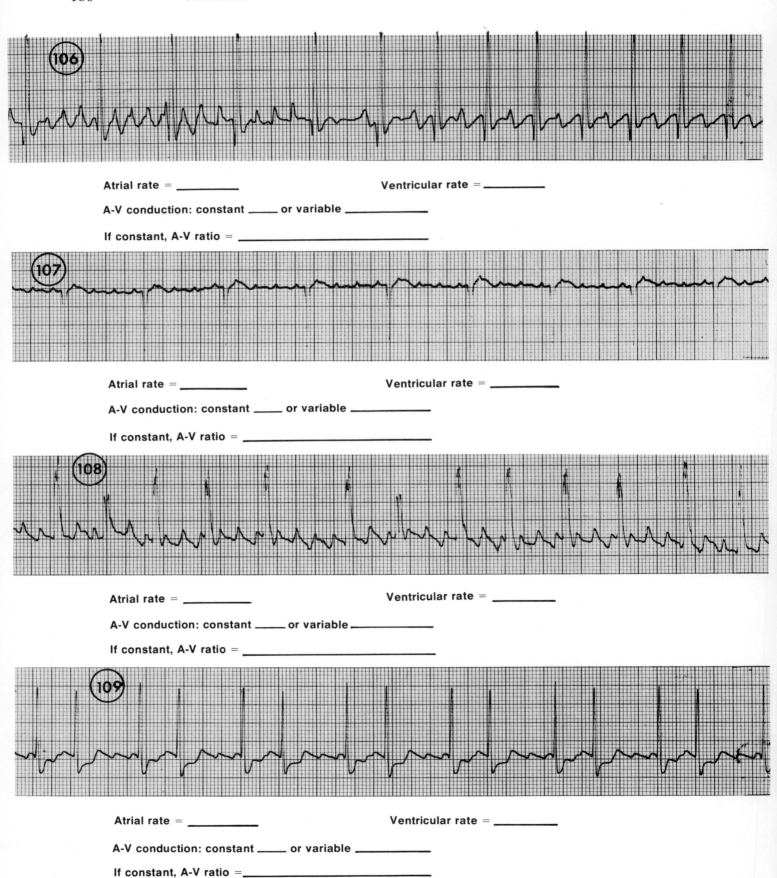

Atrial rate = _____   Ventricular rate = _____

A-V conduction: constant _____ or variable _____

If constant, A-V ratio = _____

Atrial rate = _____   Ventricular rate = _____

A-V conduction: constant _____ or variable _____

If constant, A-V ratio = _____

Atrial rate = _____   Ventricular rate = _____

A-V conduction: constant _____ or variable _____

If constant, A-V ratio = _____

Atrial rate = _____   Ventricular rate = _____

A-V conduction: constant _____ or variable _____

If constant, A-V ratio = _____

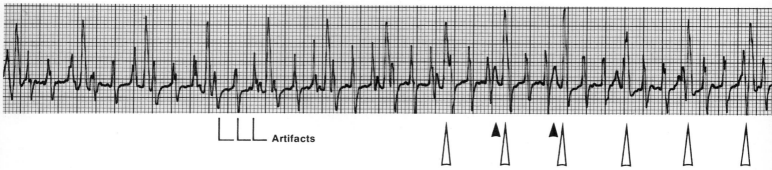

Figure 4–53. Apparent atrial flutter. An artifact due to rapid arm movement.

Figure 4–53 appears to indicate atrial flutter with a somewhat variable A-V conduction. In fact, this tracing was recorded on a telemetry unit on a patient with normal sinus rhythm, and the apparent arrhythmia is in fact produced by vigorous arm movement during brushing the teeth. Close inspection of the strip allows the interpreter to identify QRS complexes at measured intervals. Although the P waves are largely obscured by superimposed movement artifact, some isolated P waves stand out, as indicated by symbols. The tracing does reemphasize the importance of always interpreting an ECG in relation to the setting in which it was obtained.

In some instances, atrial flutter is disguised by a rapid ventricular rate response. Slowing the rate with vagal stimulation may reveal the typical pattern of atrial flutter (Fig. 4–54).

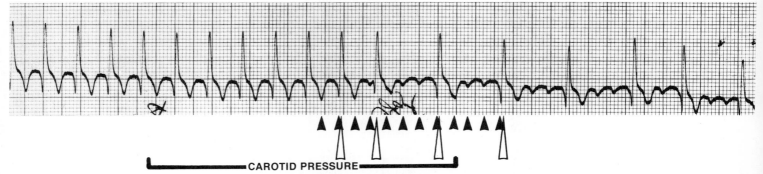

Figure 4–54. Atrial flutter demonstrated by suppression of ventricular responses with vagal stimulation.

As the ventricular rate slows with carotid pressure, atrial flutter becomes apparent. The atrial rate is 346 per minute. Not all F waves can be morphologically identified because of superimposition of the QRS complex, but they can be located by measuring out with calipers. FR intervals are variable, and it is not certain which atrial beats are actually conducted to the ventricles. In the cycles having maximum A-V block, there is a 4:1 A-V ratio.

A diagnosis of atrial flutter can now be given for the tachycardia present at the beginning of the tracing. There is a 2:1 A-V block in which the ventricular rate is 173 per minute (346 ÷ 2). Thus a difficult interpretation is clarified by increasing the degree of A-V block with vagal stimulation.

Figure 4–55 also demonstrates how a rate change can clarify the rhythm interpretation. From the earlier portion of the tracing, no precise interpretation can be made. Following carotid pressure and the resultant slowing of the ventricular rate, the pattern of atrial flutter emerges with an atrial rate of 360 per minute. On applying this infor-

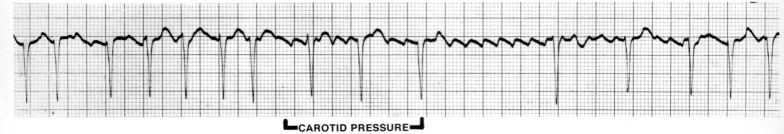

CAROTID PRESSURE

Figure 4–55. Diagnosis of supraventricular tachycardia using vagal stimulation.

mation to the beginning of the tracing, the diagnosis of atrial flutter with variable A-V block can be assumed.

The preceding two ECGs demonstrate one common feature of atrial flutter that helps to distinguish it from some forms of atrial tachycardia. Thus far, we have presented atrial flutter simply as a form of supraventricular tachycardia characterized by an extremely rapid atrial rate. In addition, the saw-toothed F wave baseline serves as a highly distinctive signature in some leads. In actuality, supraventricular tachycardias with atrial rates between 250 and 300 beats per minute dictate arbitration in diagnosis between these two types of arrhythmias (SVT and AFl), particularly in the absence of a clear saw-toothed pattern. A typical response of atrial flutter to vagal stimulation, as shown in Figures 4–54 and 4–55, is an increase in A-V block with a resultant decrease in ventricular rate; there is little change in atrial rate, and the former ventricular rate response resumes momentarily after release of parasympathetic stimulation.

Vagotonic maneuvers often produce more intense functional A-V block in atrial tachycardias as well, either of the enhanced automaticity or the reentrant forms. In the reentrant form, however, procedures such as carotid stimulation often interrupt the reentrant circuit and abruptly terminate the tachycardia, as demonstrated earlier, a result seldom observed in atrial flutter.

Now the exception must be acknowledged, shown here in conversion of atrial flutter to sinus rhythm (Fig. 4–56). Incidentally, this recording has been miniaturized photographically to preserve the continuity of transitional activity.

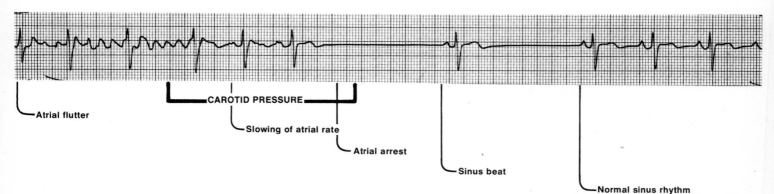

Atrial flutter

CAROTID PRESSURE

Slowing of atrial rate

Atrial arrest

Sinus beat

Normal sinus rhythm

Figure 4–56. Conversion of atrial flutter to normal sinus rhythm. Note carefully the transitional activity of impulse formation. This recording has been photographically miniaturized to avoid a break in continuity.

At the beginning of the tracing, undulating atrial activity is present in the form of a saw-toothed pattern at a rate well above 300 per minute. Carotid stimulation induces slowing of atrial rate, then momentary cessation of atrial beating. After a long pause, a sinus beat appears, then resumption of normal sinus rhythm.

Although atrial flutter may persist for weeks or even months, it is generally more short lived. The rhythm tends to revert back to a sinus mechanism spontaneously (and is therefore paroxysmal), or it eventually deteriorates into the haphazard atrial depolarization pattern of atrial fibrillation, a condition to be described shortly.

Treatment of Atrial Flutter

The object of treatment of atrial flutter lies in either inducing reversion to a sinus rhythm or increasing the intensity of A-V block, thereby decreasing the ventricular rate response. As in other forms of supraventricular tachycardia, various modalities may be enlisted.

The following series shows atrial impulse formation responses to autonomic control in a 46-year-old man following neurosurgical decompression of the cervical spine. The patient had no history of cardiac disease, and the preoperative ECG was within normal limits.

1. Sustained excitation of atrial impulse formation appears during the recovery room period. It was interpreted as atrial flutter with variable A-V block and rapid ventricular rate response.

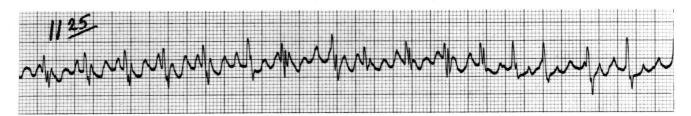

2. An attempt was made to suppress the atrial arrhythmia by a vagotonic maneuver. Carotid pressure could not be performed because of the surgical procedure. Instead, pressure on an eyeball, which also exerts strong vagal stimulation, was applied. Atrial flutter is promptly converted to sinus tachycardia by reflex parasympathetic stimulation.

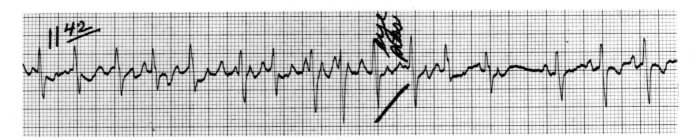

3. Continued excitation of atrial automaticity is expressed by frequent atrial premature contractions following conversion to a sinus rhythm.

Locate each APC: _____ , _____ , _____ .

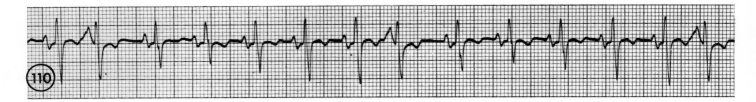

4. Note that atrial flutter begins with an APC (arrow). An important feature is that the APC is closer to the preceding normal beat than are those APCs in the previous tracing. The sequence demonstrates a general principle: The greater the degree of prematurity of an ectopic beat, the more likely it is to induce a repetitive ectopic rhythm. This phenomenon will later be encountered repeatedly.

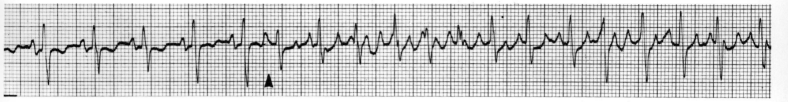

More likely than vagotonic procedures to reestablish a sinus rhythm in atrial flutter is electrocardioversion. Indeed, this technique has become firmly established in a clinician's armamentarium for the initial approach to treatment of atrial flutter. This application of electric shock is demonstrated in the next series of tracings.

1. Atrial flutter with variable A-V conduction is evident. The ventricular response is at a moderate rate, ranging between 70 and 120 per minute.

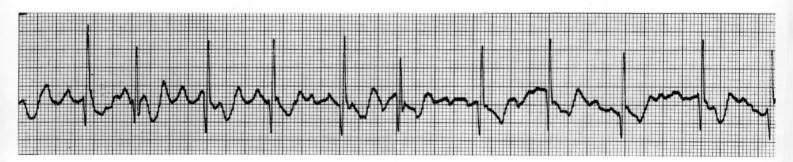

2. Precordial shock of 75 joules is applied. Note that the shock occurs at the termination of ventricular depolarization. After the expected period of electrical blackout, a brief period with indistinguishable deflections occurs, probably the result of the patient's movement. Sinus beats at a slow rate then appear but are interrupted by a ventricular complex of different origin (arrow).

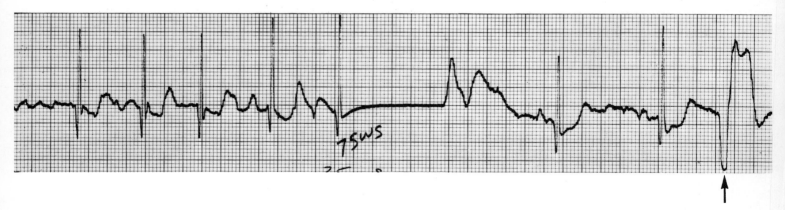

3. A stable normal sinus rhythm then supervenes, except for an atrial premature beat (located at _____ mm). The first cardiac cycle on the tracing possibly is also a premature beat, based on P wave configuration and the relatively long RR interval following this beat.

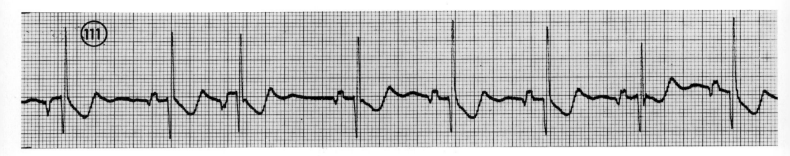

Ordinarily, relatively small amounts of electrical energy are required to convert atrial flutter to a sinus rhythm if indeed it will convert at all. It is common to use 50 joules or less for the initial attempt, as demonstrated in Figure 4–57.

The patient whose rhythms are seen in Figure 4–57 had a long history of cardiovascular disease, including surgery for myocardial revascularization 5 years before this admission. He had visited his cardiologist for his annual physical examination and was found to be in atrial flutter during the routine ECG. After 6 days in the hospital and

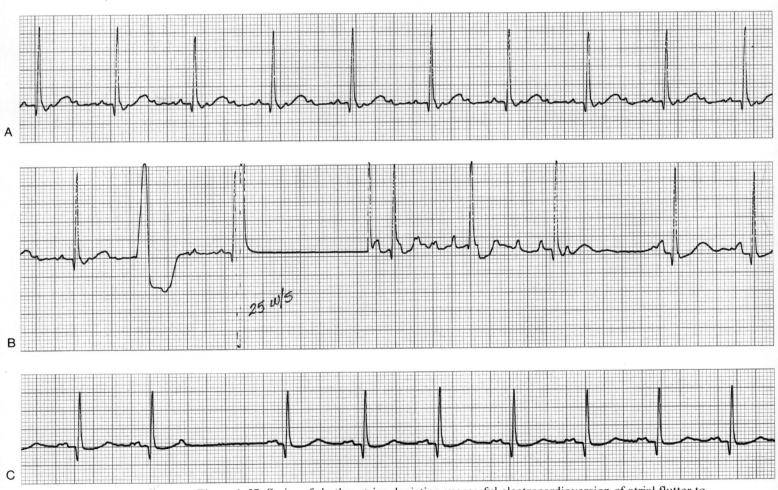

Figure 4–57. Series of rhythm strips depicting successful electrocardioversion of atrial flutter to normal sinus rhythm with a small amount of energy.

unsuccessful attempts to convert his flutter rhythm (Fig. 4–57A) with various drugs, he was cardioverted to normal sinus rhythm with only 25 joules (Fig. 4–57B). He remained in sinus rhythm with rare APCs and blocked APCs (Fig. 4–57C) until discharged.

An alternative strategy for managing atrial flutter is to maintain a suitable ventricular rate response, neither too fast nor too slow, for support of the patient's everyday activity. This approach is often chosen in those who have long-standing atrial flutter when it is unlikely that a sinus rhythm will be sustained even if reestablished. Such a controlled ventricular rate may be provided with a drug that slows A-V conduction. Most commonly, digitalis is used, as demonstrated in the serial tracings in Figure 4–58.

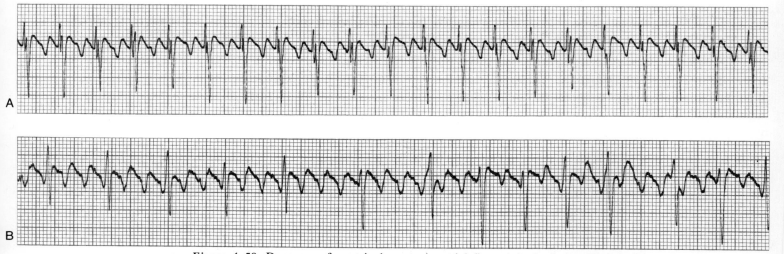

Figure 4–58. Decrease of ventricular rate in atrial flutter obtained through administration of digitalis.

The initial tracing in Figure 4–58 shows atrial flutter with 2:1 A-V conduction resulting in a ventricular rate of 155 per minute. The patient received two doses of 0.25 mg of Lanoxin intravenously. An hour after the second dose, the second strip was recorded. The atrial rate has slowed from 310 to 290 per minute, and the ventricular rate has decreased to 110 per minute as the frequency of A-V conduction has diminished.

To recapitulate, atrial flutter has been presented as a tachyarrhythmia in which

- The atrial beating is extremely rapid.
- The atrial pacemaker exhibits strict rhythmicity.
- The mechanism may have either an automatic focal origin or a reentrant impulse circuit.
- Some degree of A-V block is almost always present, the atrial rate exceeding the capacity of the A-V node to conduct impulses.

These concepts of atrial flutter are kept in mind as we now introduce another tachyarrhythmia: atrial fibrillation. Again, the interplay between atrial rate and A-V conduction is the basic determinant of electrocardiographic and clinical features. Similarities are self-evident, yet differences have critical implications. These comparisons will be explored next in some detail.

ATRIAL FIBRILLATION

When an atrial pacemaker emits impulses at a rate that exceeds the capacity of the adjacent atrial myofibrils to conduct them, a functional conduction block is created. The critical determinant for the frequency at which individual atrial myofibrils can respond is the refractory period (i.e., the time required for the cell to recover from one depolarizing stimulus before responding to another). Myofibrils distributed throughout the atrial mass do not have the same refractory period. Consequently, functional conduction block will occur at some point in various sites within the atria as the pacemaker accelerates. The result is a breaking up of the propagated wave front in some portions, with development of reentrant microcircuits and a multitude of colliding, disorganized small wave fronts. Naturally, the atria can no longer function as a pump in the presence of such electrophysiological chaos. All this leads to a conceptual basis for the condition of **atrial fibrillation**, one of the most common arrhythmias, particularly in the elderly.

Atrial fibrillation, then, is described as a disorder in which minute areas of the atrial wall are in various stages of depolarization and repolarization without coordination and, therefore, without any resemblance of wave front propagation. On direct observation, the atria appear to quiver continuously rather than to have an intermittent, forceful contraction. With loss of the muscular propulsive action, the atria do not contribute to ventricular filling, and the ventricles then fill only passively (through the sucking action of ventricular diastole) (Fig. 4–59).

The typical pattern of atrial fibrillation on the 12-lead ECG is represented as a continuous and irregular undulating baseline (Fig. 4–60). Small atrial complexes (called

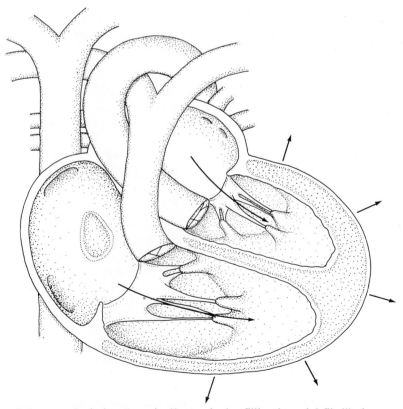

Figure 4–59. Schemata depicting "passive" ventricular filling in atrial fibrillation.

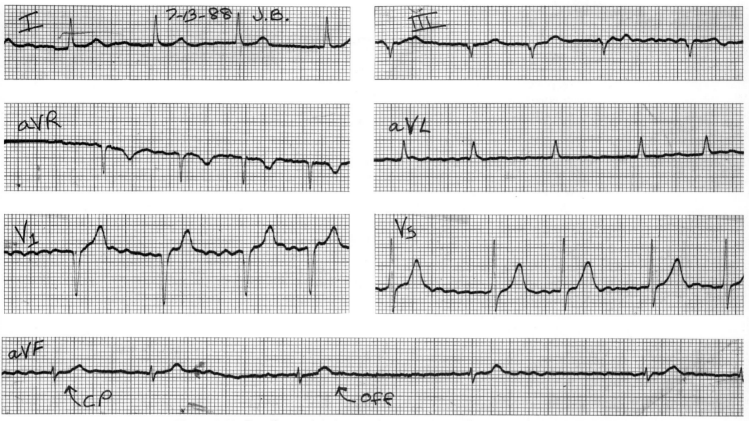

Figure 4-60. Baseline undulations typical of atrial fibrillation as seen in selected leads from a standard 12-lead electrocardiogram.

f waves) reflect fragmented depolarization-repolarization activity or, more properly, the summation of a swarm of wave fronts at any instant in time. Ventricular depolarization, on the other hand, remains normal, and QRS complexes do not ordinarily change in form or duration.

Representative leads demonstrating atrial fibrillation are shown in this ECG (Fig. 4-60) obtained from an active 83-year-old gardener who had no symptoms and was taking no medications.

Note the following features:

- The ventricular rate response is grossly irregular.
- The ventricular rate is moderate. Because a more rapid rate is expected (more than 150 per minute) if the A-V node is normal, one suspects that the A-V node conduction apparatus is compromised. (Of course, the disturbance benefits the patient in this case by maintaining a slower rate without drug therapy.)
- The fibrillation pattern varies from coarse to fine, even in the same lead. In some areas, the pattern appears to be atrial flutter, but the waveforms are somewhat irregular.
- The long strip, aVF, demonstrates that the A-V node is still sensitive to vagal stimulation, responding to carotid pressure by slowing markedly for several seconds.

This same 12-lead ECG (Fig. 4-60) demonstrates classical characteristics of atrial fibrillation. The atrial undulations are more obvious in some leads than in others. Yet even where it is most evident, the pattern exhibits periods in which atrial complexes are barely distinguishable owing to the complexity of atrial activity and the ever varying relationships of many individual wave fronts.

Also note the second cardinal feature of atrial fibrillation: the totally irregular ventricular rate. Measure all intervals between ventricular beats; the ventricles appear to respond to signals from the fibrillating atria with a wholly random timing. The mechanism for this irregular response appears to be a form of concealed conduction, an electrophysiological phenomenon that can be explained as follows.

In atrial fibrillation, the atria bombard the A-V node with as many as several hundred impulses a minute. The ventricles are protected against such a dangerous rate by the A-V node, which blocks most of the impulses. It will be recalled from the description of the A-V node in Chapter 2 that its fibers lie in a meshwork rather than in the more or less parallel arrangement of myofibrils found in the atrial and ventricular walls. This interlacing structure of conduction fibers in the A-V node slows impulse propagation in the A-V node, allowing for a momentary delay between atrial contraction and ventricular contraction. In addition, the A-V node represents the slowest part of the entire conduction system, where a limit to transmission is imposed on excessively rapid impulse formation in the atria. This limit is roughly 150 to 180 transmissions per minute in a resting individual (Fig. 4–61). As will be seen, the transmission frequency may be altered markedly by autonomic forces, by the action of drugs, and by various diseases.

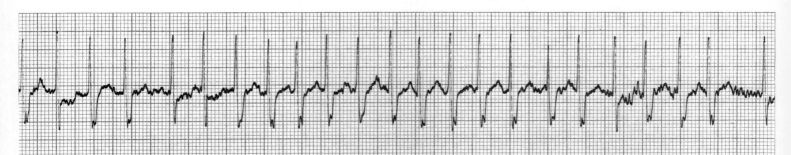

Figure 4–61. Transmission rate of impulse conduction through the A-V node is limited to less than 180 per minute.

Considering the high frequency of impulses striking the A-V node, it can be expected that most will be blocked. Immediately after atrial to ventricular transmission has occurred, fibers within the A-V node begin their recovery, and during this functional refractory period no further impulses can be conducted. As fibers in the proximal A-V node recover, an impulse is conducted into this complex structure, only to dissipate somewhere in the network of crossing and incompletely recovered more distal fibers. Of course, this impulse depolarizes the responsive fibers, rendering them momentarily refractory to subsequent impulses. As a new impulse gains entrance, its penetration may proceed an even shorter distance until it, too, is blocked. Thus, a series of blocked impulses at progressively shorter degrees of penetration allow the more distal fibers to recover their resting membrane potentials. Enough fibers in the A-V node eventually attain responsiveness to provide a complete pathway through the A-V node and thereby admit an atrial impulse into the ventricles, after which the process of progressive A-V conduction block occurs all over again.

Because of the variability of atrial impulses entering the A-V node and because of the heterogeneity of refractory periods of individual conduction fibers and their arrangement in the A-V node itself, the repetitive sequences of penetration in atrial fibrillation vary from beat to beat. Consequently, the ventricular response rate in atrial fibrillation is predictably irregular, with notable exceptions. Indeed, a constantly changing RR interval is a characteristic feature of atrial fibrillation. When the ventricular rate is regular, an additional factor (namely, some form of A-V conduction block) has been superimposed, as will be explained later.

In the sequence of events just described as occurring within the A-V node, the action of an impulse cannot be observed directly. Instead, its effect on a subsequent impulse, altering that impulse's degree of penetration through the phenomenon of concealed conduction, can be seen. In atrial fibrillation, the nature of this phenomenon is such that the more rapidly the impulses from the atria assail the A-V node, the greater the degree of functional block developed. Paradoxically, then, the faster the impulses enter into the A-V node, the stronger the dampening effect on A-V nodal transmission and consequently the slower the ventricular rate. An analogy is a bridge snarled by heavy traffic approaching from random directions, resulting in slowed vehicular crossings.

As can be appreciated now, concealed conduction plays a critical role in determining the rate of ventricular beating during atrial fibrillation. We will later examine other conditions in which concealed conduction is an important factor in the expressions of arrhythmias.

When the ventricular rate is grossly irregular, rates must be expressed as averages. The most accurate method of determining rate, of course, is counting all the beats in 1 minute. However, this tactic is tedious and impractical. Instead, counting all of the ventricular complexes within two 3-second markers and multiplying by 10 will give a satisfactorily accurate rate (except in extreme irregularities at very slow rates). Also, the three-beat ruler is usually adequate if the interpreter selects a span that includes representative fast and slow beats (Fig. 4–62).

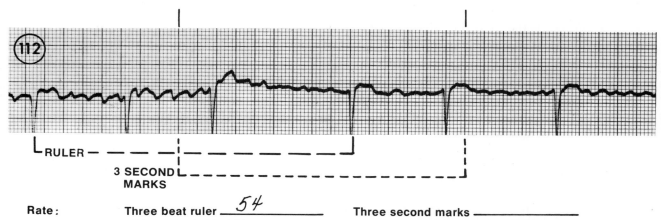

Rate: **Three beat ruler** _____54_____   **Three second marks** _____

Figure 4–62. Variable ventricular rates in atrial fibrillation require checking of the rate for a longer duration.

In each of the following examples of atrial fibrillation:
1. Determine average ventricular rate.
2. Observe the fibrillatory baseline pattern.

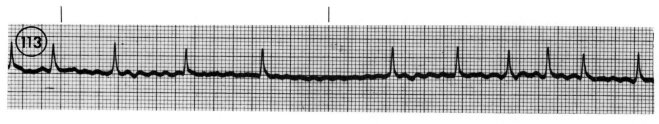

Rate: **Three beat ruler** _____   **Three second marks** _____

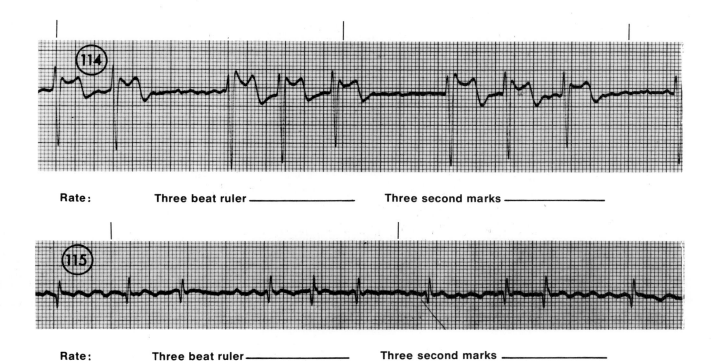

Rate: **Three beat ruler** _____   **Three second marks** _____

Rate: **Three beat ruler** _____   **Three second marks** _____

As in atrial flutter, the question of etiology involving enhanced automaticity or a reentrance mechanism again arises. This subject of intense investigation over more than half a century remains elusive. Nevertheless, it seems reasonable to conclude (from both experimental and clinical evidence) that atrial fibrillation may be precipitated by an ectopic atrial pacemaker; the arrhythmia is then sustained by multiple micro-reentrant circuits in which the structural integrity of the atrial mass has been disrupted by disease. Thus is provided a working concept that has practical application in the management of this arrhythmia.

Pointing out the crucial function of pacemaker rate in the genesis of atrial fibrillation, the tracing in Figure 4–63 is presented. Here, the rhythm reveals alternating atrial flutter and atrial fibrillation: F waves clearly evident for brief periods with other areas in which waveform contour and regularity have dissipated, leaving only low-amplitude, erratic f waves.

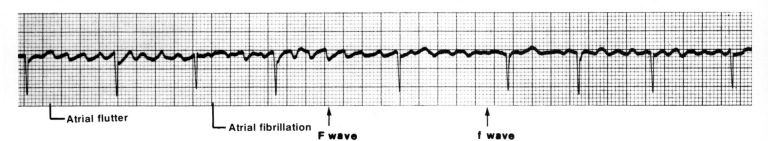

Figure 4–63. Transitional atrial flutter-atrial fibrillation pattern.

As already described, the atria are activated normally by a wave front passing along from fiber to fiber. The duration and relative homogeneity of refractory periods limit the tendency for development of micro-reentrant circuits. This mode of activation differs sharply from that of the ventricles, which enjoy a special, rapid conduction pathway (the His-Purkinje system) in which propagation along contiguous myofibrils is at most the relatively short distance from endocardial to epicardial surface. From this difference, it would be expected that the atria are more vulnerable to developing asynchronous wave fronts than are the ventricles and furthermore that the larger the atrial mass, the greater the chance of developing atrial fibrillation. This is exactly the case. An enlarged atrium in humans, as occurs in mitral stenosis, is a strong predisposing condition for atrial fibrillation. Large mammals, for example horses and cows, are exceptionally prone to this arrhythmia (Fig. 4–64). Dogs and cats, on the other hand, are particularly resistant.

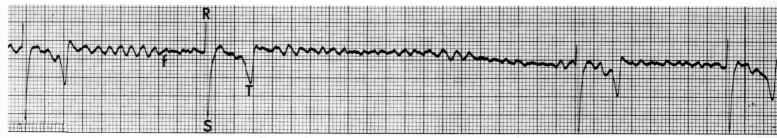

Figure 4–64. Example of coarse atrial fibrillation in a 3-year-old racehorse.

In addition to increased wall mass, conditions that interfere with the integrity of myofibrillar action potentials are causal factors in atrial fibrillation. These result in a patchy fibrosis with increased heterogeneity of electrophysiological properties. Variability in refractory periods, of course, enhances the opportunity for disorganization of a propagating wave front through micro-reentry.

To summarize the principal causes of atrial fibrillation, the following conditions are notable:

1. Atrial enlargement. The major etiologies are disorders of the A-V valves (most especially mitral stenosis), systemic and pulmonary hypertension (including pulmonary embolism), and severe ventricular insufficiency.

2. Atrial fibrosis. Degenerative disease of aging, sequelae of various forms of myocarditis, and hypertrophic cardiomyopathies or factors associated with these conditions may be responsible. The strong likelihood that persons with sinus node dysfunction will eventually incur atrial fibrillation suggests that these conditions share a common pathogenesis.

3. Atrial ischemic injury. This arrhythmia is fairly common in acute myocardial infarction, even in the absence of thrombotic occlusion of the sinus node artery.

4. Metabolic disorders. Atrial fibrillation is common in patients with hyperthyroidism. One special characteristic is the unusually rapid ventricular rate response, caused by accelerated conduction in the A-V node associated with adrenergic overdrive. The pathogenesis in hyperthyroidism has not been confirmed, but it probably relates to atrial dilation and hypertrophy. Sometimes atrial fibrillation is the outstanding clue to this condition when other signs and symptoms are unusually subtle. Atrial fibrillation complicating heavy ethanol intake may have a similar etiology.

5. Primary disorders. By this definition is meant atrial fibrillation without any underlying causal factor. It is a condition that occurs occasionally in paroxysms of widely variable duration in young and (by definition) healthy individuals. Often referred to as "lone" or "benign" atrial fibrillation, the paroxysms may appear only a few times throughout life, or transition to a permanent arrhythmia may occur.

The ECG below is from an elderly diabetic man who, 3 hours before recording, was started on digitalis (Lanoxin) for treatment of congestive heart failure after an ileofemoral bypass graft. Determine the ventricular rates in the sinus and atrial fibrillation rhythms.

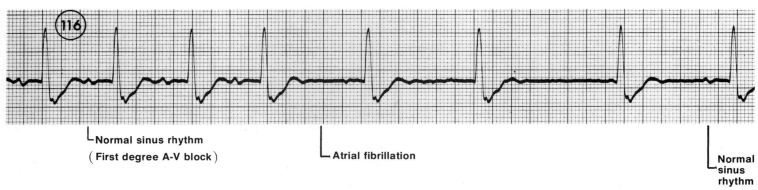

└Normal sinus rhythm
(First degree A-V block)

└Atrial fibrillation

└Normal sinus rhythm

Determine the ventricular rates in the following examples of atrial fibrillation:

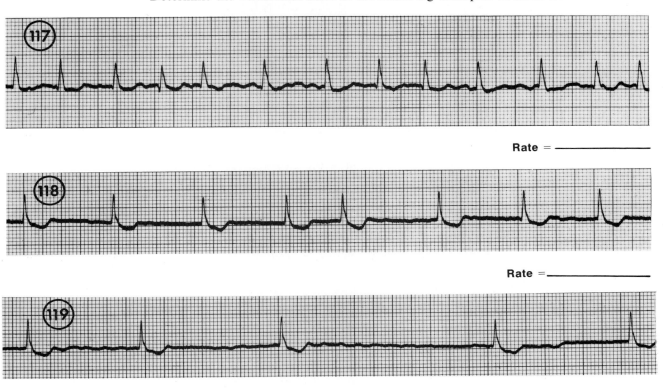

Rate = _____

Rate =_____

Rate =_____

Atrial fibrillation imposes compound disadvantages to cardiac function. Briefly, these liabilities are the result of the following:

- Loss of atrial contraction. Ventricular filling (and necessarily, ventricular ejection) is decreased when the atria fail to pump effectively. This failure may not be important in the resting heart, which is physiologically well compensated. However, loss of the atrial kick preceding ventricular contraction becomes progressively more contributory to diastolic filling as ventricular rate increases, especially in the presence of myocardial insufficiency.
- Irregular ventricular rate. Gross irregularity of the ventricular beat is associated with marked variations in stroke volume (and in the amplitude of the peripheral pulse). The determining factor is duration of diastolic filling time.
- Rapid ventricular rate. Usually, untreated atrial fibrillation is associated with a ventricular rate approximating 150 beats per minute, although the range is up

to 180 per minute (the natural capacity for A-V conduction). Such rapid rates often compromise diastolic filling time, particularly critical in the failing myocardium. Even mild exercise may induce marked acceleration of heart rate in which cardiac output is further limited at a time of increased need (Fig. 4–65).

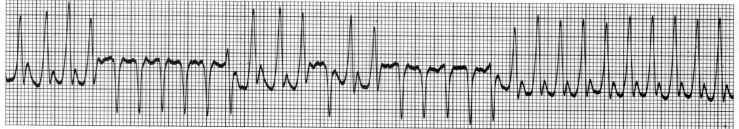

Figure 4–65. Atrial fibrillation with an extremely rapid ventricular rate response. The alteration in configuration of QRS complexes is caused by variations in impulse conduction through the ventricles (further described in Chapter 8).

- Associated diseases. These causal or concomitant disorders so commonly associated with atrial fibrillation further compromise cardiac function. Coexisting myocardial insufficiency is, of course, widely prevalent in the elderly population, in whom this arrhythmia is most common. Concurrent disease involving the A-V node and the ventricular conduction pathways is also found extensively in the elderly. Problems arising from these defects will be considered in subsequent chapters.
- Mechanical fibrillation of the atria. The noncontracting atria also pose an additional hazard. The lack of mechanical activity produces a tendency for stagnant blood to coagulate on the endocardial surface. Such mural thrombi are occasionally large enough to obstruct blood flow. Even more likely is the possibility of clot disintegration, producing fragments that embolize to distant organs. Emboli are particularly common when atrial contractions are restored, such as during electrocardioversion of atrial fibrillation. Thus, anticoagulant therapy is given to prevent embolization in selected patients with atrial fibrillation.

At the bedside examination, atrial fibrillation presents important features of hemodynamics. The variable intervals between ventricular contractions allow differences in diastolic filling, resulting in beat-to-beat variations in cardiac output. Heart tones are not only irregular in rhythm but are of changeable intensity. Similarly, the force of peripheral pulses is quite variable. Some of the weaker pulses may not be felt; this is especially true for rapid rates. The so-called radial **pulse deficit** in atrial fibrillation is largely due to changes in pulsatile force, and a large discrepancy between apparent and real cardiac rates may be present. (For this reason, the pulse of patients with atrial fibrillation should be taken by auscultation of the precordium or from the cardiac monitor, rather than by palpating the radial artery.)

In the following three strips, identify the rates before parasympathetic stimulation (Valsalva maneuver or carotid pressure) and the slower rates that resulted from stimulation. Which rate will produce the strongest peripheral pulse?

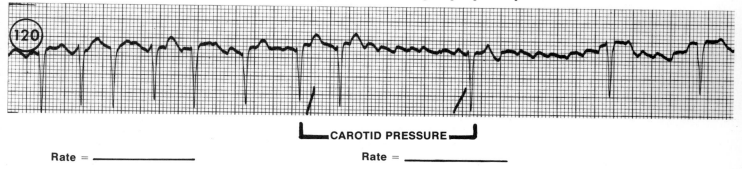

CAROTID PRESSURE

Rate = _____   Rate = _____

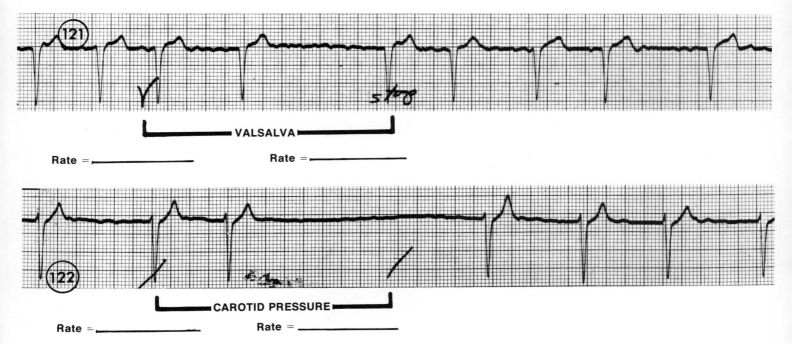

VALSALVA

Rate = _____   Rate = _____

CAROTID PRESSURE

Rate = _____   Rate = _____

Treatment of Atrial Fibrillation

Clinicians elect to treat atrial fibrillation with either of two basic strategems:

1. Convert atrial fibrillation to sinus rhythm or
2. Control the ventricular rate response to the fibrillating atria (in effect, modulate A-V conduction so that the ventricles beat neither too fast nor too slowly).

There are advantages and disadvantages to either approach, and the choice is based on the duration of atrial fibrillation, the extent of underlying cardiac disease, and a host of other clinical factors. These considerations will be discussed briefly, and a series of illustrative tracings will be presented. Through review of these examples, readers can gain excellent practice in the interpretation of atrial tachycardias as well as acquire a better understanding of the interplay between impulse formation-conduction, drug actions, and effects of the autonomic nervous system. Furthermore, the examples represent problems commonly encountered in clinical practice.

CONVERSION TO SINUS RHYTHM

Because the atrial pump contributes appreciably to ventricular filling, the goal of restoring effective beating through sinus node pacing is highly desirable. Drugs that suppress the mechanism perpetuating atrial fibrillation have been extensively used for restoring sinus rhythm. Quinidine and procainamide are prototypic agents for this purpose, although the calcium channel blocking agents have become therapeutic options. An example of this approach is demonstrated in Figure 4–66.

Most patients with atrial fibrillation require a relatively high dose of depressor agents to achieve conversion to sinus rhythm. At levels that are effective for conversion, there is a high incidence of potentially dangerous responses, such as severe depression of impulse conduction in the A-V node-His system and/or of the force of myocardial contraction. In practice, the frequency of important side effects with high-dose therapy has eliminated this approach to treatment of atrial fibrillation in favor of restoration of sinus rhythm with electric precordial shock or by controlling ventricular rate.

The advantages of electrocardioversion over drug suppression of atrial fibrillation include the instantaneous effect without the hazard of drug toxicity. That the clinician

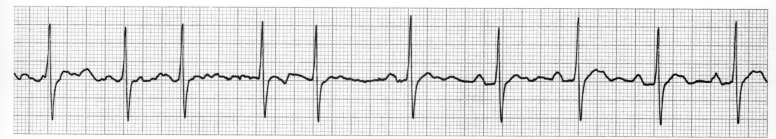

Figure 4–66. Conversion of atrial fibrillation to normal sinus rhythm by quinidine.

observes the moment of shock adds a strong measure of protection should a troublesome arrhythmia supervene. The prompt action of electrocardioversion may be a life-saving advantage when cardiac function is markedly decompensated from an extremely rapid rate response by the ventricles.

The procedure for treating atrial fibrillation with electric shock is similar to that described for atrial tachycardia and flutter. Required are sedation-anesthesia, preshock testing for proper synchronization, continuous electrocardiographic documentation, and full readiness for any serious adversity. However, two substantive differences are noted: (1) Larger amounts of electrical current are generally necessary to convert atrial fibrillation to a sinus rhythm; and (2) a suppressor drug (usually quinidine) is administered in *ordinary* clinical doses, from several hours up to 2 or 3 days before cardioversion is attempted. This preshock treatment increases the chances of successful conversion with electric shock; it may inhibit the development of ventricular tachyarrhythmias immediately after cardioversion; and it helps to maintain sinus rhythm once it is reestablished.

Electrocardioversion is presented in three case histories that follow.

A 68-year-old man with stable angina pectoris of 3 years had led a rugged life as an outdoorsman. Then, without unusual exertion, his episodes of chest pain increased in frequency, and he experienced rapid palpitations with breathlessness, even on walking. Admitted to the hospital, where acute myocardial infarction was ruled improbable, the patient was given quinidine every 8 hours for four doses, then had electrocardioversion. At the time of cardioversion, atrial fibrillation with a coarse, undulating pattern was evident (Fig. 4–67). Brief periods of atrial flutter could also be seen. A test shock of 8 joules demonstrates that the discharge is asynchronous with the R spike of the QRS. Of course, the patient was not harmed by the current because the paddles were not placed on the chest.

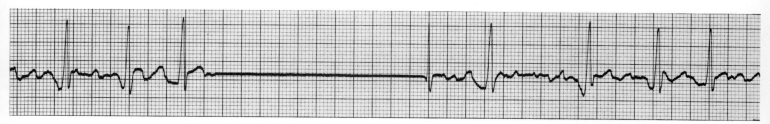

Figure 4–67. Test of synchronization of electrocardioversion discharge in atrial fibrillation.

The discharge control switch was adjusted, and having demonstrated proper synchronized function, the operator applied paddles to the chest and delivered an electrical shock of 200 joules (Fig. 4–68). After a brief period of electrical blackout, there emerged a slow sinus rhythm. Note that the actual shock occurred during the QRS complex.

The next patient was a 42-year-old man who received a prosthetic valve to correct mitral stenosis of rheumatic origin. Although atrial fibrillation had been present for several years, it was considered worthwhile to attempt restoration of sinus rhythm now

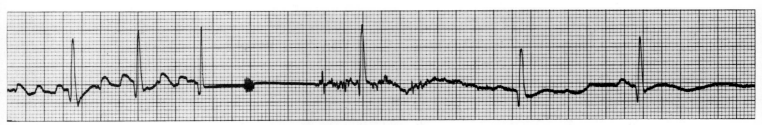

Figure 4–68. Conversion of atrial fibrillation to normal sinus with electrical current.

that high intraatrial pressure in the left atrium had been relieved by surgery. The tracing immediately preceding electric shock is atrial fibrillation with a fine baseline pattern and with a moderate, average ventricular rate response (Fig. 4–69).

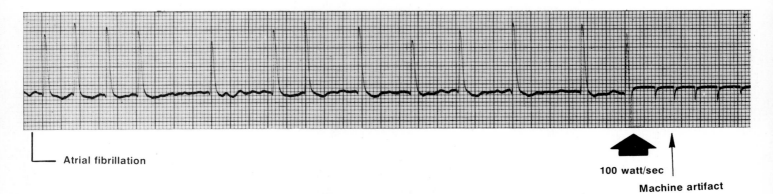

Atrial fibrillation

100 watt/sec

Machine artifact

Figure 4–69. Pattern of atrial fibrillation is present in this rhythm strip preconversion.

Normal sinus rhythm appears immediately after the period of electrical blackout (Fig. 4–70). The third beat observed in this rhythm occurs early; it has a wide QRS complex and a marked alteration in the ST segment-T wave contour. This beat represents an abnormal delay in ventricular depolarization and repolarization, as will be discussed in subsequent chapters.

The third patient was a 28-year-old school teacher who suddenly experienced severe lightheadedness, sweating, nausea, and rapid palpitations, her second such episode in as many months. When examined within 15 minutes from onset of symptoms, she was alert but very weak, dizzy on attempting to sit up, and hypotensive. Cardiac tones were distant, extremely rapid but otherwise unremarkable. Peripheral pulses were barely detectable. The ECG this time revealed atrial fibrillation with rapid ventricular response.

The typical oscillations of atrial fibrillation were present along with the irregular ventricular rhythm. Most notably, the average ventricular rate exceeded 200 per minute. With such extreme tachycardias (remember also that the atrial kick is absent), cardiac output may be markedly reduced even in persons with a healthy myocardium, accounting for the patient's symptoms.

When atrial fibrillation occurs in a person with a completely normal A-V node-His conduction system, the ventricular rate response tends to be inordinately rapid. Indeed, young and otherwise healthy people with the primary form are often severely affected by the attacks that are associated with extreme tachycardias. Atrial fibrillation often proves resistant to drug suppression and control.

Emergency electrocardioversion was deemed advisable, and its results are shown in Figure 4–71.

Within moments after electric shock, the rhythm reverted from a slower sinus

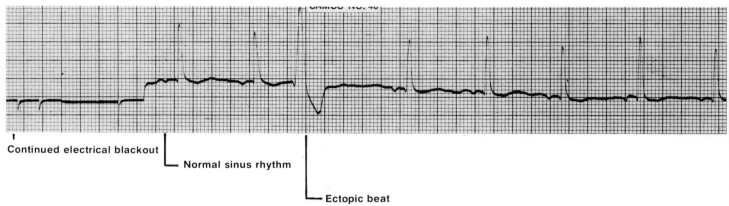

Continued electrical blackout

Normal sinus rhythm

Ectopic beat

Figure 4–70. Conversion to normal sinus rhythm following the electrical interruption of the previous atrial fibrillation.

rhythm to an even more rapid atrial fibrillation. Permanent cardioversion was achieved the next day using electrocardioversion after administering optimal doses of digitalis.

AO INSTRUMENT COMPANY

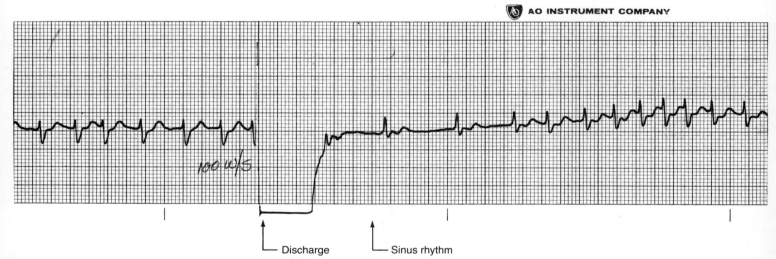

Discharge   Sinus rhythm

Figure 4–71. Temporary conversion of rapid atrial fibrillation to normal sinus rhythm.

These three patients were candidates for conversion of their atrial fibrillation to sinus rhythm. The clinical situation often precludes cardioversion as an option, however, and management of the condition is limited to controlling the frequency of ventricular response to the fibrillatory atrial activity.

VENTRICULAR RATE CONTROL

Maintaining the ventricular rate within an acceptable range with drug therapy is the preferred intervention for most patients with atrial fibrillation. This approach applies most especially to patients who have long-standing atrial fibrillation and diffuse atrial disease and in whom there is little chance of sustaining a sinus rhythm, even if restored with electrocardioversion. Further, there is an appreciable incidence of side effects of those drugs generally used to prevent recurrence of atrial fibrillation.

Of suitable drugs used for control of the ventricular rate response to fibrillating atria, digitalis has ably withstood the test over several decades, and it is still the most useful drug for this purpose. Digitalis probably acts to slow the heart rate through two mechanisms:

1. By shortening the refractory period of some atrial myofibrils, digitalis increases the extent of micro-reentrant activity. Thus, the frequency of atrial depolarization increases and the number of impulses assaulting the A-V node is intensified. We have already explained how impulse conduction in the A-V node actually decreases through concealed conduction as the arriving impulses become more frequent.

2. Digitalis has an acetylcholine-like action on the heart, most prominently on the A-V node. This indirect, or autonomic, effect augments vagal tone and in atrial fibrillation is a potent inhibitor of A-V nodal conduction.

Compare the rate change in the ventricles produced by digitalis in the example in Figure 4–72.

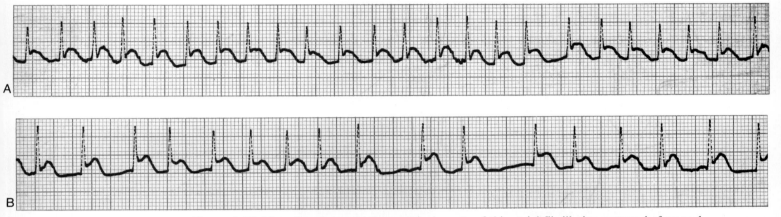

Figure 4–72. Note the change in the ventricular rate of this atrial fibrillation pattern before and after giving digitalis. $A = 150$; $B = 120$.

Notice that there are no changes in the fibrillatory baseline pattern nor in the QRS complexes. One general characteristic of atrial fibrillation is demonstrated: The slower the ventricular rate, the more pronounced is the irregularity of the ventricular rhythm (with notable exceptions).

The following two strips illustrate the effects of digitalis on reducing the ventricular rate.

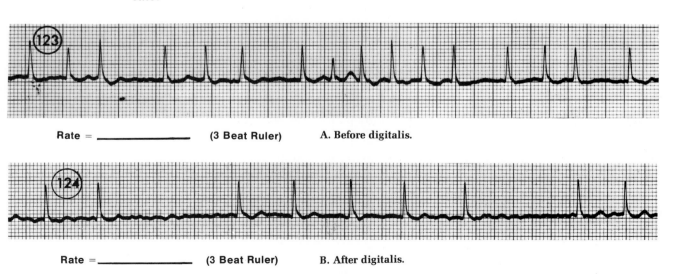

Rate = _____ (3 Beat Ruler)   A. Before digitalis.

Rate = _____ (3 Beat Ruler)   B. After digitalis.

The next clinical series illustrates the progressive changes induced by incremental administration of digitalis, including a serious complication. Test tracings 125 through

130 were obtained from an 82-year-old woman with congestive heart failure of recent onset. She had never had an ECG before this event.

1. 12/25—1:15 PM: The totally erratic, undulating baseline and the random nature of the ventricular rhythm characterize atrial fibrillation. The ventricular rate is very rapid. A proper immediate goal of therapy is to slow the heart rate while improving myocardial contractile dynamics, both of which may be achieved with digitalis.

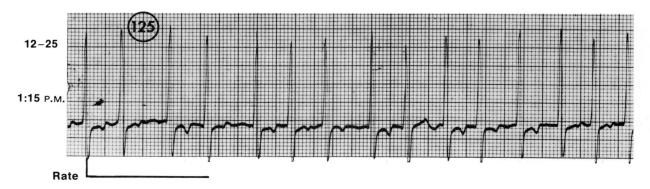

2. 4:00 PM: After administration of digoxin by mouth 2½ hours earlier, the ventricular rate is somewhat slower. Note that irregularity is more prominent.

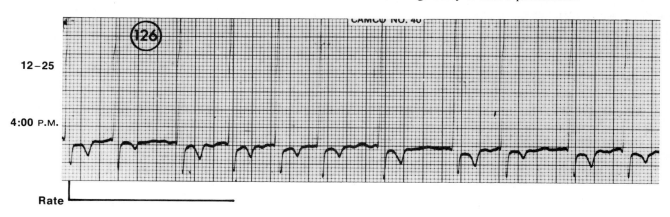

3. 10:00 PM: Four hours after an additional dose of digoxin, the ventricular response is even slower. Shortness of breath and pulmonary congestion have improved markedly. The disorganized baseline and the erratic ventricular beating persist.

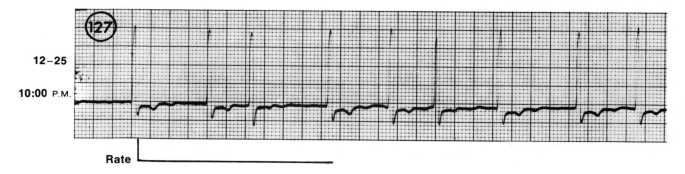

4. 12/26—2:30 AM: Digitalis effect is now very prominent as the ventricular rate has become too slow. Note that some ventricular complexes are markedly widened and the terminal portion of the QRS disfigured; this alteration represents a delay in

forces of late ventricular depolarization. Such excessive depression of impulse transmission in the A-V node and conduction velocity in the Purkinje system may be considered toxic effects of digitalis. During this time, the patient rested comfortably.

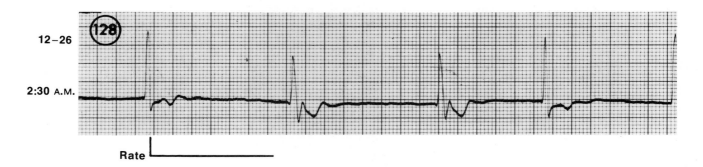

5. 12/27—10:00 AM: Digitalis is then discontinued for 1 day, during which time the ventricular rate gradually accelerates as the drug action dissipates. It is decided that electrocardioversion may be the better course of treatment. It is performed after administration of low-dose quinidine to stabilize the rhythm.

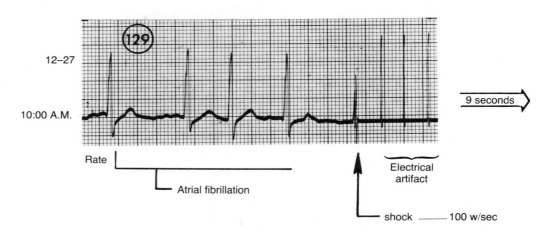

6. The tracing is shown at 9 seconds after electric shock, demonstrating restoration of a sinus rhythm. T waves are noted to be upright in this and the preceding strips. Both myocardial ischemia and digitalis effect can produce T wave inversion and were probably responsible for this abnormality in tracings taken on the previous days.

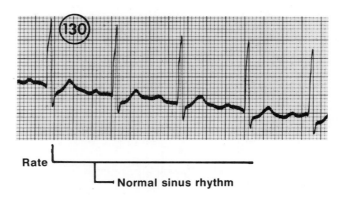

An 83-year-old woman with an acute myocardial infarction exhibited sequential changes of atrial excitation.

1. Atrial fibrillation with a moderately rapid ventricular rate.

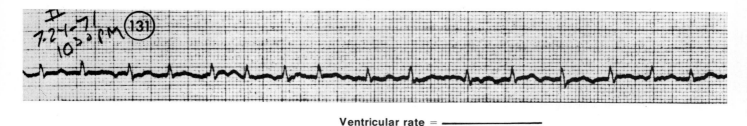

Ventricular rate = _____

2. Atrial flutter has replaced atrial fibrillation. Note the 2:1 A-V block with a constant FR interval of conducted beats. 7/25/71—9:30 AM: digitalis started.

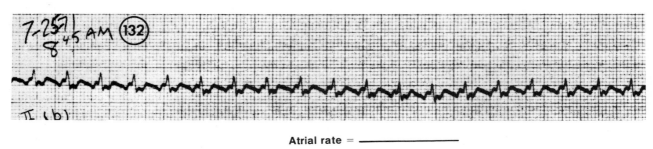

Atrial rate = _____

Ventricular rate = _____

3. Atrial flutter. The A-V ratio is now variable, and the FR interval of conducted beats is not constant. This change in A-V conduction may be due to the vagotonic effect of digitalis. Most importantly, the ventricular rate has slowed substantially because of the decreased frequency of conduction through the A-V pathways.

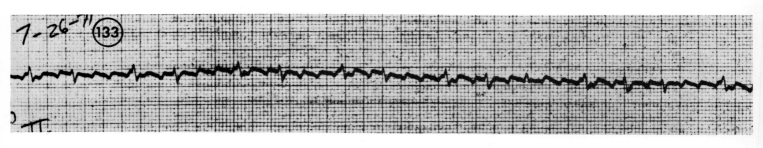

Atrial flutter   Atrial rate = _____   Ventricular rate = _____

A 54-year-old woman admitted with congestive heart failure demonstrates a rather unusual response of atrial fibrillation to digitalis.

1. Atrial fibrillation with a moderate ventricular rate response is evident. At times the fibrillatory pattern is coarse, and for brief periods it has an appearance of flutter.

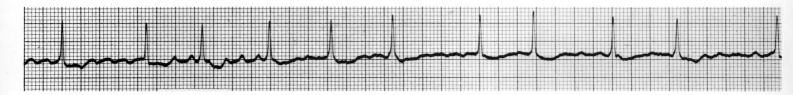

2. After administration of digitalis, atrial flutter with a 2:1 A-V block has supervened. The flutter rate has slowed considerably compared with the previous tracing. (This is an unpredictable response to digitalis.)

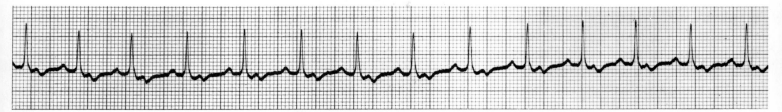

3. Carotid pressure induces marked A-V block, with a transient ratio of 8:1 in the initial period.

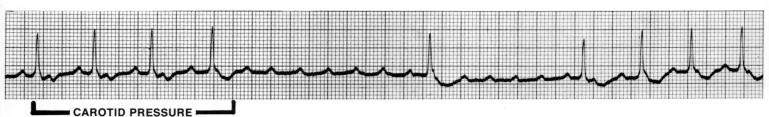

CAROTID PRESSURE

The action of this vagotonic maneuver may have been enhanced by the acetylcholine-like effect of digitalis, resulting in extreme slowing. It is interesting to observe that the atrial pacemaker itself appears to be indifferent to even this strong parasympathetic stimulation.

A pharmacological alternative to enhancement of parasympathetic tone for inhibiting A-V nodal transmission is depression of the sympathetic nervous system. A commonly used modality is beta-adrenergic blocking agents such as propranolol and timolol. These drugs do not have the propensity for causing tachycardias through enhanced ectopic pacemaker activity, as does digitalis, but they do have a greater tendency to produce autonomic-mediated side effects. By blocking adrenergic stimulation of the myofibrils in myocardial failure, these agents may further impair contractility. Used together for ventricular rate regulation in atrial fibrillation, a beta-adrenergic blocker and digitalis often prove effective. Combined drug therapy, each agent having a similar effect on a specific function (for example, A-V nodal conduction), provides additive potency while limiting the untoward effects of either by allowing smaller doses of each agent. On the other hand, the synergism from overlapping drug actions may give unpredictably intense results, as demonstrated in the situation described next.

A 79-year-old woman under treatment for atrial fibrillation complicating recent myocardial infarction had a rapid ventricular rate that was resistant to relatively large doses of digoxin. When she complained of continuous nausea (a common side effect of digitalis), it was decided to add a beta-adrenergic blocker to her regimen. The morning after propanolol was administered, the patient, on first arising, suddenly lost consciousness momentarily. An ECG obtained within 3 minutes after onset revealed marked bradycardia.

1. 11:45 AM: Atrial fibrillation with an extremely slow ventricular rate is evident. There are no ectopic beats or widened QRS complexes present (signs of digitalis toxicity).

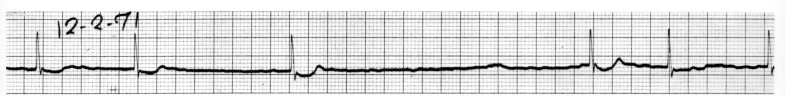

2. 11:52 AM: Isoproterenol by intravenous infusion is started. This is a purely beta-adrenergic stimulating agent that has the same effect as norepinephrine on the A-V node. By its "mass" action, it may overcome inhibition of nodal transmission by the beta-adrenergic blockers.

3. 11:57 AM: Atrial fibrillation persists, but the ventricular response has increased to a moderate rate. At this time, the patient returns to a fully alert state.

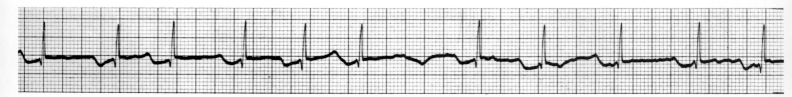

The infusion rate and concentration of isoproterenol were gradually reduced as the levels of digitalis and propanolol dissipated. Incidentally, the depressed ST segment (hammock-like shape) present on both tracings is a typical digitalis effect, although ischemia may be a cofactor. This response is not considered a toxic action of digitalis.

Another strategy was used in atrial fibrillation associated with excessively slow ventricular beating in the series shown below. The patient was a 70-year-old woman with evidence of an acute myocardial infarction of the inferior wall on evaluation in the emergency department.

1. 9:12 AM: Atrial fibrillation with a slow ventricular rate response is present in lead V_1. Because the patient is on no medication at this time, it is presumed from the depressed conduction that the A-V node (as well as the atria) is diseased. In arterial occlusion of vessels to the inferior myocardium, the A-V node is particularly prone to share the injury.

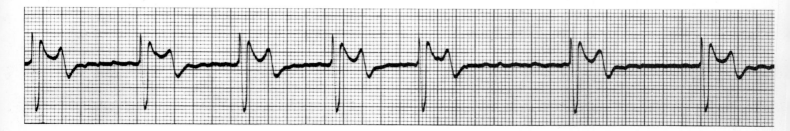

2. 9:15 AM: A decision is made to use an agent that blocks parasympathetic tone in the A-V node, thereby obliterating the inhibiting effect of vagus innervation on conduction. Atropine is the prototypic drug for this purpose. It is relatively unlikely to endanger myocardial function and the peripheral circulation. However, it has a strong tendency to produce autonomic side effects on organ systems, especially on the gastrointestinal tract. Atropine, 1 mg, is given intravenously.

3. 9:17 AM: Atrial fibrillation with a more rapid ventricular rate has supervened within 2 minutes after the injection of atropine.

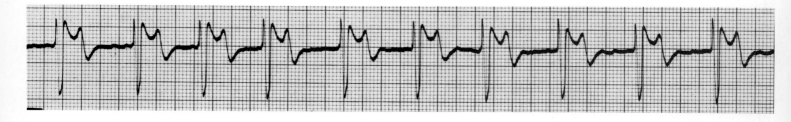

The markedly elevated ST segment in both tracings is commonly observed very early in infarction in those leads in which the positive electrode faces the site of acute injury. Its presence here suggests anterior wall infarction in the hyperacute stage.

The ventricular rate in atrial fibrillation may be altered by changing the electrical resistance to impulse transmission in the A-V node. As in atrial tachycardia and atrial flutter, increasing parasympathetic tone will retard transmission frequency, thereby decelerating the ventricular rate. This is demonstrated in the following tracings using maneuvers that enhance vagal tone.

SELF-EVALUATION: STAGE 1

On the following pages are electrocardiograms representing all the major forms of rhythms described thus far. Label components and determine rates of the basic rhythm. Be careful to look for subtle changes in rhythms, for the presence of more than one disorder, and for artifacts on each tracing. Answers are supplied in the back of the text according to the circled number. Refer to these after you have made a diligent effort to interpret each tracing thoroughly.

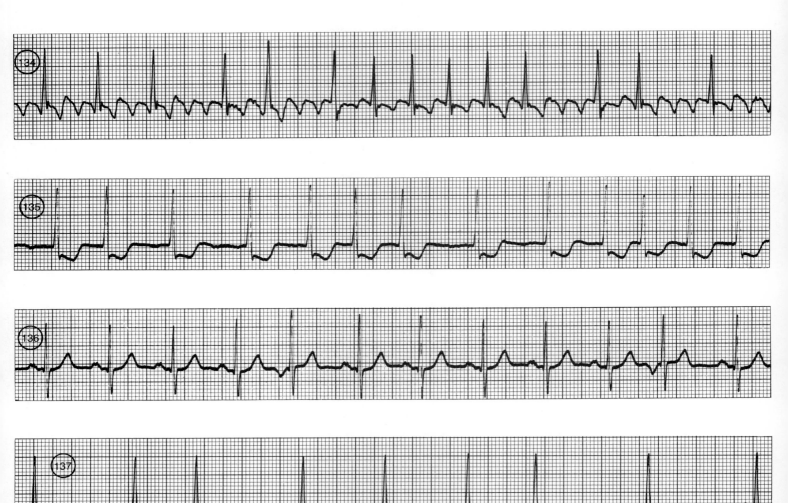

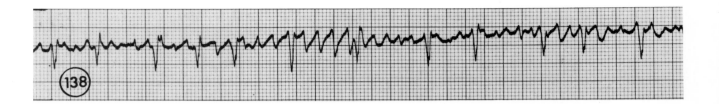

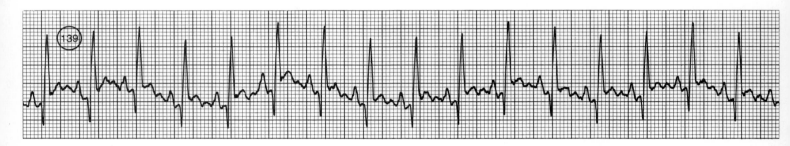

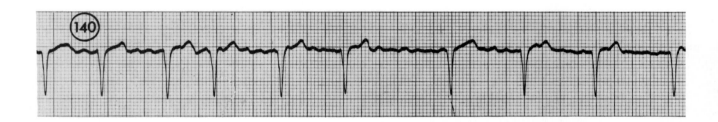

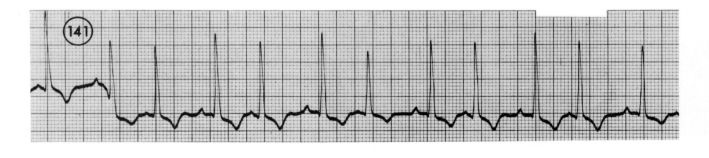

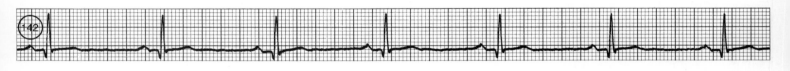

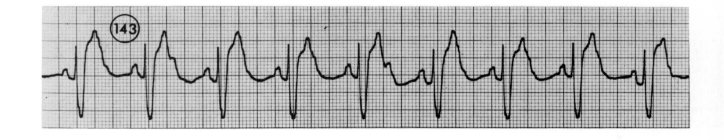

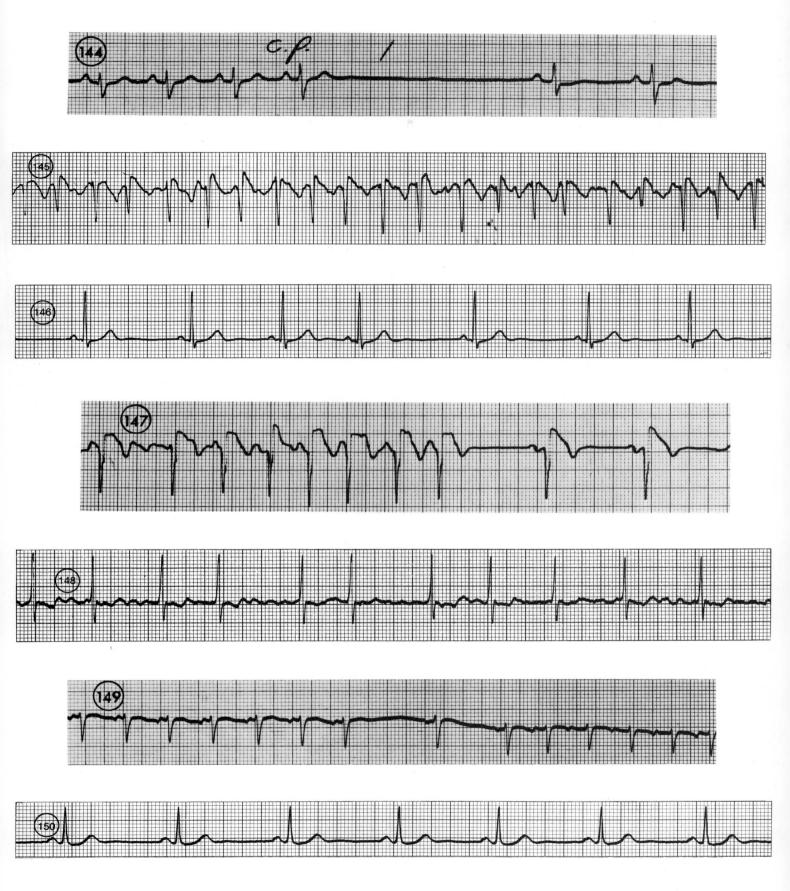

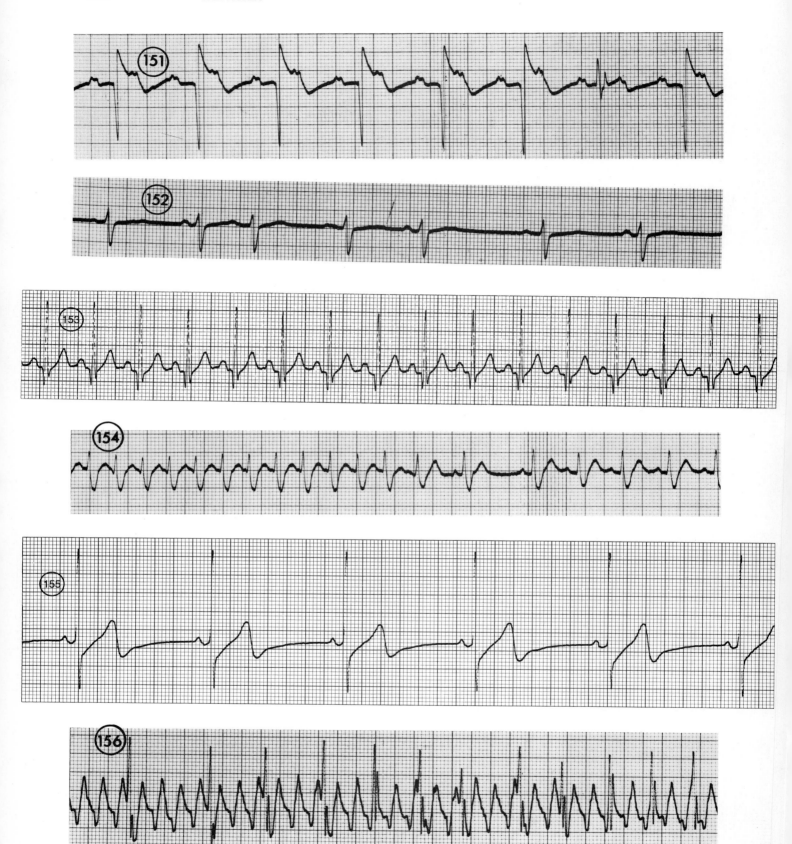

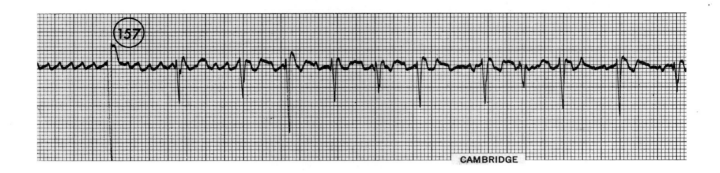

CAMBRIDGE

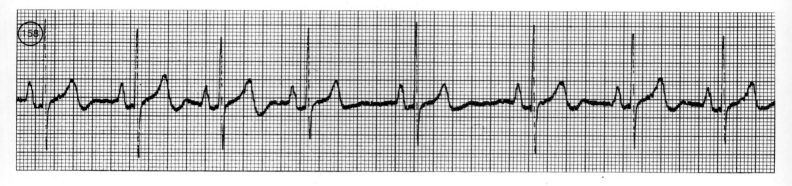

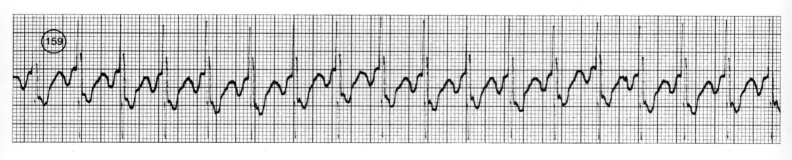

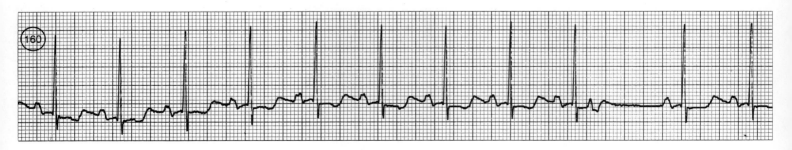

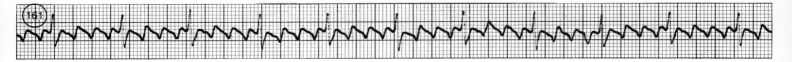

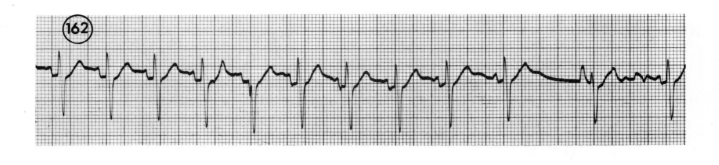

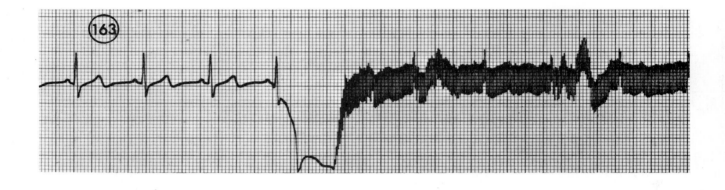

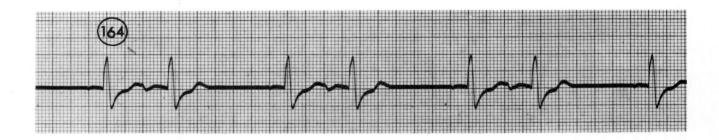

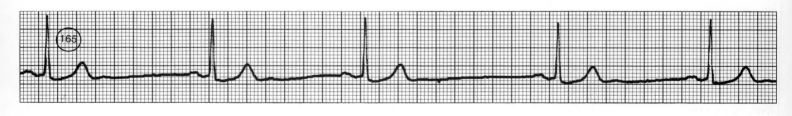

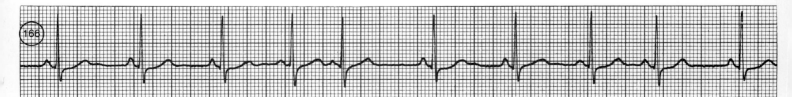

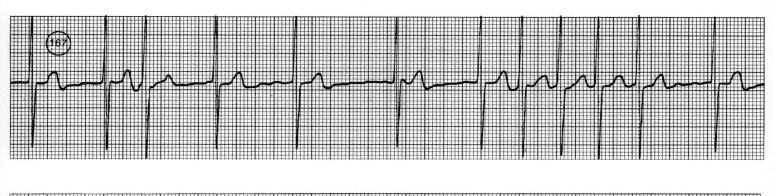

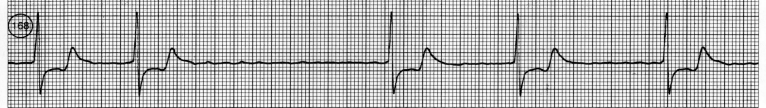

5 The Atrioventricular Node

FUNCTIONS
ANATOMICAL COMPONENTS
RECORDING ATRIOVENTRICULAR NODAL
   ACTIVITY
Electrocardiogram—PR Interval
His Bundle Electrogram
ATRIOVENTRICULAR NODE: IMPULSE
   CONDUCTION

Excitation
Ventricular Preexcitation
ATRIOVENTRICULAR NODE: IMPULSE
   CONDUCTION
Depression
First-Degree Atrioventricular Block
Second-Degree Atrioventricular Block
Third-Degree Atrioventricular Block

The atrioventricular (A-V) node serves as the sole pathway for entry of impulses from the atria to the ventricles. Composed of fibers specialized for conduction, the A-V node lies in the distal region of the intraatrial septum. Here atrial impulses are funneled and conducted to the common bundle, leading directly into the ventricles.

Although the A-V node is a specialized tissue for impulse conduction, it has the peculiar but critically important action of markedly slowing the transmission of impulses. This delaying mechanism, which provides favorable synchronization between atrial and ventricular contractions, will be explored in detail. The various electrophysiological syndromes that either intensify or offset this natural delay then will be described.

FUNCTIONS

Slow impulse conduction within the A-V node is explained by anatomical and electrophysiologic features, which are summarized as follows:

1. The action potential of A-V nodal cells has similarities to that of the sinus node cells (Fig. 5–1). The resting membrane potential of the typical fiber in the A-V node is substantially lower (about -70 millivolts) than in the ordinary contractile fibers. In addition, the rate of depolarization is considerably slower. Further, the various phases of repolarization are poorly defined. The conduction velocity in fibers of the A-V node ranges from one-fifth to one-twenty-fifth that of the working myofibril.

212

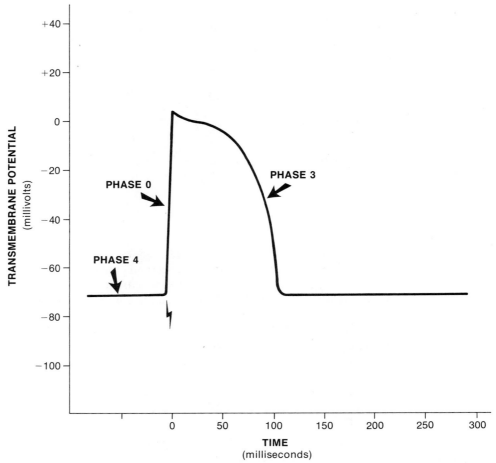

Figure 5–1. Action potential of A-V nodal fiber cells.

Like sinus node cells, the A-V nodal cells are dependent on slow channels for movement of ions, thereby assigning calcium as the preeminent cation to initiate the action potential. Those pharmacological agents that inhibit calcium transport have a preferential action on the A-V node and consequently have great therapeutic implications in diseases of the A-V node.

An essential difference between sinus node cells and A-V nodal cells relates to the virtual absence of spontaneous depolarization in the latter. This characteristic appears to exclude the A-V node as the source of automatic impulse formation.

2. An additional characteristic, related to the anatomical arrangement of fibers within the A-V node, intensifies the impulse-delaying property. Rather than being oriented in a more or less parallel direction (as is typical in specialized conduction bundles), the A-V nodal fibers are arranged at random into a meshwork (Fig. 5–2). Thus, an impulse coursing through this segment of the conduction system encounters a tangle of electrical micropathways, conjoining to impede the progression of a wave front passing through the A-V node.

The wave front eventually works its way through the A-V node and enters the common bundle and its divisions, where once again the impulse proceeds at a relatively rapid rate. In fact, impulse velocity in the His-Purkinje system may be 100 times that in the A-V node.

Cardiac performance gains two fundamental advantages by this slowing of impulse conduction in the A-V nodal system:

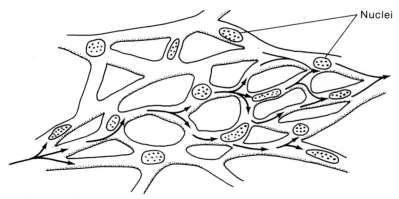

Figure 5–2. A-V nodal fibers.

1. The delay allows for complete contraction of the atria before the ventricles begin to contract. Thus, atrial emptying (and conversely, ventricular filling) approaches maximum. Furthermore, the A-V valves will close earlier in ventricular systole (thus, minimizing regurgitant flow) if the atria have already expended their contractile force.

2. The delay imposes a limit on the frequency of impulses transmitted from the atria to the ventricles. Without such a limit, the ventricles would be subject to life-threatening tachycardias should the atria develop tachycardia, flutter, or fibrillation.

Any disturbance that affects the A-V node will of course have a profound effect on the synchronization of cardiac chamber contractions. Before proceeding with a discussion of the clinical disorders of the A-V conduction system, however, it is first important to clarify the integral components of this system at which these disorders may afflict it.

ANATOMICAL COMPONENTS

The A-V nodal system can be thought of as divided into three more or less distinctive parts (Fig. 5–3).

1. **Junctional.** Also referred to as the **nodal approach zone,** the junctional tissue lying between the myofibrils of the atria and the A-V node serves to converge the wave front as it completes atrial depolarization, directing it into the A-V conduction pathway. Fibers within the A-V junctional tissue are exceptionally short, and they have an extremely slow conduction velocity (about 0.02 meters per second). The distal portions of these fibers are interwoven extensively as they penetrate into the body of the A-V node.

2. **Central.** The A-V node composes the middle portion of the atrioventricular conduction system. It contains a compact network of conduction fibers oriented in random directions so that they interlace elaborately. These fibers (called **N fibers**) are of the slow response type, being dependent on the slow calcium channels for depolarization. The paucity of collagen matrix forming the supportive tissue is similar to that found in the sinus node.

The A-V node is richly supplied with autonomic neural endings of both the adrenergic and the cholinergic systems. In most humans, this structure receives its blood supply from a branch of the right coronary artery.

3. **Penetrating.** Toward the distal portion of the A-V node, the fibers become progressively more parallel, gradually merging to form a slender tract 1 to 3 mm wide. This segment of the conduction system is referred to as the common bundle or as the

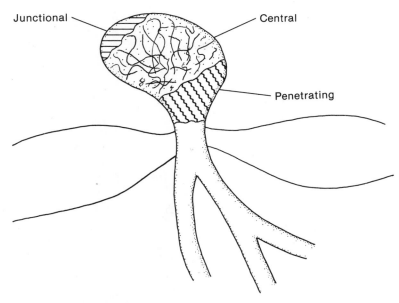

Figure 5–3. Divisions of the A-V conduction system.

bundle of His (named after Wilhelm His, a German physician and anatomist who, in the last century, described the narrow band of fibers bridging the atria and the ventricles).

During its short course of about 1 cm, the common bundle penetrates the fibrous skeleton that supports the atrioventricular valves and separates the atria from the ventricular musculature. Immediately after entering the ventricles, the common bundle divides into two main branches that straddle the intraventricular septum. Arterial branches from both the anterior and the posterior descending coronary arteries supply the common bundle, a dual source of blood flow that affords some protection in myocardial infarction.

RECORDING ATRIOVENTRICULAR NODAL ACTIVITY

Electrocardiogram—PR Interval

Because of the small size of the A-V nodal system compared with the size of the atria and ventricles, the electrical disturbances emanated during the action potential are comparatively weak. The standard electrocardiogram (ECG), in fact, reveals only an electrically silent period during A-V nodal activity, an isoelectric interval that composes the second portion of the PR interval (Fig. 5–4). The fact that the isoelectric period of this small structure takes about as long as does depolarization through the entire atrial wall reflects the relatively slow transmission of the impulse through the node.

The time required for an impulse to enter the right atrium from the sinus node and finally to emerge from the A-V node to stimulate the intraventricular septum defines the PR interval: from the beginning of the P wave to the beginning of the QRS complex. Recall that the normal PR interval ranges from 0.12 second to 0.20 second. Because the interpreter must constantly refer to the PR interval, it is imperative to remember these limits of normal.

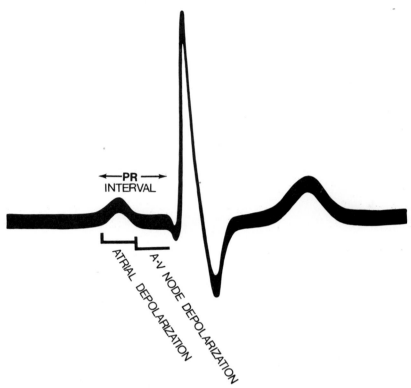

Figure 5-4. Identification of the PR interval. Normal PR interval = 0.12 to 0.20 second.

Measure the PR interval for sample strips number 169, 170, 171, and 172.

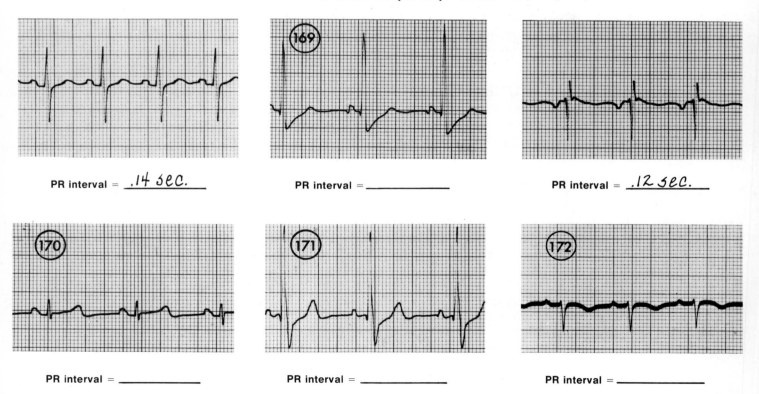

PR interval = _.14 sec._

PR interval = _____

PR interval = _.12 sec._

PR interval = _____

PR interval = _____

PR interval = _____

His Bundle Electrogram

From our brief description of the A-V nodal system, the reader can appreciate that this electrically silent period on the ECG actually represents immensely complicated activity at the cellular level. In recent years, this process has been looked at intimately using a technique in which tripolar electrodes are introduced by catheterization into the right ventricle through a peripheral vein. When the electrodes are placed directly against the septal leaflet of the tricuspid valve, they lie in close proximity to the common bundle. From this vantage point, the minute currents produced by an impulse surging through the common bundle can be recorded.

The potential recorded during depolarization of the common bundle is a very brief and small deflection. This spike can be observed in relationship to potentials recorded from the portions of the atria and the ventricles nearest to it. These consist of complex and ill-defined waveforms that are nevertheless identifiable by their timing. Thus, this intracardiac recording provides us with a view of the depolarizing activity within the intermediate conduction system: the incoming impulse from the low atrium and A-V node, the common bundle impulse, and the outgoing impulse into the high ventricle (the proximal intraventricular septum).

From this information, important conclusions have been formulated on the precise electrophysiology of these conduction pathways. In patients, this approach has disclosed the mechanism of arrhythmias in perplexing problems and has directed therapy in difficult arrhythmia syndromes.

The procedure just described provides a graphic recording known as the **His bundle electrogram**. On first appearance, it may appear strange and confusing. The reader must first realize that the speed at which the recording paper rolls is four to eight times faster than in routine electrocardiography. This more rapid movement spreads out the details of the complexes in the electrogram for easier viewing. Of course, the ECG taken simultaneously will have its waveforms stretched out as well. However, with a little practice, the reader can easily learn to recognize the components of both.

The reference point in the electrogram is the sharp, singular spike produced by a depolarizing impulse advancing through the common bundle: it is designated the **H wave** (for His) (Fig. 5–5). Note the isoelectric position of the stylus at this time in the surface ECG.

Immediately preceding the H potential lie the deflections from depolarization of the A-V node and before that those from the junctional fibers and the distal (or low) atrial tissues, all forming a complex waveform. The period from the onset of this electrical disturbance to the H wave is called the **AH interval**.

The AH interval represents the conduction time involved in transmission through the A-V node. In fact, this duration is not precise because the exact time of activation of the proximal A-V node cannot be detected in the initial deflection complex of the electrogram. Nevertheless, the measurement approximates A-V conduction time closely enough for practical purposes.

After passing through the common bundle, the impulse enters the bundle branches and begins to depolarize the ventricular septum. Those deflections that follow immediately after the H wave represent the onset of ventricular depolarization, occurring in the proximal intraventricular septum. The period between the H wave and the onset of the ventricular depolarization deflections is referred to as the **HV interval**. The waveform created by initial ventricular activation trails off as the wave front moves away from the recording electrodes.

The HV interval is much shorter than the AH interval, evidence that the conduction velocity in the common bundle is appreciably more rapid than in the A-V node.

To review, the His bundle electrogram traces the impulse wave front as it propagates through the intermediary system of conduction between atria and ventricles. During the corresponding period, the ECG records only an isoelectric line. The ECG

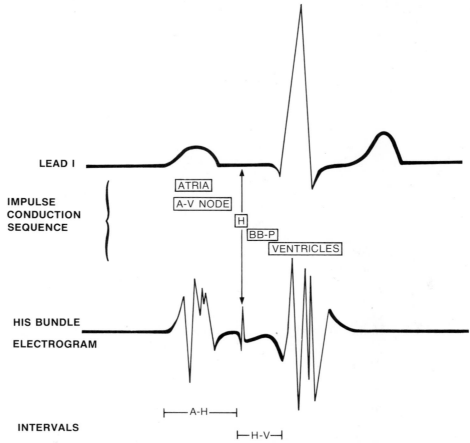

Figure 5–5. His bundle electrogram. Note electrophysiologic events in relation to the surface electrocardiogram. H = common (His) bundle; BB-P = bundle branches-Purkinje fibers.

measures changes in conduction through the A-V nodal system simply by shortening or lengthening of the PR interval, whereas the electrogram indicates where the changes occur: in the A-V node itself or in the common bundle as determined by AH and HV intervals.

The endings of autonomic neurons are much denser in the A-V node than in the common bundle. This distribution correlates with the conduction alterations induced by sympathetic and parasympathetic stimulation or inhibition. From the changes on AH and HV intervals, one concludes that the autonomic nervous system exerts its major control on the A-V node rather than on the common bundle.

The His bundle electrogram is introduced in this book because it provides valuable insight into the mechanisms of certain rhythm disorders and because the procedure is finding ever increasing clinical application. On the other hand, the reader is not expected to master interpretation of the electrogram at this stage. He or she should become acquainted enough with the fundamentals to understand the few representative electrograms that illustrate classic features of certain tachycardias and bradycardias.

ATRIOVENTRICULAR NODE: IMPULSE CONDUCTION

Excitation

Having emphasized the natural delay in impulse conduction imposed within the A-V nodal system, a number of conditions in which this delay is compromised are now presented. These conditions result in *earlier* than expected stimulation. Several distinct forms that are known collectively as **ventricular preexcitation** have been described (Fig. 5–6).

The phenomenon of preexcitation is caused by anomalous conduction pathways, in which an impulse is carried from atria to ventricles at an accelerated rate (Fig. 5–7). Such a pathway may be confined within the A-V node or, more frequently, it may pass around the A-V node, thus circumventing the normal delaying mechanism altogether.

Once thought rare, various forms of ventricular preexcitation are being recognized with increasing frequency. They may be expressed as variations in the standard ECG.

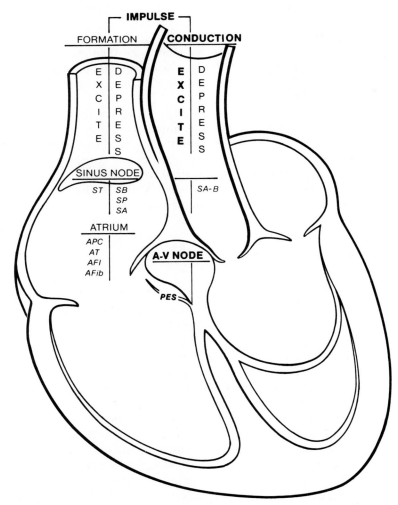

Figure 5–6. Conduction excitation in the A-V nodal area. PES = preexcitation syndrome (appearing on accessory fibers that bypass the A-V node).

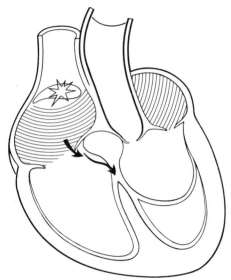

Figure 5–7. Preexcitation syndrome. Atrial impulses bypass the A-V node.

More importantly, the preexcitation *phenomenon* may be a predisposing factor for recurring tachyarrhythmias. When the electrophysiological phenonemon is associated with clinical manifestations (e.g., tachycardias), it is referred to as the *preexcitation syndrome*.

The anomalous A-V pathways that are the anatomic basis for the ventricular preexcitation phenomenon are denoted according to their site of insertion. Those pathways that lead directly to myofibrils are called **connections**. Those that are inserted directly into specialized conduction systems are designated **tracts**. The specific types of preexcitation are commonly referred to by well-accepted eponyms honoring the individuals who originally described them. Although these are pointed out here, the anatomical distinction has been chosen as the primary nomenclature.

Ventricular Preexcitation

INTRANODAL TRACT

Within the A-V node are conduction fibers that have an inherently more rapid conduction velocity than do the fibers near them (Fig. 5–8). The effects of such accelerated impulse transmission on the ECG are predictable:

1. The PR interval is abbreviated owing to a shorter A-V nodal transmission time.

2. There are *no* alterations in the sinus pacemaker rate, in the P wave, or in the QRS configuration because the sequences of atrial and ventricular depolarization are not affected.

With an intranodal bypass tract, the A-V node can be considered as having a dual pathway for transmission: one is the anomalous (**fast tract**) and the other the ordinary (**slow tract**). Another term, **longitudinal dissociation**, has been applied to this situation, emphasizing the different physiological properties of conduction in two adjacent tissues. Longitudinal dissociation in the A-V node is analogous to that described for Bachmann's bundle in the atrial tachycardia section of Chapter 4 under Intraatrial Reentry.

Ventricular preexcitation in a 6-year-old boy being examined because of episodes of fainting is revealed in Figure 5–9. Note that the PR interval is short (less than 0.12

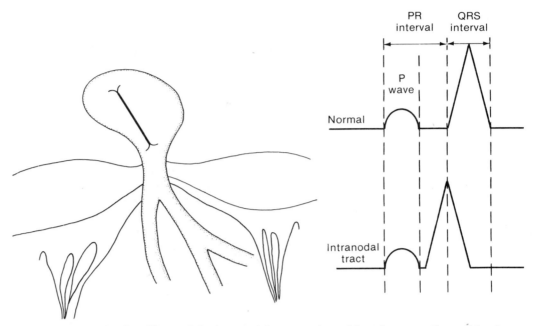

Figure 5–8. Conduction fibers of the intranodal tract and resulting electrocardiographic alterations.

second). Also note that the P waves and the QRS complexes appear normal in both contour and duration.

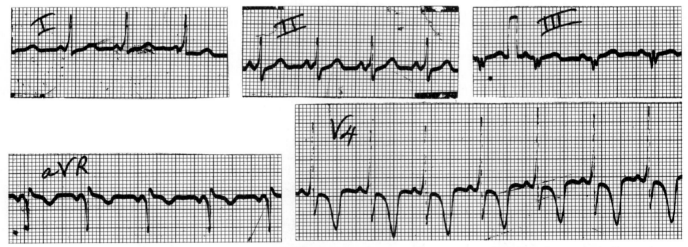

Figure 5–9. Representative leads of the electrocardiogram are selected to demonstrate the variable configuration of the delta wave in preexcitation. The PR interval, however, remains constant. An incidental feature of this tracing is the deep T waves present in lead V_4. This finding is common in healthy children.

One may make the assumption that accelerated A-V conduction (short PR interval) may be caused by a fast pathway operant within the A-V nodal system. In fact, embryologic **rests** of myofibrils have been observed in the A-V node on minute dissection. Misplaced myofibrils, which have a more rapid conduction velocity than do A-V nodal fibers, may be responsible for a dual pathway system in this instance.

One must also consider that a short PR interval by itself may be merely a variation

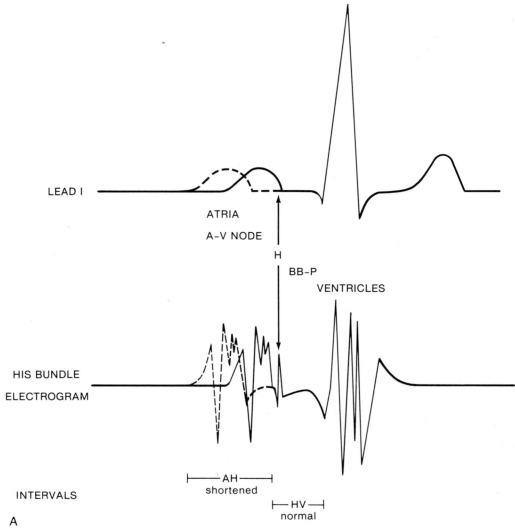

LEAD I

ATRIA

A-V NODE

H

BB-P

VENTRICLES

HIS BUNDLE

ELECTROGRAM

AH
shortened

INTERVALS

HV
normal

A

Figure 5–10. (*A*) Accelerated A-V conduction of atrial-Hisian or intranodal types with short PR interval and normal QRS interval on electrocardiogram and a short AH interval on electrogram. (Interrupted lines reflect normal activity; solid lines indicate accelerated conduction.)

out of the normal range *without* imputing a dual pathway mechanism. After all, the limits of normal for the PR interval of 0.12 to 0.20 second are arbitrary, based on population studies, akin to average height or other morphological measures. Other causes of more rapid A-V nodal transmission may be a congenital reduction in the number and size of the nodal fibers or a less woven orientation of these fibers. In addition, autonomic factors (increased sympathetic tone or decreased parasympathetic tone for whatever reason) may be responsible. Thus, the diagnosis of an intranodal dual pathway cannot be made with surety from the ECG.

The His bundle electrogram reveals details of A-V nodal accelerated conduction (Figs. 5–10*A* and *B*).

Accompanying the shortened PR interval in the ECG in Figure 5–10*A* is a shortened AH interval, indicating that the accelerated conduction occurs between the atria and the common bundle (represented by the H deflection). The anomalous pathway is

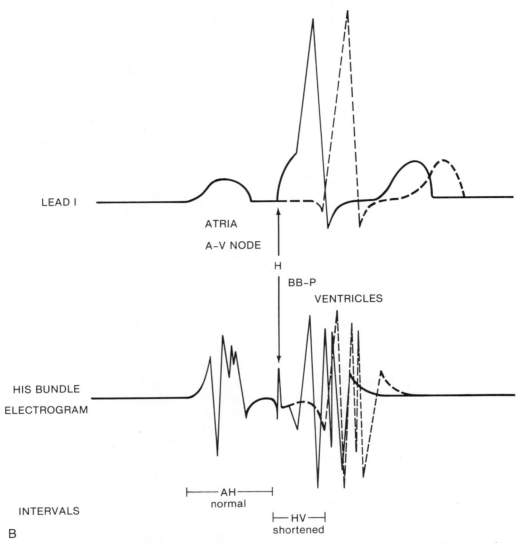

LEAD I

ATRIA

A-V NODE

H

BB-P

VENTRICLES

HIS BUNDLE

ELECTROGRAM

AH
normal

INTERVALS

HV
shortened

B

Figure 5–10. Continued (B) Accelerated A-V conduction caused by a direct A-V connection. The AH is normal, but the HV interval is markedly shortened. The accessory pathway bypasses the A-V node altogether to stimulate the ventricles before the normally conducted impulse. On the electrocardiogram, the PR interval is shortened and a slurring of the early portion of the QRS complexes (from the anomalous ventricular conduction) is present.

therefore an atrio-His* connection (James fibers) that bypasses the A-V node. Because conduction in the ventricles is normal, no QRS change is present on the ECG.

In the example in Figure 5–10*B*, the HV interval is shortened and a change in the early segment of the QRS complex is present. Thus, AH conduction is normal and a direct atrioventricular connection (Kent fibers) is present, associated with early excitation of the ventricles. Other variations of accelerated atrioventricular conduction represent different mechanisms as depicted later (see Fig. 5–19).

The presence of a dual pathway in the A-V node can be inferred from circumstantial

---

* Note that the word **His** always begins with a capital H, even in compound word forms, because it is a proper noun.

evidence, however, as recorded from the Holter monitor in Figure 5–11. The patient, a 28-year-old woman, was being studied for recurring rapid palpitations.

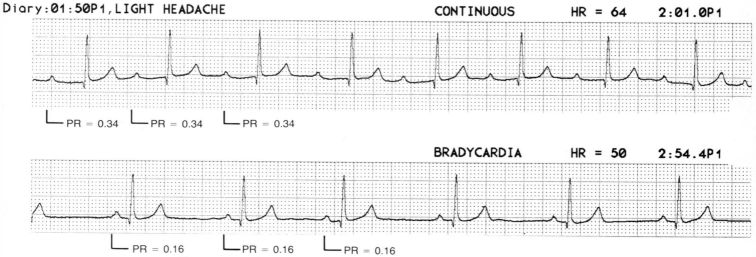

Diary:01:50P1,LIGHT HEADACHE   CONTINUOUS   HR = 64   2:01.0P1

PR = 0.34   PR = 0.34   PR = 0.34

                                                     BRADYCARDIA   HR = 50   2:54.4P1

PR = 0.16   PR = 0.16   PR = 0.16

Figure 5–11. The shift in PR interval durations indicates the presence of dual pathways that permit conduction from the atria into the ventricles.

Two strikingly different PR intervals are observed on comparing these two tracings taken a short while apart (upper = 0.36 second; lower = 0.16 second). However, the PR intervals in each tracing are constant. Because the PR interval normally tends to shorten as the heart rate increases, the exception presented here argues in favor of a mechanism other than differences in rate. It is presumed that two different pathways for A-V conduction are present, the upper tracing exhibiting a slow pathway and the lower a fast pathway.

One assumes that impulses travel through the A-V node along a slow pathway (producing a prolonged PR interval). Then the impulse diverts to a fast pathway (accounting for a shortening of the PR interval). This change in PR interval is distinct, contrasting sharply with the gradual change normally observed in the single conduction pathway in response to variations in heart rate and to autonomic stimulation.

An explanation proposed for the abrupt shifts from a fast to a slow intranodal pathway and back may involve fluctuating vagal tone. Understanding this mechanism will be helpful in learning other competitive conduction phenomena and the reentrant arrhythmias that they may generate.

As already emphasized, the anomalous (and rapid) pathway is composed of fibers having longer refractory periods than those of the slower pathway. Increased vagal tone may prolong the refractory period of the fast pathway beyond the time required for the next impulse to pass through it. With the impulse blocked along this route, it is still carried along the slow pathway (which has the shorter refractory period) to the ventricles. The switch from fast pathway to slow pathway results in a longer PR interval. This alternative tract subserves atrioventricular conduction until vagal tone is reduced sufficiently to allow recovery of the fast pathway fibers between cardiac cycles. When the prolonged refractoriness abates, the incoming impulse traverses the fast pathway again, and the PR interval shortens.

Very small changes in vagal tone may be enough to produce alternation of dual pathways in susceptible persons, even vagal influences associated with normal respiration. It should also be appreciated that the rate of the sinus pacemaker has a role in the interplay between conduction velocity and refractoriness and ultimately in which pathway an impulse will take.

The dual pathway phenomenon as the basis for reentrant tachycardias will be described in Chapter 6.

ATRIO-HIS BYPASS

A second form of ventricular preexcitation involves a rapidly conducting pathway that circumvents the proximal portion of the A-V node, thus carrying impulses received from the atria directly into a more distal segment. In some instances, the atrio-His pathway bypasses the A-V node in its entirety. The anatomical basis for this anomaly was confirmed by James and others from observations that bundles of myofibrils in the atria of some hearts insert into the distal A-V node or into the common bundle (Fig. 5–12).

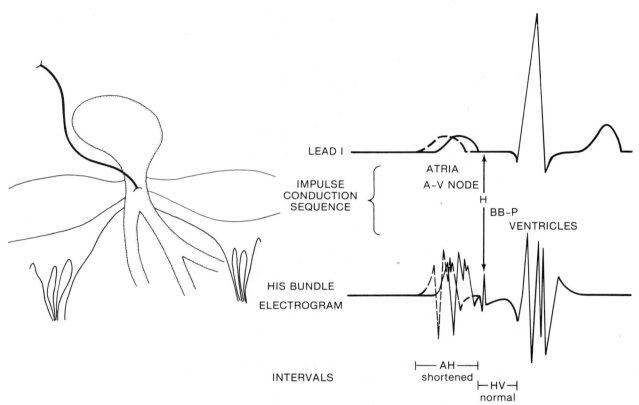

Figure 5–12. Atrial-His pathway and resultant complexes (identified by solid lines).

Just as in intranodal accelerated conduction, an atrio-His bypass tract could be responsible for producing a short PR interval but by a mechanism that allows an atrial impulse to escape the delaying action of at least a portion of the A-V node. Because both the atria and the ventricles are depolarized in their usual sequences, the P wave and the QRS complex are altered in neither duration nor configuration.

A variation of the atrio-His bypass is the atriofascicular bypass in which the tract inserts into one of the divisions of the common bundle. This form of ventricular preexcitation is rare.

NODOVENTRICULAR BYPASS

Another route by which the ventricles may undergo early excitation is through anomalous pathways that extend from the A-V node or common bundle to the proximal intraventricular septum (Fig. 5–13). Such streams of fibers, described by Mahaim in 1947, appear to act as bypasses around the distal region of the normal A-V conduction system. These fibers are designated **connections** because they insert directly into myocardial tissues rather than into conduction fibers, as do tracts.

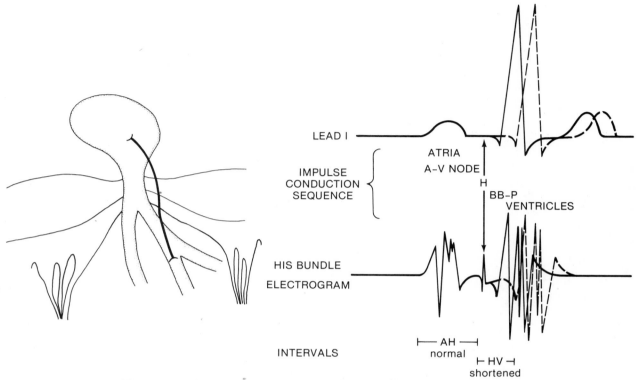

Figure 5–13. Pathway and complexes of nodoventricular connections.

As may be expected of impulse propagation that circumvents the normal delaying action of the A-V nodal system, the PR interval is shortened. The segment in the His bundle electrogram that is contracted is the HV interval, in contrast to the AH interval shortening found in the atrio-His type of bypass. The distal location of the anomalous connection makes this shortened HV predictable.

Normally, the HV interval is short compared with the AH interval, and further contraction of the HV interval through the preexcitation phenomenon generally produces only slight shortening of the PR interval. Sometimes a nodoventricular bypass causes no abnormal shortening of the PR interval and its detection by electrocardiography is possible only by changes produced in the QRS complex.

If the insertion of the nodoventricular connection is not at the site where the intraventricular septum is normally first depolarized, a wave front will take on a somewhat different direction from normal, and the wave front (proceeding through myofibrils rather than through Purkinje fibers) will be slower. These alterations may be observed as a slowly moving inscription in an aberrant direction at the onset of the QRS complex (representing septal depolarization). The slurred deflection so produced is known as a **delta wave** (Fig. 5–14).

Once this aberrant wave front has proceeded through a portion of the septal myocardium and enters the Purkinje fibers, impulse conduction becomes rapid and follows the usual sequence of ventricular stimulation. Therefore, the remainder of the QRS complex that comes after the delta wave reveals rapid depolarization and normal waveform configuration.

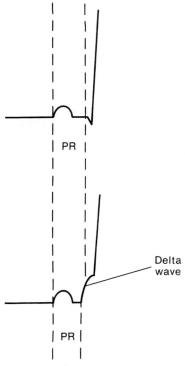

Figure 5–14. Delta wave appearance in preexcitation.

Conduction along an anomalous atrioventricular pathway may be very transitory, as demonstrated in Figure 5–15, obtained during a treadmill exercise stress test. The subject was a 36-year-old dance instructor with many episodes of rapid palpitations, sometimes associated with sudden weakness, during high levels of performance.

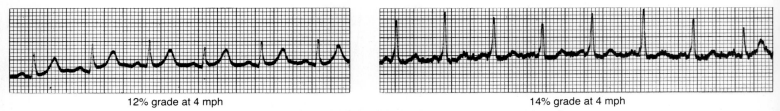

12% grade at 4 mph   14% grade at 4 mph

Figure 5–15. Electrocardiograms showing pattern of normal PR interval converting to delta wave and shorter PR interval with exercise.

The initial tracing was recorded at a speed of 4 miles per hour and a climbing grade of 12%. When the workload was increased to a 14% elevation at the same speed, ventricular preexcitation was demonstrated. The last cycle shown in the second tracing exhibits normal A-V conduction. No arrhythmia or sign of myocardial ischemia and no palpitations occurred during this study. It is presumed, however, that the transient shift in A-V conduction reveals a potential mechanism for a reentrant tachycardia.

Variants of nodoventricular bypass anatomy include anomalous connections that lead from the common bundle or from a bundle branch to insert directly into the intraventricular septum. These fasciculoventricular pathways usually exhibit minimal slurring in the initial QRS complex because of the relatively fast conduction through the normal His-Purkinje system.

ATRIOVENTRICULAR BYPASS

Thus far, the following types of anomalous pathways responsible for ventricular preexcitation have been described:

1. Pathways that bypass the normal, slower conducting fibers within the A-V node.
2. Pathwa_'s that bypass the proximal A-V nodal system.
3. Pathways that bypass the distal A-V nodal system.

The most common and most important of the types of ventricular preexcitation—those in which the A-V node is bypassed completely—are now introduced. This form involves accessory bands of fibers extending directly from the atria to the ventricles, thus eliminating the intermediary systems for impulse modulation.

In the past century, the anatomist Stanley Kent described embryonic rests of myofibril-like bands that appeared to form a direct bridge between the free wall of an atrium and the wall of the corresponding ventricle. Such tissue bands are known as bundles of Kent. Extending around the fibrous rings between atria and ventricles, these bands may insert onto the free wall of the ventricles or onto the intraventricular septum (Fig. 5–16). Because they lead directly to fibers of the working myocardium, they are termed connections, and are commonly called **accessory pathways**.

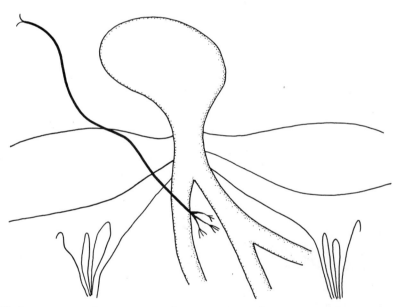

Figure 5–16. Accessory pathways connecting the atrial wall with the ventricles.

Ordinarily, the accessory pathway carries an atrial impulse more rapidly to the ventricles than does a pathway proceeding through the normal A-V nodal apparatus, so that the impulse reaches the superior ventricular wall or proximal intraventricular septum first. On stimulation, the wave front propagates through the myocardium at a relatively slow velocity. Thus, one would expect to find a short PR interval and a delta wave, similar to that associated with nodoventricular preexcitation.

Because the accessory pathway detours the A-V node completely, the resultant PR interval is usually exceptionally short (less than 0.10 second). Furthermore, the site of attachment to the ventricular myocardium is generally distant from the A-V node so that the early depolarizing wave front is long, causing a conspicuous delta wave (Fig. 5–17).

Even while the anomalous wave front is moving through the ventricular wall, an impulse is proceeding down the normal A-V nodal system to emerge eventually into

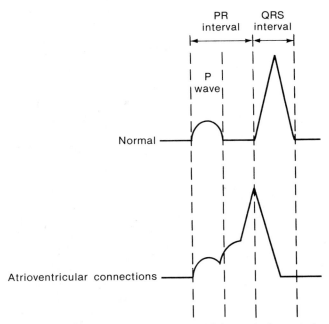

Figure 5–17. Shortened PR interval and delta wave, which result from early ventricular depolarization in preexcitation.

the Purkinje network through the endocardial walls of both ventricles. At some point, the anomalous and the normal wave fronts collide, producing a **fusion** complex. The QRS complex, then, initially represents depolarization from preexcitation (causing the change in the early portion of the QRS) and later represents depolarization from normal excitation (last segment of the QRS is unchanged).

Anomalous early ventricular conduction, represented by the delta wave, occurs during the usually electrically silent period between P wave and QRS complex (Fig. 5–18). On the His bundle electrogram, both the AH and HV intervals are normal. Stimulated prematurely, the QRS complex is prolonged, however, because it represents a fusion of premature ventricular depolarization and normal ventricular depolarization. All gradations of fusion occur (hence, varying magnitudes of delta waves), depending on the degree of penetration of the anomalous impulse into the ventricles before normal intraventricular depolarization occurs.

Restating, the initial slurring of the QRS complex in this form of ventricular preexcitation yields an overall increase in the QRS duration. This prolongation was interpreted as the result of a bundle branch block when first observed. A report published in 1930 and entitled ''Bundle-branch block with short P-R interval in healthy young people prone to paroxysmal tachycardia'' describes 11 patients with this anomaly. It was written by Louis Wolff and Paul D. White of Boston, Massachusetts, and by John Parkinson of London, England. Since this publication, the entity has been universally identified as the Wolff-Parkinson-White (WPW) syndrome. With recent differentiation of the various forms of ventricular preexcitation, it refers specifically to the form caused by accessory connections that completely bypass the A-V nodal apparatus. For interest and for practice, three cases from the original communication are presented.*

---

* The illustrations are reproduced from Wolff L, Parkinson J, and White PD: Bundle-branch block with short P-R interval in healthy young people prone to paroxysmal tachycardia. Am Heart J 5:693, 1930, with permission.

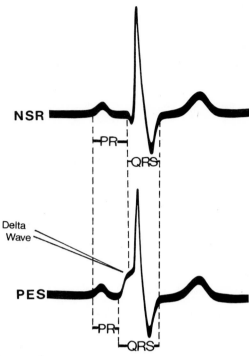

Figure 5–18. Preexcitation syndrome.

1. A preexcitation pattern is recorded following an episode of palpitations in a 21-year-old man.

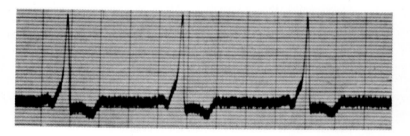

2. The transition from preexcitation pattern to normal A-V conduction and ventricular activation was recorded in a 16-year-old boy with a history of attacks of tachycardia while playing football.

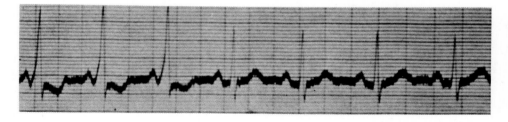

3. This example was taken from a 44-year-old widow, first examined in 1927. She had experienced attacks of palpitations since age 7. These episodes "lasted from a few minutes to several hours (intermittently) and were easily terminated by taking a deep

breath and holding it, or by lying down." An ECG taken later, during an attack, revealed auricular paroxysmal tachycardia at a rate of 230. Auricular is an older term used synonymously with atrial when referring to tachycardias, flutter, and fibrillation.

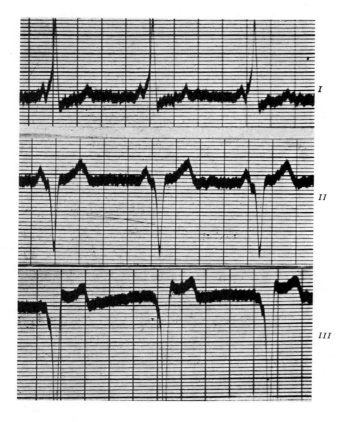

The accessory pathway in atrioventricular bypass can be on either the right or the left side. If the bypass is between left atrium and left ventricle, it is usually located in the posterior walls. The propagating wave front spreads rightward and in an anterior direction. The resultant delta wave recorded in lead I is downward, giving a reduced amplitude of the R deflection or increased amplitude of the Q deflection. In lead V_1, the same depolarizing movement will create an increased amplitude of the normal R deflection, as seen in the second strip in the preceding example. These changes, when pronounced, could result in an erroneous diagnosis of myocardial infarction, bundle branch block, or left ventricular enlargement.

When the bypass is on the right side, it usually lies within the anterior chamber walls. The resultant wave front disperses in leftward and posterior directions. The delta wave so formed is generally upright in lead I; in lead V_1, it produces reduced amplitude of the normal R deflection or it appears as a QS inscription (Fig. 5–19).

Ordinarily, an impulse passing through the A-V nodal system stimulates the right ventricle slightly ahead of the left ventricle. Consequently, there is more time for penetration of the ventricles before normally conducted intraventricular depolarization begins when the bypass connection is on the right side. The delta wave, therefore, is generally larger with right-sided accessory pathways.

The preexcitation pattern may be continuous or intermittent. Rarely, it appears in brief episodes and even in isolated beats. Increasing vagal tone may shift normal A-V node transmission to anomalous pathways in susceptible persons. In some, evidence of preexcitation on the ECG appears only on exercise; in others with the anomaly

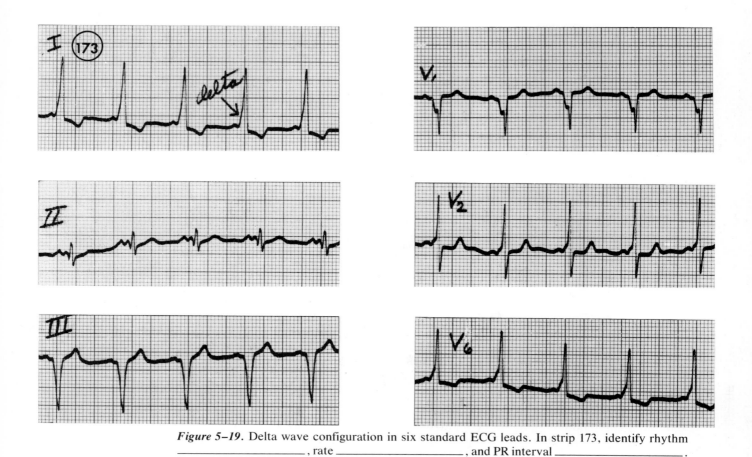

Figure 5–19. Delta wave configuration in six standard ECG leads. In strip 173, identify rhythm
_____ , rate _____ , and PR interval _____ .

at rest, it may disappear with exercise. These observations attest to the unpredictability of alternate pathways in patients with the disorder.

Tracing 174, from a 37-year-old man, was recorded with a magnetic tape recording (Holter monitor) of the cardiac rhythm over 10 hours. The ECG was then reproduced from the tape. The study was requested because of complaints of episodic rapid palpitations despite repeatedly normal resting ECGs.

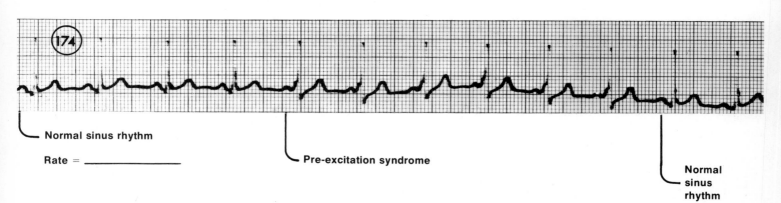

Normal sinus rhythm

Rate = _____

Pre-excitation syndrome

**Normal
sinus
rhythm**

Each of the first four cardiac cycles has a normal P wave and QRS complex configuration and a normal PR interval. (PR interval = _____ seconds).

In the fifth cardiac cycle, the PR interval is drastically shorter. (PR interval = _____ seconds).

Note particularly the slurring of the initial portion of the QRS complex, the delta wave. This abnormal sequence repeats itself up to the tenth cardiac cycle; then the original ECG pattern is resumed.

The additional but less well-known feature of the preexcitation syndrome is also illustrated in tracing 174. This alteration involves the terminal portion of the QRS complex, the result of a fusion of depolarizing wave fronts, one coming from the normal conducting Purkinje system, the other from the accessory pathway. Note that the S deflection is present only in those cardiac cycles exhibiting a short PR interval and delta wave.

Two additional practice strips (175 and 176) are provided. Indicate the rate, PR interval, and delta waves.

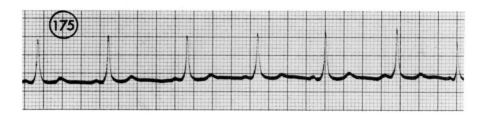

Rate = _____   **PR interval** = _____

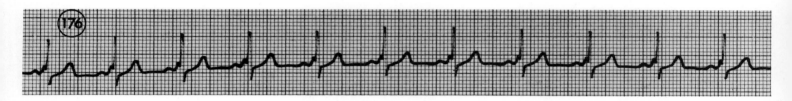

Rate = _____   **PR interval** = _____

Although anomalous A-V nodal bypass fibers are thought to be of congenital origin, symptoms of ventricular preexcitation often do not appear until early maturity. Manifestations sometimes are not expressed until even much later in life. They probably occur from intrinsic changes of impulse conduction with aging and from shifting dominance of autonomic tone or other factors that produce disproportionate alterations in normal and anomalous fibers.

Typically, persons with ventricular preexcitation phenomena have no underlying cardiac disease, consistent with the findings in the series originally described by Wolff, Parkinson, and White. However, individuals with mitral valve prolapse, malformation of the tricuspid valve, or cardiomyopathy have a greatly increased incidence.

As already mentioned, ventricular preexcitation may compromise the optimal synchronization between atrial and ventricular contraction. Furthermore, the preexcitation phenomenon confuses electrocardiographic interpretation, perhaps leading to misdiagnoses of myocardial infarction, bundle branch conduction abnormalities, or ventricular enlargement. But far more importantly, the phenomenon of ventricular preexcitation sets the stage for reentrant circuits, and these in turn predispose the heart to paroxysmal tachycardias (Fig. 5–20). Episodes of reentrant tachycardias may range from brief periods of palpitations to prolonged, recurring attacks of cardiac syncope, even with life-threatening implications. Premature beats and paroxysmal tachycardias having ventricular preexcitation as the underlying mechanism will be presented in reentrant tachycardias in Chapter 6.

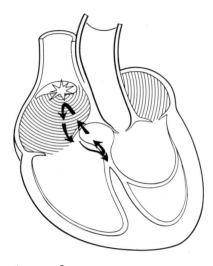

Figure 5–20. Reentry phenomenon.

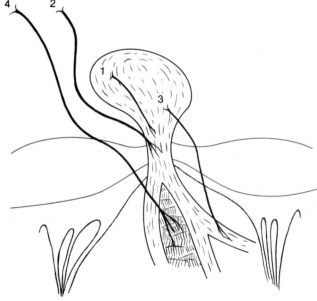

Figure 5–21. Composite diagram of anomalous pathways for A-V conduction associated with ventricular preexcitation and reentrant supraventricular tachycardias. Possible bypass tracts are (1) intranodal fibers, (2) atrial-His fibers (James), (3) nodoventricular fibers (Mahaim), and (4) A-V fibers (Kent). Fibers shown here enter to the ventricular septum. They may also connect the atria directly to the free wall of the right or left ventricle.

To review the four basic types of ventricular preexcitation, a tabular format is used to present the different pathways, terms, and electrocardiographic-electrographic distinctions (Table 5–1).

In a composite drawing, all major forms of A-V nodal bypasses are presented for comparison (Fig. 5–21).

Table 5–1. COMPARISON OF CHARACTERISTICS OF THE MAJOR FORMS OF PREEXCITATION PHENOMENA

Bypass Location	Eponym	A-V Nodal System Bypassed	Electrocardiogram PR Interval	QRS Duration	His Bundle Electrogram Intervals AH	HV
1. Intranodal	Lown-Ganong-Levine	None	Short	Normal	Short	Normal
2. Atrio-His	James	Proximal	Short	Normal	Short	Normal
3. Nodoventricular	Mahaim	Distal	Short or normal	Long (delta)	Normal	Short
4. Atrioventricular	Wolff-Parkinson-White (Kent)	Complete	Short	Long (delta)	Normal	Normal

ATRIOVENTRICULAR NODE: IMPULSE CONDUCTION

Depression

Impairment in the conduction of impulses through the A-V node results in delay of activation of the ventricles. If the impairment is severe, the impulse may fail to penetrate the A-V nodal system altogether. This group of conduction disturbances is known as **atrioventricular** (or **A-V**) **block** (Fig. 5–22). (The term **heart block** is a commonly used synonym, but it is not precisely descriptive.)

A-V block may occur in the approach fibers of the A-V node, in the A-V node itself, or in the common bundle. As will be explained in Chapter 7, similar impulse blockage may also result from a *combination* of electrical obstructions in the bundle branches.

The severity of A-V block is graded to denote the extent of conduction impairment. The mildest form is simply *prolongation* of conduction time within the A-V nodal system. This conduction defect is referred to as first-degree A-V block. When *some*

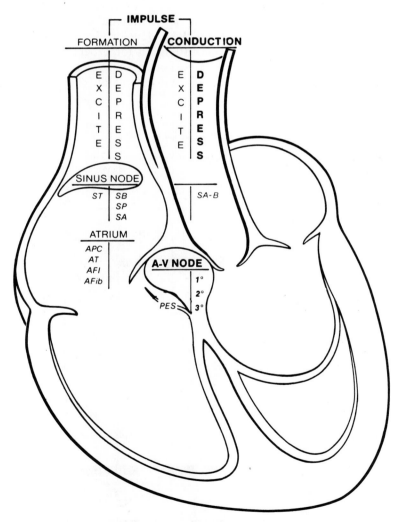

Figure 5–22. Rhythms of depression of the A-V node. 1° = first-degree A-V block; 2° = second-degree A-V block; 3° = third-degree A-V block.

but not all atrial impulses fail to penetrate the A-V nodal system, second-degree A-V block is the interpretation. Third-degree A-V block indicates that *all* impulses fail to penetrate into the ventricles.

First-Degree Atrioventricular Block

Delayed conduction velocity within the A-V nodal system of sufficient magnitude to prolong the PR interval is designated **first-degree A-V block**. This term indicates that all impulses entering the A-V node are eventually transmitted to the ventricles, however great the delay. On the ECG, first-degree A-V block is defined by a PR interval in excess of 0.20 second. The normal cardiac cycle along with first-degree A-V block is shown in Figure 5–23 for comparison.

First-degree A-V block is observed in the tracing in Figure 5–24 taken from lead V_1. Note that the biphasic P wave and the small R–large S ventricular complex are normal waveforms in this lead. The only abnormality is the markedly prolonged PR intervals, all of which are identical in length and followed by a QRS complex. (Remember that the PR interval is measured from the onset of the P wave to the onset of the QRS complex.)

First-degree A-V block may result from disease within the A-V node (ischemia, infarction) or from infections (rheumatic fever, myocarditis). Patients who are in the Coronary Care Unit and who develop delayed A-V conduction velocity should be observed with particular attention for progressive rhythms of depression. Increased parasympathetic tone slows conduction velocity in the area. Activities and drugs that intensify vagal stimulation may exaggerate the A-V conduction defect.

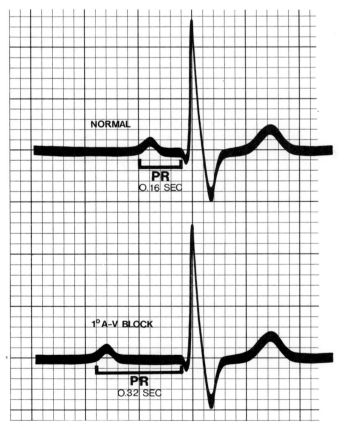

Figure 5–23. First-degree A-V block.

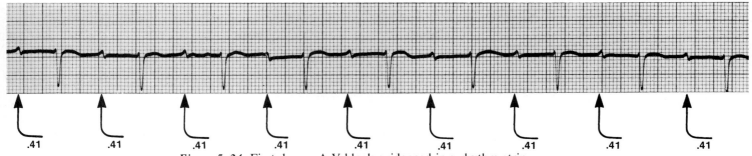

Figure 5–24. First-degree A-V block evidenced in a rhythm strip.

In the examples of first-degree A-V block that follow, (1) identify all components of a cardiac cycle; (2) determine heart rate; (3) measure PR intervals; and (4) ascertain if all PR intervals on each of the tracings remain constant.

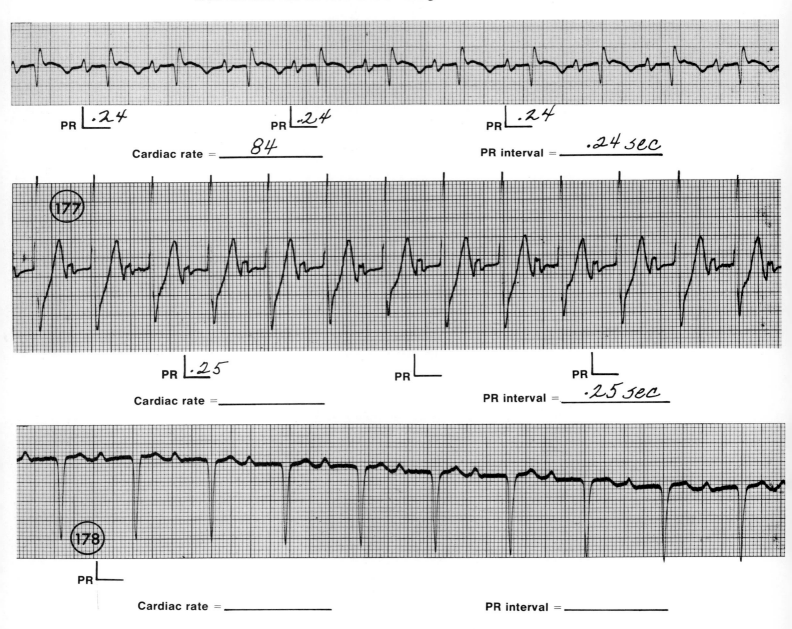

PR |.24   PR |.24   PR |.24

Cardiac rate = 84   PR interval = .24 sec

177

PR |.25   PR | PR |

Cardiac rate = _____   PR interval = .25 sec

178

PR |

Cardiac rate = _____   PR interval = _____

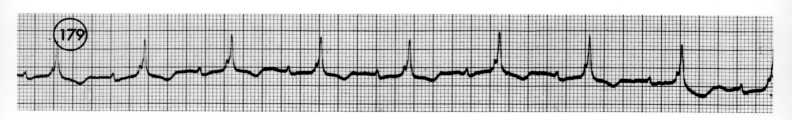

Cardiac rate = _____   PR interval = _____

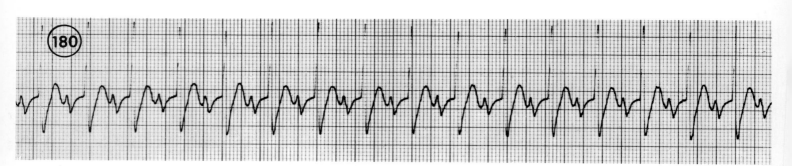

Cardiac rate = _____   PR interval = _____

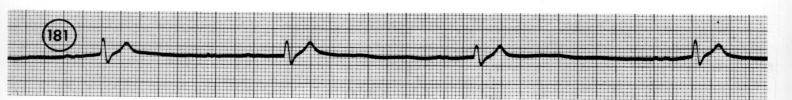

Cardiac rate = _____   PR interval = _____

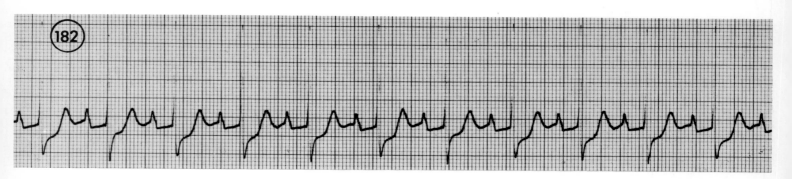

Cardiac rate = _____   PR interval = _____

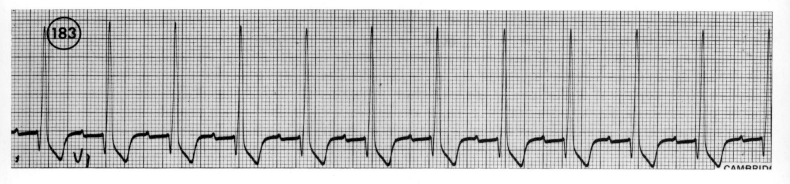

Cardiac rate = _____   PR interval = _____

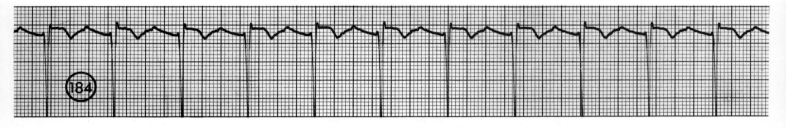

Cardiac rate = _____   PR interval = _____

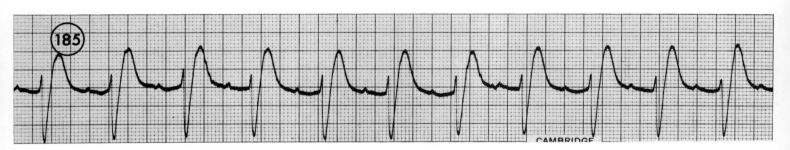

Cardiac rate = _____   PR interval = _____

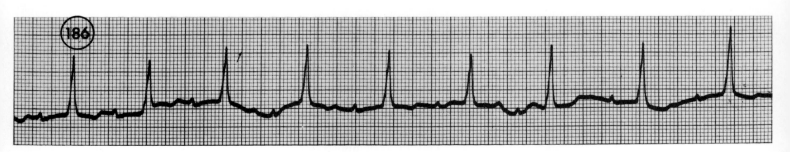

Cardiac rate = _____   PR interval = _____

For interest, an ECG strip is shown as it appeared on the front page of a newspaper, announcing the first transplant of the human heart (Fig. 5–25).

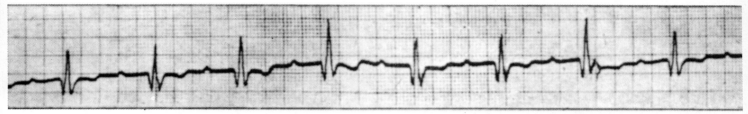

Figure 5–25. First-degree A-V block in a 54-year-old man in Cape Town, South Africa. (From New York Daily News, January 22, 1968, with permission of the Associated Press.)

As the heart rate increases or as the PR interval becomes longer, the distance between the end of a T wave and the beginning of the next P wave becomes shorter. Just as in sinus tachycardia, marked first-degree A-V block is often associated with P waves superimposed on T waves, as in practice strip 187. Because the exact time of onset cannot be distinguished here, the PR interval must be estimated.

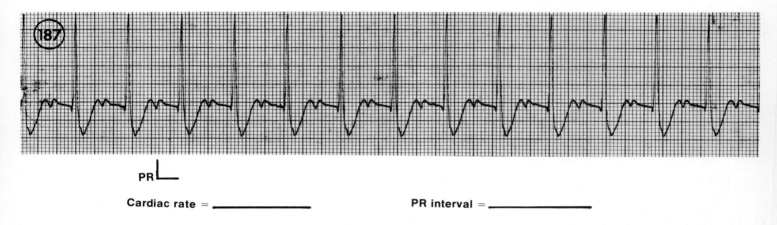

PR⌐

Cardiac rate = _____   **PR interval = _____**

Test strip 188 is an example of T-P combined waveforms that obliterate the initial portion of the P waves and therefore prevent accurate measurement of PR intervals. In such instances, the interpreter must approximate the interval by guessing where the P wave may actually begin.

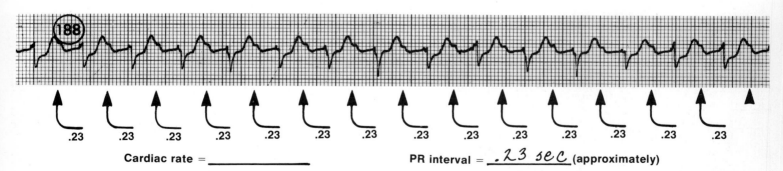

.23   .23   .23   .23   .23   .23   .23   .23   .23   .23   .23   .23   .23   .23

Cardiac rate = _____   **PR interval = _.23 sec_ (approximately)**

P waves can be identified more positively in tracing 189, although they are obscured in some cardiac cycles. This ECG demonstrates the effect that changes in heart rate can have on the timing relationship between T waves and P waves. The PR intervals appear to remain constant, but as the rate accelerates, even slightly, the P waves merge farther into the preceding T waves, making accurate measurement of the PR interval difficult.

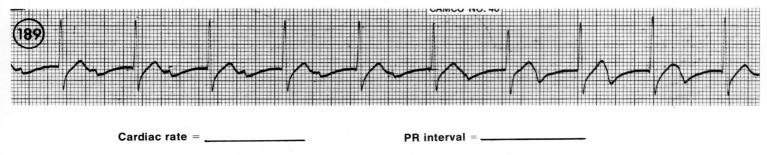

Cardiac rate = _____   PR interval = _____

Unless the PR interval is extremely prolonged, first-degree A-V block poses no hemodynamic adversity. Nor does first-degree A-V block necessarily indicate disease or an unfavorable prognosis. Indeed, it is a common finding among youths and trained athletes in excellent health, being an expression of high vagal tone. First-degree A-V block is also frequently observed in the elderly. First-degree A-V block can also occur during sleep, as shown in Figure 5–26. No abnormal findings were evident on the initial examination, and a 24-hour Holter monitor was used for further evaluation.

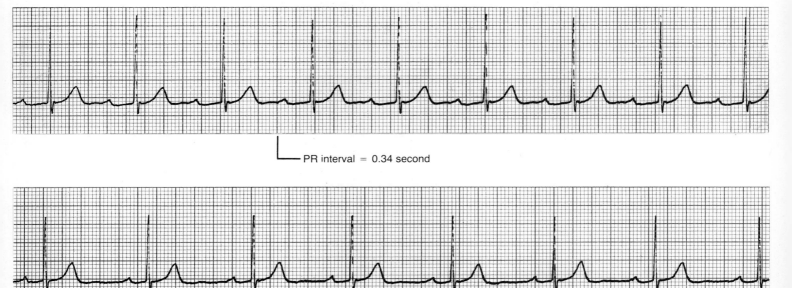

PR interval = 0.34 second

PR interval = 0.24 second

Figure 5–26. Sleep-induced worsening of first-degree A-V block. (*A*) PR interval during sleep is 0.34 second. (*B*) PR later in the morning after awakening is 0.24 second.

Although generally benign, first-degree A-V block has two important clinical implications:

1. The prolonged PR interval may be a harbinger of a progressing disturbance of impulse conduction. It should always be considered such when found in patients with acute myocardial infarction, myocarditis, drug toxicity, or other cardiac disorder of recent onset.

2. Rarely, the PR interval is so extremely prolonged as to interfere with atrial to ventricular synchronization. The ventricles may contract so much later than the atria

(because of markedly delayed A-V conduction) that the atria push against mitral and tricuspid valves, which are closed from the previous cardiac cycle. Thus is lost the advantage of the atrial kick.

Individuals sometimes exhibit prominent first-degree A-V block on vagal stimulation, owing to the inhibitory action of parasympathetic enhancement on A-V nodal conduction velocity. Carotid sinus pressure may produce not only lengthening of the PR interval but slowing of the sinus rate as well.

Probably because of the relative concentration of parasympathetic neuronal endings, right carotid sinus stimulation generally induces a stronger inhibition of sinus node activity than does left-sided stimulation. In contrast, left carotid pressure is more likely to produce a greater degree of A-V nodal impulse slowing than right.

First-degree A-V block, by itself, requires no specific treatment, except for changes in drug dosage when causally related. However, drugs of excitation can often overcome depression of A-V nodal conduction, either by augmenting sympathetic tone or by counteracting parasympathetic tone. Figure 5–27 illustrates drug treatment of marked first-degree A-V block. This action was actually taken to clarify the rhythm when the diagnosis was uncertain.

1:20 PM: On the left tracing in Figure 5–27, P waves are not found at the usual site. It was suspected that the tall T waves actually represented superimposed P waves and T waves, the former causing the sharp peak, thus representing first-degree A-V block. An alternative diagnosis (an A-V junctional rhythm) would be managed in quite another way.

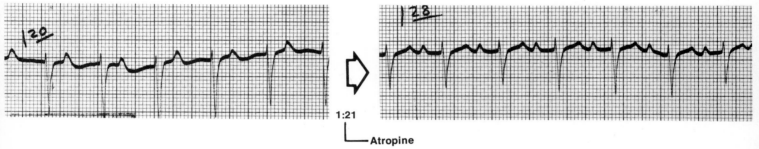

1:21
└─ **Atropine**

Figure 5–27. First-degree A-V block revealed with parasympathetic block.

1:21 PM: Atropine was given by mouth.

1:28 PM: P waves are now easily identified as they move out of the T waves. Note that the T wave amplitude is reduced and that P waves have the same contour as the peak observed in the preceding tracing. First-degree block is still present (the PR interval is 0.22 second), but it is of lesser severity. An observant interpreter will have noticed that the sinus rate did *not* accelerate concomitantly, as would be expected with atropine administration. The patient, a 60-year-old man admitted for lung biopsy, complained of dry mouth, abdominal discomfort with bloating sensation, and difficulty in urination after taking the atropine.

The causes of first-degree A-V block are numerous, but they fall into only a few general categories, which are described briefly here:

1. **Autonomic**. The A-V node is highly innervated by neural fibers of both the sympathetic and the parasympathetic nervous systems. Acting through this counterbalancing system on conduction velocity, a delay in A-V nodal conduction may be caused by a reduction in adrenergic stimulation or by accentuation of cholinergic tone.

His bundle electrography reveals that the site where the autonomic nervous system affects A-V nodal transmission is within the A-V node itself where neural fibers are most densely distributed. The graphic representation of autonomic stimulation is shown in Figure 5–28, in which vagal stimulation results in lengthening of the AH interval and no change in the HV interval.

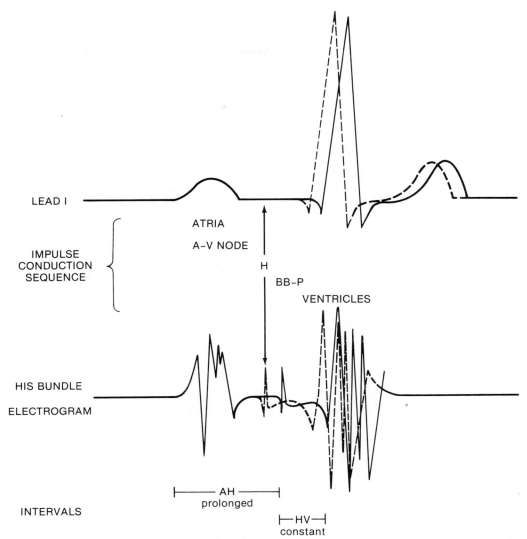

Figure 5–28. A prolongation of the AH interval results from stimulation of the parasympathetic nervous system. H = common (His) bundle; BB-P = bundle branches-Purkinje fibers. Solid lines represent the change in conduction caused by parasympathetic stimulation.

2. **Ischemic**. In about 90% of individuals, the blood supply to the A-V node and a portion of the common bundle is derived from branches of the right coronary artery. Perforator arteries from the left coronary artery supply the more distal segments of the intermediary conduction system. First-degree A-V block can be produced by occlusive disease of either major coronary artery. It is particularly common in acute myocardial infarction.

3. **Inflammatory**. Myocarditis caused by infection, autoimmune reaction, or toxic material is commonly associated with depression of A-V nodal conduction. The most noteworthy causes are acute rheumatic fever, viral myocarditis, lupus erythematosus, and bouts of alcoholic intoxication. In the diagnosis of acute rheumatic fever, first-degree A-V block is one of the important criteria. Abnormal slowing of A-V conduction is also frequently observed after cardiac surgery.

4. **Sclerodegenerative**. Some replacement of conduction fibers by fibrous tissue is a natural occurrence with aging, akin to the processes already described in the sinus node and the atria. Sclerodegenerative lesions may appear anywhere within the A-V

nodal conduction system, and they are probably the predominant cause of A-V conduction diseases. The most likely site for expression within the system is in the slender common bundle, seen as lengthening of the HV interval in the His bundle electrogram (Fig. 5–29).

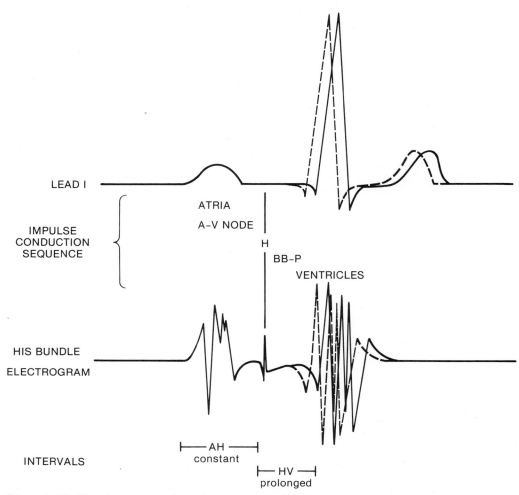

Figure 5–29. The electrogram shows lengthening in the HV interval. H = common (His) bundle; BB-P = bundle branches-Purkinje fibers.

5. **Pharmacological.** Certain drugs such as propranolol depress A-V conduction by affecting either the sympathetic or the parasympathetic nervous system. Others such as verapamil, amiodarone, and encainide have a direct action on the conducting fibers.

Drugs may depress A-V conduction through *both* autonomic and cellular mechanisms, as observed with digitalis and quinidine. Many noncardiac drugs also adversely affect A-V conduction at toxic levels; the most notable offenders are the tricyclic antidepressants, phenothiazines, and emetine (used to treat parasitic infections).

Second-Degree Atrioventricular Block

As depression of impulse conduction within the A-V nodal system progresses, impulses that originate at the sinus node may fail to reach the ventricles. When this disturbance is intermittent (i.e., some sinus impulses but not all penetrate the A-V nodal system), **second-degree A-V block** is the interpretation.

An example of second-degree A-V block is shown in test strip 190.

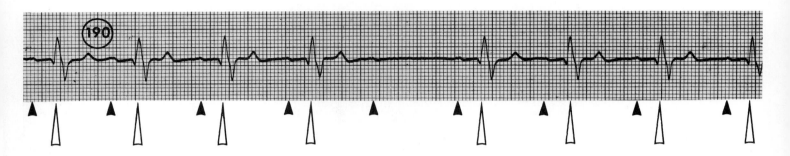

1. Basic rhythm: normal sinus rhythm (rate = _____) with prolongation of A-V conduction (PR interval = _____ second).

2. Sinus beat number 5 occurs at the expected time, but no QRS complex or T wave follows. The sinus impulse is blocked, and the ventricular beat is dropped.

3. Sinus beat number 6 is conducted, and the basic sinus rhythm is resumed without interruption of cadence (check with calipers).

4. Conclusion: second-degree or intermittent A-V block.

The prolonged PR interval in the basic rhythm suggests an adverse factor operating in the A-V node relay system. It can be appreciated that a sufficiently prolonged PR interval (delay in conduction velocity beyond a critical level) may result in dissipation of the impulse somewhere along the conduction pathways. Thus no effective ventricular stimulation will follow. This mechanism is given to explain the intermittent dropped ventricular beat.

Figure 5–30 is a tracing from a 77-year-old hypertensive woman with a history of recent onset of syncopal episodes. Her standard ECG revealed no abnormalities except borderline first-degree A-V block. Vagal stimulation was performed to evaluate the possibility of a bradycardic basis for syncope. An interpretation of the strip would be as follows:

1. *Basic normal sinus rhythm* with PR interval = 0.20 second (beats number 1 and number 2).

2. *Vagal stimulation* effected by carotid pressure causes
    a. severe slowing of sinus impulse formation.
    b. retardation of A-V node conduction velocity leading to prolongation of the PR interval (0.26 second in beat number 3) and blocked sinus impulse (beat number 4).

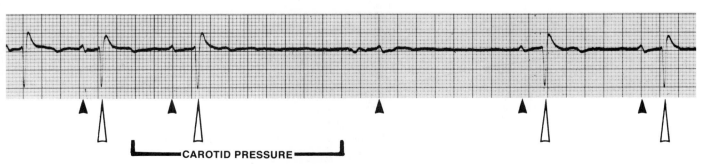

Figure 5–30. Second-degree A-V block precipitated by carotid pressure.

3. *Sinus beats* resume, with sinus bradycardia and slightly prolonged PR interval as residual effects of vagal stimulation (beats number 5 and number 6).

The tracing in Figure 5–31 was obtained during an episode of vomiting in a 52-year-old man with an acute myocardial infarction. Normal sinus rhythm had been present during his previous 2 days in the Coronary Care Unit. Intermittent failure of sinus impulse conduction is evoked by the strong parasympathetic stimulation of vomiting. Thus a defect of A-V nodal conduction is revealed.

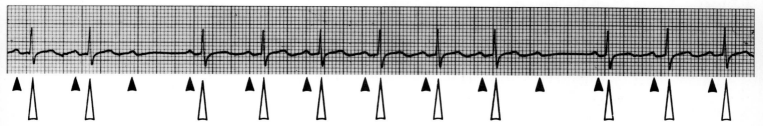

Figure 5–31. Development of second-degree A-V block with vomiting.

The vagotonic effect of vomiting or other forms of straining commonly results in a significant delay in nodal conduction velocity, particularly in the heart already affected by acute ischemic disease. Certain cardiac drugs commonly used in the treatment of myocardial infarction also enhance vagal tone. Thus the vagotonic effects of vomiting, straining, morphine, and digitalis superimposed on acute ischemic injury in the A-V nodal area may induce serious problems of impulse conduction. To anticipate development of more serious conduction defects, the PR interval should be studied in detail in the Critical Care Unit for signs of impending A-V node conduction malfunction during these provocative acts or after drug administration.

In Figure 5–32, label each P wave. Mark the blocked sinus beat and the place where the QRS should appear. Ease in interpretation of this rhythm could be enhanced if recording electrodes were reversed, producing upright P, QRS, and T waveforms.

In test tracing 191, label each P wave. Compare all PR intervals. (Are they identical?) Mark the blocked sinus beat. Indicate where the QRS complex *should have* appeared.

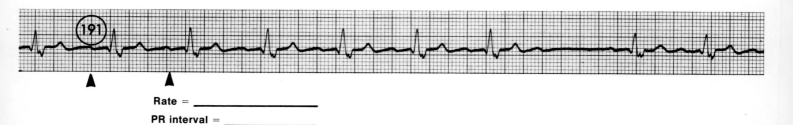

Rate = _____

PR interval = _____

The following series of rhythm strips are from a 50-year-old woman with an acute myocardial infarction. Note the changing severity of A-V block.

1. Sinus rhythm with instance of failure of A-V node conduction (Fig. 5–33). Observe that the blocked beat occurs sooner after the previous beat than conducted sinus beats. Thus, the blocked beat appears to be rate related. When the atrial rate is even slightly accelerated, the A-V node does not have sufficient time to recover from the previous beat and cannot conduct a new impulse.

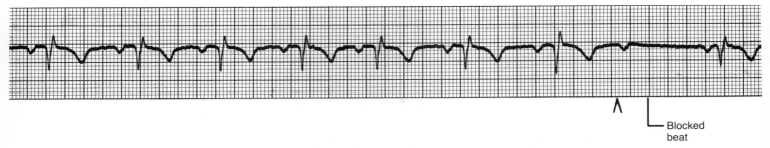

Figure 5–32. Example of second-degree A-V block.

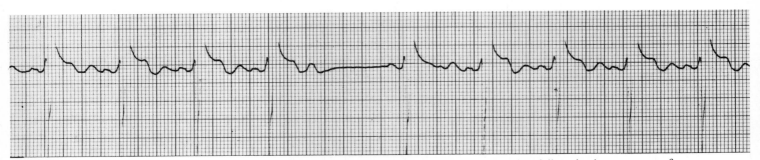

Figure 5–33. Rhythm strip with a single occurrence of conduction failure in the presence of an acute myocardial infarction.

2. The A-V conduction block has increased so that 1 hour later every other sinus beat is blocked (Fig. 5–34). This produces two atrial contractions for every ventricular contraction, a condition designated as second-degree A-V block with 2:1 A-V ratio. The atrial rate, then, is exactly twice the ventricular rate. Because of slight changes in the sinus rate from beat to beat, nonconducted P waves appear in a variable time relationship to the previous T waves.

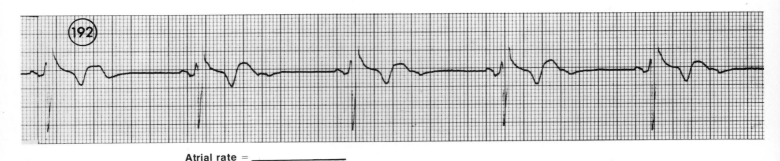

Atrial rate = _____

Ventricular rate = _____

Figure 5–34. Progression of a conduction defect causes blocking of every other sinus-initiated beat.

A rhythm with frequent blocked sinus beats is now shown in which the number of conducted beats occurring before each blocked beat varies (test strip 193).

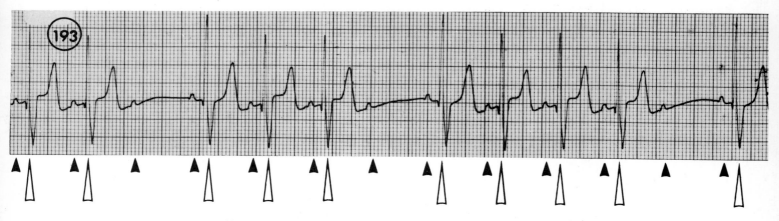

All P waves and QRS complexes in strip 193 are marked. Which sinus beats are blocked? _____

Note that each conducted sinus beat has identical PR intervals of _____ second.

In the first group of beats, the ratio of atrial to ventricular contractions is 3:2. In the second, the ratio is 4:3. In the third, the ratio is _____:_____.

Test tracing 194 exhibits second-degree A-V block of advanced severity. Mark all sinus and ventricular components. Determine the A-V ratio (_____:_____).

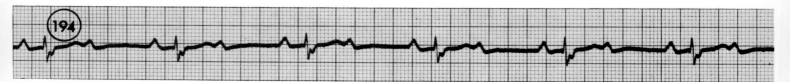

Sinus rhythm with A-V block.

Figure 5–35 is an electrocardiographic tracing from a 16-year-old boy with congenital heart disease (atrial septal defect). Variable conduction through the A-V node is observed. There are periods when every other sinus beat is blocked, and others when conduction is blocked with every third beat.

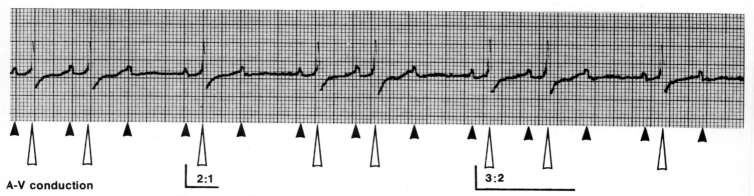

Figure 5–35. Second-degree A-V block with varying 2:1 and 3:2 A-V conduction.

Practice interpreting test tracings 195 through 197. In each, locate all conducted and all blocked sinus beats. Determine the PR intervals of conducted beats. Indicate the A-V ratio. What are the atrial rates and ventricular rates in each strip?

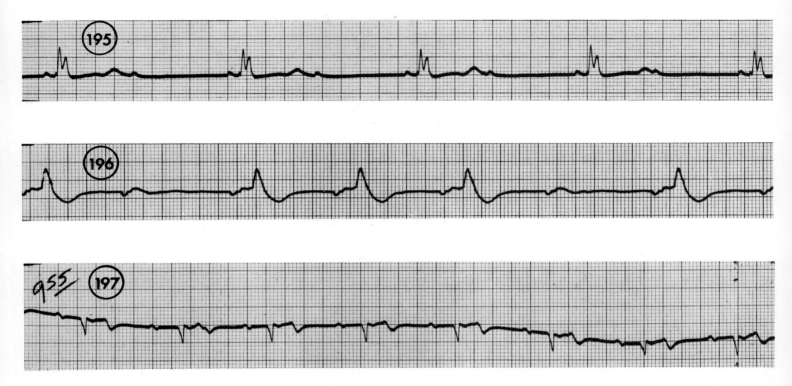

ADVANCED ATRIOVENTRICULAR BLOCK

Rhythm tracings 198 and 199 illustrate second-degree A-V block in which relatively few of the sinus-initiated impulses penetrate the A-V node to stimulate the ventricles. **Advanced A-V block**, as in these strips, results in severe slowing of the ventricular rate and often in symptomatic bradycardia (lightheadedness, weakness, fainting). In these arrhythmias, any maneuver or drug action that stimulates the vagus nerve may further increase the A-V nodal block (by increasing conduction delay) and intensify the brady-cardia.

Review the examples of advanced A-V block presented in test tracings 198 and 199. Work out the basic rhythm and the relationship between conducted and blocked beats.

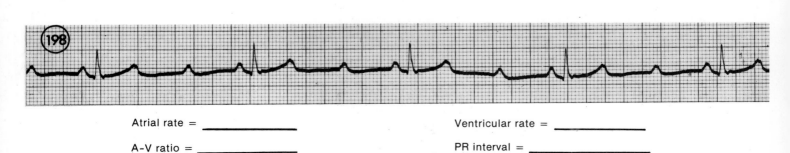

Atrial rate = _____   Ventricular rate = _____

A-V ratio = _____   PR interval = _____

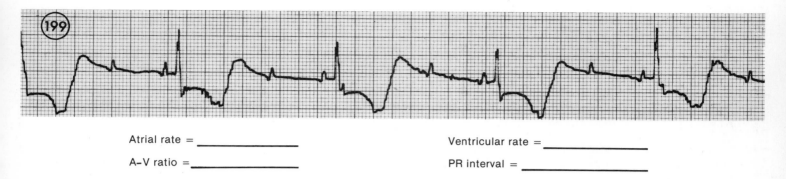

Atrial rate = _____   Ventricular rate = _____

A-V ratio = _____   PR interval = _____

  The clinical sequence that follows in test tracings 200 through 203 is included to demonstrate the progression and the unpredictability of intermittent A-V block and to illustrate the action of a drug used to control it.

  The sequential tracings are from an 81-year-old man with recurring episodes of dizziness and syncope. A cardiac arrhythmia was suspected as the cause, and the patient was admitted to the Coronary Care Unit for observation.

  1. 3:50 PM: The patient is alert and without symptoms. The cardiac monitor reveals (_____) rhythm, with a rate of _____ per minute and a PR interval at the upper limit of normal (_____ second).

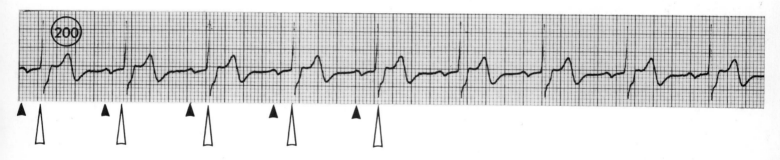

  2. 4:06 PM: The pulse detector loses the R component signal, activating the alarm system and automatic pen recorder. The next two strips (201 and 202) are continuous tracings subsequently obtained. They reveal a series of atrial waves without ventricular complexes for several seconds, during which time the patient developed the symptoms and behavior of acute cerebral circulatory arrest. With spontaneous recovery of A-V conduction, symptoms quickly disappear, and the cause of his original complaints is clarified. Note, however, that the recovery rhythm appears to be 2:1 A-V block. Also note the increase in sinus rate during the period of ventricular inactivity, presumably caused by cardiovascular reflexes. The duration of *documented* ventricular inactivity is _____ seconds.

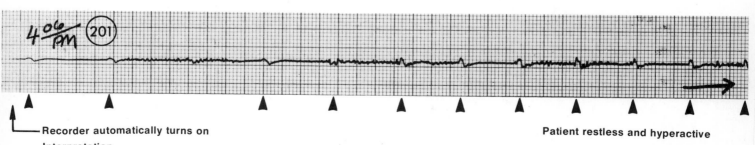

Recorder automatically turns on   **Patient restless and hyperactive**

Interpretation _____

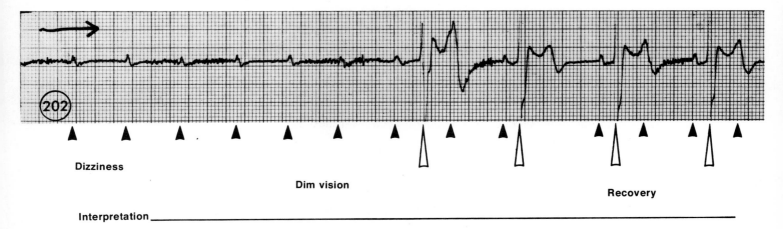

Dizziness

Dim vision

Recovery

Interpretation _____

3. By 4:08 PM, an intravenous infusion of isoproterenol is started (strip 203). Within a minute, all sinus beats are conducted. The accelerating effect of isoproterenol on sinus impulse formation is reflected in the sinus tachycardia now present (rate = _____). Explain the pharmacological action of isoproterenol in this instance.

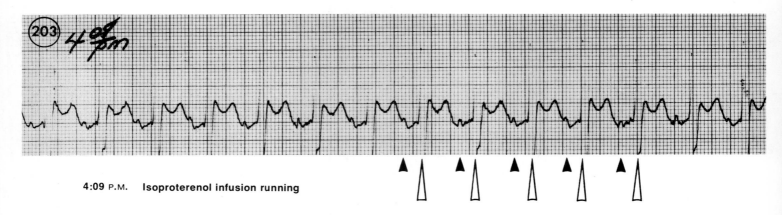

4:09 P.M.   Isoproterenol infusion running

Many patients have successfully been treated for months and even for years with long-acting oral preparations of isoproterenol to control symptomatic second-degree A-V block. However, symptoms often recurred with variations in blood levels and as the disease progressed. In addition, advances in reliability of the electronic pacemaker and the relative convenience of its insertion have rendered pharmacological treatment of this condition virtually obsolete for ambulatory patients. Administration of isoproterenol by intravenous administration remains a useful expedient in emergencies until an electronic pacemaker can be implanted.

Now that the reader has gained some experience in the concepts and interpretation of second-degree A-V block, we will introduce two basic types of intermittent A-V conduction. First of all, it will be recalled that the culpable lesion in first-degree A-V block may be located in either the body of the A-V node or in the common bundle. This distinction, however, cannot be made from the ECG (which reveals only prolonged A-V conduction in either case). First-degree A-V block with the conduction defect in the A-V node or in the common bundle was demonstrated on the His bundle electrogram, the site of block determined by a prolonged AH interval (A-V node) or by a prolonged HV interval (common bundle).

In second-degree A-V block, the location of depressed conduction is quite characteristically reflected by the pattern in which the blocked sinus beats occur. Thus, the ECG can be used to detect whether the block is in the A-V node or in the common bundle. Indeed, this distinction provides us with two basic forms of second-degree A-V block, described in 1924 by Walter Mobitz, a German physician, who classified them as Type I and Type II. His name continues to serve as an eponym for these conditions.

Although a practitioner often finds the interpretation of the specific types of second-degree A-V block perplexing, it can be mastered with good conceptual understanding and with practice. Maintaining a keen awareness in the clinical setting, an interpreter will gain the experience for detecting and differentiating these important arrhythmias. Indeed, critical decisions in management, both acute and long term, will often be determined on the basis of such interpretive skill.

TYPE I SECOND-DEGREE ATRIOVENTRICULAR BLOCK.

The electrophysiological lesion in Type I intermittent A-V block is in the A-V node (Fig. 5–36).

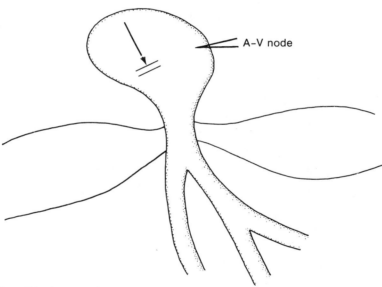

Figure 5–36. Type I lesions are located in the A-V node.

To compare the body of the A-V node with the common bundle, one should recall its special characteristics.

- The A-V node is much larger than the common bundle.
- Its fibers are oriented in a complex interweaving pattern rather than in parallel.
- It has neural endings of the autonomic nervous system concentrated in it.

When a conduction defect is present in the A-V node, successive impulses work their way through the structure with increasing difficulty, each beat taking progressively longer to penetrate the node. Obviously, the ever increasing conduction delay will be terminated at some point, and this point is identified by failure of an impulse to succeed in its penetration. Thus, a dropped ventricular complex occurs after a series of progressively increasing conduction delays.

On the ECG, this phenomenon is seen as a series of complete cardiac cycles in which the PR intervals become longer with each successive cycle until the progression is interrupted by a blocked sinus beat. After a pause, the subsequent sinus beat finds its way through the A-V node with relative ease (the PR interval is short), but the *gradual lengthening of PR intervals* thereafter begins once again. This fascinating arrhythmia is described in the point-by-point explanation that follows.

Figure 5–37 shows intermittent A-V block with lengthening PR intervals of conducted beats. The patient was a 56-year-old steelworker admitted to the Coronary Care Unit for suspected myocardial infarction. This tracing appeared on the second hospital day.

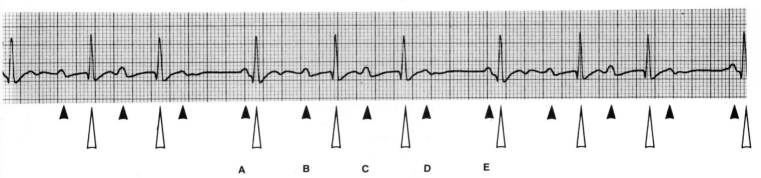

Figure 5–37. Second-degree A-V block, Wenckebach type.

Looking at the ventricular complexes of this tracing, one notices that the basic cadence is frequently interrupted by pauses. The description of events begins at the cardiac cycle that occurs immediately after the pause.

Starting with the normal cardiac cycle at A, the PR interval is 0.12 second. In the following cycle at B, the configuration of components is unchanged. However, the PR interval has increased to 0.32 second. In the next beat, C, the PR interval is now 0.41 second. There has been a progressive increase in the duration of the A-V conduction time. Certainly, this progression cannot continue indefinitely, and the following events illustrate resolution of the process.

A P wave appears at the expected time, D, but no QRS complex follows. This blocked beat establishes the rhythm as a form of second-degree A-V block. The next beat is of particular interest. Note that the sinus cadence remains constant (D-E). Then note that the PR interval at E is short, similar to that at A. In subsequent beats, the PR interval gets longer and longer. Then a blocked beat occurs. The cycle has repeated itself in four beats.

Tracing 204 is from a 58-year-old woman suspected of having myxedema. Her primary complaint on an office visit was that she always felt cold.

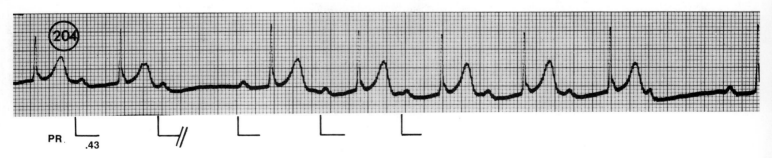

When this ECG is scanned, the pause in the ventricular rate is obvious. A blocked sinus beat seems to occur in this area. In complex rhythms, it is helpful to begin interpretation immediately after such a pause, if it is present. In this example, the first cycle after the earliest pause in the ventricular rate has a prolonged PR interval. Using a ruler or calipers, observe that this interval becomes gradually longer in subsequent beats. Then a blocked sinus beat occurs. A cycle can be recognized at the end of the strip in which the PR interval is shortened to the same length as that following the earlier blocked sinus beat and pause in ventricular complexes.

In diagrammatic form, complete the labeling of all PR intervals and blocked beats in test strip 204.

The A-V node appears to fatigue with each beat as the conduction time becomes successively longer, until one impulse fails to be transmitted. However, after a period of rest (during the blocked sinus beat), the A-V node recovers more fully. A-V conduction is improved, and the PR interval after the pause is relatively short, only to increase in subsequent beats.

Remarkably, this phenomenon (intermittent A-V block with progressing atrial to ventricular conduction times before blocked A-V conduction) was observed and correctly interpreted early in this century even *before* introduction of the ECG. One physician describing the arrhythmia was Karel Wenckebach, Professor of Medicine at the University of Groningen in Holland. With long and continued use, his name is still closely linked to this form of A-V block. Thus, the **Type I second-degree A-V block** of Mobitz is also commonly referred to as the **Wenckebach phenomenon**.

In test tracings 205 through 207, each exhibiting intermittent A-V block with Wenckebach periodicity, mark all PR intervals and determine their lengths. Do they increase in duration progressively? Indicate all blocked atrial beats. Work out the atrial to ventricular ratios.

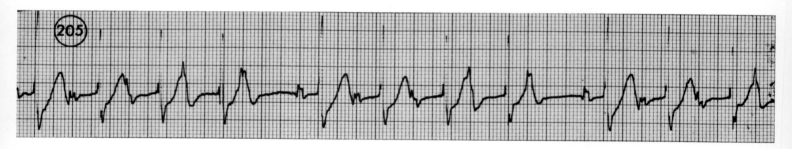

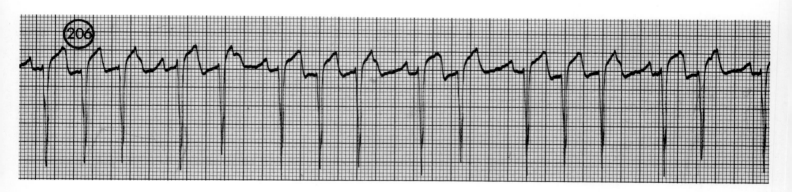

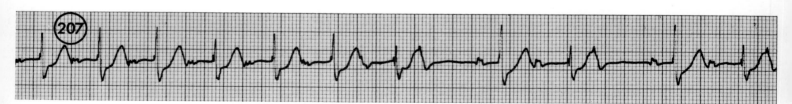

The following ECGs demonstrate the Wenckebach arrhythmia. The first strip (Fig. 5–38) is labeled for you. Complete the labeling on practice strip 208.

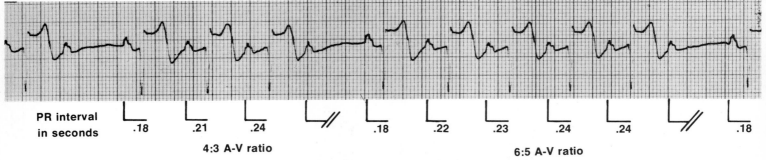

Figure 5–38. Wenckebach arrhythmia with 4:3 and 6:5 A-V block.

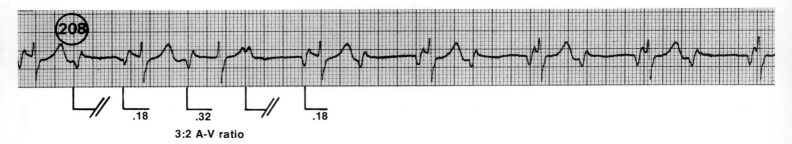

Analyze test tracings 209 through 212. In each, identify a dropped ventricular beat and, after this pause, observe the progressive lengthening of PR intervals until the next blocked sinus beat and resultant pause. In some instances, the progression is so gradual that only one blocked sinus beat (ventricular pause) is present on the tracing. Compare the shortest and longest PR intervals and determine the atrial to ventricular ratios.

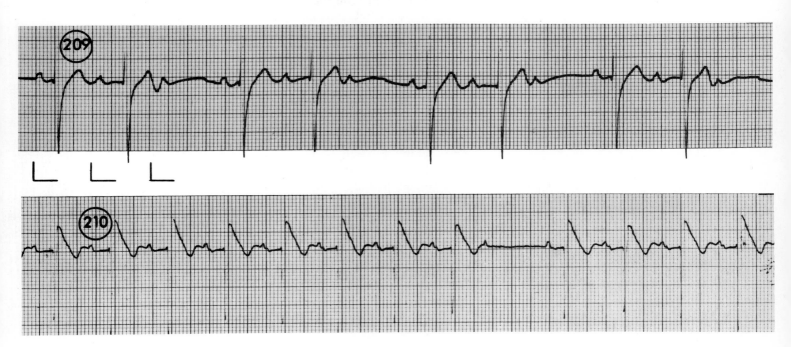

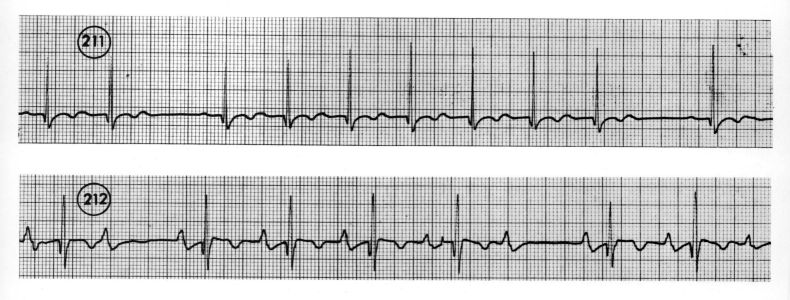

A 52-year-old man was admitted to the hospital with an acute myocardial infarction complicated by second-degree A-V block of the Wenckebach type. Spontaneous remission of the arrhythmia had already occurred at the time of this recording, although it could be elicited by application of carotid pressure (Fig. 5–39).

You can see that application of carotid pressures induces:
1. Slowing of the sinus rate.
2. Prolongation of the PR interval.
3. Temporary failure of A-V impulse transmission.

Full recovery of the cardiac rhythm occurs after the release of carotid pressure.

On the following day, carotid pressure induced similar slowing of the sinus rate and some prolongation of the PR interval, but there were no blocked beats. Further recovery was demonstrated the next day when carotid pressure again resulted in sinus slowing but no change in A-V conduction.

The effect of acute ischemic injury on the A-V node, producing Type I second-degree A-V block, has important implications in the Coronary Care Unit. As was revealed in the case just described, Type I is unlikely to progress to complete (or third-degree) A-V block, and in acute myocardial infarction it is most often transitory. Fur-

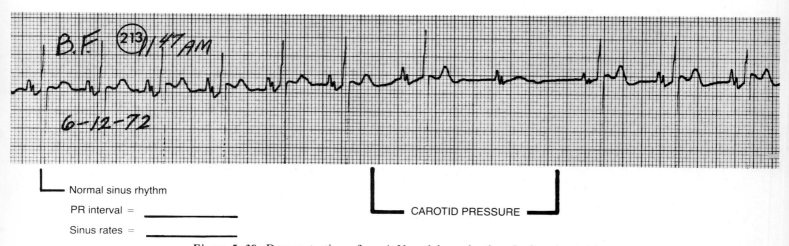

Normal sinus rhythm

PR interval =   _____

Sinus rates =   _____

Figure 5–39. Demonstration of an A-V nodal conduction dysfunction with a provocative vagotonic maneuver.

ther, hemodynamic compromise through severe bradycardia with advanced intermittent A-V block is unusual. Consequently, drug therapy or an electronic pacemaker to control Type I A-V block is seldom indicated providing that there are no concurrent complications (to be explained later).

Type I A-V block may also occur as a benign condition in otherwise completely normal individuals. This is most likely in persons with a high level of resting vagal tone, as may occur in healthy young people and especially in endurance-trained athletes.

SPECIAL FORMS OF WENCKEBACH PHENOMENON. That the Wenckebach phenomenon is a general characteristic in tissues of conduction is revealed in its occasional expression in regions of the heart beside the A-V node. Wenckebach phenomenon can occasionally be identified as the cause of rhythm irregularity in the sinus node, as a special form of sinus exit block.

Although the previous examples of the Type I intermittent A-V block pertain to sinus rhythms, the phenomenon may also occur in rhythms of atrial excitation. The following examples of atrial tachycardia present intermittent A-V block in various patterns.

In Figure 5–40, complete the labeling and indicate blocked atrial beats. PR intervals lengthen, and a pause in ventricular activity occurs after every two ventricular beats. Starting after a pause in the ventricular rate, the PR interval is 0.12 second. In the next cardiac cycle, the PR interval is 0.22 second. The atrial beat following this is blocked. The sequence then repeats itself, demonstrating the Wenckebach phenomenon in atrial tachycardia with a consistent atrial to ventricular ratio of 3:2. Atrial rate = 190. Ventricular rate = 127.

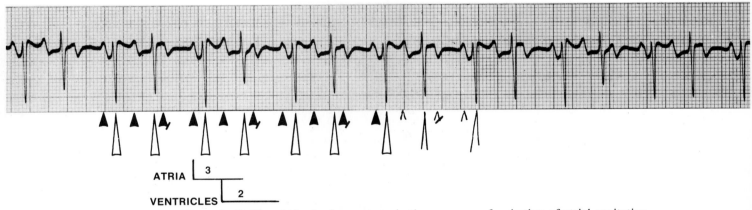

Figure 5–40. Wenckebach phenomenon in the presence of a rhythm of atrial excitation.

Figure 5–41 illustrates atrial tachycardia with Wenckebach periodicity. Identify P waves, measure PR intervals, and determine which atrial beats are blocked. Remember to begin your analysis after a pause in the ventricular rhythm. Labeling has been completed for one Wenckebach cycle. The atrial to ventricular ratio is 3:2 throughout.

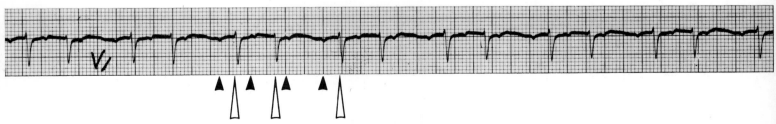

Figure 5–41. Atrial tachycardia with Wenckebach phenomenon.

The two tracings in Figure 5–42 reveal atrial tachycardia, beginning with 1:1 A-V conduction. A vagotonic maneuver is performed in an effort to restore a sinus rhythm. Observe the changes in rhythm that occur on these continuous strips.

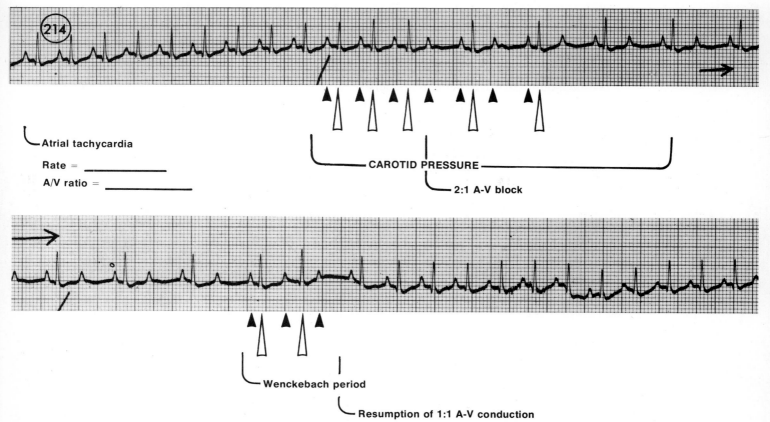

Atrial tachycardia

Rate = _____

A/V ratio = _____

CAROTID PRESSURE

2:1 A-V block

Wenckebach period

Resumption of 1:1 A-V conduction

Figure 5–42. Atrial tachycardia with varying A-V block induced with vagal stimulation.

Immediately on application of carotid stimulation, PR intervals in successive cardiac cycles lengthen gradually until a dropped beat interrupts the rhythm. There follows a short PR interval cycle with a blocked atrial beat after it, initiating a long series of beats with a 2:1 A-V block. A single set of beats then appears, exhibiting the Wenckebach phenomenon before resumption of fixed 1:1 A-V conduction. Thus, in this rhythm strip, Type I A-V block represents a transitional rhythm between 1:1 and 2:1 A-V

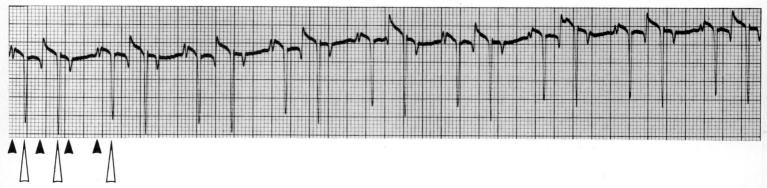

Figure 5–43. Digitalis-induced atrial tachycardia with A-V block.

conduction in both the onset and offset of parasympathetically induced intermittent A-V block.

In Figure 5–43, atrial tachycardia is present with second-degree A-V block of the Wenckebach type. The subject is a 16-year-old mongrel dog given digitalis for tachypnea in which myocardial insufficiency was the suspected cause. Each Wenckebach period is made up of three atrial and two ventricular beats. Use diagrammatic notations to label the entire tracing.

In Figure 5–44, ventricular response to atrial flutter is not random but rather occurs in groups of two and three beats. After each pause in the ventricular rate, the FR interval increases progressively in consecutive cardiac cycles. This follows the pattern of intermittent A-V block of the Wenckebach type. The A-V block is due not to an abnormality of the conduction system but rather to a physiological response to impulse overload from the atrial excitation.

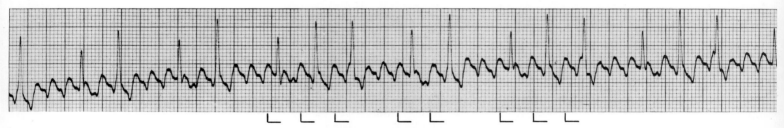

Figure 5–44. Atrial flutter with Wenckebach phenomenon.

TYPE II SECOND-DEGREE ATRIOVENTRICULAR BLOCK

Type II A-V block represents a rhythm pattern in which consecutive sinus impulses are conducted to the ventricles with nonvarying duration (*the PR intervals are constant*) but ventricular stimulation is intermittently absent (blocked sinus beats). In most instances, such a rhythm is the result of a conduction defect distal to the A-V node, somewhere in the common bundle or in its major divisions where the fibers course a narrow track, are densely packed, and have a parallel orientation.

A basic sinus rhythm is evident in Figure 5–45. However, the third sinus beat does not initiate ventricular depolarization.

In this rhythm, P waves appear normal and PR intervals are constant. The blocked sinus beat is unexpected (that is, it is not preceded by cardiac cycles with gradually lengthening PR intervals). This blocked sinus beat without gradually increasing PR

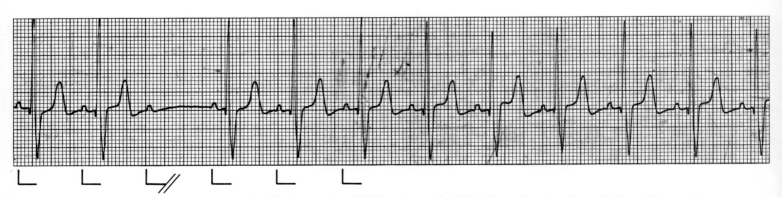

Figure 5–45. Rhythm strip exhibiting the typical blocking of a sinus beat in Type II second-degree block.

intervals preceding it defines Type II A-V block. The patient with this arrhythmia developed complete A-V block within a month. This outcome emphasizes the grave implications of the Type II intermittent A-V block.

Figure 5–46 illustrates Type II second-degree A-V block. Here, interrupted A-V conduction occurs without warning.

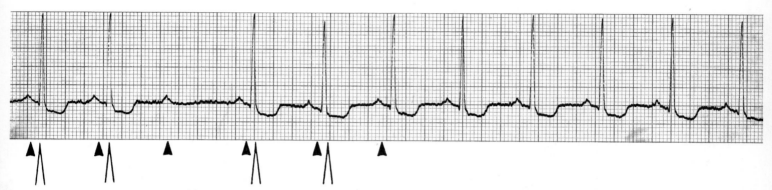

Figure 5–46. Second-degree A-V block, Type II.

Although the sinus rate is somewhat variable (changing P-P intervals), the PR intervals of all conducted beats are uniform (0.16 second). The warning of progressive lengthening in preceding cycles characteristic of Type I block is absent. Type II second-degree A-V block is an indication of disease within the His-Purkinje fibers and signals the likelihood of progression to complete A-V block. It is the form of intermittent A-V block more likely to occur in anteroseptal myocardial infarction and in degenerative diseases of the conduction system.

When second-degree A-V block has 2:1 block, Type I cannot be differentiated from Type II on the ECG. This would be the case if only the first portion of Figure 5–47 were available for analysis. The distinction, however, can be made by the His bundle electrogram.

Examples of second-degree A-V block included in the beginning of this section were chiefly of Type II. Certainly, this arrhythmia is easier to learn to identify than Type I A-V block. Yet, the unannounced blocked sinus beat associated with Type II is more often overlooked in the Coronary Care Unit because it does not give the warning signs of progressive PR interval lengthening found in Type I. Because of the gravity of this form of A-V block (which will be explained directly), precaution against such an oversight must be assured through unrelenting alertness.

A lesion depressing conduction in the slender common bundle is more likely to be expressed as Type II second-degree A-V block. (Type I is usually caused by disease more proximally in the thicker body of the A-V node.) Lesions in the common bundle are often associated with symptomatic bradycardia and usually lead to greater severity of A-V block. When encountered as a complication of acute myocardial infarction, Type II second-degree A-V block forebodes development of complete A-V block and dictates the need for intervention with an electronic pacemaker. Even with ventricular rate control by electronic pacing, Type II intermittent A-V block is commonly associated with high mortality, with myocardial failure as a sign of extensive ischemic injury.

A comparison of two distinct dysrhythmias demonstrating block is clinically important. As described under Blocked Atrial Premature Complexes, in Chapter 4, atrial premature beats occurring too early to be conducted through a refractory A-V node can become blocked. This situation is more benign than a sinus-initiated beat that fails to penetrate the A-V node because of second-degree A-V block. In Figure 5–48, these two conduction problems are contrasted.

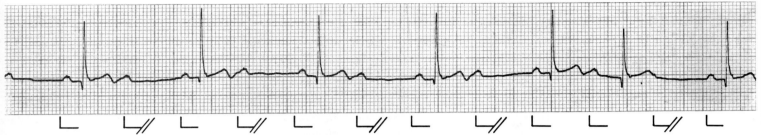

Figure 5–47. Type I second-degree A-V block is revealed when 2:1 block becomes 3:2 block near the end of the strip.

Figure 5–48*A* illustrates a sinus rhythm with first-degree A-V block (PR interval = 0.26 second). After the fifth cycle there is a pause due to absence of conduction into the ventricles. The cause of this pause can be discerned by close inspection of the T wave preceding the pause. The change in T wave configuration results from the superimposition of a premature P wave. The dysrhythmia exhibited here is a blocked atrial premature beat.

In Figure 5–48*B*, P wave number 4 is not followed by a QRS. Close inspection of the strip reveals that this P wave is related to the other P waves, indicating an origin in the sinus node. Further assessment of the strip shows that prolonging PR intervals precede the dropped beat. Thus, this strip can be labeled as Type I second-degree A-V block, a more serious situation than the blocked atrial premature complex in the first strip.

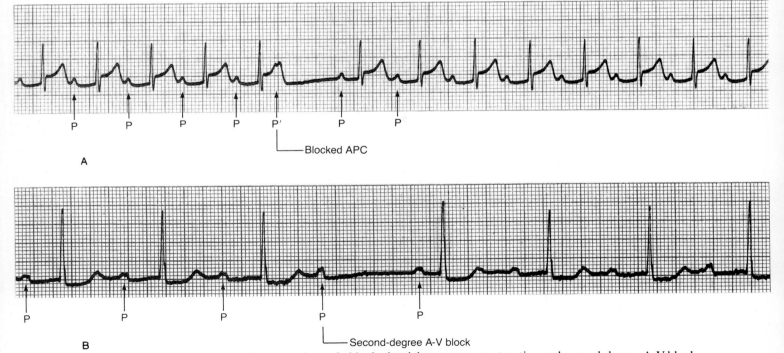

Figure 5–48. Comparison of a blocked atrial premature contraction and second-degree A-V block.

Patients with second-degree A-V block of either type are extremely susceptible to bradycardia from drugs that further suppress impulse conduction. Such drugs may act by accentuating vagal tone or by directly depressing the action potential of conductile cells. These drugs (digitalis, procainamide, quinidine, lidocaine, propranolol) may be given to treat other disorders of the myocardium or cardiac ectopic arrhythmias. Other potentially conduction-depressing drugs, such as phenothiazines (e.g., Thorazine, Compazine, Sparine) or the tricyclic antidepressants (e.g., Elavil, Tofranil, and Sinequan) may be used to treat nonrelated conditions.

Figure 5–49 contains two rhythm strips from a 62-year-old patient admitted to the hospital with complaints of intermittent syncope. On admission, she was in 2:1 second-degree block (Fig. 5–49*A*). She was experiencing lightheadedness, as well as nausea. She was given Compazine intravenously for the nausea, and within 2 minutes advanced second-degree block with 4:1 conduction was recorded (Fig. 5–49*B*).

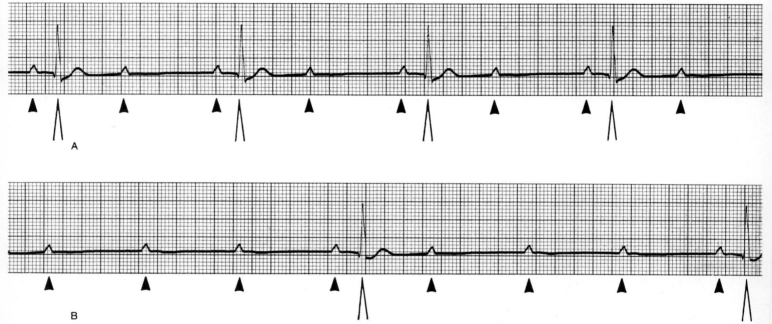

Figure 5–49. Intensification of second-degree block with intravenous administration of Compazine.

Third-Degree Atrioventricular Block

Propagation of impulses through the A-V nodal system may be so severely depressed that *no* impulses are transmitted through it. This condition is known as **complete** or **third-degree A-V block**. Because the ventricles cannot receive stimuli from the sinus or atrial pacemakers, death from ventricular standstill can only be prevented by spontaneous activation of some latent automatic cells farther along the conduction system (e.g., in the His-Purkinje apparatus).

To introduce the concept of complete A-V block, the following series of tracings is presented showing the rapid progression of A-V block from delayed A-V conduction to intermittent A-V conduction and finally to absent A-V conduction. The patient was a 56-year-old man who had incurred a massive intracerebral hemorrhage. It is suspected that the patient had a concurrent acute myocardial infarction, and the rhythm progression may have been exaggerated by severely increased intracranial pressure. The entire sequence shown here occurred in less than 1 minute.

1. First-degree A-V block.

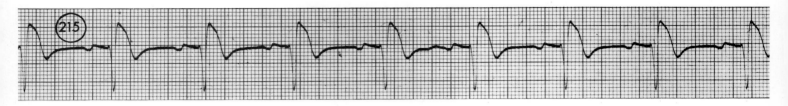

PR interval = _____

First degree A-V block.

2. Second-degree A-V block. Locate blocked sinus beats. Which type of intermittent A-V block is present?

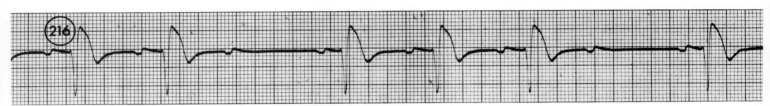

Second degree A-V block (intermittent failure of A-V node conduction).

3. Second-degree A-V block of increased severity is evident with an atrial to ventricular ratio of _____ .

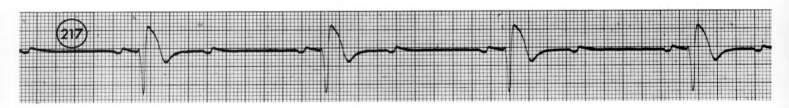

4. After a ventricular complex (evidently from an impulse conducted through the A-V node) there is cessation of further ventricular activity. Rhythmic sinus impulse formation with atrial complexes continues, but impulse transmission between atria and ventricles has become totally blocked. The patient at this point manifested signs of cardiac and respiratory arrest and could not be resuscitated.

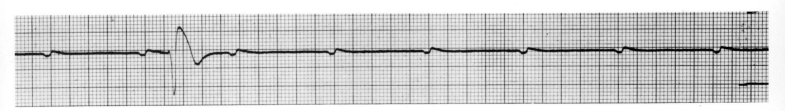

On cessation of ventricular contractions, evidence of circulatory arrest appears within a few seconds. When disease affects the A-V node and major conduction pathways between the atria and ventricles so that impulses can no longer pass, the ventricles are no longer stimulated from above. Survival then depends on the development of sustained pacemaker activity beyond the conduction disturbance.

Cardiac fibers adjacent to the A-V node and in the His-Purkinje system have the

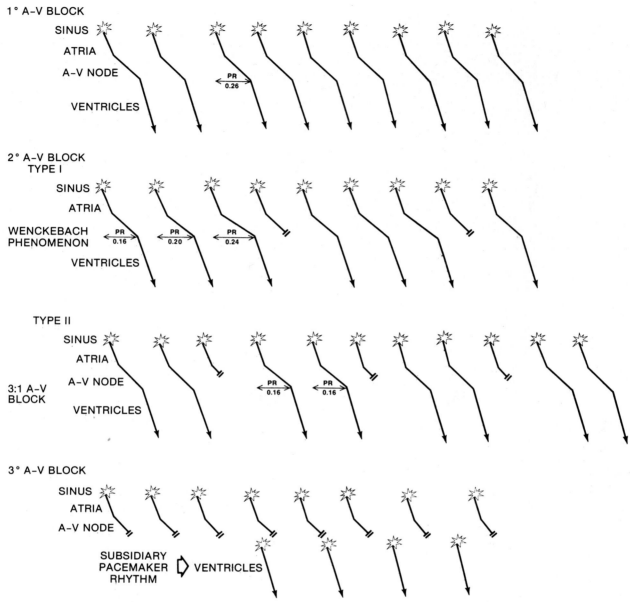

Figure 5–50. Schematic summary of forms of A-V conduction block. *First-degree A-V block:* Prolonged PR interval. All atrial depolarizations are conducted to the ventricles. *Second-degree A-V block:* Type I—Progressive lengthening of PR intervals until A-V block occurs, followed by repetition of these "Wenckebach" cycles. Type II—Intermittent A-V block with constant PR intervals. *Third-degree A-V block:* No atrial depolarizations are conducted to the ventricles. Ventricular depolarizations depend on pacemaker activity distal to the A-V node.

capability of automaticity (undergo spontaneous diastolic depolarization). As with atrial automatic cells, they generate an impulse when a naturally more rapid pacemaker impulse does not reach them within a certain time. By this mechanism, the heart is protected from standstill (absence of a pacemaker for the ventricles) when impulses from the sinus or atrial pacemakers fail to stimulate automatic tissues within the A-V junction by a given time. This interval is determined by the intrinsic rate of discharge of potential pacemakers in the A-V junction. Further discussion of third-degree A-V block will be deferred to subsequent chapters when the mechanisms of A-V junctional and ventricular escape pacemakers can be explained.

Figure 5–50 summarizes the various forms of A-V block. The slope of the conduction pathway line represents the relative velocity of impulse transmission.

6 The Atrioventricular Junction

IMPULSE FORMATION
Atrioventricular Junctional Escape Complex
Atrioventricular Junctional Rhythms with Decreased Impulse Formation
Atrioventricular Junctional Rhythms with Atrioventricular Block
ATRIOVENTRICULAR JUNCTION: IMPULSE FORMATION
Excitation
Atrioventricular Junctional Premature Complex

Retrograde Block
Atrioventricular Junctional Tachycardia
Enhanced Automaticity
Atrioventricular Independent Rhythms
Reentrant Tachycardias
Supraventricular Tachycardia
Variant Accessory Pathway Tachycardia
Treatment of Atrioventricular Junctional Tachycardias
SELF-EVALUATION: STAGE 2

IMPULSE FORMATION

Under certain conditions, automatic tissue in the region of the atrioventricular (A-V) node generates spontaneous impulses, and these impulses may assume the role of cardiac pacemaker. Thus, we introduce the important class of rhythms that originate from the intermediary zone of the cardiac conduction system.

Until recent years, electrocardiographers presumed that impulses formed in the intermediary zone arose from fibers within the A-V node itself. It is now known that the normal human A-V node does not possess the capacity for automaticity. Instead, impulses are formed in tissue near the body of the A-V node (Fig. 6–1). These automatic fibers may be in the A-V nodal approach fibers (in the vicinity of the coronary sinus where the large veins empty into the right atrium). Also, A-V nodal automatic fibers may be distal to the A-V node, in the common bundle or its divisions (where Purkinje fibers are present).

The conceptual basis for the origin of rhythms from the intermediary zone has gradually led to a shift in terminology from A-V nodal to **A-V junctional** rhythms. This more precise term is becoming well established in electrocardiography. However, rhythms arising in this region are interchangeably referred to as junctional or nodal.

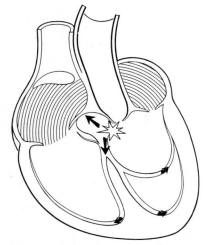

Figure 6–1. Initiation and conduction of impulses originating in A-V junctional tissue.

Latent automatic fibers in the A-V junctional tissues have properties similar to those described for potential pacemaker fibers within the atrial wall (in Chapter 4 under Atrial Escape Beats). A-V junctional rhythms may become operant under either of two general conditions:

1. Impulses generated by the sinus node and by the automatic fibers in the atria fail to stimulate the A-V nodal system within a certain interval of time.

2. Automaticity within the A-V junctional tissue is enhanced to the point of causing formation of impulses at a faster rate than that of the sinus node.

The former condition will be discussed first, explaining how A-V junctional tissues may serve as rescue (or escape) pacemakers acting as a back-up system for failure of impulse formation in proximal pacemaker regions.

Atrioventricular Junctional Escape Complex

Comparable to the mechanism already described for the atrial arrhythmias under Atrial Escape Beats in Chapter 4, escape impulses may be generated in the A-V junctional tissues. Ordinarily, these potential pacemakers are repeatedly depolarized by the more rapidly beating pacemakers in the sinus node or atria before they can undergo spontaneous depolarization. The dominance of the more proximal pacemakers is simply an expression of the inherent rate at which these various tissues normally discharge. The sinus node normally initiates conduction at a rate of 60 to 100 beats per minute, thus superseding the inherent A-V junctional impulse-forming rate, which is only 30 to 60 beats per minute.

A-V junctional beats (interchangeably also called complexes or contractions) come into play when impulses from the sinus node and atria fail to stimulate the A-V junctional tissues within the time at which these tissues remain stable at full repolarization. One cause may be slowing of either the sinus node or atrial automatic cells to less than the inherent rate of the A-V junctional tissue for self-excitation. A second cause may be the failure of an emitted impulse from these proximal pacemakers to reach the A-V junctional tissue because of depression of conduction in the intervening pathways.

Atrioventricular Junctional Rhythms with Decreased Impulse Formation

Figure 6–2 illustrates a sudden slowing of the sinus rhythm. During the pause, a QRS complex and T wave appear, identical in configurations to those of the sinus beats, thus representing usual ventricular depolarization and repolarization. However, a P wave, which normally precedes this QRS-T complex, is not present, indicating that normal atrial depolarization did not occur. Thereafter, subsequent beats suggest resumption of the normal sinus rhythm.

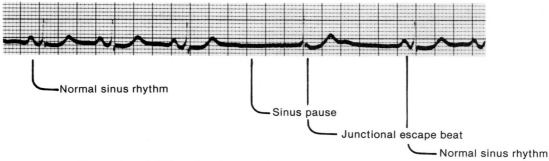

Normal sinus rhythm

Sinus pause

Junctional escape beat

Normal sinus rhythm

Figure 6–2. A-V junctional escape beat.

Using the **one-beat rate ruler**, one can reconstruct the following events. At a rate of 83 beats per minute, the sinus pacemaker controls cardiac activity. When the sinus beating slows abruptly, another usually dormant pacemaker initiates an impulse, here at a rate equivalent to 50 per minute. The impulses proceed normally into the ventricular conduction pathways. An atrial depolarization cannot be recognized as such, but the slight changes at the beginning and at the end of the escape QRS complexes may reflect simultaneous atrial depolarization proceeding in a backward (or retrograde) direction.

A-V junctional escape beating is a *normal* response to failure of ordinary pacemaker activity or impulse propagation at proximal sites. It represents another intrinsic mechanism (in addition to atrial escape beating) that protects the heart against excessive slowing.

In Figure 6–3, carotid stimulation appears to obliterate sinus node activity, resulting in the emergence of a slower rhythm having normal QRS complexes and T waves but without P waves. Thus, a series of A-V junctional escape beats has replaced the sinus rhythm on suppression of the sinus pacemaker. The presence of sinus bradycardia with first-degree A-V block at the beginning of the tracing suggests that vagal tone may be high already and that an exaggerated parasympathetic response could be anticipated.

Severe sinus bradycardia is present in Figure 6–4. The interval between beats is given in seconds above the horizontal arrows and in beats per minute below the arrows. Note that when the sinus rate slows to 28 per minute, an A-V junctional escape beat appears, sparing the heart even further slowing if it were dependent on the sinus pacemaker alone. A P wave is found immediately after this A-V junctional QRS complex; although only a portion of it is obvious, it appears to have the same configuration as P waves from sinus beats. As the sinus rate then speeds up even slightly, to 33 per minute, the next sinus beat takes over control of ventricular depolarization. Obviously, this latter rate exceeds the inherent escape rate of the A-V junctional tissue, which once again becomes dominated by the sinus pacemaker. Note, incidentally, the prominent U waves in this tracing. Do not confuse them with P waves, the U waves having a consistent time relationship with the preceding T waves even in A-V junctional beats.

In strip 218, sinus bradycardia with a junctional escape beat at number 4 is evident. Note, however, that the P waves of the preceding beats appear to be moving closer to

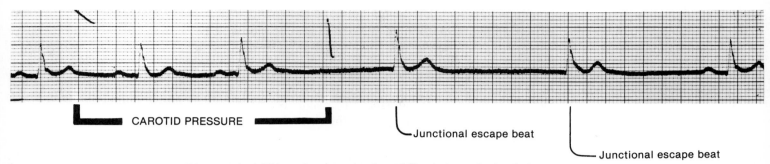

CAROTID PRESSURE

Junctional escape beat

Junctional escape beat

Figure 6–3. A-V junctional escape beat following vagal stimulation.

the QRS complexes. In beat 3, in fact, the isoelectric line produced by normal A-V nodal delay is almost nonexistent. Also note the slight slowing of the sinus rate.

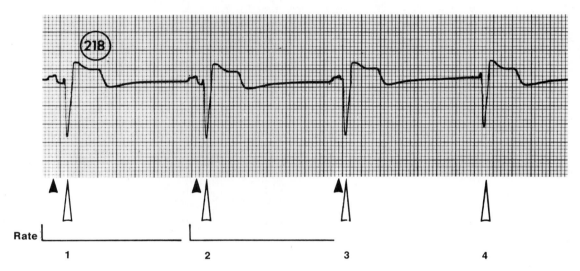

Rate

1   2   3   4

It is presumed that the slowing in sinus impulse formation, even though very slight, allowed the release of automatic firing from an A-V junctional site. This escape pacemaker rate is close to that of the sinus rate. The result, in beats 2 and 3, is a nodal

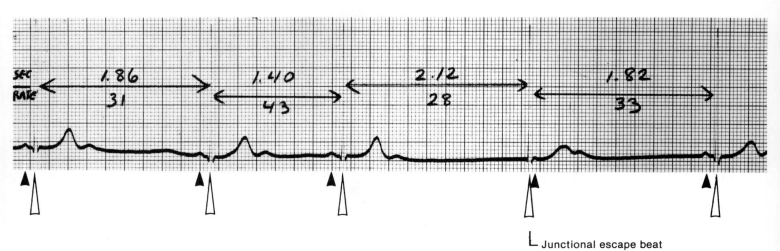

Junctional escape beat

Figure 6–4. A-V junctional escape beat.

(junctional) escape beat that begins *after* the atria have been depolarized and before this wave front can penetrate the A-V node, accounting for the changing relationship of P to QRS. In beat 4, the escape impulse begins before atrial excitation.

A sudden delay in the sinus rate occurs in test tracing 219, allowing an A-V junctional beat to escape. There is no sign of an associated P wave. In the beat that follows, a sinus P wave begins to develop, but before it can complete atrial depolarization another A-V junctional beat emerges. The sinus beating subsequently accelerates to its original rate and assumes control of the rhythm.

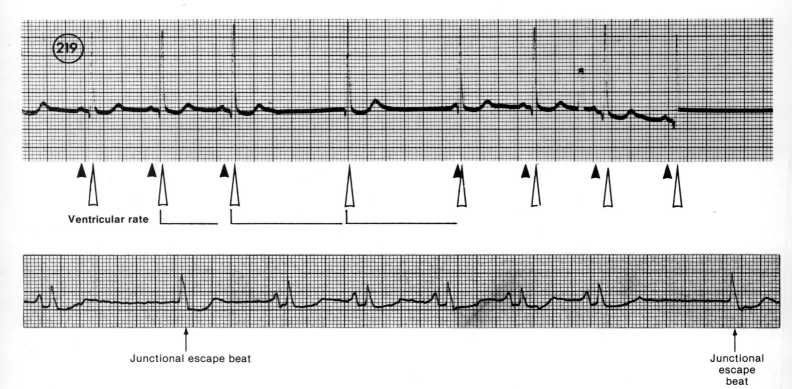

Ventricular rate

Junctional escape beat

Junctional escape beat

Figure 6–5. Two junctional escape beats interrupt pauses created by failure of the sinus node to fire.

Sinus pauses of greater than 2 seconds occur after beats 1 and 7 in Figure 6–5. The patient is prevented from fully experiencing this extended asystole by the presence of nodal escape beats (complexes 2 and 8). The inherent discharge rate for the A-V junctional tissue in this patient is 43 beats per minute. Note that the QRS complexes

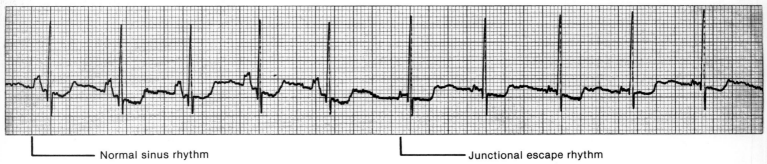

Normal sinus rhythm   Junctional escape rhythm

Figure 6–6. Assumption of rhythm control by a junctional escape rhythm.

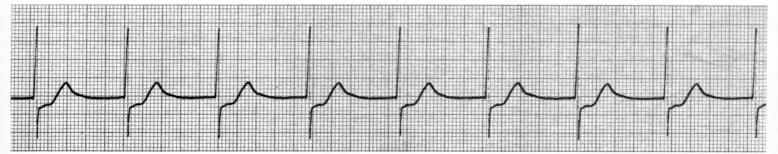

Figure 6–7. Total asystole resulting from sinus arrest is prevented by an escape junctional rhythm.

exhibit a configuration similar to the sinus initiated beats; however, there is no P wave preceding the ventricular complex.

When sinus node depression extends for a long period, junctional escape rhythms can sustain ventricular activity. In Figure 6–6, the sinus node initially shows no abnormality, firing at a rate of 83 per minute. However, the sixth complex reveals an alteration in pacemaker activity: The rate slows to 76, the P wave configuration changes, and the PR interval shortens to 0.10 second. All of these characteristics indicate the mechanism of a junctional escape rhythm.

Complete asystole was averted in Figure 6–7 through the maintenance of ventricular activity by a junctional escape rhythm at a rate of 62 beats per minute. The blood pressure during this episode dropped from 126/70 to 100/60, but the patient experienced no symptoms.

Thus far, examples of A-V junctional rhythms are relatively simple in that the A-V junctional beat stimulated only the ventricles; the atria were either under sinus node control or were at a standstill. However, a characteristic feature of impulses that originate in the A-V junctional tissues is that the impulse transmits back through the atria as well as forward to the ventricles. As already described, the forward (or **antegrade**) impulse follows the ordinary route through the His-Purkinje system, and there is no change in the resultant QRS complex. The wave front that proceeds backward (or **retrograde**) through the atria activates these chambers in reverse direction compared with sinus-originated beats. The P wave so produced exhibits altered form and is often opposite in polarity from the normal P waves in some leads (Fig. 6–8).

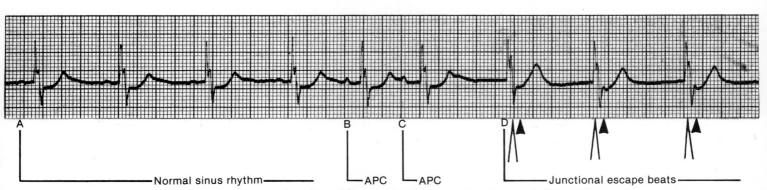

Figure 6–8. Note the altered form and polarity of the P wave in this example of retrograde conduction.

In Figure 6–8, a retrograde P wave can be identified in the terminal portion of the last three QRS complexes, all junctional escape beats. A full interpretation of the rhythm shows the following:

1. Four beats of sinus rhythm with a PR interval of 0.17 second.
2. An atrial premature complex (APC) with a PR interval of 0.17 second.

3. An APC with a PR interval of 0.20 second.

4. Junctional escape beats with retrograde P waves.

Depolarization of the atria by a retrograde wave front may occur before, during, or after depolarization of the ventricles, depending on the time relationship of conduction from the pacemaker to these sets of chambers. Accordingly, the P wave may appear before, during, or after the QRS complex initiated by the junctional impulse (Fig. 6–9).

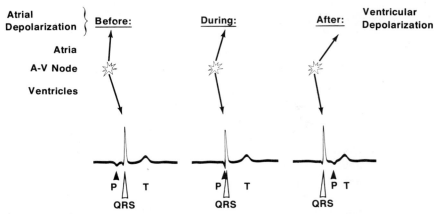

Figure 6–9. Schematic of antegrade and retrograde conduction from the A-V junction.

Because it is important to identify retrograde P waves to establish the diagnosis of A-V junctional rhythms, examples of the three possible positions relative to QRS complexes are provided.

P wave precedes the QRS complex.

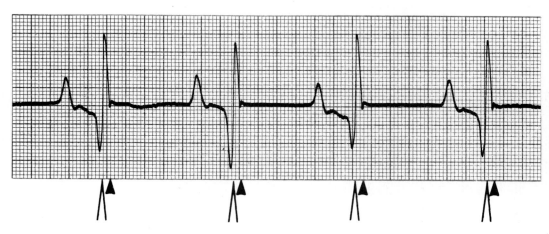

P wave is buried in the QRS complex.

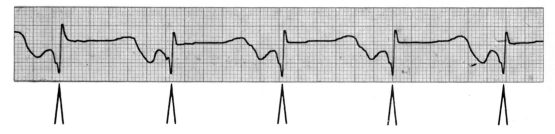

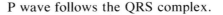

P wave follows the QRS complex.

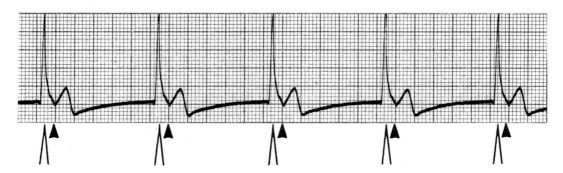

An impulse from the A-V junction sometimes fails to propagate in a retrograde direction. Consequently, atrial depolarization from this impulse is absent, and of course no retrograde P wave will be formed.

When severe slowing of the sinus rate occurs (or when sinus arrest develops), a sustained A-V junctional escape rhythm may become established. Such a rhythm exhibits the inherent periodicity of its rate of spontaneous depolarization. This rate depends on which portion of the A-V junctional tissue acts as pacemaker.

If the proximal portion of the A-V nodal system serves as pacemaker, the usual rate is between 45 and 60 beats per minute. Because this is a region where autonomic neural control is strong, the rate can be modified appreciably through autonomic stimulation or suppression. For example, vagal stimulation can be expected to slow the rate appreciably whereas atropine may increase the rate of the A-V junctional pacemaker by about 30 beats per minute.

In Figure 6–10, the effects of nausea and atropine on the sinus and junctional discharge rates are demonstrated in three rhythm strips recorded from the same patient.

The first strip shows the initial effects of retching (vagal stimulation) with intermittent severe slowing of the sinus rate (to 37 beats per minute) and a prolonged PR interval (0.24 second). The patient's blood pressure was stable at 124/74.

In the second strip, additional slowing of the sinus node discharge rate (36 and 35 beats per minute, cycles 2 and 4, respectively) allows nodal escape beats (rate of 39 beats per minute) when the patient is vomiting. The patient also complained of lightheadedness at this time, and her blood pressure dropped to 90/70. Intravenous atropine was administered.

The last strip shows the transition back to the patient's normal sinus pattern. Initially the sinus rate was only 36 beats per minute, allowing the junctional site to capture the second complex at a rate of 39 per minute. The atropine has increased both the sinus and junctional firing rates, with a lesser effect on the A-V junction. The sinus node eventually resumes normal firing at a rate averaging 60 beats per minute by the end of the series. First-degree A-V block is still present.

Rhythms emanating from the distal portion of the A-V nodal system (e.g., the common bundle) have a much slower rate, between 30 and 40 beats per minute. Autonomic control is usually lacking, and atropine causes no acceleration of rate in A-V junctional rhythms originating here. Additionally, carotid stimulation and other vagotonic interventions are likely to have little or no effect on the rate.

Analyze test tracings 220, 221, 222, and 223 and determine if the A-V junctional rhythms arise from the proximal or the distal portion of the A-V junctional tissue. Note the precise regularity of pacemaker activity in tracing 220, a typical finding when the impulse-forming tissue is not under strong autonomic control. The terminal portion of QRS complexes of A-V junctional beats in tracing 221 is more prominent than in those of sinus node origin. These inscriptions most likely represent the ends of P waves superimposed on the QRS complexes indicating that sinus-atrial depolarization started *during* ventricular depolarization.

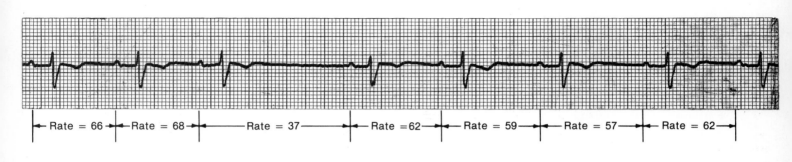

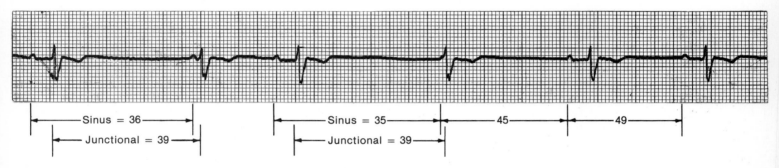

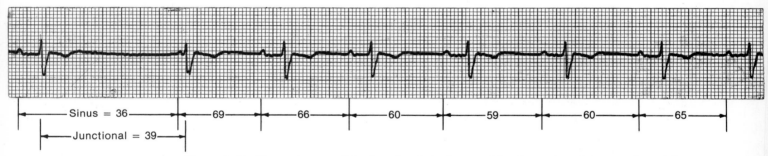

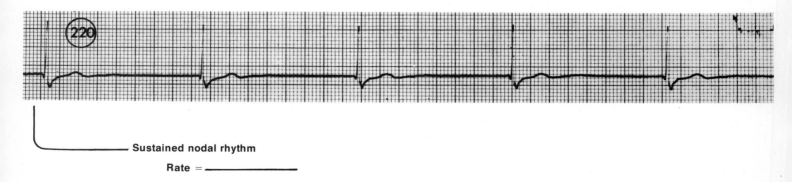

Figure 6-10. Change in rate of the junctional rhythm resulting from altered autonomic activity.

Sustained nodal rhythm

Rate = _____

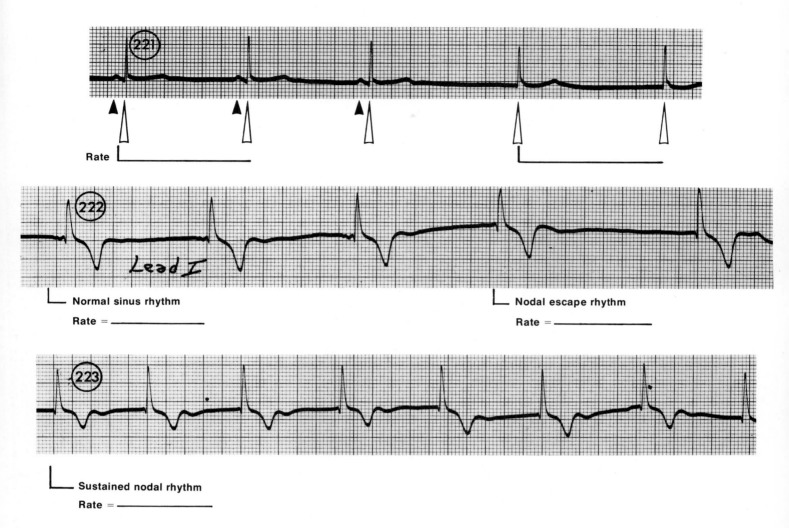

Rate

Normal sinus rhythm

Rate = _____

Nodal escape rhythm

Rate = _____

Sustained nodal rhythm

Rate = _____

Atrioventricular Junctional Rhythms with Atrioventricular Block

The preceding electrocardiograms (ECGs) demonstrate the activation of latent pacemakers in the A-V junctional tissue in response to failure or delay of impulse formation at a more proximal site (e.g., the sinus node and automatic atrial fibers). Examples will now be given of similar activation of A-V junctional pacemakers, but the underlying pathology is failure of transmission of impulses from higher centers to the A-V nodal system. By this mechanism, ventricular contractions will continue even in the presence of severe grades of sinoatrial or A-V nodal conduction block.

Figure 6–11 begins with a sinus rhythm showing first-degree A-V block. Parasympathetic stimulation converts the conduction delay into complete A-V block. After an interval of 1.74 seconds, an A-V junctional beat appears, terminating the ventricular pause. Note that vagal stimulation has slowed the sinus rate somewhat as well as increased the conduction defect. By measurement with calipers, one can determine that the change in the terminal configuration of the A-V junctional escape beat is actually due to a sinus-initiated P wave. After four blocked sinus beats, a sinus rhythm with first-degree A-V block returns.

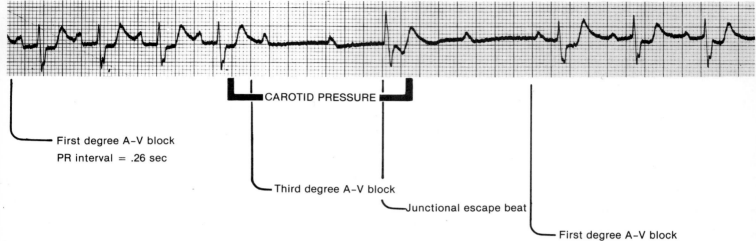

First degree A–V block
PR interval = .26 sec

CAROTID PRESSURE

Third degree A–V block

Junctional escape beat

First degree A–V block

Figure 6–11. Transitory complete A-V block with A-V junctional pacemaker.

We now encounter the condition of complete A-V block in which the ventricular rhythm is sustained by an A-V junctional pacemaker. In complete A-V block, there is no transmission of impulses between atria and ventricles; separate and wholly independent rhythms coexist in the atria and in the ventricles. Complete A-V block is illustrated in Figure 6–12, displaying regular atrial and ventricular beating but without any temporal relationship between the two.

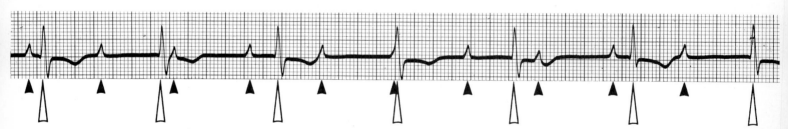

Figure 6–12. The regular atrial and ventricular complexes that have no temporal relationship indicate a junctional pacemaker maintaining ventricular activity in this sample of complete A-V block.

Interpreting this ECG step by step, the first P wave-QRS complex appears to be a normal cardiac cycle with a normal PR interval. The next cycle has an extremely long PR interval. Then, a blocked P wave occurs. Up to this point, one might suspect that second-degree A-V block of the Wenckebach type has occurred. However, this pattern does *not* recur and, in fact, no pattern can be recognized linking atrial with ventricular beating. Instead, the atrial beats are set at one rate (75 per minute) and the ventricles at another (49 per minute). The constancy of each independent rhythm and lack of relationship between the rhythms can be verified by using calipers.

We deduce the following features of this tracing:

- A pacemaker in the sinus node or atrium fires at a regular rate.
- A conduction defect in the A-V nodal system prevents all of the supraventricular impulses from reaching the ventricles.
- A pacemaker located in the A-V nodal system beyond the impulse blockade serves to drive the ventricles, in this case at a much slower rate than that of the supraventricular pacemaker.

- None of the A-V junctional impulses enter the atria, indicating that the disturbance in conduction also exists for the retrograde pathways.

The tracing below was recorded from a 52-year-old man with an acute myocardial infarction (Fig. 6–13).

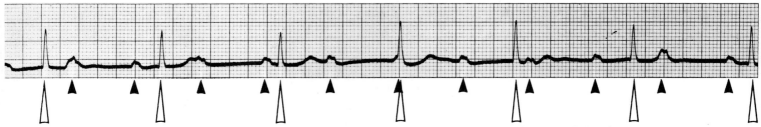

Figure 6–13. Complete A-V block in a patient with an acute myocardial infarction.

Note that the atrial rhythm is steady at 86 beats per minute. (The use of calipers will help in locating P waves even when they are superimposed on QRS complexes.) The ventricular rate is 47 per minute, and it has almost perfect regularity. Apparent PR intervals are extremely variable, and no pattern of intermittent A-V block can be recognized. Because both the atrial and the ventricular rhythms are virtually regular but at different rates, the sets of chambers must be beating independently, indicating the presence of complete A-V block. Intermittent (second-degree) A-V block also results in a faster atrial than vetricular beat. In 2:1 A-V block, the atrial rate would be exactly twice the ventricular rate. If the Wenckebach periodicity were present (accounting for the variance in PR intervals), the ventricular rhythm would be irregular owing to a recurring pause from blocked sinus impulses. Neither intermittent A-V block condition fits the pattern of the ECG shown here.

Rhythm strip 224 is aVR from the standard ECG obtained from an elderly man with a long-standing "very slow pulse" and recent postural syncope.

Sinus rate = _____   Regular? _____

Ventricular rate = _____   Regular? _____

Is there any time relationship between sinus and A–V nodal beats? **No**
Interpretation ***Complete A-V block with A-V junctional pacemaker***

Practice interpretation of A-V junctional rhythms by filling in the blanks for rhythm strips 225 to 230.

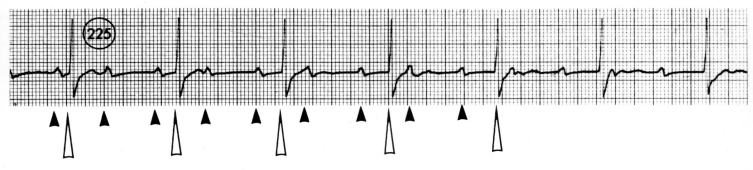

Sinus rate = _____ A–V junctional rate = _____

Is there any relationship between sinus and A–V junctional beats? _____

Interpretation *Complete A-V block with A-V junctional pacemaker*

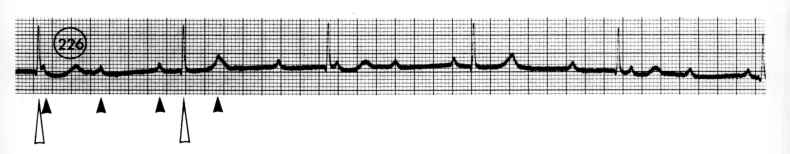

Label remaining P waves and QRS complexes.

Sinus rate = _____ A-V junctional rate = _____

Is there any relationship between sinus and A-V junctional beats? _____

Interpretation _____

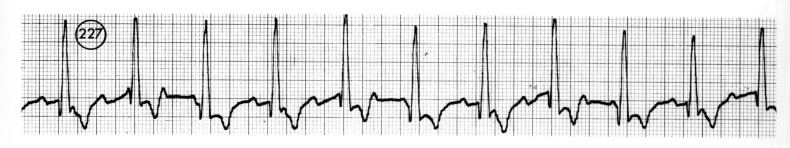

Label completely.

Atrial rate = _____ Ventricular rate = _____

Atrioventricular activity: Related? _____ Unrelated? _____

Interpretation _____

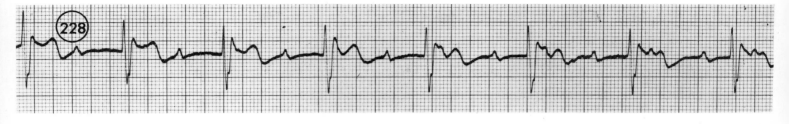

Atrial rate = _____ Ventricular rate = _____
Atrioventricular activity: Related? _____ Unrelated? _____
Interpretation _____

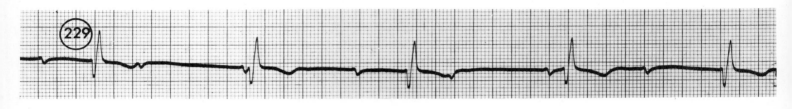

Atrial rate = _____ Ventricular rate = _____
Atrioventricular activity: Related? _____ Unrelated? _____
Interpretation _____

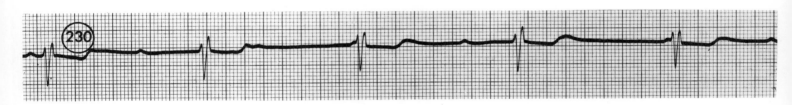

Atrial rate = _____ Ventricular rate = _____
Atrioventricular activity: Related? _____ Unrelated? _____
Interpretation _____

Complete A-V block may occur with various supraventricular rhythms. In examples already provided, sinus tachycardia, sinus bradycardia, and atrial tachycardia were present. Figure 6–14 reveals atrial fibrillation with complete A-V block.

Examine the ventricular rhythm, measuring out with calipers, and note that it is precisely regular. The only mechanism by which the ventricular rhythm could remain regular in the presence of a totally irregular atrial rhythm is by electrical isolation of the chambers with an independent pacemaker distal to the block controlling the ventricles.

In the tracing in Figure 6–14, third-degree A-V block was induced by digitalis. Such pharmacological block is an important sign of digitalis toxicity in atrial fibrillation. Hence, when a patient who has atrial fibrillation and who is on digitalis develops a regular ventricular rate (or a regular apical heartbeat), one should suspect this serious form of drug toxicity.

The following series demonstrates progression and regression of various forms of A-V block in acute myocardial infarction and the responses of impulse formation and conduction to a sympathetic stimulating agent.

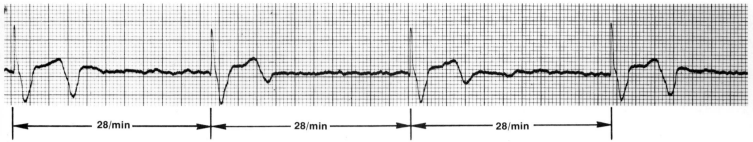

Figure 6–14. Atrial fibrillation with slow ventricular rate.

1. 6/9/71—12:45 PM: Portions of the standard ECG taken in the ER of a 54-year-old man with chest pain and the electrocardiographic pattern of acute myocardial infarction reveal intermittent A-V conduction with 2:1 A-V block. The ventricular rate was 47 per minute. The wide Q waves in leads II and III indicate transmural myocardial necrosis, probably in the inferior wall. The prominent ST segment elevation present in these leads is characteristic of injury of recent origin (the so-called hyperacute stage).

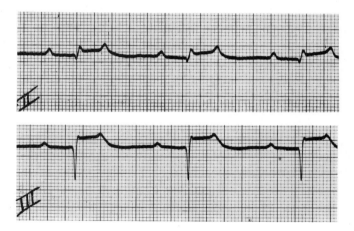

In 2:1 A-V block, one cannot be certain if the pathology is of the Type I or the Type II mechanism. As explained in Chapter 5, Type I A-V block is more likely to be located in the A-V node and to be temporary; Type II, located in the more distal portion of the A-V nodal system, tends to be irreversible and often progresses to higher degrees of block.

2. 1:15 PM: On transfer of the patient to the Coronary Care Unit, the cardiac monitor disclosed complete A-V block with an A-V junctional pacemaker having a rate of 46 per minute. Although the atrial rhythm is somewhat irregular, the ventricular rhythm is almost exactly regular. There are no pauses in the ventricular beat, and PR intervals are grossly variable. Only a dissociation of atrial and ventricular rhythms could produce this pattern. Note that ST segment elevation has become more marked in this lead (lead III). T waves have become inverted, a sign of ischemia that often occurs shortly after the onset of acute myocardial infarction.

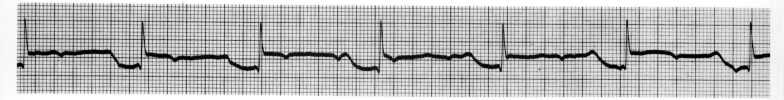

3. 1:20 PM: Isoproterenol was given by intravenous infusion, 1 mg/1000 ml 5% D/W at 50 drops per minute.

4. 1:27 PM: Second-degree A-V block has been reestablished, but the rhythm is now of the Wenckebach type with an atrial to ventricular ratio of 3:2. The ventricular rate is 76 per minute.

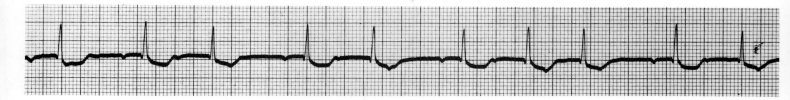

5. 2:12 PM: Complete A-V block has reappeared, even though the concentration of isoproterenol has been increased to 2 mg/1000 ml 5% D/W, and the infusion rate sped up to 100 drops per minute. The A-V junctional rate has increased from 46 to 64 per minute.

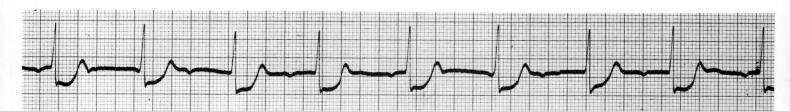

Complete A-V block persisted through the subsequent 2 days, while the infusion of isoproterenol was continued at 50 drops per minute at the same concentration. An interesting development during this time was the transient appearance of atrial fibrillation, demonstrated in the next ECG.

6. 6/11/71—8:45 AM: Complete A-V block is evident. After the sixth ventricular beat, atrial fibrillation emerges. Note that there is no change in the ventricular rate or regularity because of the conduction abnormality.

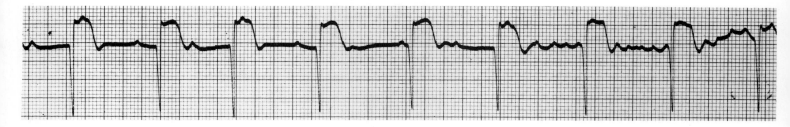

7. 12:45 PM: Second-degree A-V block has reappeared and is again of the Wenckebach type with an atrial to ventricular ratio of 3:2. The isoproterenol is still being infused at 2 mg/1000 ml 5% D/W at 50 drops per minute.

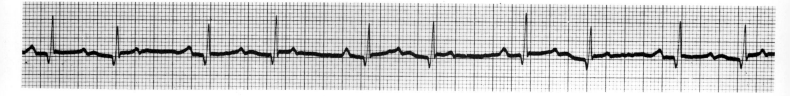

8. 12:52 PM: The rate of the infusion is increased from 50 to 100 drops per minute. Continuous tracings reveal improvement in A-V conduction.

The severity of second-degree A-V block decreases from a 3:2 to an 8:7 atrial to ventricular ratio because of the increased adrenergic stimulation, observed in the middle of the upper tracing below.

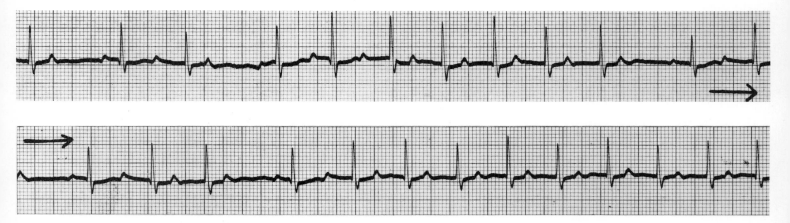

Then a 4:3 ratio appears, followed by complete sinus capture, in which the PR interval is prolonged. The sinus rate is 117 per minute, and the PR interval 0.33 second. This first-degree A-V block persists, even as the isoproterenol concentration and infusion rate are gradually reduced.

9. By 6/12/71, the isoproterenol concentration has been reduced to 1 mg/1000 ml 5% D/W and the infusion rate slowed to 25 drops per minute.

10:30 AM: The PR interval has been decreased to within normal limits (0.19 second). An APC occurs and is blocked. The PR interval immediately following the resultant ventricular pause is even shorter (0.13 second).

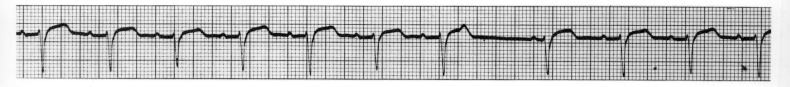

Isoproterenol was discontinued at 2:00 PM after gradually decreasing its infusion rate.

10. 3:00 PM: Stable normal sinus rhythm is maintained without pharmacological agents.

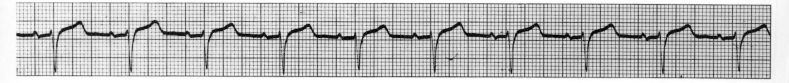

The subsequent course of recovery from acute myocardial infarction remained entirely uneventful. The patient has withstood a serious arrhythmia complicating acute myocardial infarction with support by an adrenergic agent given to prevent symptomatic bradycardia. The temporary nature of this arrhythmia is entirely consistent with a Type I lesion, and indeed, the Wenckebach phenomenon appeared as a transitional rhythm both entering into and emerging from complete A-V block. Furthermore, inferior myocardial infarction is more commonly associated with Type I A-V block than are infarctions in other locations.

Because of highly predictable recovery from Type I second-degree A-V block in acute myocardial infarction, specific treatment is often not necessary except to protect against severe, associated bradycardias. Isoproterenol may serve as an effective expedient in such bradycardic emergencies, although it has the undesirable effects of increasing myocardial work and metabolic requirements as well as enhancing ectopic automaticity. Today, a temporary electronic pacemaker would probably have been inserted in this patient at the time complete A-V block was recognized.

ATRIOVENTRICULAR JUNCTION: IMPULSE FORMATION

Excitation

The escape beat from the A-V junctional region was described as a *normal* response to failure of a higher-order pacemaker to function within a critical time or of failure of impulses from such pacemakers to reach the A-V node. In contrast, A-V junctional tissue may be excited so that impulses are emitted at a faster rate than the normally dominant pacemaker. The result is ectopic beats occurring singly or in succession: A-V junctional (nodal) premature complexes (NPC) or A-V junctional (nodal) tachycardia (NT) and accelerated rhythms (Fig. 6–15).

Atrioventricular Junctional Premature Complex

Impulses arising from excited automatic fibers in the A-V junction typically produce beats that have the following features:

1. They occur prematurely.

2. Depolarization of the ventricles takes place by forward (or antegrade) propagation through the usual pathways of the His-Purkinje system. Hence, activation of the ventricles occurs in the normal sequence, and QRS complexes are altered in neither form nor duration from those produced by impulses originating in the sinus node.

3. Depolarization of the atria is caused by backward (or retrograde) conduction of the impulse from the discharged A-V junctional site. The sequence of activation of the atrial chambers occurs in *reversed* order.

4. The sinus node is eventually depolarized by the invading retrograde impulse. Because the action potential of the sinus node is interrupted prematurely, it must undergo repolarization anew before it again can discharge spontaneously. Thus, the cadence of the normally beating sinus node may be reset, reflected in a slight change in its rhythmicity.

5. The time relationship between retrograde atrial and antegrade ventricular depolarization determines the position of the P wave and the QRS complex relative to each other. Because an A-V junctional impulse is usually carried much more rapidly through the His-Purkinje fibers than through the A-V node fibers, the QRS complex usually falls *before* the P wave or the P wave will be at least partially superimposed on it.

These characteristics describe the physiological and electrocardiographic activity of premature junctional beats. As with atrial premature beats, they are also referred to as complexes or contractions.

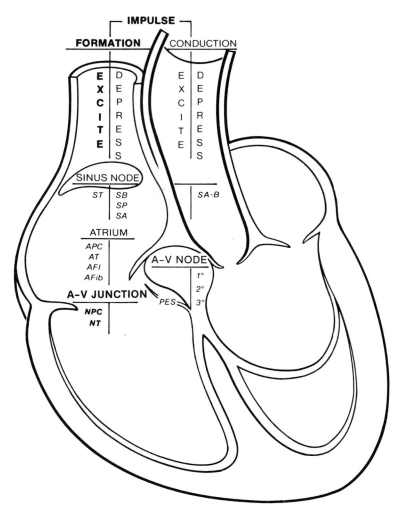

Figure 6–15. Excitation of A-V junctional tissue. NPC = nodal premature contraction; NT = nodal tachycardia.

All of these characteristics can be observed in the ECG in Figure 6–16.

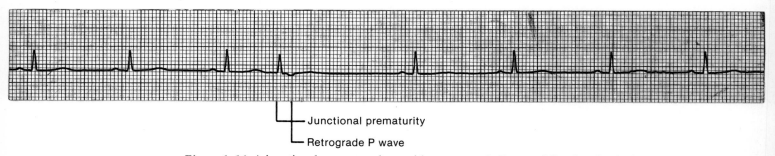

└── Junctional prematurity

└── Retrograde P wave

Figure 6–16. A junctional premature beat with a retrograde P wave following the QRS complex.

The premature beat shown appears *earlier* than the expected sinus beat, not later as occurs with escape beats. In addition, the premature beat alters the established rhythmic pacing of the sinus node. The QRS complex of the premature beat is similar in every way to QRS complexes produced by the sinus node impulse. The P wave of this beat is inscribed *after* the QRS. Furthermore, the direction of the P wave is opposite in direction from P waves resulting from the sinus impulse. In these latter features (QRS appearance and P wave locations and configuration), the premature cycle resembles escape beats already described.

The different timing relationship between antegrade QRS complexes and retrograde P waves from an impulse arising in an A-V junctional pacemaker are exemplified in the three tracings that follow. Accompanying laddergrams will help to clarify these events. Remember that A-V nodal fibers conduct more slowly than fibers in the His-Purkinje system, whether in a forward or reverse direction. An additional determinant of the time of onset of atrial and ventricular depolarization is the proximity of the ectopic pacemaker to these chambers.

1. The retrograde P wave is inscribed just before the QRS complex and can be recognized as a deformity in the initial portion of the QRS (Fig. 6–17).

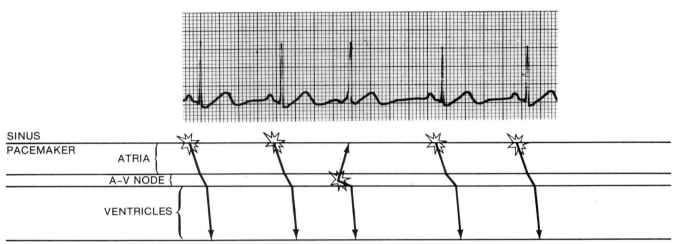

Figure 6–17. Nodal premature contraction with retrograde P wave distorting the initial portion of the QRS complex.

2. The retrograde P wave begins *during* the inscription of the QRS complex and is observed as a slight deflection on the initial portion of the waveform (Fig. 6–18).

3. The retrograde P wave occurs in its entirety *after* the corresponding QRS com-

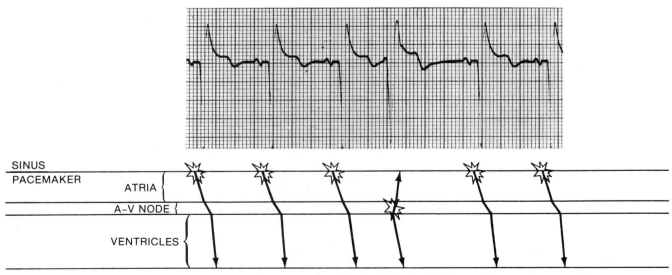

Figure 6–18. Retrograde P wave inscribed within the QRS complex.

plex, reflecting relatively slow conduction through the A-V node to the atria (Fig. 6–19). One can then refer to an R-P interval, in this instance measured at 0.10 second. It is interesting to note that the duration between corresponding points of consecutive sinus P waves is almost precisely that between the *end* of the retrograde P wave and the beginning of the next sinus P wave. This period corresponds to the normal cycling time of the action potential of the sinus node.

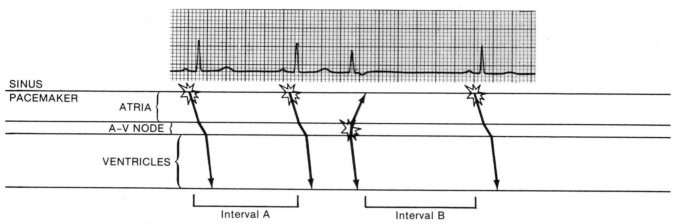

Figure 6–19. Retrograde P wave visible following the QRS complex.

Retrograde Block

Impulses that arise in the A-V junctional tissue are readily carried into the ventricles by the Purkinje fibers. They propagate more slowly and more tortuously through the proximal A-V nodal system toward the atria. When the A-V junctional pacemaker rate exceeds the capacity of the A-V node to respond to these retrograde impulses, the beat is blocked. This capacity is further limited by all those physiological influences that inhibit impulse conduction and were noted at the end of the section entitled First-Degree A-V Block in Chapter 5. These factors include augmented parasympathetic tone and direct conduction fiber inhibitors such as ischemia, inflammation, and depressor drugs.

Recognition of an A-V junctional beat with retrograde block will be explained using the ECG in Figure 6–20.

A premature beat is identified. Although the QRS complex appears normal in form and in duration, there is no evident P wave, either before or after the QRS complex.

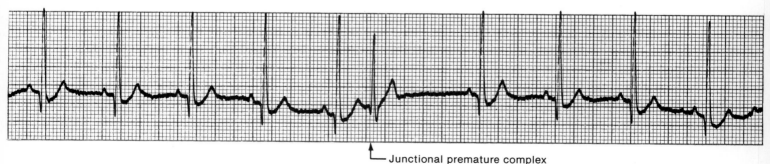

Figure 6–20. An A-V junctional beat with retrograde block.

Of course, atrial depolarization could occur simultaneously with ventricular depolarization and therefore be entirely masked. However, the premature QRS complex is similar to those of sinus beats, weighing against the likelihood of a hidden P wave. Hence, there is no evidence of atrial depolarization from the premature beat, and it can be presumed that the retrograde impulse dissipated somewhere in the A-V nodal system. The normal on-time blocked sinoatrial depolarization is obscured by the T wave of the premature beat.

Supporting the assumption that retrograde block has occurred is the absence of change in sinus node rhythmicity after the premature beat (confirm with calipers). Remember that retrograde conduction ordinarily depolarizes the sinus node, resetting its cadence and producing a pause in the cycling of sinus-originated P waves.

Additionally, blockage of impulse conduction can occur in just the region of the sinus node itself. Figure 6–21 demonstrates premature nodal complexes (beats 2, 5, and 8), which have the following characteristics:

1. Prematurity.
2. Normal QRS complexes.
3. Abnormal P waves (P′) preceding early QRS beats with PR intervals of 0.10 second.
4. P waves (P) following early QRS complexes with configurations that resemble sinus P waves and that are in cadence with other sinus P waves.

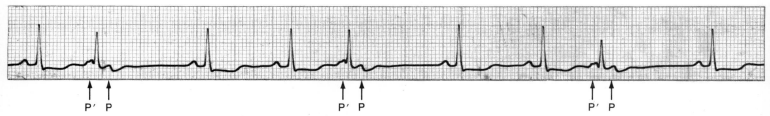

Figure 6–21. Failure of a premature junctional beat to depolarize the sinus node through retrograde conduction.

These apparent sinus P waves indicate that the P′ that resulted from the premature junctional beat failed to depolarize the sinus node. The sinus P is unable to produce a subsequent QRS complex because the ventricles have not recovered from the junctional activation. (Note that repolarization, as indicated by the T wave, occurs after the sinus P wave.)

Atrioventricular Junctional Tachycardia

When excitation of automatic tissue within the A-V junction is sustained, tachycardia results. Just as atrial premature beats are the progenitors of atrial tachycardia, so may A-V junctional premature beats be isolated expressions forerunning A-V junctional tachycardia. In both instances, the underlying mechanism may be either enhanced automaticity or a reentrant circuit movement. Recognition of these different mechanisms is crucial because of the different requirements for effective clinical management.

Two episodes of A-V junctional tachycardia interrupting a sinus rhythm are shown in the next tracing (Fig. 6–22).

Cardiac cycles occurring during the tachycardia exhibit the same characteristics as A-V junctional premature beats. To review, the QRS complexes are normal in morphology and duration; the P waves cannot be clearly identified.

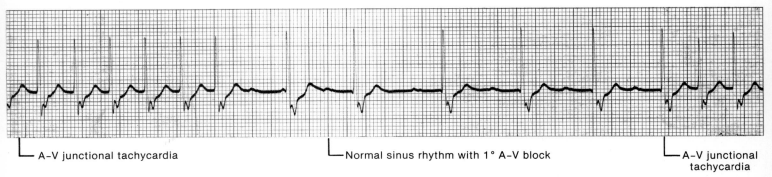

└─A-V junctional tachycardia   └─Normal sinus rhythm with 1° A-V block   └─A-V junctional
                                                                                       tachycardia

Figure 6–22. Interruption of sinus rhythm by two episodes of A-V junctional tachycardia.

Before proceeding further, we should clarify a point in terminology. A rhythm of A-V junctional origin is designated A-V junctional **tachycardia** when the rate is 100 beats per minute or faster. You will recall that the inherent rate of automatic tissue within the A-V node varies from 30 to 60 beats per minute, depending in part on which portion of the A-V junctional tissue acts as an escape pacemaker. When a pacemaker in the A-V junction is excited so that it produces a rhythm faster than 60 but less than 100 beats per minute, it is designated an **accelerated** A-V junctional rhythm. These limits are arbitrary, and some variations in limits exist among authorities. The terms *accelerated* and *tachycardic* rhythms, incidentally, define an accepted rate; they do not imply whether the causative mechanism is from enhanced automaticity or is of the reentrant circuit type.

Enhanced Automaticity

When automatic fibers within the A-V junction undergo changes that accelerate the rate of spontaneous depolarization, A-V junctional tachyarrhythmias may arise. Disturbances that cause this enhanced automaticity are the same as those also known to produce atrial tachyarrhythmias: ischemia, inflammation, anesthesia, trauma, drug toxicity, and adrenergic stimuli. Persons without cardiac disease or drug influence occasionally develop A-V junctional tachyarrhythmias. Whether an atrial or an A-V junctional pacemaker becomes activated under automaticity-provoking circumstances depends on a complex interplay of many factors on the action potentials of these tissues.

A-V junctional tachyarrhythmias caused by enhanced automaticity may be revealed by characteristics of their onset and offset. Specifically, the ectopic rhythm replaces the dominant sinus rhythm, taking over in a gradually accelerating rate until a steady rate is reached. The end of the tachycardia is conversely a gradual, rather than abrupt, slowing of rate until the sinus pacemaker once again controls the heartbeat. (The gradual acceleration and deceleration of ectopic pacemakers resulting from enhanced automaticity have already been described for the atrial tachycardias.) Detecting such details, so important in differentiating this type of arrhythmia from those of reentrant mechanisms, emphasizes the value of recording and carefully examining the beginning and the end of these tachycardias.

Although there are no fixed limits for rates of A-V junctional tachyarrhythmias from enhanced automaticity, the upper range seldom exceeds 130 beats per minute. Accelerated A-V junctional rhythms may be as slow as 70 per minute.

Examine the tracing in Figure 6–23, which exhibits typical features of an A-V junctional tachyarrhythmia due to enhanced automaticity.

From a monitoring lead, Figure 6–23 reveals an abrupt change in P wave contour accompanied by a slight increase in heart rate. Beginning with normal sinus rhythm

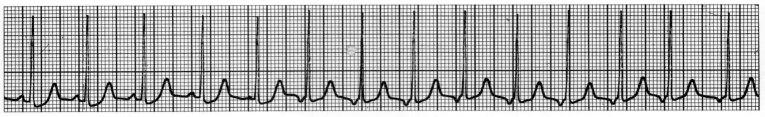

Figure 6–23. A-V junctional tachycardia resulting from enhanced automaticity.

and upright P waves, there is a transition to inverted P waves. The change indicates that the atria are being depolarized from a different direction, presumably from a focus originating at the lower portion of the atria. This rhythm is identified as nodal (or more properly as A-V junctional), in which retrograde conduction through the atria precedes antegrade conduction through the ventricles. Because the rate of this rhythm is faster than the sinus rate that it replaces, it is referred to as an accelerated nodal or A-V junctional rhythm.

Drug toxicity must be considered as a possible cause of A-V junctional tachyarrhythmia that has the characteristics of enhanced automaticity. Of all the drugs that have the potential for inducing these rhythms, digitalis is by far the most commonly encountered and is the most important. Indeed, A-V junctional tachycardia in a patient on digitalis should be judged to be a form of digitalis toxicity until proven otherwise. In patients already compromised by cardiac disease, development of such a tachycardia may itself present an additional serious threat and also may be the harbinger of an even more dangerous arrhythmia.

Readers should appreciate at this point that digitalis has complex actions on impulse formation and conduction in various cardiac tissues. Briefly, digitalis accelerates the decay of the resting membrane potential (Phase 4), leading to its more rapid approach toward spontaneous discharge (probably through inhibition of the sodium-potassium exchange pump activity). It reduces the upstroke velocity as well as the amplitude of the action potential (Phase 0). Digitalis also prolongs the refractory period (Phase 3), thereby delaying the return to full polarization. In addition, digitalis accentuates vagal tone, as the increased acetylcholine released promotes more rapid movement of potassium to the cell exterior. This effect alone alters excitability of both conduction and automatic fibers.

One further action of digitalis on automatic fibers has only recently been recognized by the use of intracellular recordings. It involves the tendency of digitalis to exaggerate the minute increase in excitability that normally occurs immediately after completion of the major action potential. This effect is referred to as **oscillatory afterpotentials**, among several other descriptive terms. If this enhancement is sufficient to cause the fiber to reach threshold for spontaneous depolarization, an impulse is generated. The electrophysiological explanation may be fluctuations in sodium-potassium transport across the cell membrane at the time of restoration of resting membrane potential, but the release of calcium ions from the sarcoplasmic reticulum is also held responsible.

Not surprisingly, disorders of body cation concentration affect the propensity of digitalis to produce tachyarrhythmias. For example, hypokalemia is a notorious cofactor in the genesis of digitalis toxicity, as illustrated in Figure 6–24.

The patient is a 56-year-old man with congestive heart failure under treatment with digoxin and a thiazide diuretic. On 3/9/70, tachycardia with a precisely regular rate of 162 per minute was recorded. P waves cannot be identified. QRS complexes are of normal duration. A-V junctional tachycardia was suspected, perhaps with a retrograde P wave occurring at the terminal portion of the QRS complex. Blood chemistries at this time reveal a serum potassium of 3.2 mEq/liter. Other major electrolytes were found to be within normal limits.

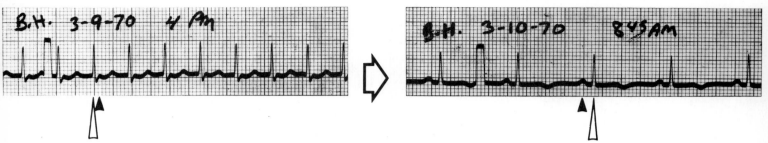

Figure 6–24. A-V junctional tachycardia due to hypokalemia and digitalis.

Although the hypokalemia is only of a moderate degree (and presumably caused by the thiazide), this condition was thought to be a contributing factor in a digitalis-induced tachycardia. Consequently, digitalis was withheld and a preparation of potassium chloride was administered orally.

By 3/10/70, normal sinus rhythm replaced the tachycardia. P waves were then obvious. The S wave present in the previous tracing disappeared, suggesting that it represented a retrograde P wave. These changes then establish the original rhythm as an A-V junctional tachycardia with digitalis toxicity certainly culpable.

Figure 6–25 compares two monitor strips from the same patient. This teenager had complained of recurrent episodes of lightheadedness. The top strip shows normal sinus rhythm with a rate of 90 beats per minute and a PR interval of 0.14 second. The second pattern is typical of junctional tachycardia with a rate of 116 beats per minute and a PR interval of 0.06 second. Ironically, this patient had been taking digitalis for control of symptomatic paroxysmal atrial tachycardia.

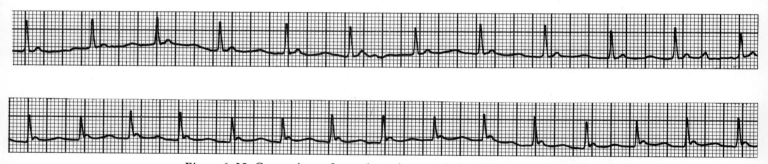

Figure 6–25. Comparison of complexes in normal sinus rhythm and junctional tachycardia.

Clinicians learn to suspect digitalis as a cause of any tachyarrhythmia, particularly when potentially contributing conditions such as hypoxia or low serum potassium or magnesium or high calcium are also present. Blood levels of digoxin are useful for confirmatory evidence of toxicity, but a host of other factors must be taken into account as well, including individual sensitivity. Certainly, there is no arrhythmia unique to digitalis toxicity, including A-V junctional tachyarrhythmias, and definitive diagnoses must be based on circumstantial findings.

In Chapter 5, we explored in detail the effect of digitalis in slowing conduction within the A-V node, even to the point of blocking it altogether. Purkinje cells, which make up the bulk of the common bundle, are of course specialized fibers for impulse conduction, but they are also capable of initiating impulses. It is on these cells that digitalis appears to exert its excitatory action on automaticity.

This dual action of digitalis on the A-V nodal system—inhibition of conduction in the A-V node and stimulation of automaticity in the common bundle and adjacent fibers—provides strong grounds for incriminating digitalis in A-V junctional arrhythmias. Thus, the finding of A-V junctional tachyarrhythmias combined with retrograde A-V block is a powerful sign of digitalis toxicity. Such disorders fall within a special group of arrhythmias under the heading of A-V dissociation. It is appropriate to introduce this subject here because of its close association with digitalis-induced tachyarrhythmias.

ATRIOVENTRICULAR INDEPENDENT RHYTHMS

Thus far, rhythms presented have been produced by a single pacemaker—from the sinus node, atria, or A-V junction—that controls both chambers of each cardiac cycle. When the pacemaker is located midway in the electrical system (e.g., in the A-V junction) *and* retrograde block is present, the atria are isolated and fall under control of a local pacemaker (ordinarily, the sinus node). The rhythms of each set of cardiac chambers become independent, the atria controlled by one pacemaker and the ventricles by another.

THIRD-DEGREE ATRIOVENTRICULAR BLOCK. One such form of separated atrial and ventricular beating results from a complete conduction block in the A-V node in which sinus impulses are unable to penetrate into the ventricles. The ventricles then come under control of a rescue pacemaker, which may be located in the A-V junction. This subsidiary pacemaker produces an escape rhythm, and its rate is *slower* than that of the dominant sinus pacemaker. This arrhythmia is classified as **complete—or third-degree—A-V block**.

Characteristics of third-degree A-V block can be seen in Figure 6–26, recorded from a postinfarction patient who experienced a syncopal episode while vomiting. The sinus rate is 96 beats per minute, and the ventricular rate is 52 beats per minute. Further evidence of the independence of atrial and ventricular activity is the variability of the relationship of the P to QRS. In actuality there is no measurable PR interval because there is no atrial-to-ventricular conduction as a result of the complete A-V block. The ventricles are presumed to be depolarized by a stimulus arising in the A-V junction because of the rate of 52 beats per minute and the normal duration of the QRS complex (less than 0.12 second).

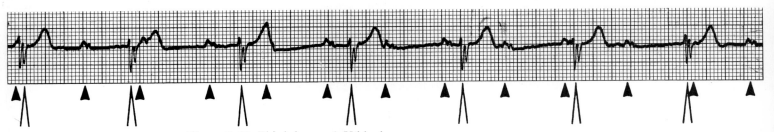

Figure 6–26. Third-degree A-V block.

In Figure 6–27, independence (dissociation) of atrial and ventricular activity is also present, with a sinus rate of 135 beats per minute and a ventricular rate of 75 beats per minute. The regularity of the QRS complexes and their normal duration of 0.08 second implicate the A-V junctional tissue as the focus for the escape rhythm mechanism. The patient experienced no adverse effects of this dysrhythmia, perhaps because of the rate of the escape rhythm.

The following two strips further illustrate third-degree A-V block. The first reveals a sinus rate of 72 per minute and a ventricular rate of 29 per minute. Although the rate

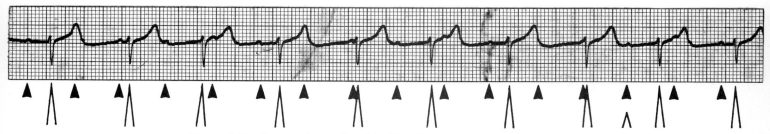

Figure 6–27. Sinus tachycardia with third-degree A-V block.

is slower than would be expected from a rhythm originating in the A-V junction, the narrowness of the QRS complex indicates a starting point near the A-V junction.

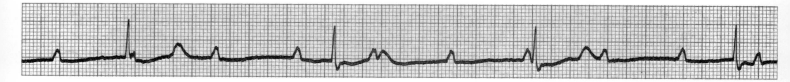

The last example of complete A-V block exhibits nonconduction of a sinus rhythm. Initial inspection may lead a clinician to interpret the strip as 3:1 advanced second-degree A-V block. Closer inspection, however, reveals variability in the P to QRS relationship. An additional finding, sinus tachycardia, is a frequent occurrence in third-degree A-V block. The reduced cardiac output due to the slow ventricular rate and the absence of A-V sequencing results in a normal physiological response of increased rate of sinus node firing.

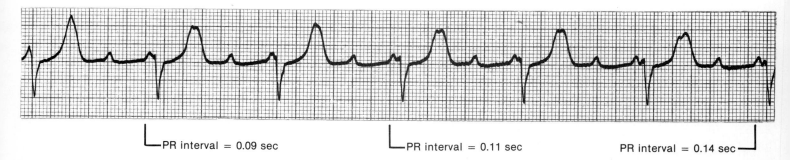

PR interval = 0.09 sec   PR interval = 0.11 sec   PR interval = 0.14 sec

ATRIOVENTRICULAR DISSOCIATION. A second form of independent atrial and ventricular beating results from an excited pacemaker in the A-V nodal system attended by antegrade conduction to the ventricles but with blocked retrograde conduction.

The atria, receiving no impulse from the A-V junctional pacemaker, are electrically isolated. Yet, the sinus node remains intact and continues to beat in its usual manner. In turn, the atria respond to the sinus rhythm. Hence, two coexisting pacemakers become operative. The A-V junctional rhythm will be *faster* than the sinus rhythm owing to excitation of its pacemaker. This dual rhythm is the form referred to as **A-V dissociation.**

Because the independent pacemakers are almost always beating at different rates, atrial and ventricular contractions are asynchronous. This ever-changing time relationship can be detected on physical examination, reflected in beat-to-beat variations in the intensity of the first heart sound (representing onset of ventricular contraction) and in variations of the pulsatile amplitude of the jugular vein "a wave" (caused by atrial contraction).

Figure 6–28 supplies an example of A-V dissociation in which the pacemaker controlling the atria and that controlling the ventricles are set at slightly different rates.

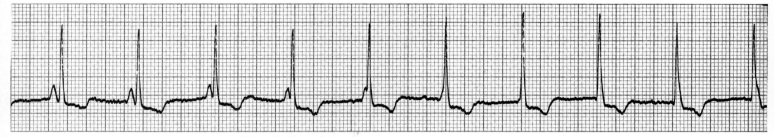

Figure 6–28. A-V dissociation.

At first glance, normal sinus rhythm appears to be present at the beginning of the tracing. Gradually, however, the PR interval shortens until, near the middle of the tracing, the P wave actually merges into the QRS complex and emerges behind the last QRS. Obviously, conduction through the A-V node could not have taken place. Indeed, careful measurement of rates reveals that the atria and the ventricles differ slightly; the ventricular rhythm is regular (at 75 beats per minute), and the atrial rhythm (72 per minute) nearly so. The only explanation for these findings is that each set of chambers is stimulated independently. The contour of P waves, their moderate rate, and the slight variations in cadence suggest that a sinus pacemaker controls the atria. The regularity of ventricular beating and the narrow QRS complexes indicate that the ventricles are paced from the A-V junction.

The diagnosis is established as A-V dissociation due to an accelerated A-V junctional rhythm (rate more than 60 but less than 100 per minute) with retrograde block and an independent sinus rhythm. Remember that an A-V junctional escape rhythm would be slower than the sinus rhythm if the independent rhythms were caused by antegrade block of impulses from the sinus node (i.e., complete A-V block).

The two independent rhythms (one controlling the atria and the other controlling the ventricles) often occur when the inherent depolarization rates of the sinus node and the A-V junction are almost identical. Such a situation is illustrated in Figure 6–29.

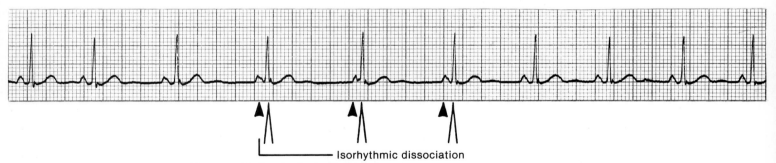

Isorhythmic dissociation

Figure 6–29. Isorhythmic dissociation.

In this example, the patient initially is in a sinus rhythm with a rate in the 70s and a PR interval of 0.14 second. The influence of respiratory activity on the cycling variance of the sinus node causes the sinus node gradually to slow its rate of discharge. This normal slowing becomes evident in the fourth cycle where the P wave rate drops to the low 60s. Note that the PR interval for this beat is only 0.10 second. The following P wave occurs at a rate of 59 beats per minute. The PR interval for this fifth beat is even shorter (0.08 second). The QRS complexes of beats 4 and 5 can be measured at a rate of 60 beats per minute. It is evident from the difference in rates of the atrial and ventricular complexes and the shortening of the PR intervals that the firing rate of the sinus node has slowed below the inherent rate of discharge of the junctional tissue. Thus, the junction controls depolarization of the ventricles. With the sixth beat, the sinus rate has begun a gradual increase in the rate of discharge. The short PR of 0.10 second indicates that the QRS is still under the influence of the A-V junctional tissue. The sinus regains control with the seventh beat and maintains control for the remainder of the example.

Rhythms in which separate atrial and ventricular beating occur at nearly the same rate (as in the two preceding ECGs just described) are referred to as **isorhythmic dissociation**. Although this phenomenon may be purely coincidental, it can also be the result of synchronization from nearby pacemakers without direct connecting tracts. This form of A-V dissociation can be misinterpreted because of the nearly constant time relationship between P waves and QRS complexes (mimicking a true PR interval). Isorhythmic A-V dissociation often exhibits an extremely short PR interval or the P wave actually merges with the QRS complex. Eventually, some variation in the P wave-QRS complex relationship will divulge the true nature of the arrhythmia.

Isorhythmic dissociation most often occurs when the natural variance in cadence of sinus node cycling results in an intermittent discharge rate that is below the inherent rate of the junctional tissue. Because the A-V junction has an escape rate that can provide impulses at a rate of 60 per minute, this form of A-V dissociation typically occurs when the patient has sinus activity that varies between the high 50s and low 60s. When the sinus is firing in the 60s, the patient is in normal sinus rhythm that exhibits all of the usual characteristics including respiratory influence on cadence and normal PR intervals. As the sinus gradually slows into rates in the 50s, the A-V junctional tissue assumes control of the ventricular activity at its inherent rate. With return of faster sinus discharge, the rhythm again comes under complete control of the sinus node.

Patients with isorhythmic dissociation typically experience no symptoms, although both rate and atrial-ventricular sequencing are disturbed. A clinician is most likely to see this dysrhythmia when a patient has the slowest sinus firing rates, such as during sleep.

In Figure 6–30, the slowing of sinus node discharge is more severe, resulting in a rate of 51 beats per minute for the P waves. Note with beat 3 that the shortening of the PR interval becomes apparent. The P waves of subsequent beats (where the sinus P waves emerge behind the QRS complexes) reveal even more clearly the fact that the

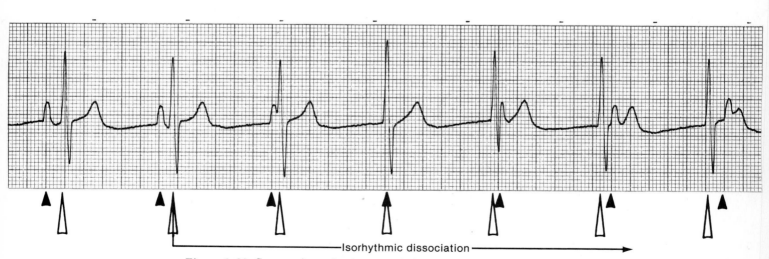

Figure 6–30. Severe sinus slowing reveals isorhythmic dissociation.

slowing of the sinus rate has allowed the A-V junction to assume control of the ventricular activity. The duration of isorhythmic dissociation for this patient during sleep, when his sinus rate typically slowed into the low 50s or high 40s, often was more than 5 minutes. The nursing staff was unable to determine clinical symptoms during these episodes because disturbing the patient to assess changes in mentation or blood pressure resulted in sympathetic stimulation to the sinus node and his sinus rate increased to 75 beats per minute, eliminating the dissociation.

A-V dissociation with A-V junctional tachycardia may occur in the presence of sinus or atrial tachycardias. In the following tracings, the typical features of sinus tachycardia are found; yet, this sinus rhythm is totally out of synchrony with the narrow QRS tachycardia also present.

The strips were recorded from a 17-year-old youth hospitalized for a gunshot wound to the chest. The bullet entered the right atria and followed a path through the tricuspid valve and lodged in the apex of the right ventricle. Surgery was required to recover the bullet and determine damage to cardiac structures. Fortunately, minimal trauma to the myocardium was discovered. However, edema from the injury and surgery resulted in intermittent episodes of junctional tachycardia. During his early recovery phase, the patient also had sinus tachycardia. The presence of these concurrent tachycardias often resulted in A-V dissociation.

For the first 6 days of hospitalization, sinus tachycardia was the usual rhythm as seen in the following strip. Only during sleep did the rate occasionally drop below 100 beats per minute.

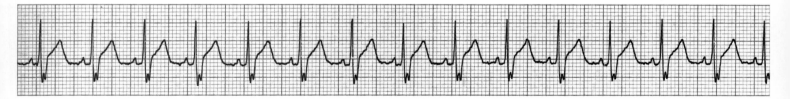

The junctional tissue intermittently superseded the rate of the sinus node, resulting in simultaneous sinus and junctional tachycardia. The next tracing demonstrates the assumption of ventricular control by the A-V junction (note the disappearance of the P wave as the PR shortens). These episodes of concurrent tachycardias often lasted for several minutes.

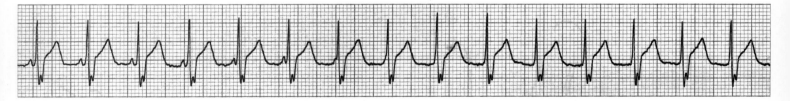

Conversion back to sinus tachycardia is revealed in the following strip.

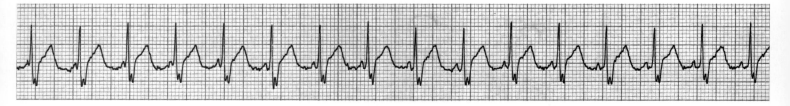

On the last day of hospitalization, the patient was in a normal sinus rhythm with a rate of 95.

Digitalis is particularly suspect in rhythms with both atrial and junctional tachycardias and is characterized by the following:

1. Excitation of an atrial pacemaker.
2. Excitation of an A-V junctional pacemaker.
3. Functional block between atria and ventricles, either in an antegrade or a retrograde direction.

In the following strip of A-V dissociation, identify the rates for the two pacemakers and note the independent atrial and ventricular activity.

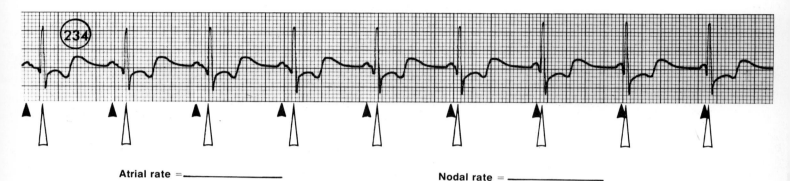

Atrial rate = _____   Nodal rate = _____

Reentrant Tachycardias

In the previous chapter, we presented four situations in which anomalous fibers, within the A-V node or around it, provide a pathway for early entry of impulses from the atria to the ventricles. These anomalous, fast-conducting fibers are responsible for shortening of the PR interval and/or for deforming the initial portion of the QRS complex. These same fibers may also serve as one limb of a closed electrical circuit, thus acting as a potential cause for reentrant beats and reentrant tachycardias.

The physiological basis for these arrhythmias is similar to that described for reentrant arrhythmias of the atria, except that the A-V node (and in some forms, a portion of the common bundle, the bundle branches, or the ventricles) makes up the circuit. As in the intraatrial type of reentrance, the heterogeneity of electrophysiological properties of adjacent conducting fibers—a fast pathway and a normal (or slow) pathway—is the substrate for these arrhythmias.

We have emphasized the important of enhanced automaticity in the etiology of A-V junctional tachyarrhythmias because of the high likelihood that it is an expression of myocardial injury or toxic effect of a drug. Yet, for patients with recurring episodes of A-V junctional tachyarrhythmias, the reentrant mechanism is a far more common cause. Although attacks may be asymptomatic or produce little more than an occasional annoyance, episodes with rapid rates and long duration may be severe enough to result in acute cardiac failure.

That anomalies within the A-V nodal system may have clinical implications was suggested as early as 1938, when the association between short PR intervals (with normal QRS complexes) and the tendency for palpitations was identified. This relationship was more precisely defined in 1952 in a published summary of patients who had short PR intervals and who were subject to recurring bouts of ''atrial'' tachycardia, flutter, or fibrillation. This syndrome is still referred to by the names of the authors, Drs. Lown, Ganong, and Levine, of Boston, Massachusetts.

To return to the four anatomical forms of ventricular preexcitation, we will now describe the role of each in the production of A-V junctional tachyarrhythmias.

INTRANODAL REENTRANT TACHYCARDIA

At relatively slow heart rates, an anomalous fast pathway within the A-V node conveys impulses preferentially from the atria to the ventricles. When the rate increases above a critical level, however, the oncoming impulse arrives at the fast pathway *before* it has recovered from the preceding depolarization and therefore is unresponsive; at the same time, the ordinary fibers of the A-V node (the slow pathway) have already recovered from the previous depolarization owing to their shorter refractory period. Consequently, the impulse is carried along the slow pathway into the ventricles. Such an event may attend sudden acceleration of the sinus pacemaker or, more commonly, a premature atrial beat. Indeed, it is not infrequently observed that such a premature beat is associated with prolongation of the PR interval (Fig. 6–31). In any case, this alternate route of conduction forms the descending limb of a potential reentrant circuit.

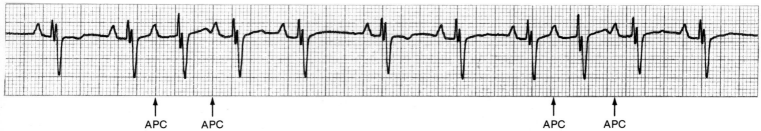

APC   APC   APC   APC

Figure 6–31. Altered PR intervals of atrial premature complexes produced by conduction through an alternate pathway to the ventricles.

The tracing in Figure 6–31 demonstrates the altered transmission through pathways that are influenced by the speed with which impulses reach them. Beats 3 and 4, as well as beats 9 and 10, are APCs. The sinus complexes at a rate of 80 beats per minute are conducted with a PR interval of 0.18 second. The premature atrial beats, however, demonstrate prolonged PR intervals. The earlier the APC, the longer the PR intervals. Thus beats 3 and 9, with firing rates of 140 beats per minute, have PR intervals of 0.29 second; the slower rates of beats 4 and 10 (discharge rates of 90) have PR intervals of 0.24 second.

As an impulse penetrates the slow pathway of the A-V node, it may reach the distal end of the fast pathway after it has fully recovered from the earlier depolarization cycle. The impulse can then enter the fast pathway (as well as continue on into the ventricles) and ascend through it in a retrograde direction. The atria sometimes are restimulated by this echo impulse, depending on the duration of the refractory period in atrial fibers. In this sequence (Fig. 6–32), an inverted P wave is found immediately after the QRS complex of an atrial premature beat.

The fourth cycle in this example is produced by an atrial premature beat (note the more intense peaking of the T wave). After this APC, a P wave indicates retrograde activation of the atria. It can be presumed that this P wave was initiated in the junctional tissue because it has a reversed polarity from all other P waves in the strip.

If the retrograde impulse in the fast pathway exits at the proximal end at a time when the slow pathway has also recovered, the impulse can then reenter the slow pathway, thus completing one reentrant cycle. Should the cycle repeat itself, a circus rhythm is established. The repetitious circuit acts as a pacemaker, driving both atria and ventricles, usually at a very rapid rate. Figure 6–33 illustrates such a tachycardia, which begins with an atrial premature beat.

A review of the events leading to A-V junctional beating from intranodal reentry follows:

- A premature atrial beat occurs.
- Its atrial wave front finds the anomalous fast tract refractory, and the impulse

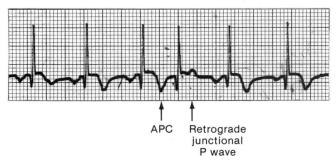

APC   Retrograde
junctional
P wave

Figure 6–32. Atrial premature beat with a nonconducted junctional P wave following the premature beat.

descends the normal, relatively slow, pathway. (Remember that fibers of the fast pathway have *longer* refractory periods than do those of the adjacent conducting system so that they block more readily as rapid stimuli encroach on the limit of responsiveness.)

- The descending impulse enters the His-Purkinje system to the ventricles *and* it enters the now responsive fast pathway at its distal end.
- The impulse ascends the fast pathway to enter the atria *and* to reenter the slow pathway.
- The circuit completed, a repetitive series of firings occurs, each acting as a pacemaker, establishing an ectopic tachycardia.
- The tachycardia continues until the reentrant circuit is interrupted somewhere along either limb.

Because the reentrant impulse is coming from midway between the atrial and ventricular conduction systems, the antegrade impulse usually initiates ventricular depolarizational about the same time that atrial depolarization from the retrograde impulse begins. Consequently, the electrocardiographic pattern in intranodal reentrant beating generally contains a P wave that is superimposed on the QRS complex and is therefore at least partially obscured. Sometimes, however, the retrograde P wave occurs shortly after the QRS complex or (probably less commonly) in front of it. The determining factor for this relationship is the velocity of the ascending impulse in the fast pathway compared with that of the descending impulse in the common bundle and bundle branches. As expected, very rapid reentrant A-V junctional rhythms frequently exhibit A-V dissociation, the retrograde impulse being blocked altogether in the A-V transitional tissue or the proximal A-V node.

The characteristics of P wave contour cannot be used to distinguish A-V junctional reentrant arrhythmias from those caused by enhanced automaticity. In both instances,

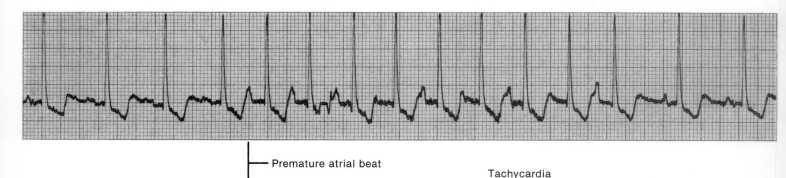

└─ Premature atrial beat

Tachycardia ────────────────►

Figure 6–33. Tachyarrhythmia initiated at cycle 5 by an atrial premature beat.

the atria are depolarized by a reverse flow wave front, moving upward and predominantly leftward. The resultant P waves are inverted in those limb leads with the positive electrode away from the wave front movement: leads II, III, and aVF. Lead I, with its positive electrode in the left lateral axis, often inscribes a diphasic retrograde P wave, the negative component initiating the waveform.

The most important electrocardiographic clue distinguishing reentrant from enhanced automatic A-V junctional tachyarrhythmias is the sudden appearance and the sudden cessation of the reentrant form, each change usually preceded by a premature atrial beat. There are no warm-up or cool-down periods as are commonly observed with enhanced automaticity. These features (which are shared with reentrant atrial tachycardias) are also referred to as **paroxysmal**, alluding to the abrupt changes in rhythm (see glossary). Conversely, tachyarrhythmias resulting from enhanced automaticity (having a gradual acceleration at onset and a gradual deceleration at offset) are known as **nonparoxysmal**.

Alternating fast-slow pathway conduction in which changes in vagal innervation appear responsible for sequential impulses jumping from one A-V nodal route to the other were discussed in Chapter 5 under Ventricular Preexcitation. Along similar lines of reasoning, we deduce that variations in parasympathetic tone could also be a provoking factor in the onset and termination of A-V junctional tachyarrhythmias. For example, ablation of vagal tone by administration of atropine occasionally leads to transient A-V junctional rhythms, presumably of reentrant etiology (Fig. 6–34).

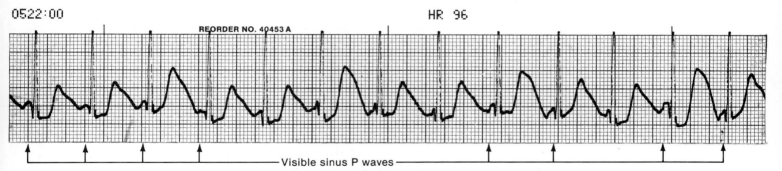

Figure 6–34. Junctional rhythm produced by administration of atropine.

The rhythm in Figure 6–34 occurred when a patient who had experienced cardiac syncope was given atropine to reverse severe sinus slowing. As anticipated, the atropine reversed the decreased sinus firing rate and the P waves are now seen at a rate of 99 per minute. The unexpected effect of the atropine was the simultaneous development of A-V junctional tachycardia at a slightly faster rate of 100 per minute.

Although the emergence of an A-V junctional pacemaker after atropine is decidedly unusual (acceleration of sinus pacemaker rate is the typical response), this response points out the inhibitory influence that normal vagal tone has on modulating the complex activity of the A-V nodal system.

The sympathetic nervous system also plays a prominent role in conduction velocity and the refractory period of conducting fibers. Its influence may certainly affect neighboring fibers to different degrees. By increasing velocity or by decreasing the refractory period in one limb of a potential reentrant circuit more than in the other promotes the likelihood of reentrance. Hence, strong sympathetic reflexes (as with severe emotional reactions or strenuous exercise) may sometimes trigger a paroxysm of A-V junctional tachycardia.

A 32-year-old woman who was taking a sustained-release theophylline preparation for asthma developed dyspnea, palpitations, headache, and nausea. At a nearby emergency room, no signs of bronchospasm were found, although her blood pressure was

86/50 supine and her heart rate was rapid. The ECGs seen on the left in Figure 6–35 are from the initial evaluation.

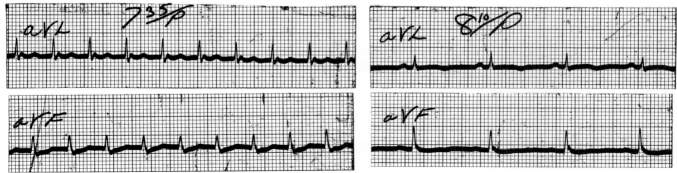

Figure 6–35. Changes in complex configuration are seen in selected electrocardiogram leads of a patient who converted to normal sinus rhythm from junctional tachycardia.

Supraventricular tachycardia in which P waves cannot be identified is evident. Arterial blood gases were within normal limits. A theophylline blood level was 26 μg/liter, within the range of toxicity. Before any therapeutic intervention was initiated, the rhythm converted spontaneously, her blood pressure increased to 100/60, and her symptoms disappeared. Comparing the tracings recorded immediately after conversion, shown on the right, with the initial tracings, one can conclude that the terminal portion of the earlier QRS complexes actually represented retrograde P waves. The original rhythm, then, is diagnosed as A-V junctional tachycardia. The arrhythmia was assumed to be a complication of theophylline, which has adrenergic properties.

Pharmacological agents having adrenergic stimulating properties are often found to underlie recurrent attacks of tachycardia in susceptible persons. Caffeine, theophylline, phenylephrine, and isoproterenol are a few examples. Another, phenylpropanolamine, is found in a variety of prescribed and over-the-counter preparations for upper respiratory infections and weight control.

The intranodal form of A-V junctional reentrant beating is probably the predominant cause of paroxysmal tachycardias. The rate is highly variable among different individuals but tends to be relatively constant for the same individual (suggesting that the reentrant circuit is the same). Rates are generally quite rapid and may exceed 200 per minute.

Treatment of intranodal A-V junctional tachycardia is directed at interrupting the reentrant circuit in either of its limbs. By increasing the conduction velocity or by prolonging the refractory period of either the fast or the slow pathway fibers, the reverberating wave front eventually confronts nonresponsive fibers, and the tachycardia stops abruptly.

The heavy concentration of parasympathetic terminals in the A-V node renders it exceptionally sensitive to vagal stimulation. This effect increases the refractory period of fibers within the slow pathway (fast pathway fibers are relatively resistant) and is often of sufficient magnitude to break up the tachycardia. Vagal stimulation produced by carotid pressure, gag reflex, Valsalva maneuver, or cold water on the face often aborts intranodal reentrant tachycardia precipitously, as demonstrated in Figure 6–36.

If the reentrant circuit is located in the His-Purkinje portion of the A-V nodal system (where autonomic control is absent), vagal stimulation produces no change in the reverberating circuit or in the ventricular rate. However, it may lead to retrograde impulse blockade, causing A-V dissociation and termination of the tachycardia.

The same result may be attained using a drug with parasympathetic enhancing properties. Edrophonium (Tensilon) has been used for many years with much success, even in patients in whom vagus-stimulating maneuvers have failed. However, this drug

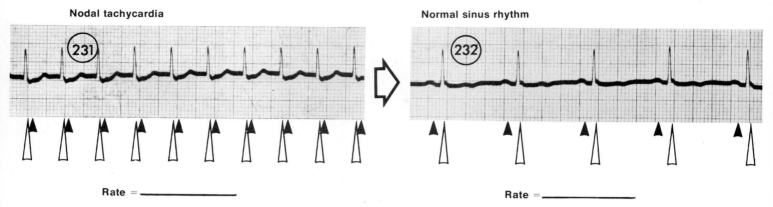

Figure 6–36. Termination of reentrant tachycardia from vagal stimulation.

is attendant with numerous disturbing cholinergic effects, which include abdominal cramping, nausea, and sweating. Newer nonautonomic agents, specifically the calcium channel blockers, have replaced edrophonium as the drug of choice for treating this form of A-V junctional tachycardia. Of those currently available, verapamil is generally the most effective. Normal fibers in the A-V node (which compose the slow pathway of the circuit) are much more dependent on calcium channel activity than are anomalous fibers, and verapamil quite effectively preferentially prolongs the refractory period of the normal pathways. The rapid action of verapamil when given intravenously, coupled with its high degree of safety in properly selected patients, has ensured this drug a major therapeutic role in terminating the common form of A-V junctional tachycardia.

Digitalis, which also prolongs the refractory period of slow conduction fibers, has long been used to control this arrhythmia. However, its beneficial parasympathetic-enhancing effect is complicated by the tendency to augment ectopic automaticity. The drug is generally more useful in preventing recurring tachycardias than in terminating them in patients with anomalous intranodal bypasses.

Some of the beta-adrenergic blocking agents provide an additional option for inhibiting a circus impulse, the target site again being the slow fiber pathway. Their mode of action is probably also on the refractory period. By blocking sympathetic tone, these drugs leave parasympathetic tone relatively unopposed and consequently more intense.

All of the drugs just mentioned exert their therapeutic action on the A-V node itself and are reflected in lengthening of the AH interval on His bundle electrography. They have little effect on the His-Purkinje system and therefore produce no appreciable change in the HV interval.

An alternative approach to the reentrant circuit in intranodal tachycardias is to interrupt the impulse in the fast fiber pathway (the retrograde limb). Many of the beta-adrenergic blockers have a preferential action on the fast tract fibers. Drugs that directly affect the action potentials of conduction fibers are used to advantage because of their disproportionate effect on the fast fibers, slowing conduction velocity and prolonging the refractory period to a greater degree than in the slow fibers. Quinidine, procainamide, and disopyramide have such actions. Unfortunately, fairly large (and potentially toxic) doses are often required for conversion of these tachycardias to a sinus rhythm. Their chief value lies in preventing paroxysmal tachycardias in susceptible persons.

Amiodarone, a drug having vasodilating properties, can be highly effective in suppressing reentrant tachycardias, including those proven resistant to conventional drugs. Its pharmacological action appears to prolong the effective refractory period of the anomalous fibers of the reentrant circuit. The drug can be useful for either interruption or prevention of tachycardias, although side effects (involving the cornea, liver, thyroid gland, neuromuscular system, and alveoli) may limit its use.

Electrocardioversion is an additional option for treatment of reentrant intranodal tachycardias (Fig. 6–37). This procedure is almost always successful in interrupting the circus loop, even when low-energy discharges of 25 to 50 watt-seconds are applied. Electrocardioversion is administered with precordial paddle electrodes, and the technique is identical to that described for treatment of atrial tachycardias in Chapter 4.

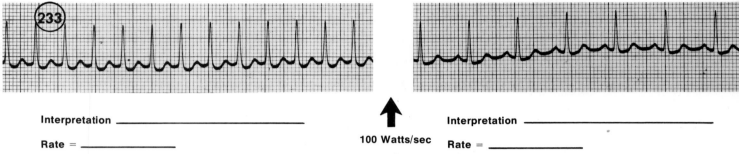

Interpretation _____

Rate = _____

100 Watts/sec

Interpretation _____

Rate = _____

Figure 6–37. Electrocardioversion of a reentrant intranodal tachycardia.

The moments immediately following electrocardioversion of reentrant tachycardias are commonly complicated by ectopic arrhythmias from enhanced automaticity. This tendency is most notable if the patient is on digitalis. Using an alternative approach to cardioversion is preferred if there is any danger of digitalis toxicity. Unfortunately, signs of toxicity may be masked in patients with reentrant tachycardia, only to appear after cardioversion.

Beta-adrenergic blockers also present a potential complication in electrical treatment of these arrhythmias. Patients with sinus node dysfunction or with defective A-V conduction may incur extreme degrees of bradycardia after cardioversion, owing to the action of adrenergic depressor drugs.

Drugs used in combination (such as verapamil or propranolol, with quinidine) to suppress or to prevent a reentrant tachycardia are sometimes required for drug-resistant patients for their synergistic actions. Together, they may result in severe postconversion bradyarrhythmias.

Reentrant intranodal tachycardias may also be terminated in the electrophysiological laboratory, using intracardiac stimulation. A wire electrode is introduced into the right atrium by intravenous cannulation, and it is positioned near the A-V node. A small current of electricity is given, and when properly timed it will impinge on the reentrant loop. This discharge acts as a premature impulse, which may then enter the loop. If the impulse produces a new wave front that arrives too early for the entire loop to conduct it, the circuit is obliterated, and the tachycardia stops sharply.

Rarely, reentrant tachycardias of intranodal origin occur so frequently and are so disabling and resistant to standard treatment that physical ablation of the A-V nodal bridge is justified. Such a drastic measure can be accomplished by surgical transection or by percutaneous, transvenous procedures of electrocoagulation or cryoablation. Thereafter, permanent stimulation of the ventricles with an electronic pacemaker is required.

ATRIO-HIS REENTRANT TACHYCARDIA

Anomalous fibers passing from the atria around the A-V node and entering either its distal portion or the common bundle directly defines the atrio-His form of ventricular preexcitation. As in the intranodal form, preferential conduction follows the anomalous fibers (also known as James fibers), which act as an extranodal fast pathway. The anatomical differences notwithstanding, these two forms of ventricular preexcitation are alike in producing a shortened PR interval but without causing any deformity or change in duration of the QRS complex. They also share the tendency toward paroxysmal reentrant tachycardia through a similar mechanism. Again a fortuitously timed stimulus (such as an atrial premature beat) or disproportionate changes in action potential dynamics in the fast or the normal pathway can result in unidirectional A-V block and a situation favoring reentrance.

In the ordinary type of atrio-His reentrant tachycardia, the normal A-V nodal fibers serve as the alternate conduction route and the extranodal anomalous fibers as the retrograde limb of the circuit (Fig. 6–38).

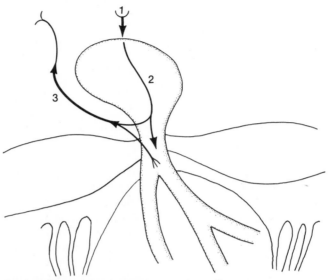

Figure 6–38. Conduction through extranodal anomalous fibers.

Although the retrograde P wave may occur simultaneously with the QRS complex, it usually falls well after it, creating a relatively long R-P interval (Fig. 6–39). The retrograde P waves have a negative polarity in leads II, III, and aVF, as in intranodal bypass tracts. Lead I and MLI (as shown) often have upright P waves.

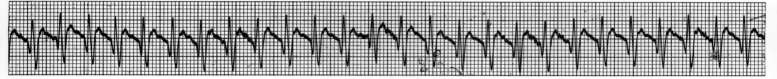

Figure 6–39. Junctional tachycardia with an R-P interval of 0.12 second as recorded in the standard monitoring lead.

Actually, these intranodal and extranodal forms of ventricular preexcitation and reentrant tachycardias cannot be distinguished by electrocardiographic signs. The atrio-His bypass usually produces the shorter PR interval (when it skirts the A-V node altogether), but this differentiating feature is not reliable. Distinction can only be made by electrophysiologic studies involving intracardiac recordings, and even here there is often much uncertainty.

In a variant of atrio-His bypass, the anomalous fibers extend from the atria directly to one of the major bundle branches; it is known as the atriofascicular bypass tract (Fig. 6–40). In sinus rhythms, the PR interval is abnormally short, and in addition, the initial inscription of the QRS complex is deformed because of a brief period of direct myocardial fiber propagation of the wave front. Paroxysmal tachycardias typically exhibit loss of the aberrant configuration of the QRS complex because the ventricles are now activated entirely by the A-V nodal route.

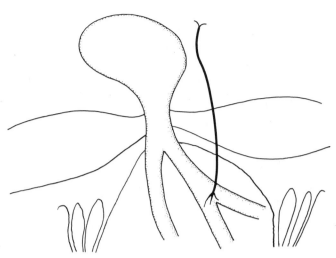

Figure 6–40. Atriofascicular anomalous bypass tract.

Because one limb of a reentrant circuit courses the entire A-V node, atrio-His bypass tachycardias are usually highly susceptible to interruption by autonomic influences. Consequently, a therapeutic strategy centers on this feature: vagotonic maneuvers (e.g., carotid stimulation), parasympathetic-stimulating drugs (e.g., edrophonium and digitalis), or sympathetic-inhibiting agents (e.g., propranolol). The calcium antagonists (notably verapamil) act preferentially on the slow channel-dependent fibers within the A-V node. All exert their antiarrhythmic effect by slowing conduction velocity and by prolonging the refractory period of the normal fibers that serve as the intranodal descending limb of the circuit.

Other agents that are useful in atrio-His bypass tachycardias act primarily on the anomalous fibers, prolonging conduction as well as the refractory period, through direct cellular mechanisms (not autonomic). Quinidine, disopyramide, and procainamide exert this mode of action. Electrocardioversion is a further therapeutic option, eminently suited for patients with circulatory failure. These various approaches are precisely those already described for intranodal reentrant tachycardias.

NODOVENTRICULAR REENTRANT TACHYCARDIA

When anomalous fibers connect the distal A-V node or common bundle to the ventricular myocardium (usually the intraventricular septum), the normal His-Purkinje entry into the ventricles is circumvented. Referred to as a nodoventricular bypass, this form of ventricular preexcitation produces a normal PR interval (or only a very slightly shortened one) because the supraventricular pacemaker must first penetrate most of the A-V node. To review, preexcitation occurs by way of fast fibers around the already rapidly conducting common bundle. As anticipated, the His bundle electrogram exhibits a normal AH interval and a contracted HV interval. The early impulse depolarizes a small portion of the ventricular myocardium until the normally timed impulse (descending the His-Purkinje system) enters the ventricles to complete depolarization. This sequence of activation creates an initial deformity of the QRS complex (a delta wave); the remainder of the QRS complex is normal. Because there is little difference in timing between the anomalous fiber impulse and the normal fiber impulse, the degree of preexcitation is slight and the size of the delta wave tends to be small.

Once again, the anatomical potential for alternative pathways in sinus rhythms presents the opportunity for generating reentrant tachycardias. For example, a premature beat may find the anomalous pathway blocked but the normal His-Purkinje fibers responsive. The circuit is completed if the impulse enters the distal portion of the anomalous connection and ascends it to reenter the His-Purkinje system.

Reentrant tachycardias of nodoventricular type are relatively uncommon. One explanation is that there is little difference in either conduction times or refractory periods between the two competing pathways. Thus, those physiological characteristics that favor reentrant rhythms are less pronounced than in the other forms of ventricular preexcitation.

Treatment of nodoventricular tachycardias usually requires agents that affect the action potentials of anomalous fibers directly, such as quinidine and procainamide. Because the anomalous connection does not pass through the A-V node, vagotonic maneuvers and drugs that act through the autonomic neurons are generally ineffective.

ATRIOVENTRICULAR REENTRANT TACHYCARDIA

The classic form of ventricular preexcitation depends on an anomalous fiber pathway that directly connects the atria to the ventricular myocardium, thus bypassing the A-V nodal system altogether. The strong association between atrioventricular preexcitation and the tendency for recurring tachyarrhythmias was pointed out in the landmark article by Wolff, Parkinson, and White in 1930, and the clinical syndrome still bears their names.

Atrioventricular connections are inserted directly into the myocardium of either the free ventricular wall or into the intraventricular septum. In contradistinction, other forms of preexcitation have anomalous fibers that include at least a portion of the A-V nodal system and are limited to a relatively small area (or **microcircuit**). Atrioventricular connections, on the other hand, may extend across a large area of the ventricles (forming a potential **macrocircuit**). This long pathway exaggerates the discrepancy between conduction velocities and refractory periods of the anomalous pathway and those of the normal A-V nodal pathway, thus favoring development of the reentrance phenomenon and tachyarrhythmias.

Atrioventricular preexcitation in sinus rhythms is recognized by an abnormally short PR interval and by a delta wave, inscribed by a depolarizing wave front in a portion of the myocardium. About half of those who have the atrioventricular form of preexcitation, a relatively rare condition, are not bothered by any symptoms of tachycardias. Others may have short-lived episodes of palpitations or weakness from recurring tachycardias, although some have very frequent attacks characterized by acute circulatory failure. In all individuals who are subject to severe recurring tachycardias, the incidence of atrioventricular preexcitation is fairly common. Young persons (including infants and children) with paroxysmal tachycardias should be especially suspected of having preexcitation.

Reentrant tachycardia involving an atrioventricular connection typically begins with a functional antegrade block in the extranodal pathway, permitting impulse transmission through the A-V nodal system and retrograde conduction in the anomalous connection. As in the other forms of reentrant tachycardias, a series of reverberating beats is thereby established. It is important to note that the delta wave is lost with the onset of tachycardia because conduction to the ventricles is entirely dependent on the A-V nodal system (Fig. 6–41).

The two strips in Figure 6–41 above were obtained from a patient who had complained of palpitations for several years, beginning during her late teens. The delta wave during the sinus rhythm example is most obvious in beats 3, 5, 7, and 8. The patient often exhibited APCs (some blocked as in this tracing) during sinus rhythm. With the onset of tachycardia, the initial portion of the QRS has a straighter upstroke.

With the onset of tachycardia, the His electrogram reveals prolongation of the AH

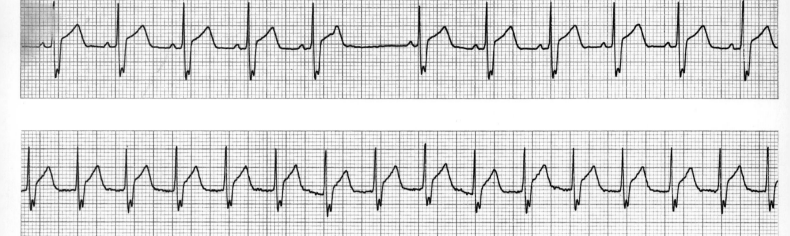

Figure 6–41. The delta wave present in sinus rhythm disappears with the onset of tachycardia.

interval, reflecting a shift of the antegrade impulse from the fast (anomalous) to the normal (A-V nodal) pathway. The retrograde impulse then reenters the atria by the anomalous bundle. Because the ventricles of each reverberant cycle begin depolarization before the atria, the P wave is usually found after the QRS complex or the P wave is obscured by the QRS (at least in part). On right-sided anomalous pathways, the P wave is inverted (upright) in lead aVR. If the anomalous fibers bridge the left-sided chambers, the P wave is characteristically inverted (downward) in lead I. (The wave front proceeds away from the positive electrode of these leads.) These waveforms are seen only during sinus rhythm and reverse with the onset of tachycardia.

Although the rates of reciprocating atrioventricular bypass tachycardias have a wide range, they tend to be faster than those caused by intranodal reentrant mechanisms, commonly greater than 220 beats per minute and sometimes as fast as 250 per minute (Fig. 6–42). In the tracing, P waves are not clearly distinguishable and the possibility of 2:1 A-V block cannot be excluded. Tachycardias associated with ventricular preexcitation that exceed this rate are likely to coexist with atrial flutter or fibrillation. Precise regularity distinguishes atrioventricular bypass tachycardias, although irregularity may occur by the Wenckebach phenomenon or in the presence of atrial fibrillation.

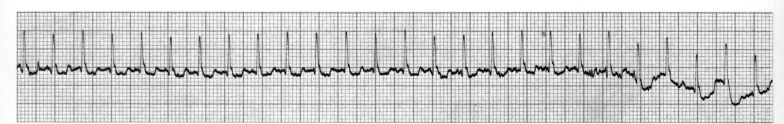

Figure 6–42. A-V bypass tachycardia.

Supraventricular Tachycardia

The term *supraventricular* is used to embrace all those rhythms driven by a pacemaker located above the common bundle branches even if its precise location—sinus node, atria, A-V junctional system—cannot be ascertained. P waves are obscured, either wholly or in part, by simultaneous ventricular activity, thus obliterating the major diagnostic clues. A clinician very often does not have the advantage of observing the onset of a tachyarrhythmia to study the character of premature beats that may have preceded the tachycardia, so the general designation of supraventricular tachycardia is handy and commonly used. It is not an entirely accurate term for all tachyarrhythmias of reentrant mechanism, however, because the reentrant circuit may incorporate a portion of the ventricles (e.g., in nodoventricular, fasciculoventricular, and atrioventricular bypasses).

Any rhythm in which the QRS complexes are narrow (less than 0.12 second) can be classified as supraventricular. This criterion indicates that the ventricles are depolarized by the usual His-Purkinje conduction system, and therefore the pacemaker must be located above the bifurcation of the common bundle. Supraventricular rhythms also may be associated with wide QRS complexes caused by aberrant conduction within the ventricles. The subject of wide QRS rhythms will be considered in Chapter 8.

Figure 6–43 is an example of a narrow QRS tachycardia. P waves cannot be identified. (They may be present at the peak of the T waves, buried in the QRS complexes, or absent altogether.) The rhythm exhibits perfect regularity, and the configuration of QRS complexes is normal for lead V_1. Certainly, no origin for the tachycardia can be determined. Here, the diagnosis of supraventricular tachycardia is clearly appropriate. The patient complained of palpitations and lightheadedness.

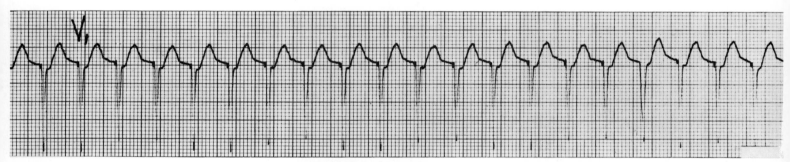

Figure 6–43. Supraventricular tachycardia.

Another example of tachycardia of uncertain origin is shown in test tracing 235, but this time the QRS complex is abnormally long. A vagal stimulating maneuver is used to alter the pacemaker dynamics, if possible, thereby disclosing the site of its origin.

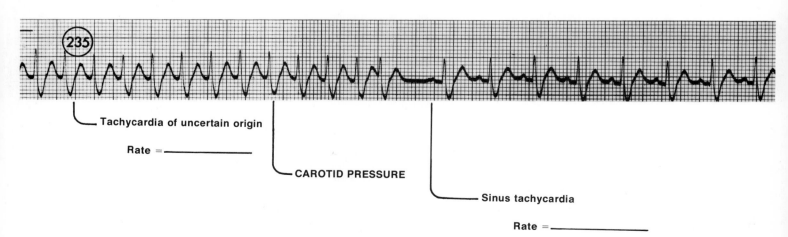

Tachycardia of uncertain origin

Rate =

CAROTID PRESSURE

Sinus tachycardia

Rate =

Carotid pressure resulted in abrupt slowing of the rate and the emergence of a well-defined sinus rhythm. Note that the last beat of the ectopic tachycardia is early. This finding almost certainly identifies the tachycardia as reentrant in mechanism. It is assumed that the premature beat interrupted the circus movement in either the antegrade or the retrograde limb. The cardiac cycle that immediately follows the premature beat at the transition is evidently an atrial escape beat, the P wave morphology differing from that present in the sinus rhythm. Observe also that there has been no change in the duration or the form of the QRS complexes as the sinus node takes over. This finding confirms that ventricular depolarization occurs in the same sequence for both the normal and the reentrant tachycardia, establishing that the latter is of supraventricular origin, as well.

A later ECG contains the clue to a precise interpretation. Tall, peaked T waves preceding the early cycles suggest an atrial focus. The frequency of atrial premature beats and the slightly sharper T wave form during the tachycardia suggest the probability of sustained atrial beats.

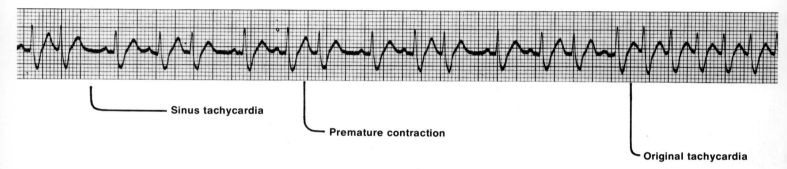

Sinus tachycardia

Premature contraction

Original tachycardia

Jim R. visited the emergency department when he experienced his third episode of palpitations in a week. His strip on admission revealed a tachycardia with a regular ventricular rate of 186 beats per minute. A QRS of 0.12 second indicates a supraventricular origin despite the inability to identify a P wave.

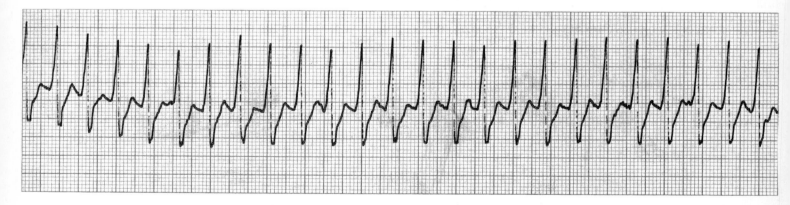

SHORT REFRACTORY ACCESSORY PATHWAYS. A special problem complicates the unusual form of accessory pathway in which the refractory period is very short, thereby endowing the anomalous fibers with the capacity for transmitting impulses at an extremely rapid rate. The danger lies in spontaneous development of atrial flutter or atrial fibrillation in which the ventricles are bombarded with stimuli in excess of 300 times a minute. Ordinarily, of course, the A-V node protects the ventricles from such extreme stimulation by filtering out most of the impulses. The presence of a highly reactive accessory pathway, however, eliminates this natural defense.

When the ventricles beat faster than 220 times a minute, cardiac output declines as a result of decreased diastolic filling; at 300 beats per minute or greater, weakness or syncope can be expected in an adult. (These events occur at much slower heart rates if there are concurrent cardiac disorders such as myocardial or valvular disease.) In addition to the hemodynamic burden, such rapid rates also lead to instability of the electrical dispersion system in the ventricles. Ventricular tachyarrhythmias thus generated are thought to be responsible for a sizable proportion of sudden death syndrome among individuals with ventricular preexcitation. Exercise may contribute to this phenomenon because it increases the rate at which the accessory pathway can conduct impulses.

Development of atrial flutter or fibrillation is estimated to occur in about 20% of persons with symptomatic paroxysmal tachycardia of A-V junctional origin. It may be more common in those with concurrent sinus node dysfunction and/or atrial sclerodegenerative disease. Atrial flutter or atrial fibrillation complicating ventricular preexcitation is particularly suspect in youths in apparent excellent health but subject to frequent attacks of tachycardia-related syncope. This mechanism may be, in fact, a preeminent cause of the sudden cardiac death syndrome in this age group.

One outstanding caution must be kept in mind when using digitalis to treat persons who have documented or suspected accessory pathways and who experience episodic atrial flutter or fibrillation. Among the multiple actions of digitalis is the propensity for *shortening* the refractory period of accessory pathway fibers, thereby *increasing* the rate at which impulses can be transmitted. Furthermore, by decreasing the conduction capacity of the A-V node (mediated by increased vagal tone), digitalis reduces the frequency of potential reentrant impulses (which interfere with antegrade conduction in the accessory fibers). In addition, digitalis tends to convert atrial tachycardia and flutter into atrial fibrillation, as already explained in the drug treatment of atrial tachycardia in Chapter 4.

All too frequently, clinicians are faced with treating narrow QRS tachycardias in which the mechanism is uncertain and in which digitalis may provoke accelerated conduction over an accessory pathway from fluttering or fibrillating atria. It is a commonly accepted practice to begin therapy with a drug that counteracts this potential threat, a beta-adrenergic blocker or calcium channel blocker often the preferred options before digitalis is administered. (Of course, the presence of congestive heart failure may contraindicate using either drug.) Electrocardioversion handily circumvents this therapeutic quandary.

This precaution with digitalis also holds for patients who have ventricular preexcitation and who are in a sinus rhythm but are known to have episodic atrial flutter or fibrillation. Individuals with concurrent valvular disease producing atrial enlargement, with atrial sclerodegenerative disease, or with sinus node dysfunction must also be suspected of having such paroxysms. In any case, digitalis may precipitate a more serious tachycardia owing to the increased ventricular rate response.

Before proceeding to an overview of therapeutic approaches to the different A-V junctional tachycardias, an important subtype of accessory bypass mechanism—variant bypass tachycardias—will be examined.

Variant Accessory Pathway Tachycardia

The typical bypass phenomenon in which anomalous fibers provide entrance of impulses into the ventricles more readily than do those of the A-V node has been described. **During sinus rhythms** there results an electrocardiographic pattern characterized by a short PR interval and/or a wide QRS complex (caused by the delta wave). Four such types of ventricular preexcitation have been presented. Reentrant tachycardias developing from this anomaly undergo altered impulse conduction so that the normal A-V nodal system transmits impulses to the ventricles while the accessory pathway serves for their return to the atria. **During the tachycardia**, the QRS complexes are narrow (reflecting normal A-V nodal:intraventricular conduction).

In a special form of reentrant tachycardia, the directional pattern for impulse conduction is reversed. This variation results because some anomalous fibers conduct impulses poorly (or not at all) from the atria to the ventricles. Such fibers, of course, will not participate in ventricular preexcitation in sinus rhythms, and in fact, the typical ECG exhibits a normal PR interval and a narrow QRS complex (no delta wave).

However, these variant fibers have the capacity for readily transmitting impulses from ventricles to atria, a property referred to as **unidirectional** conduction. A stimulus distal to the A-V nodal system can enter the anomalous pathway and propagate to the atria. Timed fortuitously, this infranodal impulse may then return through the normal A-V nodal:His-Purkinje pathway to the ventricles, thus completing a reentrant circuit.

Enough of the ventricles is depolarized by the infranodal stimulus to produce an initial deflection in the ECG before the reentering impulse returns to the ventricles through the normal A-V conduction route. Consequently, the QRS complex in reentrant beats from A-V junctional mechanisms involving variant anomalous fibers displays fusion of a delta wave of ventricular origin and the normally conducted depolarization sequence within the ventricles. In contrast to those of typical anomalous pathway reentrant tachycardias, those of the variant form have abnormal QRS complexes during the tachycardia, whereas in sinus rhythms the QRS complexes are narrow.

Variant accessory bypasses are a form of concealed conduction, so designated because they remain inoperative during normal rhythms but reveal themselves only during reentrant tachyarrhythmias. They constitute an important group of tachycardias, occurring nearly half as commonly as the typical form of A-V junctional tachycardias. Notoriously they evade detection, owing to the normal ECG in the absence of tachycardia. Further, the wide QRS complex during the tachycardia often obscures the patterns of myocardial infarction, bundle branch block, ventricular enlargement, and, most importantly, tachycardias of ventricular origin. The subject of variant accessory bypass tachyarrhythmias will be discussed in more detail in Chapter 8 under Preexcitation Syndrome.

Treatment of Atrioventricular Junctional Tachycardias

In most instances, treatment of A-V junctional tachycardias follows those measures outlined for atrial tachycardias in Chapter 4. These are reviewed here briefly, and a few special considerations are noted.

If enhanced automaticity of fibers within the A-V junctional complex is suspected as the cause of tachycardia, treatment is directed at controlling the inciting factor: hypoxia, acidosis, ischemia, hypokalemia, catecholamine stimulation (endogenous or administered), and drugs. Of the latter, digitalis is held culpable until established otherwise. Drugs (quinidine and procainamide) to suppress the ectopic focus may also be indicated, but their effects may further depress the normal pacemaker-conduction system or the failing myocardium.

For A-V junctional tachycardia of the reentrant type, a clinician has a number of options, as described in the paragraphs that follow.

If the ventricular rate is extremely rapid, resulting in hypotension, chest pain, dyspnea, or other indicators of circulatory distress electrocardioversion under intravenous sedation is probably the most effective (as well as the fastest and safest) modality. It is useful even if the tachycardia is complicated by atrial flutter or fibrillation, A-V dissociation, or wide QRS complexes. Should a wide QRS complex tachycardia actually be of ventricular origin (these rhythms are commonly confused), this mode of treatment is ordinarily effective and, in fact, indicated.

The procedure for electrocardioversion of A-V junctional tachycardias differs in no way from that for atrial tachycardias. One precautionary point deserves a reminder. If the A-V junctional tachycardia is not of the reentrant mechanism but instead has resulted from enhanced automaticity, electrical shock could precipitate a more serious ventricular rhythm (most especially when digitalis is the precipitating factor).

If the tachycardia does not compromise adequate major organ perfusion, a series of interventions can be introduced as needed until a sinus rhythm is established. Although a large number of interrelated factors must be considered as one proceeds in treatment, the following sequence will usually serve:

VAGAL STIMULATION. The standard vagotonic maneuvers are performed (carotid pressure, Valsalva maneuver, exposure of the face to cold) as already described in Chapter 4. In the presence of atrial flutter or fibrillation (obvious or obscure), vagal stimulation is most likely to slow the ventricular rate response temporarily but not result in conversion.

If these maneuvers are ineffective or only transiently so, one may choose to use a parasympathetic stimulating drug, of which edrophonium is the prototypic agent (see drug therapies in the Atrial Tachycardia section of Chapter 4). However, the expected and often disturbing side effects of edrophonium and the minimal symptoms produced by certain calcium channel blockers (namely, verapamil) have generally given priority to the latter as the therapeutic intervention.

CALCIUM CHANNEL BLOCKADE. The rapid action, the relative freedom from side effects, and the high likelihood of terminating reentrant tachycardias have raised this group of drugs to preeminent status in the antiarrhythmia armamentarium. Their predominant site of action within the reentrant circuit appears to be on the fibers of the A-V node, prolonging both the conduction time and the refractory period. These synergistic actions on fibers (primarily dependent on slow channel ionic movement) is usually enough to interrupt the reverberating impulse. The calcium antagonists have little effect on the action potential of the accessory pathway fibers. The most useful drug of this class is verapamil, although diltiazem has similar actions (less intense on conduction fibers but stronger effects on the vasculature). Verapamil, incidentally, sometimes increases the ventricular rate response if atrial fibrillation is present, and the drug is usually withheld in this situation. It is particularly dangerous in the form of ventricular preexcitation, which exhibits broad QRS complexes, and therefore the drug should be withheld in this situation.

ADRENERGIC BLOCKADE. The beta-adrenergic blocking agents are often effective in terminating reentrant A-V junctional tachycardias of all types, their principal action mediated by prolonging the refractory period of fibers in the A-V nodal loop. They have no effect on the accessory bundle component of the circuit. Several drugs within this class are now available; propranolol has enjoyed the longest and most extensive use. Should conversion of the reentrant tachycardia to a sinus rhythm fail, a second agent, which acts directly on the accessory fibers, can be added.

DIRECT CONDUCTION FIBER DEPRESSION. Quinidine, disopyramide, and procainamide are drugs that slow conduction velocity and the refractory period of specialized fibers without mediation by autonomic neurotransmitters. They tend to affect anomalous fibers disproportionately to normal fibers, and by this action interrupt a reverberant circuit responsible for A-V junctional tachycardia. Long the classic drugs used for supraventricular tachycardias, they also present important potential liabilities. They can depress myocardial contractility (especially if the myocardium is already compromised). In addition, they have vagolytic effects and may increase the ventricular rate response in atrial flutter or fibrillation. To circumvent the latter hazard, a drug in this group is administered after sympathetic blockade with propranolol or another beta-adrenergic blocker.

ELECTROCARDIOVERSION. Electrocardioversion is generally preferred over drugs when the tachycardia is rapid enough to cause circulatory insufficiency. This intervention may be efficacious when drugs have failed to control A-V junctional paroxysmal tachycardia. However, it must be remembered that there is a high incidence of postshock arrhythmias when drugs (and especially digitalis) have been recently administered. Electrocardioversion is eminently safer than drug treatment in the life-threatening form of ventricular preexcitation in which atrial fibrillation with wide QRS complexes is present.

ELECTRONIC PACING. A properly timed electrical stimulus even from an external source can terminate reentrant A-V junctional tachycardias. This intervention is finding increased application for drug-resistant tachycardias, using intravenously threaded electrode wires into the right ventricle. The technique is especially effective when a macro-reentrant pathway is incorporated into the circuit. Implanted electronic pacing instruments that emit intracardiac impulses during a tachycardia are now available. The emissions may be triggered by patients when they perceive symptoms or by automatic sensors. Such instruments are reserved for patients with severe paroxysms of reentrant tachycardias that prove highly drug-resistant.

SELF-EVALUATION: STAGE 2

Label each tracing completely: components, rate(s), rhythm(s).

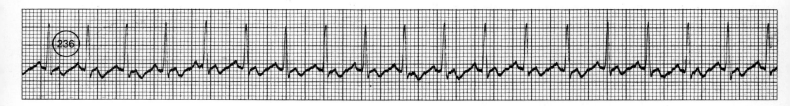

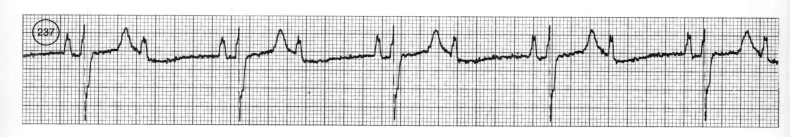

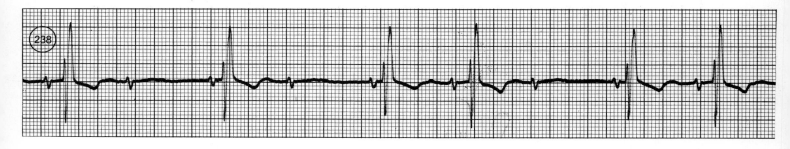

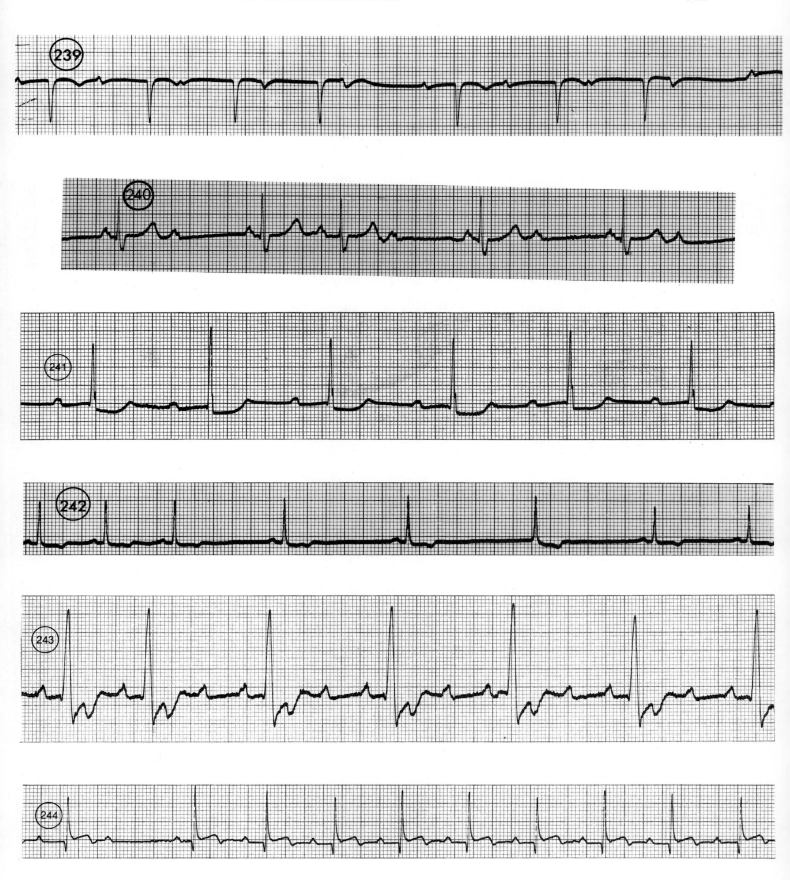

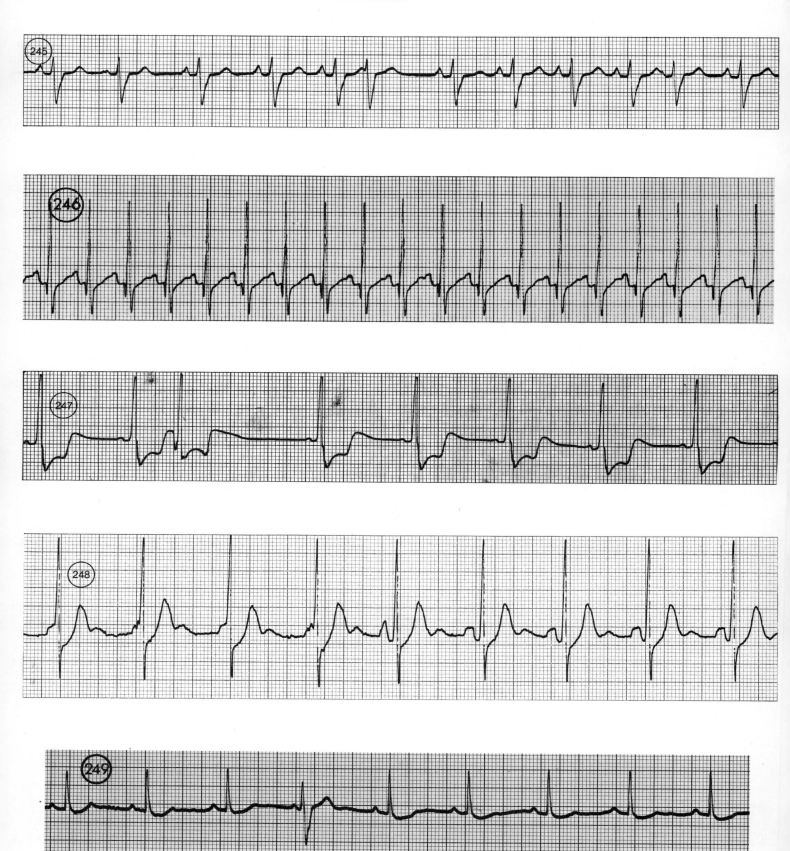

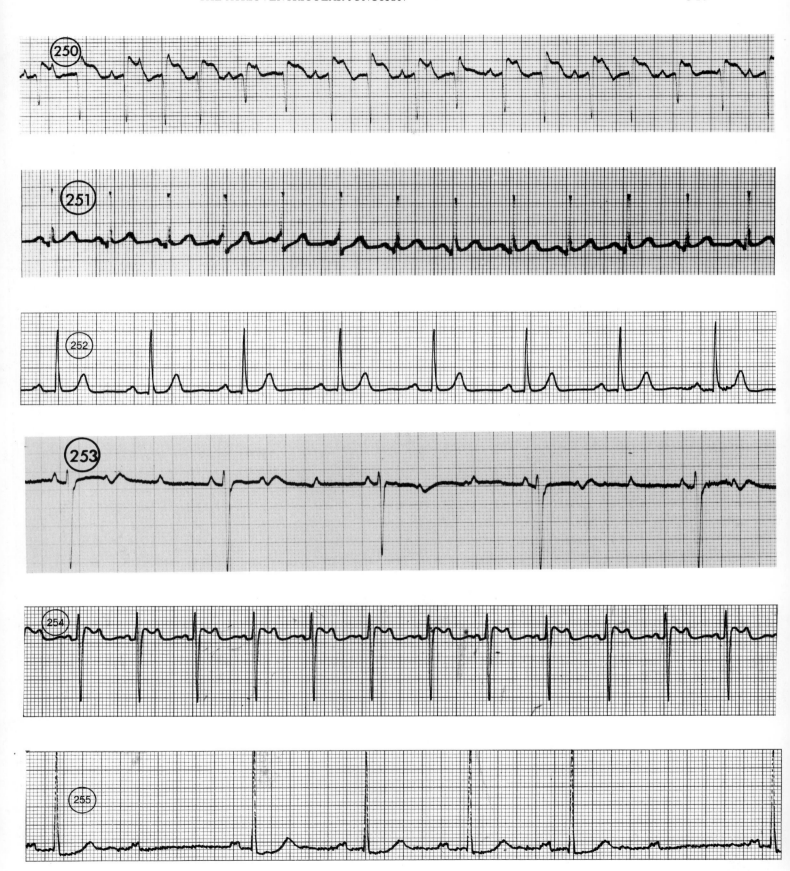

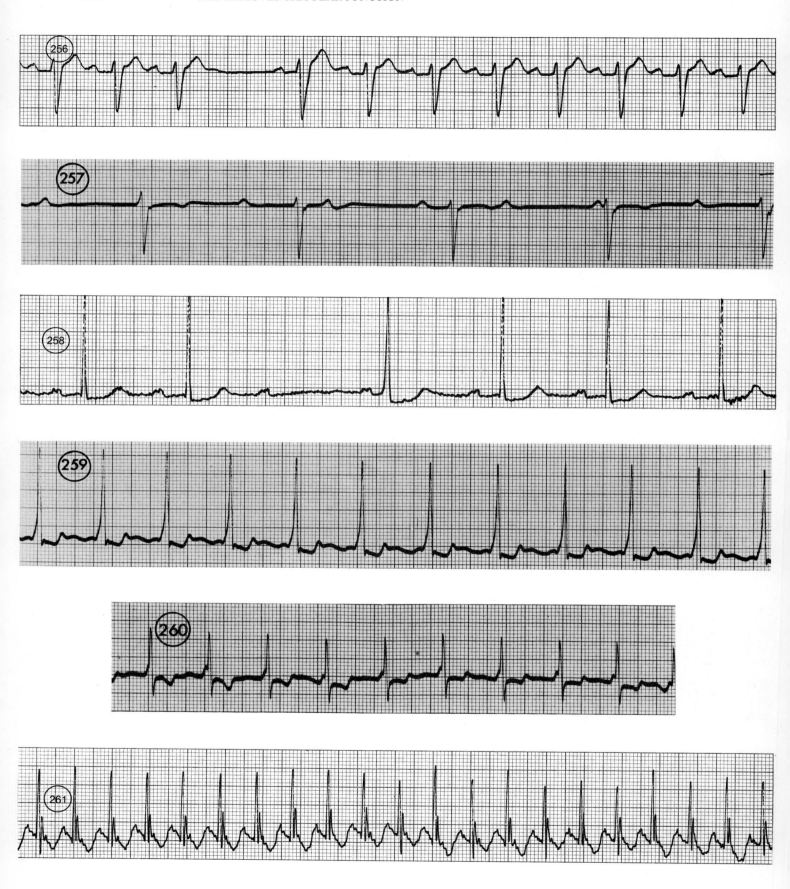

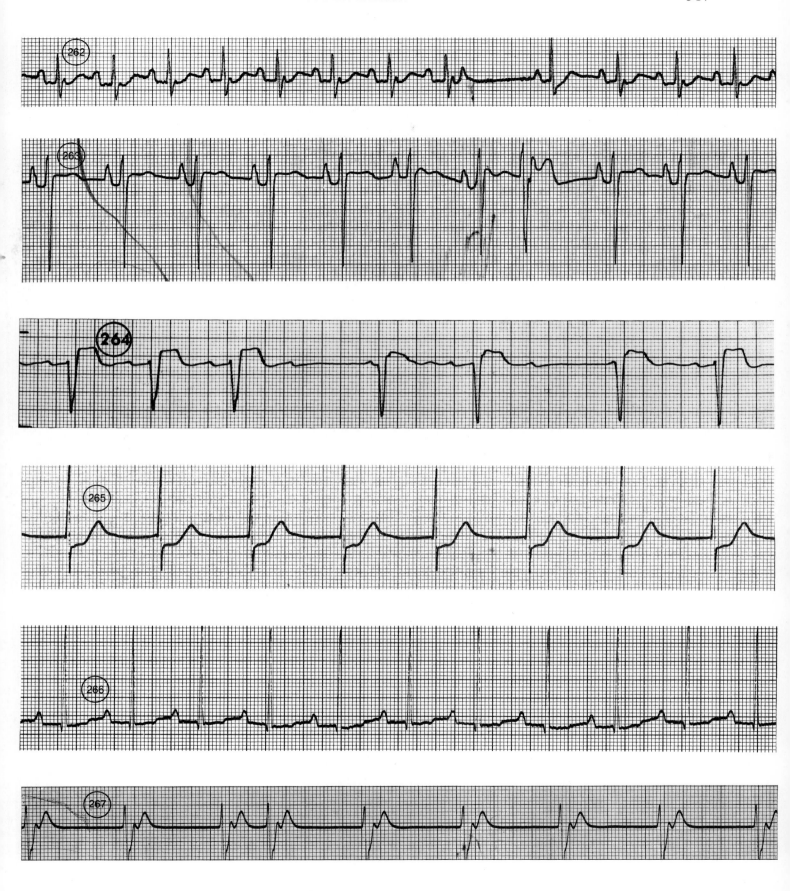

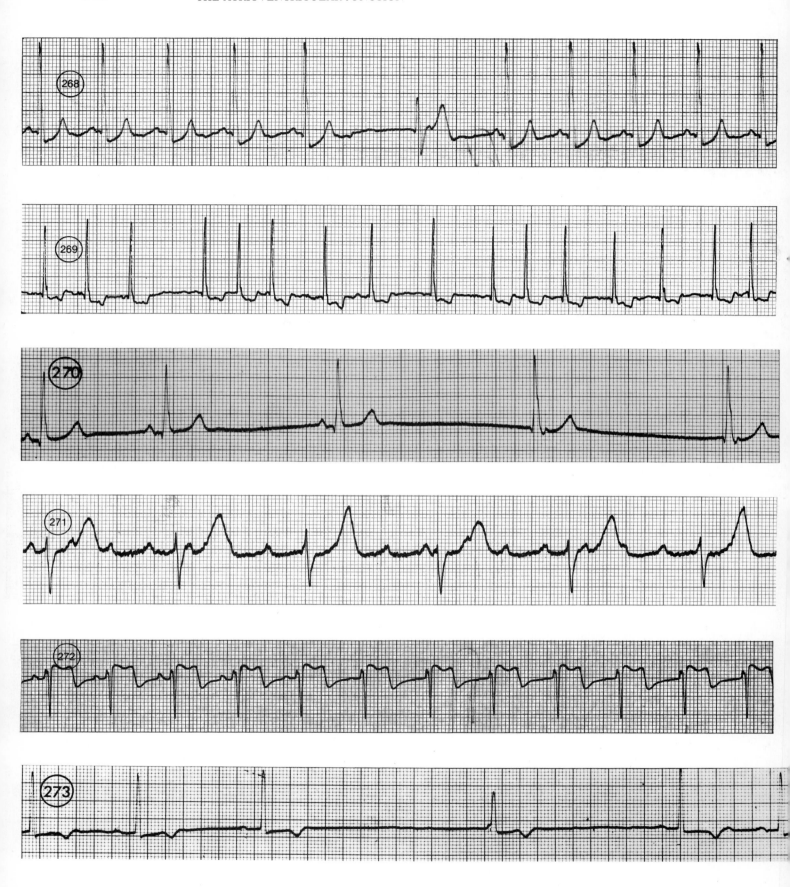

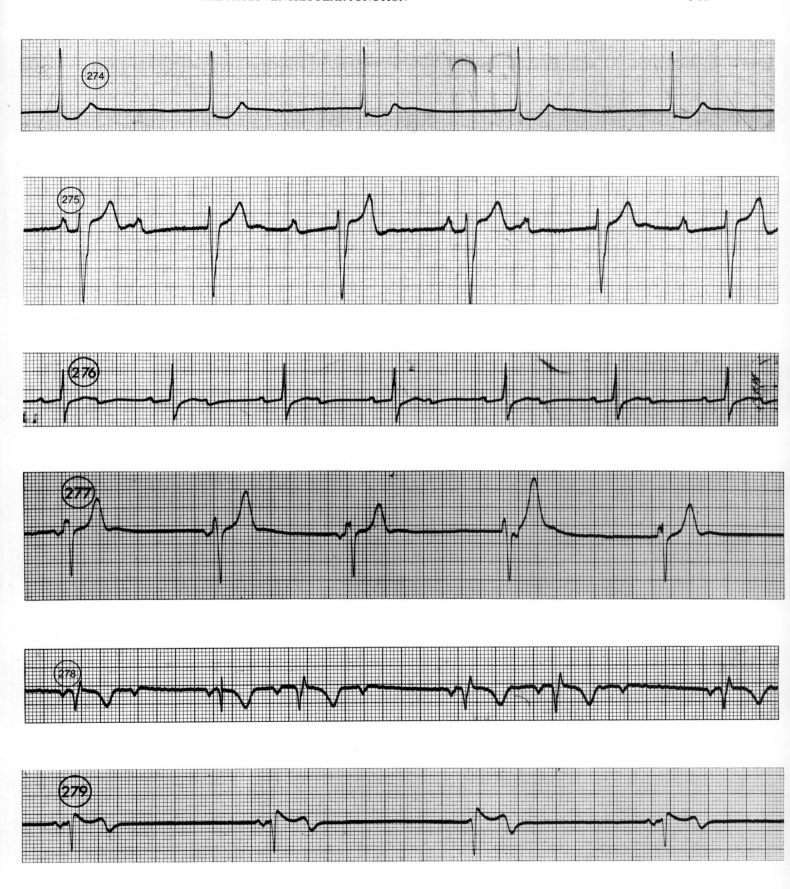

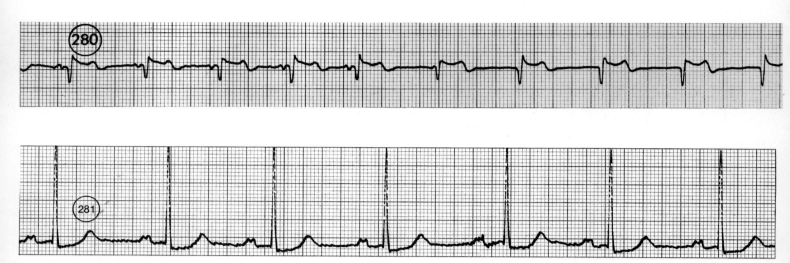

7 The Bundles

IMPULSE CONDUCTION
Depression
Right Bundle Branch Block

Left Bundle Branch Block
The Hemiblocks
Combined Conduction Defects

IMPULSE CONDUCTION

At the crest of the intraventricular septum, the common bundle divides in two, forming the right and left bundle branches. These are the pathways through which impulses from the atria are distributed to the ventricles (Fig. 7–1).

The **right bundle branch** begins as a slender cord that courses down the right surface of the intraventricular septum just beneath the endocardial layer. There are no branches from it until it reaches the distal portion of the septum and the apex of the right ventricle. At these regions, the right bundle branch divides extensively to form a diffuse neural network, distributed to the entire inner wall of the ventricle.

In sharp contrast, the **left bundle branch** begins as a broad band that splits almost immediately into two major divisions: (1) an anterior-superior bundle or fascicle and (2) a posterior-inferior fascicle. A number of smaller divisions may be present, and considerable variation in this anatomical pattern is found among individuals. Each of the fascicles leads to a papillary muscle in the left ventricle, where it then disperses throughout the subendocardial surface of this chamber. The terminal fibers of this network penetrate the myocardium to about one-third of its thickness. Impulses arriving at these Purkinje terminals then proceed outward through the myocardium without a specialized conduction system. The wave front that spreads from myofibril to myofibril toward the epicardium does so at about one-tenth the velocity of that in the Purkinje fibers.

Because of the minute electrical disturbance produced by an impulse moving in the common bundle and in the peripheral Purkinje system, there is no recordable deflection on the standard electrocardiogram (ECG). The first electrical activity in the ventricles represents a depolarizing wave front in the myocardial wall. Normally, the initial deflection of the QRS complex results from depolarization of the myocardium from the endocardial surface of the left ventricle through small branches of the left bundle branch that penetrate the septal wall, proceeding toward the right ventricle. This direction of wave front in the septum is determined by a more rapid conduction

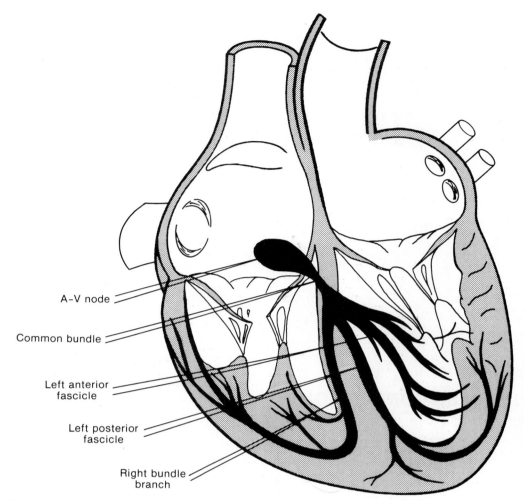

A-V node

Common bundle

Left anterior
fascicle

Left posterior
fascicle

Right bundle
branch

Figure 7–1. Major ventricular conduction pathways.

velocity than on the right; in addition, fibers from the left bundle branch divisions may enter the septum at a more proximal level.

Together, the bundles compose a trifascicular system: (1) the right, (2) the left anterior, and (3) the left posterior fascicles. They provide the pathway from the atria to the ventricular myocardium. These fibers conduct impulses more rapidly than those of the atrioventricular (A-V) node. This extremely rapid transmission contributes to both ventricular chambers being simultaneously activated near the apices. This conduction system favors synchronous contraction of the ventricles as well as transmission of the contractile wave from apex to base, where blood is ejected into the great vessels.

Just as in the common bundle, the cellular elements here are almost entirely made up of Purkinje fibers, arranged in parallel pathways, nearly devoid of myofibrillar (contractile) material, and notable for their rapid conduction. Indeed, conduction velocity is 50 to 100 times that of the A-V node. An additional distinguishing feature is the virtual absence of autonomic influence on the His-Purkinje fibers by either sympathetic or parasympathetic activity.

The action potential of the His-Purkinje conduction cell features a high resting transmembrane potential of −90 millivolts. The upstroke, Phase 0, is exceedingly rapid, and the overshoot is even greater than in the working myofibril (Fig. 7–2). Another important quality of His-Purkinje cells is their relatively long Phase 2 repolarization.

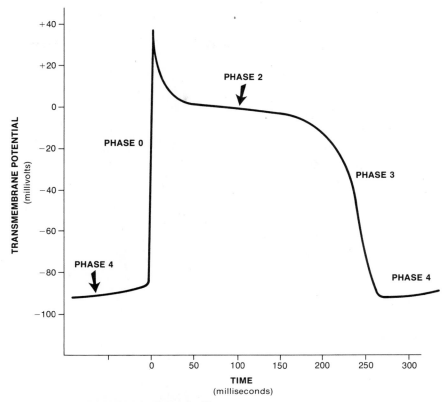

Figure 7-2. Action potential, His-Purkinje fiber.

Thus, the major conduction pathways are protected against reverberating impulses in the myocardium, leaving them clear for subsequent antegrade impulses from normal pacemakers. In other words, the rapid excitation of the conduction system together with its slow recovery reduces the chances for development of reentrant arrhythmias.

Depression

The conduction sequence and resultant ECG activity of ventricular activation are reviewed below (Fig. 7-3):

A. Initial conduction proceeds from the septal region of the left ventricle toward the right side of the septum, producing an upright deflection as it is directed toward V_1 and a downward deflection in leads I and V_6 as it moves away from the left ventricle.

B. Conduction is rapidly transmitted through the bundle branches in the septum toward the apex, resulting in a negative deflection in V_1 and an upright deflection in V_6.

C. The impulse bifurcates at the apex, spreading toward the free walls of the right and left ventricles and contributing to the downward deflection in V_1 and the upright configuration in V_6.

The ECG deflections in various leads reveal the **vector** (**direction** and **magnitude**) of ventricular conduction. Because the left ventricle is larger and denser, left ventricular conduction often dominates in electrocardiographic recordings.

Normally, ventricular depolarization is completed within 0.12 second. Any prolongation of the QRS duration beyond this interval defines depression within the ventricular conduction system.

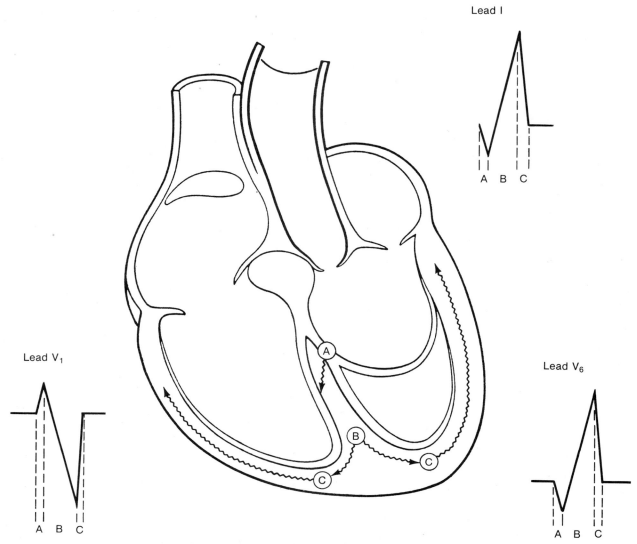

Figure 7–3. Conduction schemata and vectors in various leads.

Although the His-Purkinje system is relatively protected against intrafascicular reentrance, it is commonly affected by lesions that either delay impulse propagation or block it altogether. The defect may be caused by an anatomical disruption (ischemic or inflammatory) or by a physiological or pharmacological influence (hypoxia or quinidine). Conduction block has already been described in the common bundle; it may also occur in the right bundle branch, in the left main bundle branch, or in either of its major divisions (Fig. 7–4).

Actually, bundle branch block when uncomplicated does not fall within the definition of an arrhythmia because there is no change in cardiac rhythm. All portions of the heart are activated by the same pacemaker. Only the route of activation is altered. Nevertheless, a conduction defect in a major branch distorts the configuration of the QRS complex and prolongs its duration. Such beats simulate those arising from impulses formed within the ventricles themselves so that an interpreter must learn to recognize bundle branch blocks. Furthermore, multiple lesions producing block in all three fascicles (or both major branches) do occur, and in effect this condition is clinically indistinguishable from complete A-V block due to a lesion in the common bundle or the A-V node (which are, of course, arrhythmias) (Fig. 7–5).

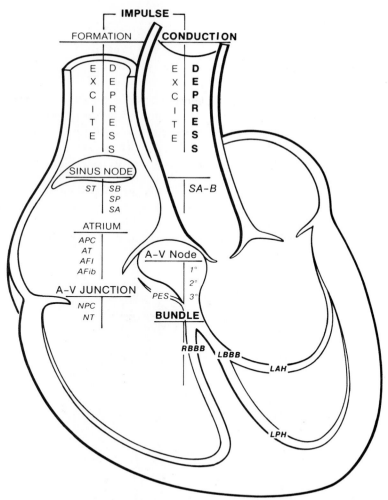

Figure 7–4. Depression of ventricular bundle conduction. RBBB = right bundle branch block; LBBB = left bundle branch block; LAH = left anterior hemiblock; LPH = left posterior hemiblock.

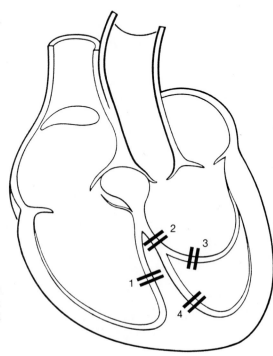

Figure 7–5. Composite drawing of bundle branch blocks. 1 = Right bundle branch block; 2 = left bundle branch block; 3 = left anterior hemiblock (or fascicular block); 4 = left posterior hemiblock (or fascicular block).

325

Right Bundle Branch Block

When transmission of an impulse is prevented somewhere along the right bundle branch, alteration in the sequence of depolarization in the ventricles takes place. Activation of the right ventricle originates entirely from the left bundle branch. This change produces a recognizable pattern in the ECG (Fig. 7–6).

Formation of the QRS complex in right bundle branch block is described in three sequential steps:

1. **Early depolarization: the intraventricular septum.** Ventricular depolarization from an impulse traversing the A-V nodal system begins at the normal site—that is, at the left surface of the septum where innervation by the left bundle branch remains intact. The wave front proceeds from the left epicardical surface to the right. Thus,

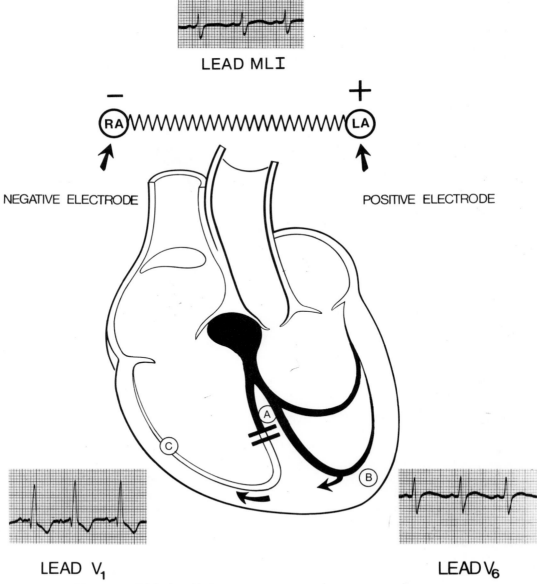

Figure 7–6. Right bundle branch block.

the usual initial phase of activation is preserved and the early portion of the QRS complex is unchanged.

2. **Intermediary depolarization: the left ventricular wall.** Normally, activation of the free walls of the right and the left ventricles begins virtually simultaneously, first at the apical regions and then proceeding toward the bases. The absence of stimulation from the right bundle branch results in unopposed left-sided depolarization midway in the development of the QRS complex. Leads I, V_6, and MLI, having leftward positive electrodes, exhibit a taller and broader R wave, whereas leads aVR and V_1 have a more prominent S wave.

3. **Terminal depolarization: the right ventricular wall.** Here, the major changes in right bundle branch block occur, producing the typical configuration of the QRS complex. A depolarizing wave front from the *left* ventricle now enters the right, proceeding relatively slowly along contiguous myocardial fibers. The direction of this slow wave front is sometimes from apex to base so that the last portion of the QRS complex reflects the following:

Prolongation. The overall duration of the QRS complex is 0.12 second or longer.

Vector shift. A radical alteration in the terminal deflection occurs toward the right ventricular base, the left ventricle having already been depolarized.

These combined factors produce a broad and downward deflection at the end of the QRS complex (S wave) in leads I, V_6, and MLI, having leftward positive electrodes. As expected, leads V_1 and aVR display a prolonged and upward late deflection of the QRS complex (referred to as R prime or R').

Because alterations in the *depolarization* sequence of the ventricles occurs in right bundle branch block, the overall electrical forces of *repolarization* are usually affected. The T waves are often reduced in amplitude or become reversed in polarity. Deviation of ST segments from the isoelectric line can sometimes be observed as well.

Review the configurations of the QRS complexes in three different leads in the following example of right bundle branch block.

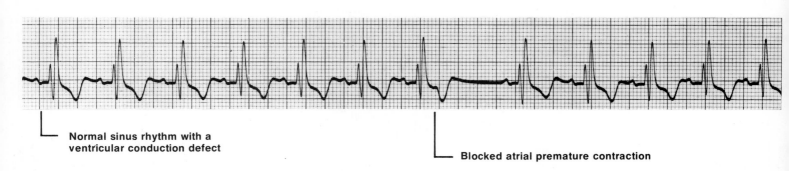

Normal sinus rhythm with a
ventricular conduction defect

Blocked atrial premature contraction

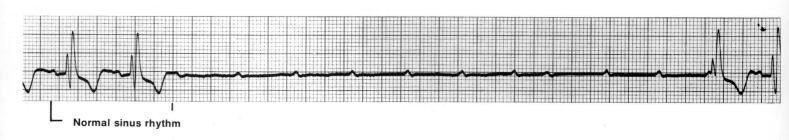

Normal sinus rhythm

Continued sinus rhythm with absence of ventricular response

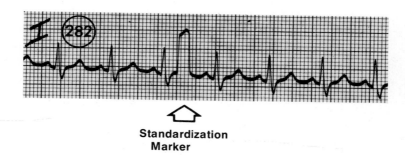

Standardization
Marker

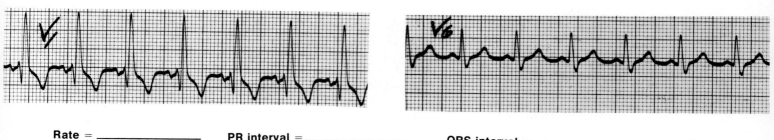

Rate = _____   PR interval = _____   QRS interval = _____

The slender configuration of the right bundle branch renders it vulnerable to anatomical lesions, most commonly sclerodegenerative, ischemic, and inflammatory disorders. Furthermore, the Purkinje cells of the right bundle branch have a longer refractory period than do those of the left, so that it is more susceptible to physiological block induced by premature beats and tachycardias. It is also one of the earlier signs of drug toxicity by those agents that depress impulse conduction. Indeed, bundle branch block is a common clinical finding, of which several examples are included here.

Although quite common as a permanent complication of diffuse diseases of diverse etiology, right bundle branch block may appear transiently in pulmonary embolism (evidently as a result of sudden right ventricular overload). Developing in acute myocardial infarction, it signifies that injury of the intraventricular septum has occurred, a complication with a high incidence of subsequent complete A-V block. Right bundle branch block, on the other hand, may be found in individuals with no history or physical findings suggesting heart disease nor with any abnormal exercise stress tests or coronary angiograms. In these persons, the condition can be considered benign, although it may be the first expression of an underlying disease.

Cardiac rhythms are commonly monitored using an arrangement of electrode placement that simulates lead V_1. This selection is favored in many cardiac care units because of the distinctive rSR′ pattern exhibited in lead V_1 in right bundle branch block. One must remember, however, that a conduction defect is evident in *all* leads, and the bundle branch blocks can generally be identified in each. Of course, learning the characteristic pattern of these blocks in one's customary monitoring lead is imperative. In MLI, right bundle branch block is typified by a small Q, an R (of highly variable amplitude), and a revealing deep and wide S deflection.

The following tracings from leads I and V_1 exhibit right bundle branch block (Fig. 7-7). They are from a 58-year-old man who sustained a recent inferior wall myocardial infarction. Inspection reveals that apparent PR intervals vary from beat to beat, and in actuality, the atria and ventricles have independent pacemakers.

The presence of right bundle branch block in this rhythm indicates that the pacemaker driving the ventricles arises from A-V junctional tissue. It cannot be located in the atria, because the atria are under the control of the sinus pacemaker. The sequence of depolarization of the ventricles places the secondary pacemaker high in the ven-

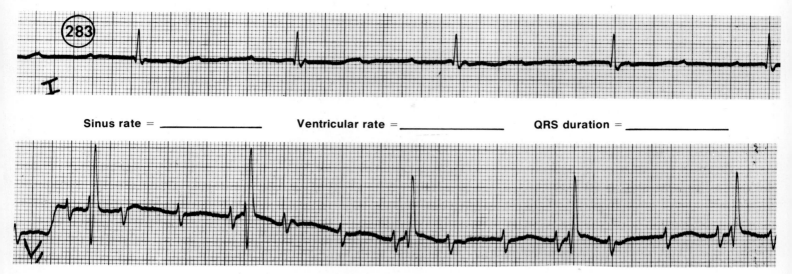

Sinus rate = _____   **Ventricular rate** = _____   **QRS duration** = _____

Figure 7–7. Compound arrhythmia (having more than one electrical disturbance) taken from leads I and V₁.

tricular conduction system near the A-V node. Thus, identification of a bundle branch block pattern is helpful in establishing the origin of ventricular beats.

Thus, Figure 7–7 provides an example of **compound arrhythmia**, defined as a rhythm with more than one electrical disturbance. The interpretation includes the following:

1. Sinus tachycardia.
2. Complete A-V block.
3. A-V nodal (or junctional) rhythm.
4. Right bundle branch block.

Rhythm strip 284 (Fig. 7–8) was recorded from a student nurse who complained of a frequent flip-flop sensation in her chest. The symptom was particularly noticeable after drinking coffee.

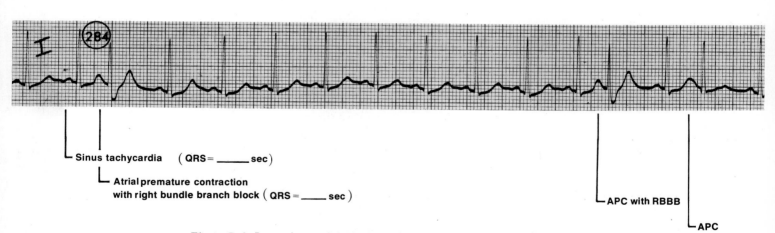

Sinus tachycardia (QRS = _____ sec)

Atrial premature contraction with right bundle branch block (QRS = _____ sec)

APC with RBBB

APC

Figure 7–8. Intermittent right bundle branch block.

In this tracing from lead I, premature contractions having aberrant ventricular conduction are evident. Note the first and second atrial premature complexes (APCs); each is characterized by the following:

1. Prolonged QRS complex.

2. Initial QRS complex similar to that of normally conducted beats (small Q waves), while the terminal portion consists of a widened and deeper S component.

3. Altered contours of ST segment and T wave.

Compare these forms with the third APC, in which the QRS complex is similar to that of the sinus beats. This APC occurs at a slightly longer interval after the previous beat, which evidently allows just enough additional time for the right bundle branch to recover and conduct the atrial impulse normally.

Figure 7–9 is a tracing from a 32-year-old marathon runner in excellent physical condition. Here a premature beat takes place before full recovery of the conduction pathways from the previous beat (e.g., during the refractory period). Such a conduction defect, particularly right bundle branch block, is commonly associated with atrial and nodal premature contractions. In this tracing, determine the basic rate and locate the APC with right bundle branch block. Again note that the onset of the QRS complex (early septal depolarization) is not changed, but that the QRS prolongation in its terminal portion results from delayed ventricular depolarization due to right bundle branch block. Identify the location and type of premature beat.

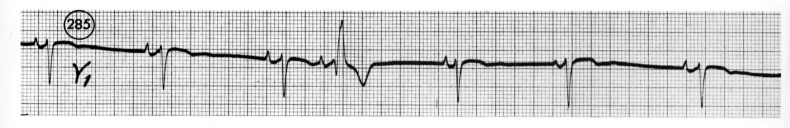

Rate = _____

Figure 7–9. Premature contraction with conduction defect.

In Figure 7–10, atrial fibrillation with intermittent right bundle branch block (rR′ in lead V_1) is evident. Locate the abnormally conducted ventricular beats. The bundle branch block pattern appears with the more rapidly occurring beats, suggesting a relationship of bundle branch conduction to rate. Evidently, the earlier beats are formed while the right ventricular conduction fibers are still in a refractory state. This is analogous to the failure of conduction in the A-V node after some APCs (see Blocked Atrial Premature Complexes in Chapter 4). Note the change in ST segment and T wave configuration caused by the bundle branch conduction defect. Identify the beats with right bundle branch block.

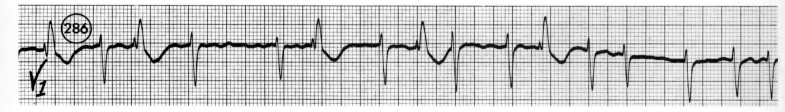

Figure 7–10. Normal and abnormal ventricular conduction as determined by rate.

Right bundle branch block produced by deep breath holding (Valsalva maneuver) is revealed in tracings 287 and 288. Notice that increased vagal tone has reduced the sinus rate and decreased conduction velocity in both the A-V node and the right bundle branch, producing transient lengthening of the PR interval and bundle branch block. The patient had sustained an anteroseptal infarction 3 days previously, accounting for the QS form (absence of a small septal R deflection in monitoring lead V_1). Note these

effects with deep breath holding:
1. Slowing of the sinus rate.
2. Development of right bundle branch block.
3. Prolongation of A-V conduction; this is progressive and results in a sequence
of second-degree A-V block of the Wenckebach type.
4. Recovery of A-V and right bundle conduction.

Measure unlabeled PR and QRS intervals and identify the location of nonconducted
sinus beats.

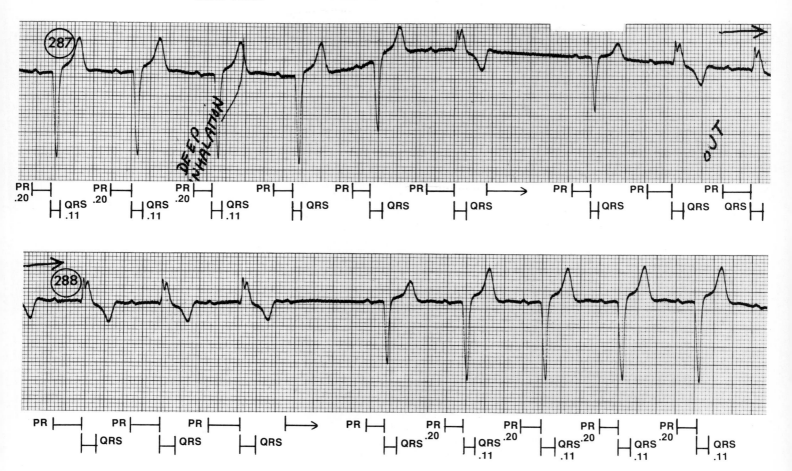

Tracing 289 reveals intermittent right bundle branch block in the presence of atrial
tachycardia with Wenckebach phenomenon and a regular 3:2 atrial to ventricular ratio.
The arrhythmia is recorded from special monitoring lead MLI.

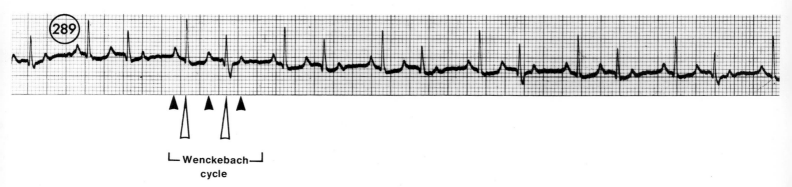

For test strip 289:

1. Determine PR intervals.
2. Complete the diagram.
3. Label all beats with right bundle branch block located at ____ mm, ____ mm, ____ mm, ____ mm.

Each instance of right bundle branch block appears in the second beat of the three-beat Wenckebach series. It is at this time that the ventricular conduction pathways have had the least time for recovery, and the impulse reaches the right bundle during its refractory period.

In this example of atrial flutter (Fig. 7–11), the tracing is taken from the standard ECG of a 66-year-old grocer who complains of occasional lightheaded episodes, especially tending to occur while lifting heavy boxes.

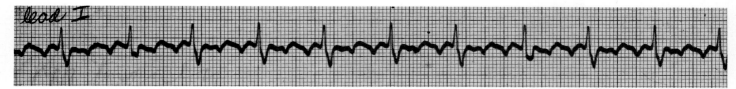

Figure 7–11. Right bundle branch block in the presence of atrial flutter.

The presence of a consistent 3:1 atrial to ventricular ratio and the constant FR intervals establishes the diagnosis of a supraventricular rhythm. The atrial rhythm controls the ventricular; the rhythm is not a form of A-V dissociation. The prolonged QRS complexes (0.13 second) have the configuration of right bundle branch block. However, note that the first F wave of each cardiac cycle falls in the terminal portion of ventricular depolarization. Because the F waves are predominantly downward in this lead, the prolonged S deflection may be at least in part caused by superimposed atrial activity. Thus, the reader cannot be certain if right bundle branch block is present or if it merely appears to be so.

Left Bundle Branch Block

Although the origin of the left bundle branch is a very broad, almost sheet-like band of conduction fibers, its continuity for impulse transmission can be damaged by extensive anatomical lesions. The end result is a characteristic change in ventricular activation, more profound than in right bundle branch block and of greater clinical importance (Fig. 7–12). The aberrant ventricular conduction is summarized as follows:

1. **Early depolarization: the intraventricular septum.** With loss of conduction at the common left bundle branch, the intraventricular septum becomes activated from the right bundle branch. The septum undergoes depolarization from *right to left*, contrary to the normal direction. In addition, the waveform spreads across adjacent myofibrils, beginning at the lower septal innervation; it does not use the rapid conduction fibers from the left bundle that serve the septum. Consequently, the initial portion of the QRS complex in left bundle branch block is drastically altered. The normal Q wave observed in leads I, V_6, and MLI is obliterated and replaced by a slowly developed, slurred R wave. Conversely, a Q wave (or small R followed by a deep S wave) is recorded in leads V_1 and aVR.

These changes in the initial deflection of the ECG are also found in myocardial infarction. The presence of left bundle branch block seriously interferes with the electrocardiographic diagnosis of infarction.

2. **Intermediary depolarization: the right ventricular wall.** The dominant electrical activity occurring during mid-QRS complex evolution is right ventricular depolariza-

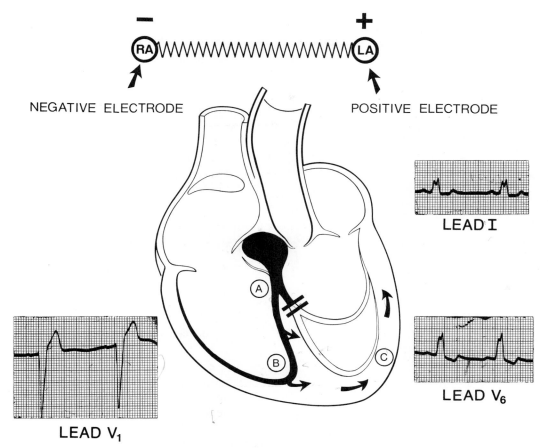

Figure 7–12. Left bundle branch block.

tion, initiated by the normal conduction system to that chamber and unopposed by the unstimulated left ventricle. Because the right ventricle normally contributes a relatively small and brief electrical force to the midportion of the QRS complex (owing to its thin wall), the resultant vector plays but a minor role in the final development of the QRS complex when depolarization in the left ventricle dominates.

3. **Terminal depolarization: the left ventricular wall.** Formed solely by a wave front arising at the lower end of the intraventricular septum or at the apex of the right ventricle and moving laterally toward the left and upward toward the base of the left ventricle, the final portion of the QRS complex is written as a wide, often "feathered" deflection that is upright in leads having left-sided positive electrodes. The wave front, invading from the right, may enter the distal Purkinje fibers of the left bundle branch distribution (beyond the conduction block), and the heterogeneity of depolarization gives the notched appearance to the resultant deflection. The thickness of the left ventricle undergoing aberrant depolarization produces a markedly delayed deflection in which the overall QRS duration may be as long as 0.18 second. Because the wave front proceeds toward the left shoulder, an upward terminal QRS deflection is found in leads I, V_6, and MLI. A deep Q wave or small R-deep S wave is usually present in leads V_1 and aVR. In most examples of left bundle branch block, the initial QRS deflection appears to merge with the terminal portion so that the complex often appears monophasic in these leads.

ST segment and T wave deviations usually result from this conduction defect, and often they are marked, as can be noted in the illustrations presented here.

The features of left bundle branch block can be observed in Figure 7–13, recorded from lead V_1 in a patient with an acute myocardial infarction. The conduction defect was intermittent. The beats to the right of the tracing are normal in respect to QRS duration and configuration. Those to the left exhibit typical left bundle branch block, coincident with a very small increase in rate.

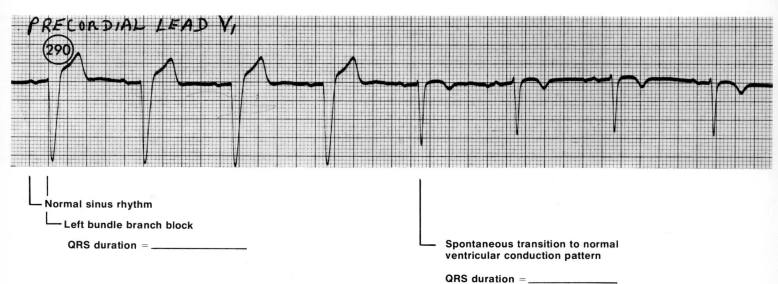

Normal sinus rhythm

Left bundle branch block

QRS duration = _____

Spontaneous transition to normal ventricular conduction pattern

QRS duration = _____

Figure 7–13. Transient rate-related left bundle branch block.

Note the absence (or virtual absence) of the R wave in left bundle branch block in addition to the abnormally wide QRS duration. In these beats, the ST segment is markedly elevated and the T wave upright, in sharp contrast to the form associated with normal ventricular activation. Measure the durations of the normally conducted ventricular complex and the QRS during left bundle branch block.

The causes of left bundle branch block are almost always anatomical and permanent rather than physiological and temporary. The condition should always be considered pathological, and in fact, it generally indicates extensive pathology. Clinicians should also appreciate that left bundle branch block may reflect a combination of lesions involving both anterior and posterior divisions of the bundle branch, a condition that would be indistinguishable from a single block in the main stem.

A comparison of the characteristics of the QRS complex in monitor lead MLI for left bundle branch block and right bundle branch block is presented below.

	Initial Portion	*Terminal Portion*
Right bundle branch block:	Normal depolarization of ventricular septum: **Usually small Q**	Delayed right ventricular depolarization: **Wide S**

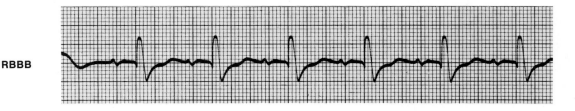

RBBB

	Initial Portion	*Terminal Portion*
Left bundle branch block:	Reversed depolarization of ventricular septum: **Absent Q**	Delayed left ventricular depolarization: **Wide R**

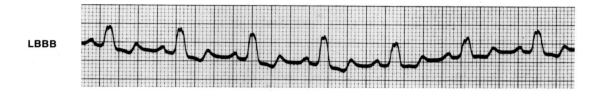

LBBB

The Hemiblocks

As the trunk of the left bundle branch block flares out, it forms two major divisions and often a number of minor ones. Highly variable anatomically, these divisions may incur a disturbance in conduction, either singularly or in combination. Such segmental blocks affect only a portion of the left ventricle so that the alteration in depolarization is more restricted than in main stem left bundle branch block. The area of the left ventricle subtended by the blocked segment receives a propagating waveform from the normally innervated right ventricle or another portion of the left ventricle. This aberration of conduction produces a modest prolongation and deformity of the QRS complex and a shift in the mean electrical axis of ventricular depolarization.

Failure of conduction in either of the two main divisions, or fascicles, is referred to as a hemiblock (a not quite accurate term denoting "half-block"). Like right and left bundle branch block, these lesser conduction defects do not fall within the definition of an arrhythmia, yet they produce electrocardiographic changes that are extremely helpful to recognize when interpreting rhythms. Although it is beyond the intent of this text to present the hemiblocks in detail, a brief description is provided.

The anterior limb of the left bundle branch subserves the midportion of the intraventricular septum as well as the anterior, lateral, and superior portions of the free wall of the left ventricle. In **left anterior hemiblock**, these areas are stimulated last by wave fronts coming predominantly from the posterior and inferior wall, where impulses from the intact posterior limb are received. The alteration in sequence produces a deeper Q wave in leads I and MLI owing to slower septal depolarization from the more distal branches of the posterior limb. More conspicuous is the delayed terminal force, which is oriented toward the anterior and superior ventricular wall, resulting in a deep S deflection and marked left axis deviation as seen in the lead II strip of Figure 7–14 (see the section on Component Abnormalities in Chapter 2). Although the duration of the QRS complex may be prolonged, the conduction delay is usually slight.

More slender than its counterpart posteriorly, the anterior limb is far more susceptible to adversities affecting impulse conduction. The prevalent causes are ischemic heart disease, sclerodegenerative fibrosis, and left ventricular enlargement (associated with hypertension and aortic valvular obstruction). The electrocardiographic diagnosis of left anterior hemiblock may be obscured in myocardial infarction of the inferior wall, and vice versa.

The posterior limb of the left bundle branch is distributed to the septum and to the posterior and the inferior free walls of the left ventricle. In **left posterior ventricular hemiblock**, early septal depolarization is altered, causing loss of Q waves in leads I and MLI and replacement by a small R wave (Fig. 7–15). The most striking feature, however, is a marked shift of electrical axis in the terminal deflection as the wave front proceeds from the end of the anterior limb toward the inferior and posterior wall. These

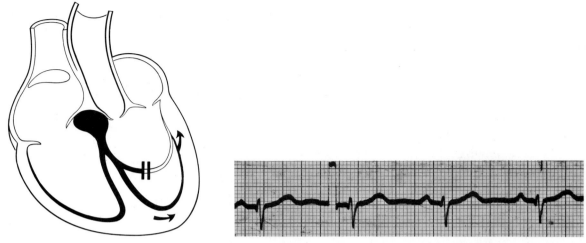

Figure 7–14. Left anterior hemiblock. Lead II in an asymptomatic patient with left anterior hemiblock. (The generally downward deflection of QRS in this lead indicates marked left axis deviation.)

leads then exhibit a prominent S wave often associated with terminal slurring. Right axis deviation is characteristic (see the section in Chapter 2 entitled Component Abnormalities), and the QRS complex is sometimes prolonged beyond the limits of normal.

As an isolated lesion of conduction, left posterior hemiblock occurs rarely. More likely, it reflects diffuse disease in which other defects of the A-V node and His-Purkinje systems are also present. Furthermore, it may simulate the electrocardiographic pattern of right ventricular hypertrophy and a vertical heart configuration.

The criteria given above for both anterior and posterior hemiblock are not always adequate for definitive diagnosis. Even so, the reader should be aware of the possibility that these more distal defects in impulse conduction may explain a shift in electrical axis and in lengthening of the QRS complex when the characteristics of the major bundle branch blocks are incompletely represented.

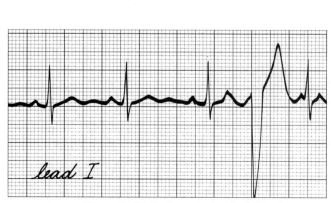

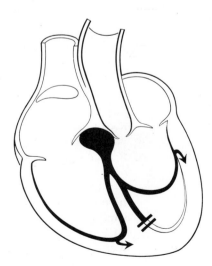

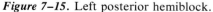

Figure 7–15. Left posterior hemiblock.

Combined Conduction Defects

It is most probable that the majority of hemiblocks represent diffuse involvement of the defective pathways rather than a single lesion. It can be readily appreciated that such microconduction disturbances at multiple sites may be associated with disease in other regions of the conduction system. Combined fascicular block, in fact, is a common clinical entity. Indeed, left bundle branch block is more likely to be caused by **bifascicular block** (left anterior hemiblock plus left posterior hemiblock) than by singular disease of the left bundle main stem. Bifascicular block may occur also as a combination of right bundle branch block with block of either of the left fascicles.

The combination of left anterior hemiblock with right bundle branch block is a frequent complication of extensive ischemic heart disease; its presence indicates that both ventricles are supplied by the left posterior branch alone. Although this form of conduction disease may be clinically stable for a number of years, progression to complete A-V block should always be expected eventually as the left posterior fascicle becomes involved in the disease. Appearing in acute myocardial infarction, left anterior hemiblock with right bundle branch block is a valid indication for the prophylactic use of an electronic pacemaker because of the high incidence of development of complete A-V block.

An example of progression to multiple fascicular block is demonstrated in Figure 7–16. In the top row of selected leads, normal sinus rhythm and PR and QRS intervals of normal duration are evident. Left axis deviation is present (the QRS complex in lead II is nearly equal in positive and negative deflections, indicating an electrical axis of about −30°).

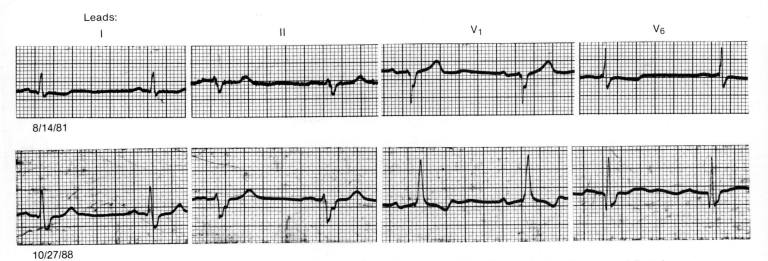

Leads:

I II V₁ V₆

8/14/81

10/27/88

Figure 7–16. Electrocardiograms from the same individual showing development of first-degree A-V block and combined ventricular conduction defects.

Without any symptoms suggesting cardiac disease, a routine ECG taken several years later and shown in the bottom row of Figure 7–16 reveals the typical pattern of right bundle branch block (widened terminal negative deflections in leads I and V₆ and positive deflection in lead V₁). In addition, the electrical axis of the QRS complex has rotated appreciably more leftward (predominantly negative QRS complex in lead II). This latter finding is indicative of left anterior hemiblock. Also note that the PR interval has become prolonged, pointing to a conduction defect within the A-V node-common bundle. The P waves have also become prolonged and multiphasic (best seen in lead II), which may represent disturbed conduction within the atria. The overall impression is that of diffuse conduction disease developing during the years between ECGs. The patient is at high risk of developing complete A-V block.

Trifascicular block consists of right bundle branch block, left anterior hemiblock, and left posterior hemiblock. Actually, this is another form of complete A-V block, and the electrocardiographic pattern cannot be distinguished from that of a single lesion in the A-V node or in the common bundle. The progressive development of conduction defects from mono- to bi- to trifascicular block is sometimes documented by serial ECGs in the same patient.

Persons with bifascicular blocks have a high incidence of progression into complete A-V block. This is particularly true if prolongation of the PR interval is also present. A patient who complains of periods of syncope, lightheadedness, or other manifestations of sudden circulatory depression and who, in addition, has multiple electrocardiographic conduction disorders should be suspected of having periods of intermittent third-degree A-V block, causing transient symptomatic bradycardia.

An example of multiple conduction pathway defects can be seen in the case of a 56-year-old baker who had increasingly frequent episodes of unexplained lightheadedness for several weeks (Fig. 7–17). A standard ECG revealed normal sinus rhythm with right bundle branch block and left anterior hemiblock. During the recording of lead V₁, an arrhythmia appeared, disclosing the cause of the symptoms.

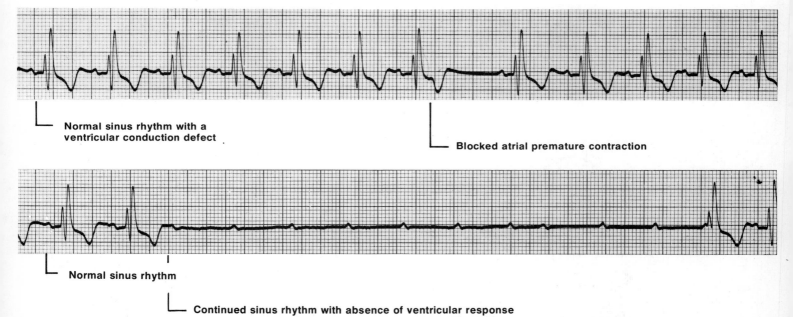

Normal sinus rhythm with a
ventricular conduction defect

Blocked atrial premature contraction

Normal sinus rhythm

Continued sinus rhythm with absence of ventricular response

Figure 7–17. Multiple bundle branch blocks progressing to ventricular asystole.

During this recording time, the patient felt faint. A 6-second period of ventricular asystole is ended with a nodal escape beat, after which the sinus rhythm is resumed. At this instant, the patient recovered fully.

Note that the PR interval of conducted beats is normal, suggesting that impulse transmission through the A-V node is unimpaired. As the patient was known to have complete block of two of the major bundle branches (bifascicular block), it was presumed that the third bundle (left posterior branch) was diseased and temporarily incapable of transmitting impulses, producing intermittent trifascicular block. A poorly functioning escape mechanism led to a period of symptomatic ventricular asystole.

The extensive nature of the cardiac disease is thus revealed. Insertion of an electronic pacemaker prevented further episodes of presyncope.

These segmental bundle branch blocks can be suspected from a single monitoring lead by documenting widening of the QRS complex and a marked shift in its electrical axis. However, the accurate diagnosis of a specific hemiblock pattern requires the use of several leads. Inferior myocardial infarction and conditions that produce left ventricular hypertrophy may simulate left anterior hemiblock. Conditions associated with right ventricular hypertrophy, such as cor pulmonale, may resemble the typical pattern of left posterior hemiblock.

8 The Ventricles

IMPULSE FORMATION
Ventricular Escape Beat
Idioventricular Rhythm
Ventricular Rhythm in Complete Atrioventricular Block
VENTRICLE: IMPULSE FORMATION
Excitation
Ventricular Premature Complexes
Ventricular Tachycardia
Ventricular Flutter
Ventricular Fibrillation
VENTRICLE: IMPULSE FORMATION
Depression
Ventricular Bradycardia
Ventricular Pause
Ventricular Arrest
DIFFERENTIATION OF SUPRAVENTRICU-
LAR RHYTHMS WITH ABERRANT VENTRICULAR CONDUCTION FROM VENTRICULAR RHYTHMS
Relationship Between Atrial Beats and Ventricular Beats
QRS Complex Morphology
Post-Extrasystolic Pause
Regularity of Rhythm
Onset of a Tachycardia
Captured Beat
Fusion Beat
The Ashman Phenomenon
T Waves
Rate Changes
Preexcitation Syndrome
Atrial Fibrillation
SELF-EVALUATION: STAGE 3

IMPULSE FORMATION

Impulses formed within the ventricular mass constitute an extremely important group of arrhythmias in clinical practice. Spontaneous impulses may arise in the common bundle, in the major intraventricular fascicles, anywhere along the branches of the Purkinje system, and in the termini of these fibers as they intermingle with the myofibrils of the ventricles (Fig. 8–1).

A representative action potential for the major fascicles has already been discussed in Chapter 7, The Bundles. Noteworthy characteristics of this action potential are

1. Rapid velocity of upstroke.
2. Long refractory period.
3. Slow, spontaneous diastolic depolarization.

Figure 8–2 demonstrates how the property of automatic depolarization leads to a succession of automatic beats if the ventricles become isolated from control by higher impulse-forming centers. What distinguishes spontaneous discharge of ventricular tissue from the sinus node, the atrial tissue, and the atrioventricular (A-V) junctional tissue is its comparatively *slow* rate of spontaneous decrement in resting membrane

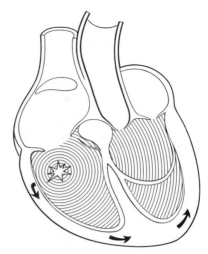

Figure 8–1. Ventricular impulse formation.

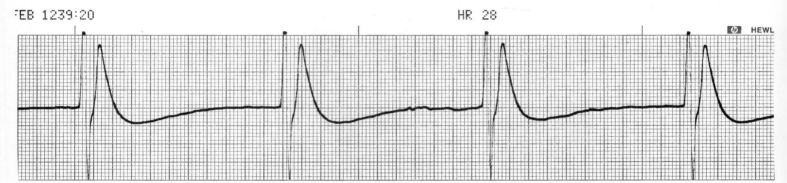

FEB 1239:20   HR 28

Figure 8–2. Ventricular escape beats occur when sinus node activity is absent.

potential. Under normal circumstances, the sinus node (and, in its absence, the atria or the A-V junctional tissue) beats at a more rapid rate. Its discharge reaches the ventricles *before* the ventricles themselves can undergo great enough diastolic depolarization to generate a discharge.

Ventricular Escape Beat

When impulses from higher pacemakers fail to stimulate the ventricles within a certain period (determined by the natural cycling time of the action potential), the ventricles emit a spontaneous impulse. The responsible mechanism is precisely that described for atrial and A-V junctional escape beats. This situation may occur ① when the sinus pacemaker slows to below the intrinsic rate for automatic firing of the ventricles and ② when subsidary pacemakers in the atria and A-V junctional tissues remain quiescent. Such a ventricular escape beat is illustrated in Figure 8–3. It was recorded as an unexpected result of carotid pressure stimulation on a 52-year-old longshoreman who presented without symptoms or findings of clinical heart disease except for first-degree A-V block.

A mild A-V conduction defect is evident at first, with a PR interval of 0.24 second. On carotid pressure, the sinus pacemaker slows somewhat and its impulse fails to stimulate the ventricles. There follows a delay in ventricular activity of 1.98 seconds, interrupted by a QRS complex that is grossly altered in configuration and markedly

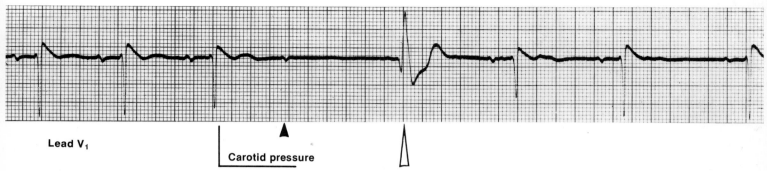

Lead V₁

Carotid pressure

Figure 8–3. Ventricular escape beat.

prolonged to 0.21 second (normal QRS duration should not exceed 0.12 second). Note that its initial deflection is changed, a deep Q wave replacing the normal small R wave in lead V_1. The major prolongation of the complex is created by widening of the terminal deflection, forming a wide S wave.

The altered form and lengthening of the QRS complex are characteristic of ectopic ventricular beats. These changes represent a slow propagation of wave front from the automatic focus, coursing through contiguous myocardial fibers and spreading radially through the ventricular shell. This sequence contrasts sharply with ventricular impulses that follow the normal, rapidly conducting Purkinje fiber pathways to the entire endocardial surface and then have but a short distance to travel through the myocardium to the epicardial surface.

The disturbances revealed by vagal stimulation in Figure 8–3 are (1) that marked hypersensitivity of the sinus node is present and (2) that secondary potential pacemakers above the ventricles are depressed. Even so, a latent pacemaker in the ventricles is operative, and it prevents excessive slowing of the heart. For lead V_1, the QRS complex does not exhibit the pattern of right bundle or left bundle branch block. Thus, one is persuaded that the beat does not arise from the A-V junctional tissue or from the common bundle, then encountering a conduction defect in a large intraventricular conduction pathway. The initiating impulse arises from within the ventricular tissue itself.

The tracing in Figure 8–4 is from an 86-year-old man whose activity is limited only by arthritis of the hip. He has no symptoms attributable to cardiovascular disease nor any pertinent physical findings. The electrocardiogram (ECG) (lead II is shown here) was taken during a routine periodic examination.

Two consecutive escape beats appear after the first sinus pause. Each beat has an anomalous form with changes in initial and terminal deflections and lengthening to 0.16

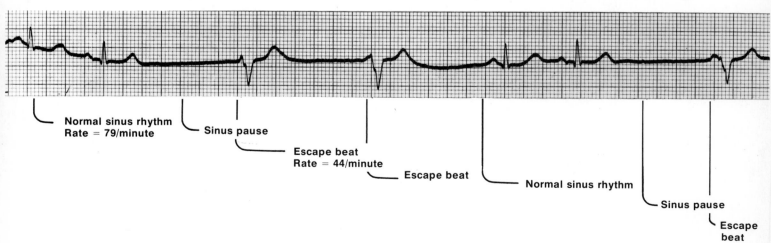

Normal sinus rhythm Rate = 79/minute

Sinus pause

Escape beat Rate = 44/minute

Escape beat

Normal sinus rhythm

Sinus pause

Escape beat

Figure 8–4. Ventricular escape beats interrupting sinus pauses.

second. The intrinsic rate is slow (44 if projected to 1 minute). A P wave can be identified, partially inscribed immediately preceding the second escape beat. The absence of any recognizable time relationship of atrial to ventricular activity, the absence of a bundle branch block or hemiblock pattern, the deformed, wide QRS complexes, and the slow rate lead one to conclude that these beats arise from a pacemaker within the ventricles.

At the end of this tracing, observe another sinus pause. The pause is now broken by a P wave that is completely inscribed (proving that the atria had fully depolarized before the QRS complex began). However, the PR interval appears too brief to permit impulse transmission through the A-V node. Furthermore, the QRS complex resembles in every way the previous escape beats, already identified as ventricular in origin. The P wave and the QRS complex in question are then presumed to arise from independent pacemakers (sinus node and ventricular) firing almost simultaneously.

From this tracing, we may conclude with reasonable surety the following:

1. The sinus node pacemaker is erratic, with spontaneous and marked slowing (probably a form of sinus node dysfunction).

2. Subsidiary pacemakers in the atria and the A-V junctional tissues fail to emerge (normally triggered by the sinus node at a rate faster than 44 per minute).

3. A ventricular pacemaker assumes control at a rate (for two consecutive beats) that is slow but entirely within the range of the natural automaticity in ventricular tissue. This pacemaker rescues the heart from more profound slowing or even asystole. When the sinus node pacemaker speeds up, it again resumes control of the heartbeat, and the ventricular pacemaker once again becomes dormant (at least temporarily).

When unstimulated by a higher pacemaker, the inherent rate of the ventricles is between 20 and 50 beats per minute. In general, the more distal the ventricular pacemaker, the more slowly it beats.

The tracing in Figure 8–5 from the monitoring lead (simulating lead I) is from an elderly man with a recent history of brief lapses of consciousness.

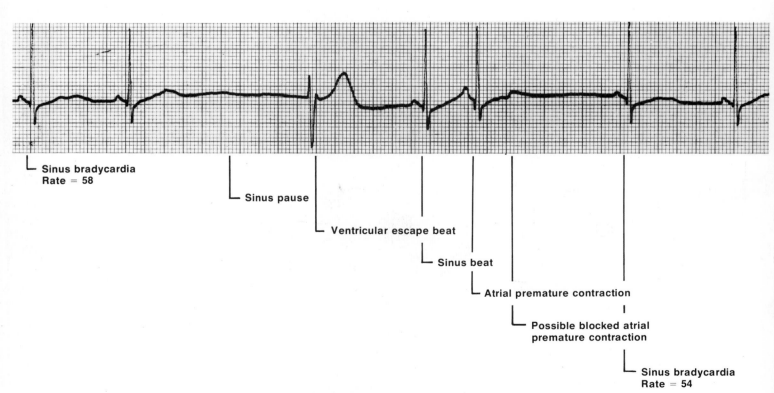

Figure 8–5. Compound rhythm with ventricular escape beat.

The escape QRS complex that appears after a pause of 1.88 seconds is altered in morphology and is increased in duration, from 0.08 to 0.13 second. Both initial and terminal components of the complex are changed. No P wave is observed before it nor identified within or shortly after the QRS complex. In addition, neither the pattern of right nor left bundle branch block is recognized. All these points establish that the beat does not arise from the sinus node, atria, or the A-V junction, but rather from a ventricle. An atrial premature beat is noted, incidentally, in this tracing.

An additional feature that is common in beats that originate in the ventricles is a change in ST segment and T wave contour. The altered waveforms represent an anomalous sequence of repolarization after an abnormal sequence of depolarization. Figure 8–6 illustrates an idioventricular rhythm, in which the distinguishing features for interpretation of ventricular initiated rhythms (prolonged QRS interval, no atrial activity/ relationship, T wave and ST segment changes) can be observed.

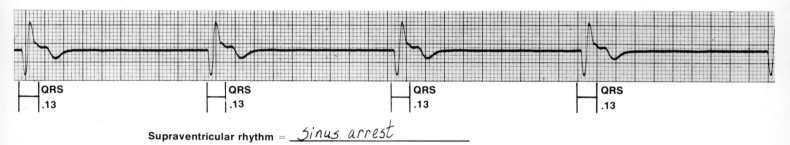

Supraventricular rhythm = *Sinus arrest*

Ventricular rhythm: Rate = *31* QRS duration = *.13 sec.*

Figure 8–6. Ventricular rhythm with characteristic QRS changes of beats originating in the ventricle.

Idioventricular Rhythm

The tracings that follow illustrate sustained ventricular escape rhythms. They appear with sinus arrest in the absence of functioning escape pacemakers in the atria and the A-V junction. Designated idioventricular rhythm (referring to its self-induced property), it maintains the heartbeat while all other pacemakers have failed. Look for the typical features of this rhythm in each of the examples. Complete the labeling of the following examples of idioventricular rhythm.

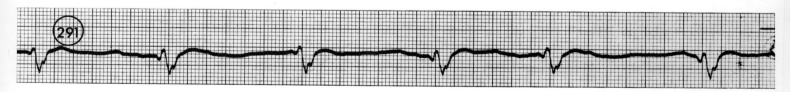

Supraventricular rhythm = *Atrial activity indistinct*

Ventricular rhythm: Rate = *43* QRS duration = _____

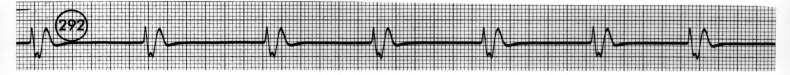

Supraventricular rhythm = _____

Ventricular rhythm: Rate = _____ QRS duration = _____

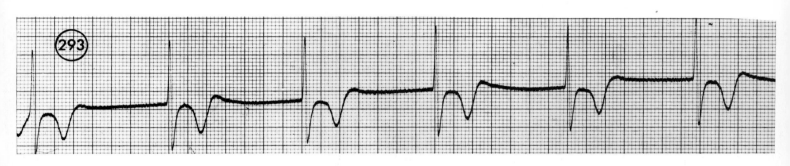

Supraventricular rhythm = _____

Ventricular rhythm: Rate = _____ QRS duration = _____

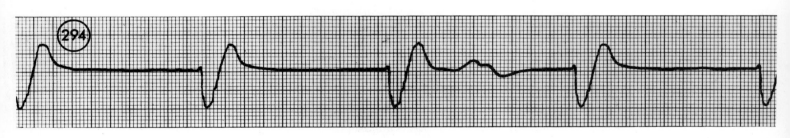

Supraventricular rhythm = _____

Ventricular rhythm: Rate = _____ QRS duration = _____

Rhythm strip 295 was obtained from a 28-year-old woman several hours after she had taken an overdose of a barbiturate. There is no evidence of sinoatrial activity, and the idioventricular rhythm is extremely slow. Furthermore, the rate of depolarization of the ventricles is markedly retarded, as indicated by the severely prolonged QRS complexes. All these findings are caused, presumably, by prolonged hypoxia and acidosis. Under such conditions, it is expected that the force of myocardial contractions is seriously compromised as well.

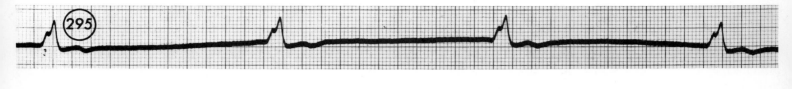

Supraventricular rhythm =_____

Ventricular rhythm: Rate = _____ QRS duration =_____

Ventricular Rhythm in Complete Atrioventricular Block

The previous examples demonstrate emergence of a pacemaker within automatic tissue of the ventricles after delay or cessation of activity in higher pacemaker centers. The same escape mechanism can become operative when impulses from these higher pacemakers fail to reach the ventricles. Such an idioventricular rhythm is established in complete A-V block. It may also occur in intermittent A-V block when the rate of transmitted impulses through the A-V node is slower than the inherent rate of any of the potential pacemakers within the ventricles.

Figure 8–7 reveals complete A-V block with a slow ventricular rhythm that is, by definition, entirely independent of the atrial rhythm. The recording is from a monitoring lead.

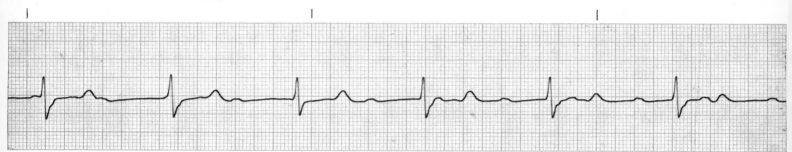

Figure 8–7. Complete A-V block with QRS complexes originating from an independent ventricular focus.

Note that the atrial rhythm is almost precisely regular, as is the ventricular rhythm. However, there is no relationship of timing between P waves and QRS complexes. QRS complexes are markedly deformed and widened; their morphology is uniform, but not the configuration of a major bundle branch type. These characteristics place the pacemaker in the ventricles, and the conduction defect distal to the common bundle.

Except for the site of origin of the subsidiary pacemaker, this rhythm is similar in mechanism to that described in Chapter 6 under complete A-V block with an A-V junctional pacemaker. One difference, however, is the slower inherent cycling of automatic pacemakers in the ventricles. Those in the proximal His-Purkinje system are usually expressed at rates of 35 to 40 beats per minute. Furthermore, these pacemakers usually beat at very regular intervals. In contrast, pacemakers located in the distal Purkinje system generally form impulses at much slower rates, about 20 to 30 per minute and sometimes even slower. In addition, these distal pacemakers tend to have an irregular cadence, as demonstrated in Figure 8–8.

Here, there is no sign of A-V transmission. Blocked atrial beats are glaringly

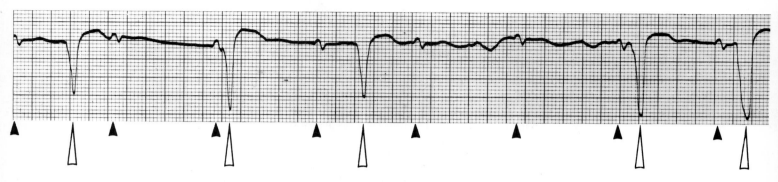

Sinus rhythm: Rate = 58   **Ventricular rhythm, extremely irregular: Rate = approximately 30**

Figure 8–8. Irregular ventricular rhythm in the presence of complete A-V block.

evident, while those that immediately precede a QRS complex have variable PR intervals. The extremely wide QRS complexes (0.16 second) identify a ventricular origin. Because the rate is very slow and very irregular, varying from an extrapolated 21 to 43 beats per minute, this rhythm probably arises from the distal conduction system of the ventricles.

Tracings 296 and 297 are examples of complete A-V block with escape rhythms. Check each with calipers for independent atrial and ventricular activity and for distinguishing features of the secondary pacemaker.

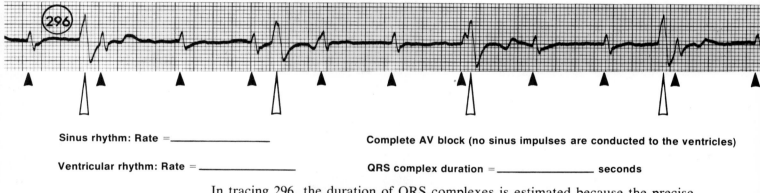

Sinus rhythm: Rate =_____   **Complete AV block (no sinus impulses are conducted to the ventricles)**

Ventricular rhythm: Rate =_____   **QRS complex duration =_____ seconds**

In tracing 296, the duration of QRS complexes is estimated because the precise point at which ventricular depolarization ends cannot be determined.

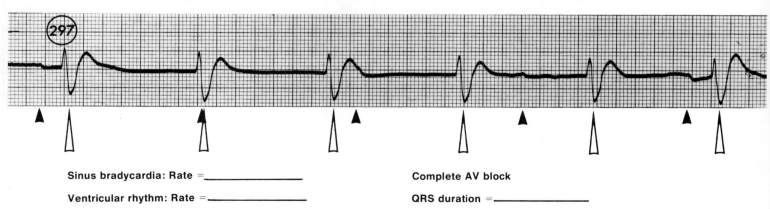

Sinus bradycardia: Rate =_____   **Complete AV block**

Ventricular rhythm: Rate =_____   **QRS duration =_____**

The ventricular rhythmicity in tracing 297 is regular. Taken from lead I of the standard ECG, the pattern has the appearance of right bundle branch block. This finding places the pacemaker either in the A-V junctional tissue or high in the intraventricular conduction system, near the origin of the bundle branches. (For typical right bundle branch block to become manifest, the depolarization impulse must course through an intact left bundle branch system.) The pacemaker rate favors its location in the A-V junction or common bundle.

Label all pertinent details in test tracings 298 through 300, working out their full interpretations. Include the designation of both supraventricular and ventricular rhythms with their respective rates and determine the duration of QRS complexes.

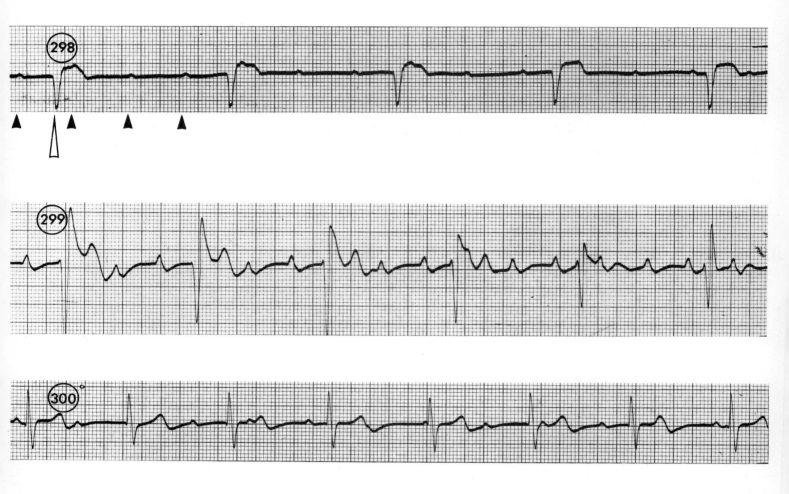

VENTRICLE: IMPULSE FORMATION

Excitation

The inherent rate of automaticity of pacemakers within the ventricles can be increased by a large number of highly varying factors so that it exceeds the rate of usually dominant pacemakers. The result is development of (1) ventricular premature complexes (VPCs) or, if sustained, (2) ventricular tachycardia. More advanced stages of excitation lead to (3) ventricular flutter and (4) ventricular fibrillation. These four rhythm disturbances are depicted in Figure 8–9.

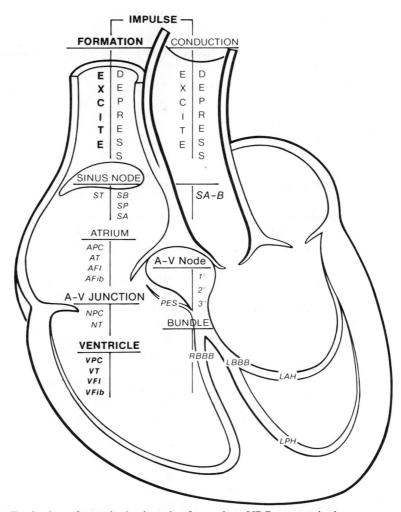

Figure 8–9. Excitation of ventricular impulse formation. VPC = ventricular premature complex; VT = ventricular tachycardia; VFl = ventricular flutter; VFib = ventricular fibrillation.

Ventricular Premature Complexes

Figure 8–10 illustrates normal sinus rhythm interrupted by anomalous beats. Features that distinguish these beats are as follows:

1. Prematurity (accelerated impulse formation).

2. Wide and distorted QRS complexes. It is assumed that the sequence of ventricular depolarization is altered by aberrant impulse conduction of slow velocity.

3. Altered ST segment and T wave contours.

4. Absence of retrograde conduction. The cadence of sinoatrial activity is undisturbed. This finding suggests that the premature beat originates below the A-V nodal system and that there is no conduction from ventricles to atria.

Cardiac cycles having these characteristics are designated ventricular premature complexes (VPCs). The excited impulse-forming site that is responsible may be in the common bundle, in the major bundle branches, or in the Purkinje termini within the free wall of either ventricle or within the intraventricular septum.

The terminology used for these premature cardiac cycles of ventricular origin is comparable to that described for supraventricular cycles. The word *contraction* denotes

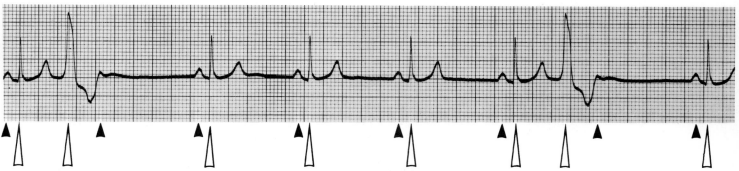

Figure 8–10. Normal sinus rhythm with ventricular premature beats.

a mechanical event, which, of course, is not detectable on the ECG. The words *beat, depolarization,* and *complex* imply an electrical event only and are often applied interchangeably in electrocardiography. Of these, we have chosen the term *ventricular premature complex* as most useful when referring to the ECG.

One feature of the previous tracing deserving further explanation is the blocked sinoatrial complex that follows each of the VPCs. Such an incomplete cardiac cycle is often identifiable after VPCs. Atrial depolarization from the normal sinus pacemaker occurs so soon after ventricular depolarization from the premature pacemaker that it finds the ventricular conducting system still depolarized or in the refractory state, and stimulation of the ventricles does not take place. Here, the nonconducted P waves are clearly identified. Use caliper measures of intervals to confirm that no disruption of sinus pacemaker rhythmicity occurs despite the VPC and the blocked atrial beat.

Ventricular beats that begin in the common bundle travel into both the right and left bundle branches and into the normal rapid conduction system of the ventricles. Retrograde conduction is often present so that P wave contour is altered and the sinus node is reset. Premature beats of this origin are identical to those from the A-V junctional sites when the surface ECG alone is used.

Ventricular beats from more distal sites inscribe a "negative" HV interval by electrogram. That is, the H spike occurs after the high ventricular depolarization because of reverse direction of the wave front; it is more properly called the VH interval (Fig. 8–11).

The interval between the VPC and the subsequent sinoatrial conducted beat is longer than the RR interval between normal cardiac cycles (owing to both prematurity of one beat followed by failure of ventricular stimulation by the next sinus beat). This longer interval is known as the *compensatory pause,* alluding to the delay in ventricular beats without change in sinus node rhythmicity. (The pause appears to compensate for the early cardiac cycle.) On taking the peripheral pulse, one may feel the premature beat very weakly or not at all; both prematurity and absent atrioventricular synchronous contraction contribute to decreased stroke volume. When the peripheral pulse generated by the early ventricular stimulus cannot be palpated, the accompanying pause is double that of the normal pulse interval. On the ECG, the interval between the complete cardiac cycles that flank the VPC is precisely twice the RR interval between two adjacent normal beats (Fig. 8–12).

Note that the simultaneously displayed rhythms remain in phase, even though an early ectopic beat has occurred.

Figure 8–13 is another example of a VPC in which the basic rhythm continues without any disruption of the dominant sinus pacemaker.

Recognizing the compensatory pause after premature ectopic beats is important to an electrocardiographer. Its presence demonstrates that the premature beat is electrically isolated from the sinus node and the atria; in other words, the excited impulse-forming site is distal to the A-V nodal system, and its wave front is not carried into the atria by retrograde conduction.

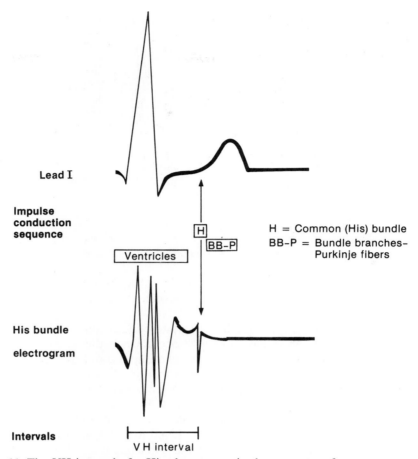

Figure 8–11. The VH interval of a His electrogram in the presence of a premature ventricular beat.

At the same time, the reader must be aware that the A-V nodal fibers usually conduct impulses in both directions, although retrograde conduction is often much slower than antegrade conduction. Also protecting the atria from stimulation by impulses originating in the ventricles is the relative refractoriness in the A-V node rendered by the supraventricular beat that immediately precedes the ventricular one. Thus both properties contribute to the dynamics of the compensatory pause.

The compensatory pause by itself has no important clinical implications. However, patients may experience palpitations from VPCs because of the long pause. Although the VPC may generate a relatively small stroke volume, the complete cardiac cycle

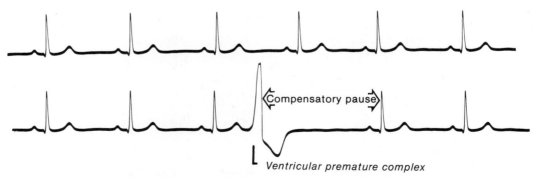

Figure 8–12. Compare the compensatory pause with normal sinus rhythm cycling intervals.

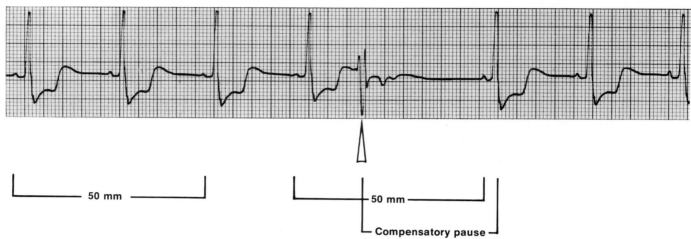

Figure 8–13. Ventricular premature beat that does not alter sinus node cycling.

that follows it will have a long ventricular filling time and inordinately strong ejection dynamics and large stroke volume. Patients often describe the sensation as a sudden ''kick'' inside the chest.

A VPC in which retrograde conduction can be identified is occasionally noted. This event is most likely to occur when the sinoatrial rhythm is slow, thus allowing sufficient time for the ventricular impulse to traverse the A-V node before it is blocked by an oncoming atrial impulse. In this instance, an aberrantly conducted atrial complex is found immediately after the premature beat, as shown in Figure 8–14.

This tracing exhibits a VPC in every way typical except that it is followed by a deformed P wave due to retrograde atrial depolarization.

A VPC is commonly referred to as an **extrasystole**. However, the typical dropped ventricular stimulation of the subsequent sinoatrial beat results in *no additional* (or extra) systole. For this reason, many authorities object to the long-used term extrasystole for this phenomenon.

A VPC in which the subsequent sinoatrial beat *is* conducted sometimes occurs, however, leading to ventricular stimulation, as demonstrated in Figure 8–15.

As is distinctive for ventricular premature beats, the early cardiac cycle has a wide and deformed QRS complex and altered ST segment and T wave configurations; in addition, the sinus pacemaker cadence is *not reset* by this beat. The unusual feature is that the sinus impulse that immediately follows the premature beat is conducted to the ventricles. (A slight prolongation of the PR interval reflects some delay in A-V

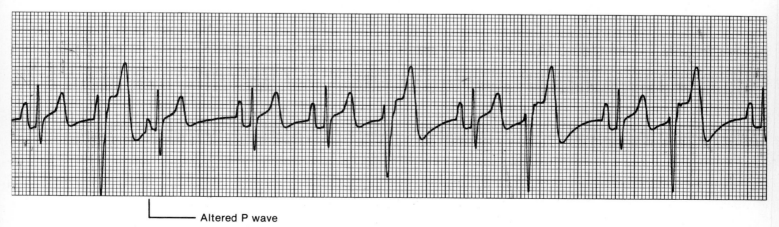

Figure 8–14. Aberrant atrial initiated cycle following a premature ventricular beat.

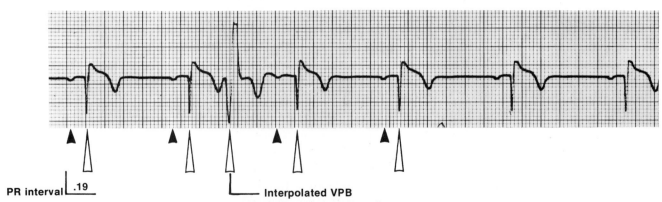

Figure 8–15. Interpolated ventricular premature beat.

conduction time due to relative refractoriness.) Such a VPC, which is not followed by a blocked sinoatrial beat, is termed an *interpolated beat*.

The interpolated VPC *does* add an extra beat to the pulse and therefore can properly be termed an extrasystole.

Several independent factors determine if the sinoatrial beat that follows a VPC will be conducted or blocked (e.g., whether the premature beat will result in a compensatory pause or it will be interpolated). Factors promoting conduction of the subsequent sinoatrial impulse are a slow sinus rate, very early prematurity, and rapid recovery of the A-V nodal system. Those factors that favor blocking of the subsequent sinoatrial impulse are a rapid sinus rate, very late prematurity, and delayed recovery of the A-V nodal system.

The interplay of factors influencing A-V nodal conduction after VPCs is observed in Figure 8–16.

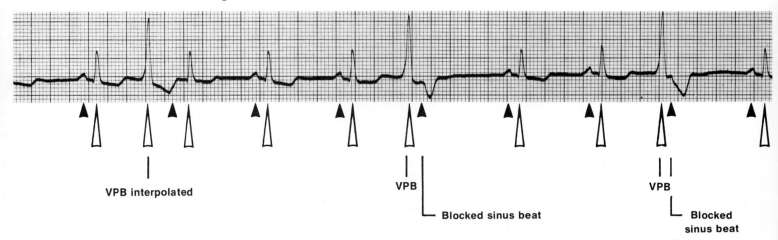

Figure 8–16. The compensatory pause.

In this tracing, VPCs are identified by timing, by QRS widening and deformity, and by lack of change in the sinus pacemaker cadence. After identifying the VPCs, note that *both* interpolated beats and compensatory pauses are present. The deciding factor appears to be the degree of prematurity of the ectopic ventricular beat. Those VPCs associated with a blocked sinoatrial beat following them occur somewhat later than the interpolated beat; the earlier of the VPCs allows the A-V nodal system to recover in time for transmission of the subsequent normal sinus impulse to the ventricles.

To review, compare now the compensatory pause associated with VPCs with the noncompensatory pause typically produced by premature beats originating in the atria or the A-V junction, as represented in the pictogram Figure 8–17.

Both depicted forms of supraventricular premature beats usually stimulate and discharge the sinus node before it reaches its natural time for spontaneous discharge. This premature stimulation resets the sinus node timer. At this instant, the sinus node begins a new action potential. The sinus beat that ensues occurs at a time determined by the natural cycling duration, usually the same as that between adjacent normal sinus beats that precede the premature beats. This change in cadence is displayed in the pictogram. The VPC, on the other hand, is followed by sinus beats that align with the matched undisturbed sinus rhythm.

The differences between compensatory and noncompensatory pauses are also demonstrated in the laddergram in Figure 8–18. Observe how the two types of premature stimuli affect the sinus beating that follows. To summarize, the depicted atrial premature beat resets the sinus node pacing; the VPC leaves the subsequent rhythm unaltered (including the single blocked sinoatrial wave front).

In rhythm strips 301, 302, and 303, examples of VPCs with compensatory pauses are demonstrated. Label the premature contraction, the blocked sinus beat, and the compensatory pause.

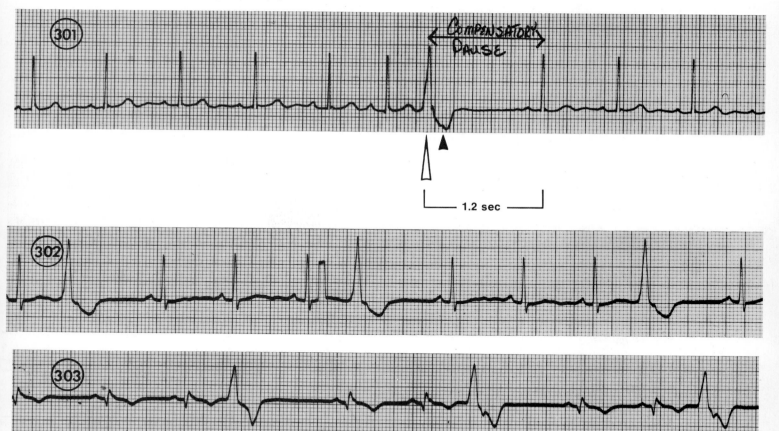

PREMATURE COMPLEXES IN SINUS NODE DYSFUNCTION. To expand briefly on the noncompensatory pause, we point out that the interval between supraventricular premature P waves and the next sinus P wave is usually not precisely equal to the PP interval between normal sinus beats. In fact, the shock sustained by the premature stimulation commonly results in some delay in the recovery phase of the sinus node cells, thus retarding the ensuing spontaneous discharge. The degree of lengthening of the noncompensatory pause is unpredictable.

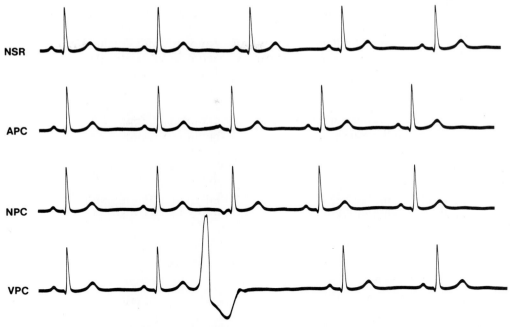

NSR

APC

NPC

VPC

Figure 8–17. Compensatory and noncompensatory pauses.

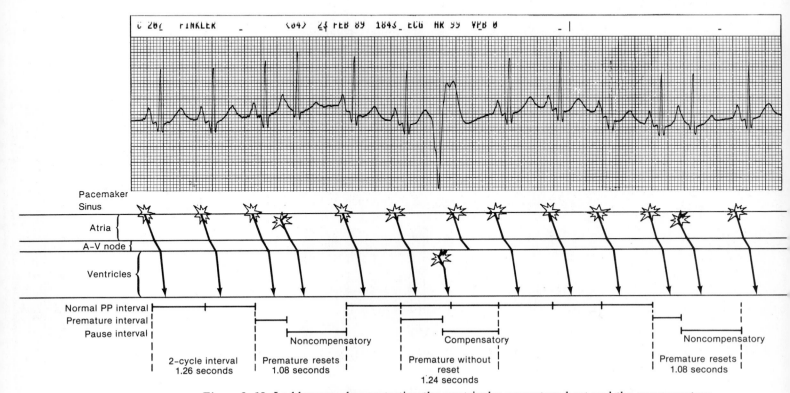

Figure 8–18. Laddergram demonstrating the ventricular premature beat and the compensatory pause. Retrograde conduction into the A-V node prevents the sinus beat from entering the ventricular conduction pathways. The result is a delay (compensatory pause) but *not* a loss of cadence.

As already described, patients with sinus node dysfunction tend to have an exaggerated delay of sinus rhythmicity after a supraventricular premature beat. Indeed, a very long noncompensatory pause is quite common and sometimes can be striking, as observed in the tracing in Figure 8–19, where the pause is terminated by an atrial escape beat. Had the escape beat not occurred, the pause could have exceeded 3 seconds.

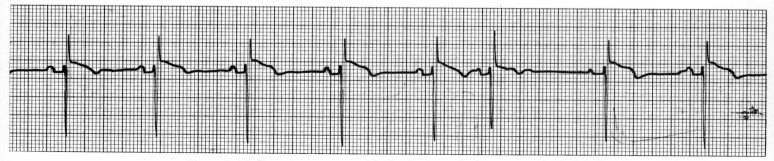

Figure 8–19. Premature supraventricular beat results in an excessively long noncompensatory pause.

Such long periods of sinoatrial arrest may result in presyncopal symptoms when atrial, A-V junctional, and the ventricular escape mechanisms are also defective. The finding of an unusually prominent noncompensatory pause should alert an electrocardiographer to the presence of underlying sinus node dysfunction. This phenomenon may be, in fact, the earliest clue to the disorder.

TIMING OF VENTRICULAR PREMATURE COMPLEXES

Ventricular premature beats are found at varying time relationships to the previous beats. Some occur early in the cardiac cycle; others appear very late. There are, of course, beats with intermediary timing. This relationship is one of the factors that determines if the beat will be interpolated or if there will be an associated compensatory pause—that is, whether or not the subsequent P wave will be blocked.

EARLY VENTRICULAR PREMATURE COMPLEX. The VPC appears *before* the normal P wave. There most often is enough time for the ectopic wave front to enter the A-V nodal system and block the entrance of the subsequent atrial impulse through it. Consequently, early VPCs are usually associated with a compensatory pause, as is evident in the following tracings.

On strips 304 to 308, label the VPC, the nonconducted P wave, and the compensatory pause. Is there a change in cadence of the sinoatrial rhythm?

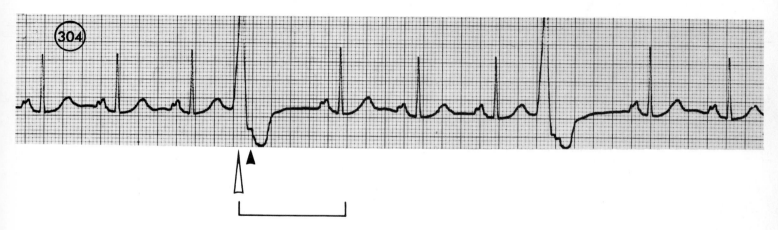

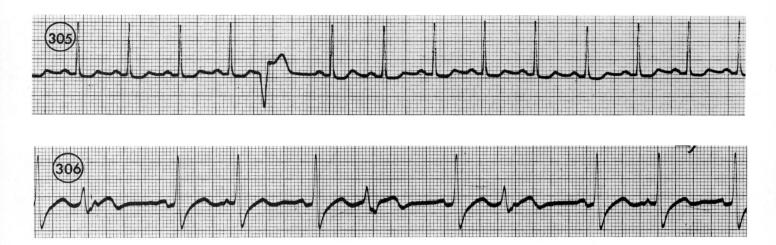

Tracing 306 illustrates a complicated arrhythmia exhibiting (1) normal sinus rhythm, (2) right bundle branch block, (3) atrial premature complexes, and (4) ventricular premature complexes. Locate all ectopic beats. The sinus rate may appear difficult to determine because there are no two consecutive sinus beats. Determine with calipers the interval from sinus P wave to blocked P wave appearing at the end of QRS of the VPCs. The next sinus P wave should occur precisely on time. Now use this interval to compare with cardiac cycles interrupted by the atrial premature beats, and a slight change in cadence becomes evident.

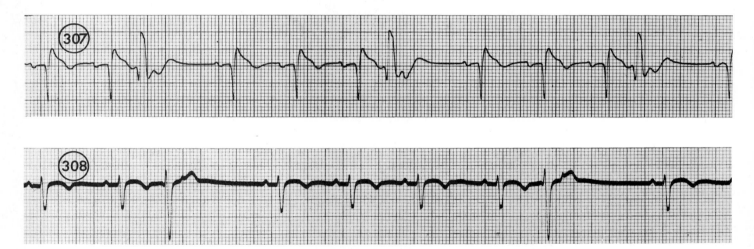

INTERMEDIARY VENTRICULAR PREMATURE COMPLEX. When the timing of a VPC is such that it occurs simultaneously with normal atrial depolarization, the P wave is generally obscured. Only a small portion of it may be detectable either at the onset of the QRS complex or at its terminus. Often, no P wave at all can be identified.

The tracing in Figure 8–20 was obtained from an anxious 26-year-old new mother who was worried about the recent onset of a thumping sensation in her chest, occurring several times a day during the preceding month. Cardiovascular history, physical examination, standard ECG, chest x-ray, complete blood count, electrolyte panel, and thyroxin blood level were entirely normal. The VPC recorded here was coincidental with her chest symptoms; the ECG was left on lead I after a 12-lead tracing, and the ectopic beat appeared just before venipuncture for the various blood tests.

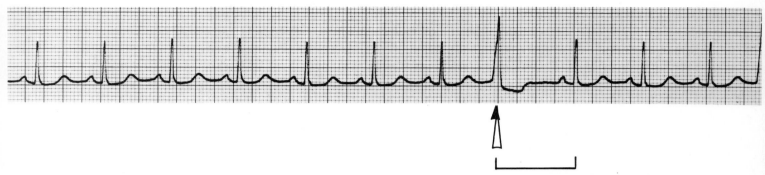

Figure 8–20. Ventricular premature contraction with P wave buried within the QRS.

Lead V_1 of an ECG from a 56-year-old man with a recent myocardial infarction is shown in Figure 8–21. The wide, uniphasic premature beat occurs at precisely the same time that a P wave is expected from plotting out with calipers, but there is no evidence of a P wave. Of course, a blocked sinoatrial impulse could have occurred precisely during inscription of the ectopic QRS complex, but it is more likely that the latter completely obscures the activity of atrial depolarization.

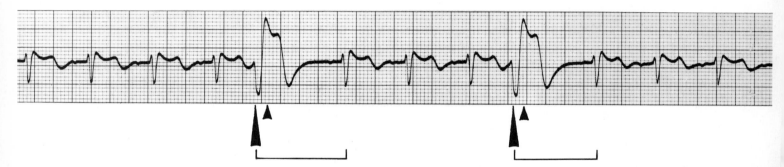

Figure 8–21. Sinus P wave occurring during the QRS.

The 82-year-old man from whom tracing 309 was obtained was completely asymptomatic. Identify the ectopic beat and the nonconducted P wave.

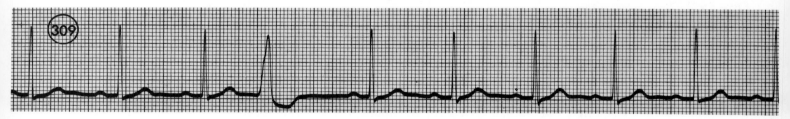

LATE VENTRICULAR PREMATURE COMPLEX. VPCs sometimes occur so late in the cardiac cycle that the sinus P wave appears *before* the ectopic QRS complex. The entire sinus P wave may be inscribed before the premature QRS complex begins. When the VPC occurs simultaneously with atrial activation, only the initial portion of the P wave may be recognizable, the remaining being lost in the QRS complex.

In the tracings in Figure 8–22, VPCs occur late in the cardiac cycle. The P waves in each tracing have already formed before the VPC begins. The degree of prematurity is very slight, so that the compensatory pause would be barely perceptible on auscultation of the heart or palpation of the pulse.

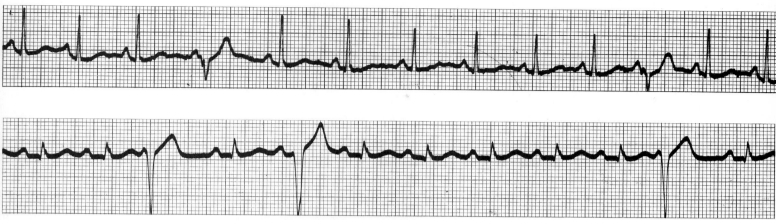

Figure 8–22. Late ventricular premature beats where the normal P wave precedes the QRS.

In test tracings 310 and 311, label all VPCs, nonconducted P waves, and compensatory pauses.

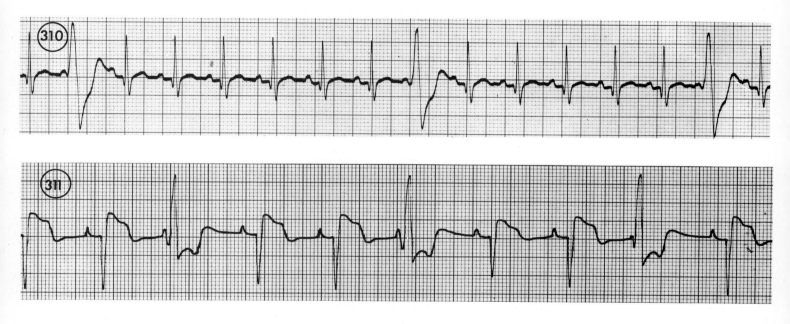

In Figure 8–23, three VPCs, occurring with slightly increasing intervals after the respective normal beat, are identified. In this single tracing, the P waves of associated blocked sinus beats can be located after, during, and before the ectopic QRS complex, according to the degree of prematurity.

THE FUSION BEAT. A VPC may occur so late in the cycle that a normal sinus pacemaker or ectopic atrial or A-V nodal pacemaker impulse has already penetrated the A-V node and started to depolarize the ventricles. Before depolarization is completed, however, a ventricular ectopic focus fires at a more distant site and initiates a wave of depolarization. These two wave fronts (one proceeding downward in a normal direction and the other moving toward the atria) collide. Thus, a hybrid QRS complex is inscribed, initially representing ventricular depolarization from a supraventricular focus and concluding with depolarization activity from an ectopic ventricular focus. Such a combination of polarizing forces is known as a fusion beat (Fig. 8–24).

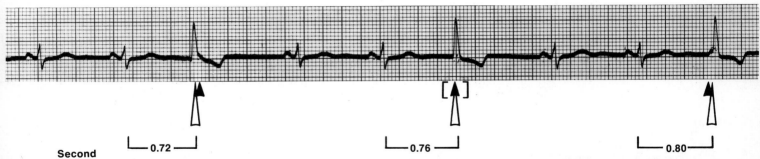

Second   └─ 0.72 ─┘   └─0.76─┘   └─0.80─┘

Figure 8–23. Comparison of ventricular premature complexes with varying degrees of prematurity.

In the pictogram in Figure 8–25, a ventricular complex is formed from two impulses, one from the sinus node and one from the ventricle. The resultant waves of depolarization fuse to produce a complex cardiac cycle. The fusion beat in this example begins with a normal sinus complex then takes on the form of a VPC. It occurs much later in the cardiac cycle than the previous one (which is not fused). The later the VPC, the greater is the penetration of the supraventricular impulse into the ventricles and, consequently, the greater is the likelihood for fusion of both wave fronts.

In Figure 8–26, compare ventricular premature beats. Each appears after a P wave has already begun to form. The second VPC occurs so late that the preceding P wave is completely inscribed. There follows an isoelectric period and the beginning of a QRS complex that is similar to that of the normal beats. Then the QRS complex takes on the form of the VPCs. This beat represents the fusion of normal ventricular depolarization from supraventricular stimulation with depolarization of ectopic origin.

One general characteristic of a fusion beat formed by collision of a supraventricular and a ventricular wave front is that the QRS complex is *narrower* than those produced by ventricular beats without fusion. This narrowing may be striking in the presence of a bundle branch block on the same side as the ectopic beat; the antegrade supraventricular impulse penetrates the ventricle in the normal bundle branch while the premature ectopic beat depolarizes the ventricle that has the conduction defect. A large portion of the complex is inscribed by the rapidly conducting supraventricular impulse along normal pathways.

Rarely, fusion beats are produced by two supraventricular foci, one of which is

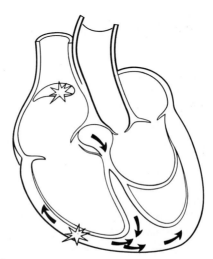

Figure 8–24. The fusion beat.

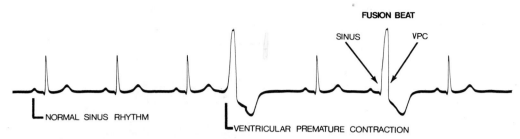

Figure 8–25. Comparison of fusion and nonfusion ventricular premature complexes.

usually the sinus node. The resultant P wave reflects the morphological characteristics of its double origin. More frequent are fusion beats from dual foci within the ventricles. Such beats tend to be of hybrid configuration and narrower than ventricular beats from a single site. A biventricular fusion complex can only be recognized on the ECG by identifying it as a composite made up of two independent VPCs.

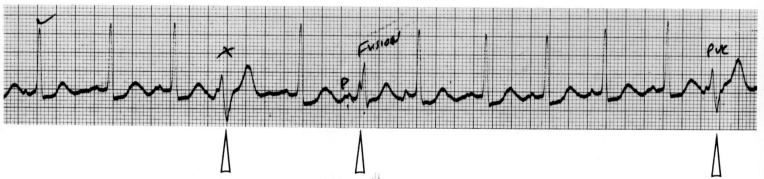

Figure 8–26. Examples of fusion beats.

The various timing relationships of VPCs which interrupt the normal rhythm are depicted for comparison in the pictorial summary in Figure 8–27. It will serve to review all details described in the various relationships of timing.

VPCs are found in entirely healthy individuals, or they may be the expression of underlying cardiac or systemic disease. In persons who are free of structural heart disease or disorders of the lungs, autonomic system, and metabolism, their presence is seldom of medical consequence. The sensation of ventricular premature beats is usually announced as a thump in the chest, probably the result of greater ejection volume in the beat *following* the premature beat (the compensatory pause allows increased ventricular filling). Uncomplicated VPCs occur at all ages and are generally innocent. An exception to this rule is middle-aged men, in whom the presence of VPCs presents an independent risk factor for coronary atherosclerotic disease.

Adrenergic stimulation is a common cause of ventricular premature beats to which individuals vary markedly in susceptibility. Strong emotional challenge, physical exertion, hypoglycemia, and adrenergic drugs and stimulants (nicotine, caffeine, and alcohol) are such provokers. Of the serious causes of ventricular ectopy, myocardial ischemia is certainly preeminent. The frequency of ventricular premature beats has a positive correlation in acute myocardial infarction with the size of the injury and the functional capacity of the left ventricle. Inflammatory conditions of the heart, hypertrophic cardiomyopathy, and mitral valve prolapse predispose to ventricular ectopy. Digitalis is an important cause, probably through enhancement of sympathetic tone. Cardiac trauma (blunt or surgical), hypoxia, and anesthetic agents commonly incite ventricular premature beats.

Ventricular premature beats are caused by (1) enhanced automaticity or by (2)

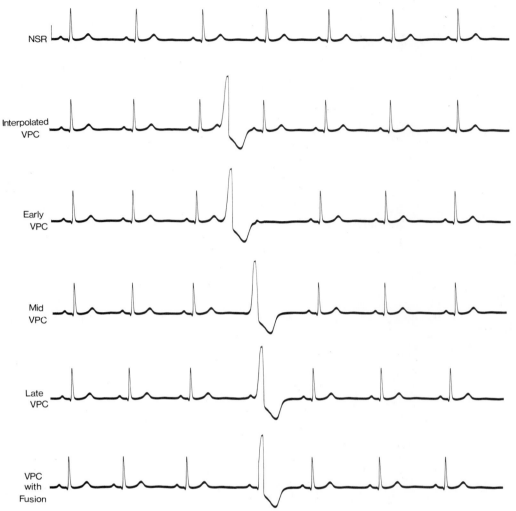

Figure 8–27. Ventricular premature complexes.

reentrant circuits. These mechanisms cannot be distinguished on the ECG, except by circumstantial evidence.

1. **Automaticity.** A potential pacemaker within the ventricles may discharge before the normally controlling wave front from higher pacemakers causes it to fire. Premature impulses can result from accelerated spontaneous depolarization, as is typically evoked by increased sympathetic tone. When ventricular premature beats are causally related to stimulation of the adrenergic system, enhancement of automaticity is the more likely mechanism. They may also arise from a reduction of the resting transmembrane potential, such as produced by hypoxia and hypothermia. These electrophysiologic events have been described for the atria (see Chapter 4), in which the same principles are operant.

2. **Reentrance.** Differences in conduction velocity and refractory period in adjacent fibers of the ventricles set up the circumstances favoring the reentrance phenomenon. The essential feature is functional longitudinal dissociation with unidirection block, as already explained for atrial ectopic beating (see Chapter 4), allowing completion of a reentrant loop with a resultant premature beat.

Reentrant beating probably occurs predominantly in the bundle branches and their major division. However, it may originate from the termini of Purkinje fibers or even at the Purkinje-myocardial junction. Normally, the Purkinje fibers enjoy protective isolation against forming reentrant circuits with the contractile fibers into which they interdigitate because of their substantially longer refractory periods.

PATTERNS OF VENTRICULAR PREMATURE COMPLEXES

VPCs often appear in recurring relationship to the dominant rhythm, for which specific terminology is assigned. (These terms, incidentally, are also applicable to premature beats of atrial and A-V junctional origin.)

VENTRICULAR BIGEMINY. This rhythm consists of a basic supraventricular rhythm (sinus, atrial, or A-V junctional) in which VPCs alternate with the supraventricular beats in a repetitive pattern. Figure 8–28 presents ventricular bigeminy in which the dominant sinus rhythm is interrupted by a VPC after every sinus beat.

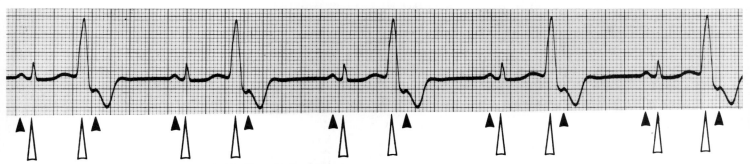

Figure 8–28. Ventricular bigeminy.

A nonconducted P wave can be identified and measured out after each ectopic QRS complex. The typical compensatory pause is evident.

Figure 8–29 is an especially interesting example of ventricular bigeminy. The rhythm could be interpreted as severe sinus bradycardia with VPCs in a bigeminal pattern. However, the true nature of the sinus rate is revealed when ventricular ectopy that had previously obscured nonconducted P waves has subsided.

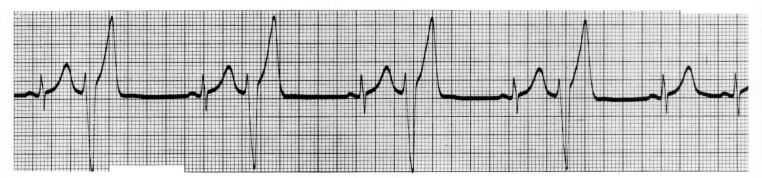

Figure 8–29. Transient ventricular bigeminy.

Figure 8–30 was obtained from a 13-year-old beagle, Candy. Late VPCs in a consistent bigeminal pattern appear after completion of atrial depolarization. The VPC (having a wide QRS complex and deep T wave) occurs soon after complete inscription of a nonconducted P wave. Note that the initial portion of QRS complexes in the supraventricular beats differs from that of ventricular beats, indicating that normal intraventricular septal depolarization is replaced in the ectopic beats.

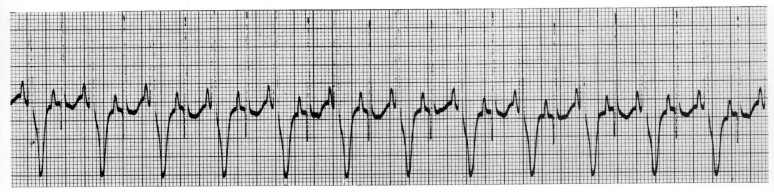

Figure 8–30. Atrial tachycardia with ventricular bigeminy.

VENTRICULAR TRIGEMINY. This pattern consists of two VPCs following each supraventricular beat in a recurring pattern (Fig. 8–31).

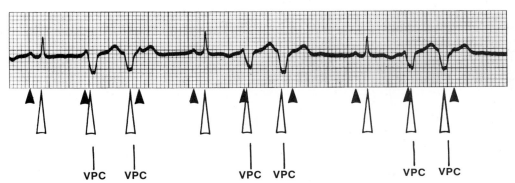

VPC VPC   VPC VPC   VPC VPC

Figure 8–31. Ventricular trigeminy.

Many clinicians use the term **ventricular trigeminy** to include not only the pattern in which one sinus beat is followed by two ventricular beats (S-V-V-S-V-V...) but also the pattern in which the VPCs occur regularly after two normal sinus beats (S-S-V-S-S-V...). The latter pattern may be found in individuals with relatively stable cardiac function, and it may continue without adversity for long periods. In contrast, the former pattern is an extremely unstable condition and is most often seen in acute myocardial infarction. It is a likely forerunner of ventricular tachycardia and fibrillation, malignant rhythms to be described later.

Based on the principle that it is undesirable to apply the same terminology to different rhythm patterns of vastly different importance, the term **ventricular trigeminy** is here restricted to the pattern in which two VPCs follow each normal beat in a recurring sequence. This convention has historical precedence, having been defined by Wenckebach in 1914.*

UNIFORM. When VPCs are similar in configuration, it is assumed that they arise from a common site and that the same aberrant pathways of depolarization are involved. In the following tracings, compare the configurations of QRS complexes, ST segments, and T waves for each ectopic beat. Minor differences are encountered in some because of the varying relationship with coincidental atrial activity.

---

* Sherf E, Schott A: Extrasystoles and Allied Arrhythmias. William Heinemann Medical Books, London, 1953, pp. 193–194.

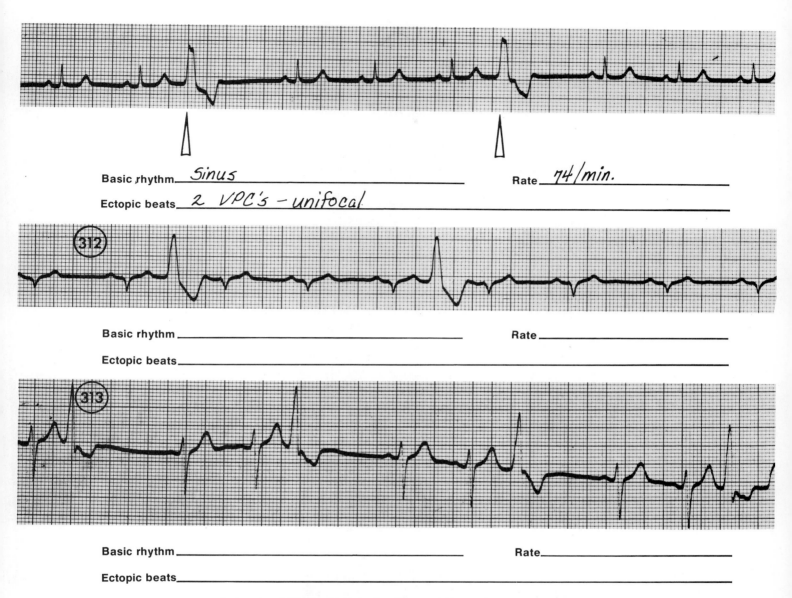

Basic rhythm *Sinus* **Rate** *74/min.*

Ectopic beats *2 VPC's - unifocal*

In tracing 313, the ventricular beat at 127 mm is slightly later than preceding ectopic beats, and the nonconducted P wave that follows is more obscured by the QRS complex.

In rhythm strips 314 and 315, compare configurations of the QRS complexes of the VPCs. Can sinus P waves be identified?

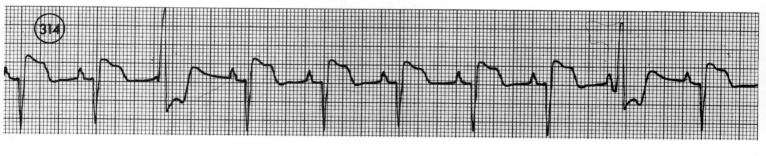

Basic rhythm _____ **Rate** _____

Ectopic beats _____

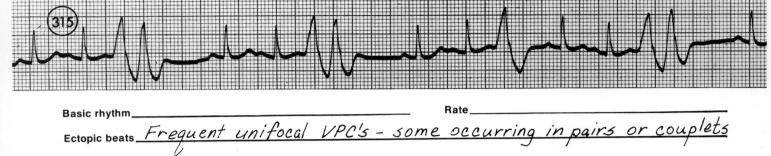

Basic rhythm_____   **Rate**_____

Ectopic beats *Frequent unifocal VPC's - some occurring in pairs or couplets*

Figure 8–32 contains three selected leads from the standard ECG of an 84-year-old man who was symptom free. VPCs are present in a bigeminal pattern. In each lead, all components of the ectopic beats are identical.

Also note that the nonconducted P waves found immediately after the ectopic QRS do not measure out to one-half the interval between conducted P waves, indicating that the sinus rhythm is irregular or interrupted. Two possible explanations are forwarded:

1. The nonconducted P waves may actually represent premature atrial depolarizations that occur so soon after the ectopic beats that entry into the ventricles is blocked by refractoriness in the A-V nodal fibers.

2. The impulse from the VPC is conducted through the A-V node and stimulates the atria, producing a retrograde P wave. The appearance of left bundle branch block of ectopic QRS complexes may represent a site of origin in the common bundle or in the A-V junctional tissue, from where retrograde conduction typically occurs.

The terms **unifocal, monomorphic,** and **monophasic** are synonymous with **uniform** and refer to a common site of origin of ectopic beats.

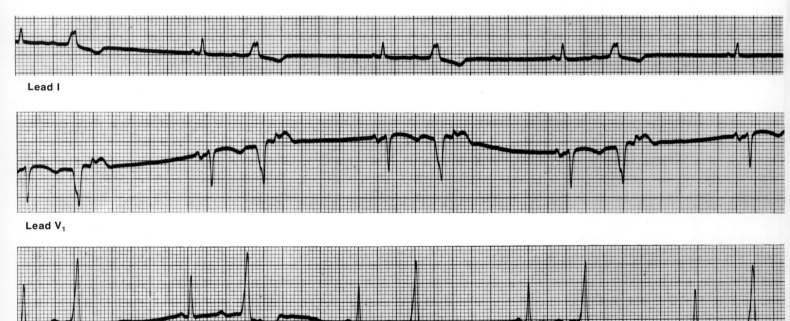

Lead I

Lead V₁

Lead V₆

Figure 8–32. Bigeminy with monophasic ectopic complexes.

MULTIFORM. When ectopic beats are dissimilar in waveform they are referred to as multiform or multiphasic. Figure 8–33 contains VPCs that exhibit this characteristic.

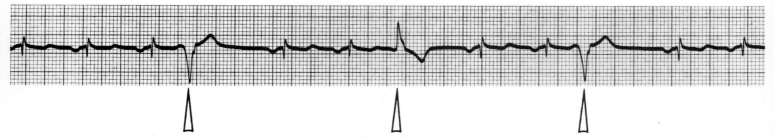

Figure 8–33. Multiphasic ventricular premature beats.

Note that the two VPCs with identical configurations flank one that is in no way comparable except for prematurity and wide QRS complex. One assumes that two automatic foci (or sites of reentry) are initiating these beats and that the similar beats arise from the same site. In fact, this concept was the basis of the older term **multifocal**. However, this term—still applicable for some rhythms—has been largely replaced by the term **multiform**, which simply describes the ECG finding. Multiphasic is a broader designation to cover those arrhythmias in which a single ectopic pacemaker is propagated through varying pathways (to produce QRS complexes of differing shapes) as well as ectopic beats from many pacemakers. Such a distinction cannot be made with certainty from the ECG.

In the electrocardiographic tracings 316 to 319, interpret the basic rhythm and rate. Locate VPCs and compare configuration and duration. Can "families" of similar VPCs be found in the same strip?

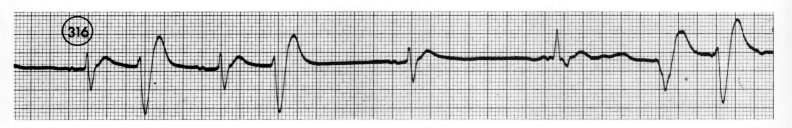

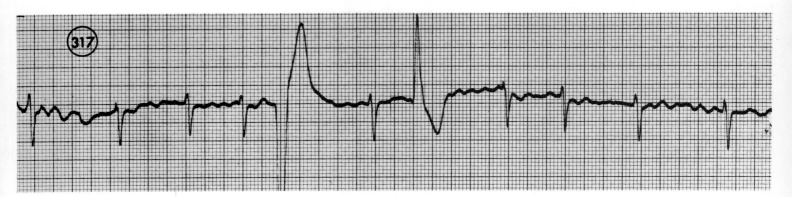

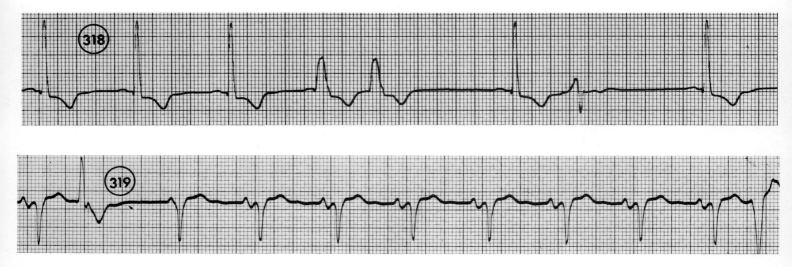

In strip 316, note that the first, second, and fourth VPCs are similar and are probably from the same site of origin.

The terms **multiphasic, polymorphic,** and **pleomorphic** are, incidentally, synonyms for **multiform.**

SITE OF ORIGIN. Electrophysiological evidence indicates that most VPCs arise from the free wall of the left ventricle. Of the remainder, most are generated in the intraventricular septum, and only a small portion come from the right ventricle. To some extent, these sites of origin can be identified on the ECG.

An impulse formed near the apex of the left ventricle spreads from the left lower chest region toward the right ventricle. Because the right ventricle is last to be depolarized, such an ectopic beat resembles right bundle branch block. In lead aVR and lead V_1, the terminal portion of the QRS is delayed and accentuated in the positive direction, whereas lead I and lead V_6 exhibit a delayed and negative terminal deflection. Of course, the premature beat from the left ventricle differs from typical right bundle branch block because the initial portion of the QRS complex has aberrant conduction as well.

Those ventricular beats that arise from the distal intraventricular septum or from the apex of the right ventricle are characterized by a wave front that propagates leftward and hence simulates left bundle branch block. Lead I and lead V_6 have QRS complexes that are predominantly upright and are markedly delayed (owing to the relatively large muscle mass of the left ventricle). QRS complexes in lead V_1 are strongly negative and very wide.

Two forms of VPCs are illustrated in Figure 8–34.

During normal sinus rhythm, a premature beat is identified as ventricular by the compensatory pause, by the absence of an ectopic P wave, and by the altered QRS complex configuration and prolonged duration. A second similar beat is found on this

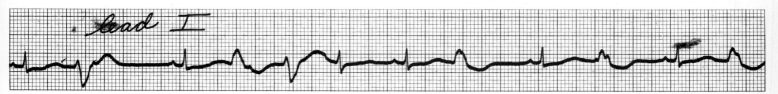

Figure 8–34. Ventricular premature complexes exhibiting the appearance of origins in the right and left ventricles.

tracing. Because the QRS deflection is largely negative in lead I (which has its positive electrode on the left), nearly the entire depolarization sequence is seen to be carried *away* from the region of the left ventricle toward the right. The configuration in this lead suggests that the automatic focus arises from the left ventricle.

Four premature beats of a second form are also present. These are entirely upright, indicating that the sequence of depolarization moves *toward* the left in head I. One presumes that this set of ectopic impulses is generated in the intraventricular septum or in the right ventricle. However, the possibility of A-V junctional premature contractions with left bundle branch block and failure of retrograde conduction cannot be excluded.

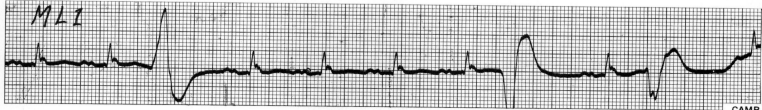

Figure 8–35. Two sites of origin for ventricular premature complexes.

In the example in Figure 8–35, VPCs are recorded from lead I with chest electrodes for monitoring. The first VPC has a QRS complex that is positive and is directed in its entirety toward the positive (left-sided) electrode. It is most likely derived from an impulse originated in the intraventricular septum or in the right ventricle. The two VPCs that follow are similar to each other and have negative polarity, indicating a wave front directed away from the positive electrode. The responsible pacemaker is therefore probably in the left ventricle. An incidental finding in this tracing is the bipeaked and widened P waves, suggesting left atrial enlargement. In this case, P wave changes were caused by mitral stenosis. QRS complexes originating from sinus beats are also widened and exhibit aberrant conduction in their terminal development.

Although these criteria are fallible (because of the intricacies of ventricular depolarization), they are nevertheless helpful as clues to the importance of ventricular premature ectopic rhythms. It is generally agreed that those originating from the left ventricle carry a more serious prognosis.

FIXED COUPLING. VPCs occurring at a constant interval after preceding cardiac cycles are said to exhibit **fixed coupling.** Figure 8–36 reveals normal sinus rhythm with uniform premature beats and wide QRS complexes in a bigeminal pattern. Each ectopic beat appears at precisely the same duration after the QRS complex before it. This constancy is maintained despite some variation in the sinus pacemaker rate.

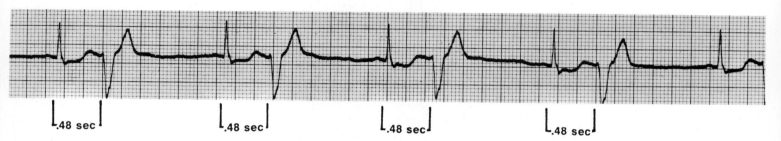

.48 sec   .48 sec   .48 sec   .48 sec

Figure 8–36. Fixed coupling.

Determine the basic rhythm and rate in tracings 320, 321, and 322. Locate the VPCs and measure the coupling interval of each with the respective preceding beats.

It is usually easiest to measure from the beginning of the normal QRS complex to the corresponding point of the ectopic beat. Does tracing 320 show ventricular trigeminy?

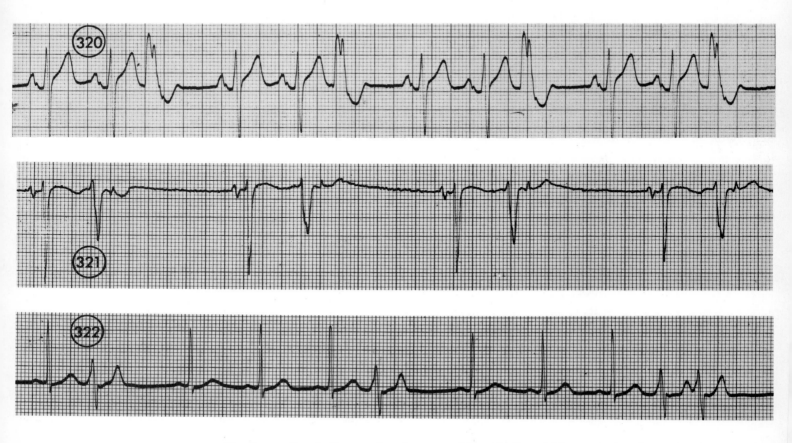

Fixed coupling indicates that the second beat is formed in some way by a circuit linkage with the first beat. Therefore, an interpreter can presume that a reentrant mechanism is involved when VPCs occur at constant intervals after a normal beat.

VARIABLE COUPLING. When VPCs appear at differing intervals after the preceding normal beats, they are said to exhibit variable coupling, as demonstrated in the ECG in Figure 8–37.

In tracing 323, monophasic VPCs occur late in the cardiac cycle, with slight variations in the coupling intervals. The variations are enough to provide entirely different degrees of exposure to the partially superimposed nonconducted P waves. Measure the coupling intervals and identify the origin for the underlying rhythm. Are the VPCs of similar appearance.

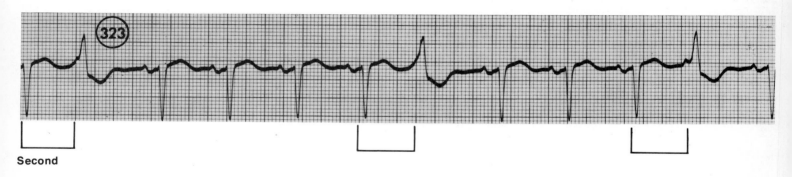

Second

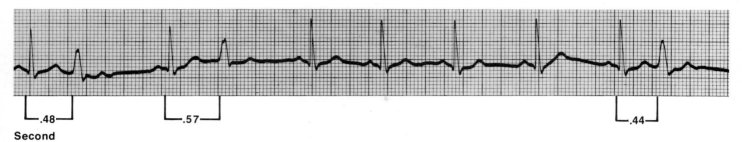

Second   .48   .57   .44

Figure 8–37. Variable coupling.

Tracing 324 reveals frequent VPCs that are monophasic and that have varying coupling intervals. Verify the coupling intervals of each VPC. Are the VPCs uniform? What is the underlying rhythm?

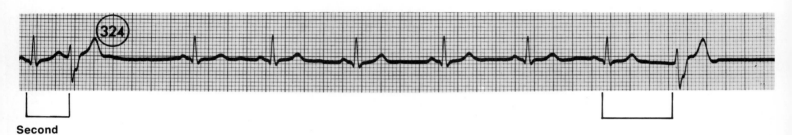

Second

The next six tracings are examples of various forms of VPCs. Label the basic rhythm and rate. Identify VPCs and describe them fully. The first one is completed for you.

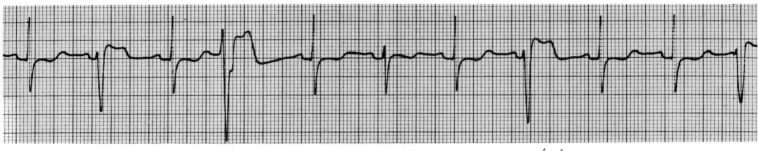

Basic rhythm _*NSR*_   Rate _*78/min.*_

Ectopic beats _*VPC's – multifocal; variable coupling*_

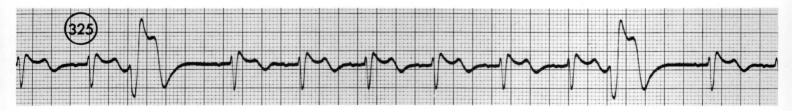

Basic rhythm _____   Rate _____

Ectopic beats _____

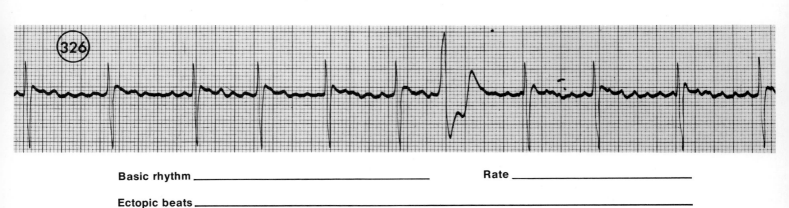

Basic rhythm _____ **Rate** _____

Ectopic beats _____

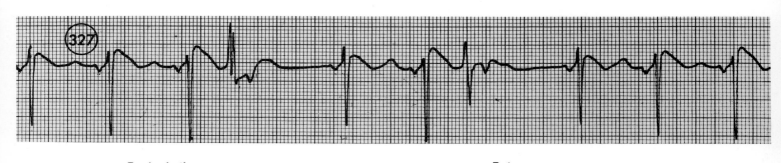

Basic rhythm _____ **Rate** _____

Ectopic beats _____

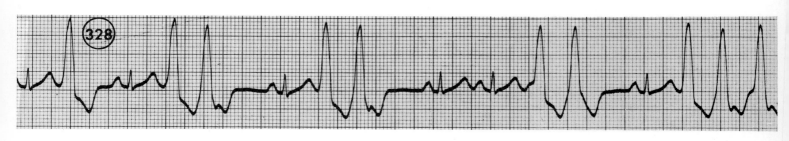

Basic rhythm _____ **Rate** _____

Ectopic beats _____

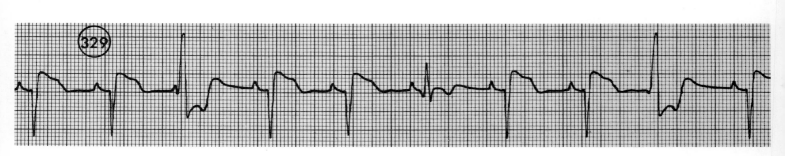

Basic rhythm _____ **Rate** _____

Ectopic beats _____

Variations in the coupling intervals of premature beats may occur with reentrant mechanisms, owing to change in routing of reentrant circuits. However, this relationship usually results from enhanced automaticity. Indeed, an automatic mechanism should be suspected in any arrhythmia that displays variable coupling of premature beats. Of possible causes, drug excitation is notoriously common, with digitalis heading the list.

The following serial tracings from the ECG of a 66-year-old man with a recent subendocardial infarction demonstrate an untoward drug effect. Distinguish the type of coupling intervals.

1. 10:30 AM: The patient is admitted to the Coronary Care Unit. The ECG shows atrial fibrillation with moderate ventricular rate response.

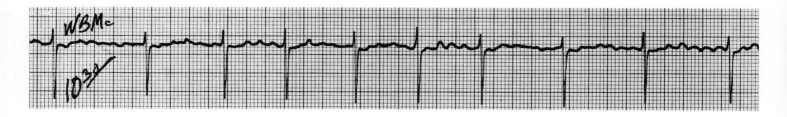

2. 10:55 AM: The ventricular rate has slowed, and escape beats of ventricular origin have appeared. The ectopic beats occur only after a long delay in the normally conducted beats.

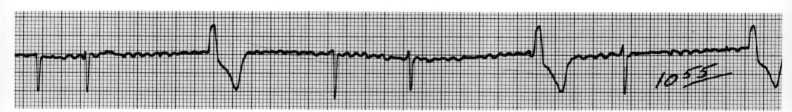

3. 11:12 AM: A sustained ectopic ventricular rhythm has replaced the usual response to atrial fibrillation. Note that the ectopic rhythm appeared after a pause in conducted beats and was slower than the preceding rhythm. At this point, the clinician elected to control the ectopic beats with a depressor agent.

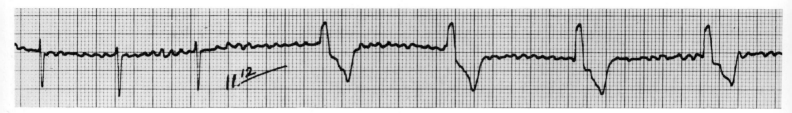

4. 11:15 AM: Lidocaine, 80 mg, was given by intravenous injection.

5. 11:22 AM: Ventricular escape beats have been eliminated. However, there are now long pauses between some ventricular beats, all of which are conducted from the atria. The drug has suppressed the ventricular escape mechanism that had previously protected the heart against excessive ventricular slowing.

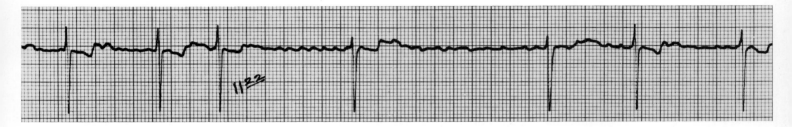

6. The reappearance of ventricular escape beats was noted about 15 minutes after stopping the lidocaine infusion.

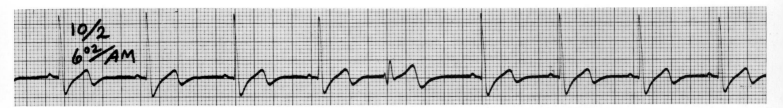

PARASYSTOLE. An automatic focus within the ventricles can establish a continuous ectopic rhythm that occurs concurrently with but independently of the natural sinus rhythm. One then finds beats with normal P-QRS-T components and beats with wide ventricular complexes alone, sustained at different rates. Such a dual rhythmicity is known as parasystole, literally a beat *beside* (or *para-*) the dominant beat. This form of arrhythmia is distinguished by the regularity of the ventricular pacemaker, which has no time relationship with the sinus pacemaker. In practice, one finds that the ventricular beats can be measured out with constant intervals and that the coupling interval with the sinus beats varies markedly from beat to beat. In the diagrammatic representation of a parasystolic rhythm in Figure 8–38, note that each pacemaker drives at a constant rate. Differences in ventricular rate, however, result in a changing relationship between each ectopic beat (closed symbol) and the preceding dominant and faster beat (open symbol).

PARASYSTOLE

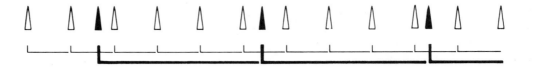

Open symbols—dominant rhythm

Closed symbols—parasystolic rhythm

Figure 8–38. Graphic representation of a parasystolic rhythm.

Observe that both the dominant and parasystolic rhythms have separate and independent cadences.

Electrophysiological properties of the parasystolic focus permit it to discharge at its inherent rate and to exit, stimulating the ventricles, as does the ordinary ventricular beat. What appears to set it apart, however, is the protection enjoyed from oncoming impulses of the dominant pacemaker. In other words, an impulse discharged by the isolated pacemaker exits and propagates further, whereas the wave front from the dominant pacemaker does not enter the area of automaticity. It is a form of undirectional block involving a small area of automatic tissue.

In Figure 8–39, a ventricular ectopic beat is seen in a 25-year-old medical student in good general health and without symptoms or findings of a cardiac disorder except for occasional palpitations often associated with anxiety, drinking coffee, or smoking. Only one ectopic beat occurring during 2 minutes of continuous recording has the typical characteristics of a VPC.

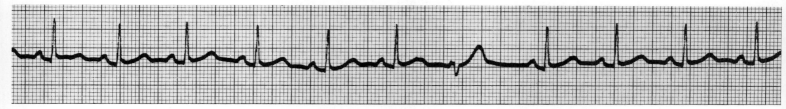

Figure 8–39. Normal sinus rhythm with one late ventricular premature beat.

Immediately after she rapidly smokes half a cigarette, VPCs become much more frequent (Fig. 8–40). Note that the ectopic beats themselves appear in a perfectly regular cadence and that the coupling interval with normal beats varies somewhat. It appears that an impulse-forming center in the ventricles has been activated, producing an entirely independent and slower rhythm than that of the sinus node.

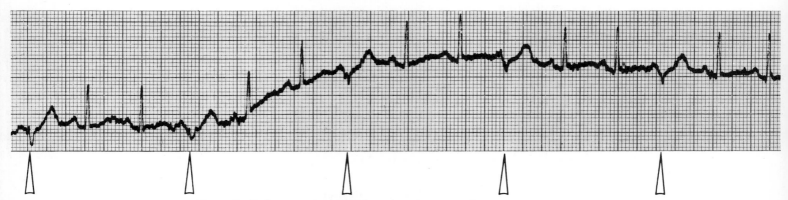

Figure 8–40. Increased ventricular premature complexes.

A break in the parasystolic rhythm now occurs (Fig. 8–41). The QRS complex symbol with brackets indicates the site where a parasystolic beat would occur if the regular cadence were not interrupted. Even though no ectopic beat appears at this point, the subsequent ventricular beat occurs at a predictable measured interval. It is assumed that the parasystolic center fired, but the impulse occurred so soon after the previous normal beat that no ectopic beat was generated. The ventricles were refractory to the parasystolic impulse at this time, indicating transient interference with the ventricular pacemaker.

This interference results in a VPC-to-VPC interval of precisely twice that of the basic parasystolic rhythm interval. Interference at two or more consecutive parasystolic beats produces higher multiples of interparasystolic intervals, as shown in the follow-up tracing, recorded about 15 minutes after the smoking provocation (Fig. 8–42).

Two consecutive blocked parasystolic impulses can be measured out above. Here, the interval between one set of VPCs is exactly three times the basic parasystolic interval. Again, measured parasystolic impulses occur very soon after a normal beat, and no ectopic depolarization results. Note also the marked variability in the sinus beat-ventricular beat coupling intervals. This random relationship in timing is characteristic of a parasystolic rhythm.

Parasystolic activity is usually in the ventricles, where the rate is generally less

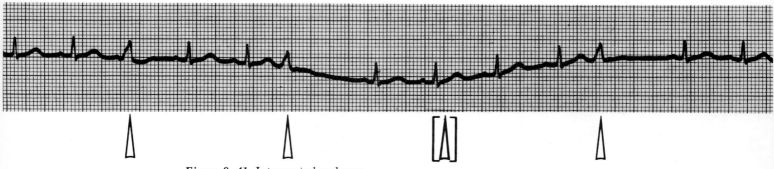

Figure 8–41. Interrupted cadence.

than 60 beats per minute (and may be as slow as 20 beats per minute), corresponding to the inherent rate of ventricular automaticity. However, a parasystolic focus sometimes operates at a much faster rate and even resembles ventricular tachycardia. Parasystolic rhythms can also become evident in the atria, A-V junctional tissue, and, rarely, the sinus node.

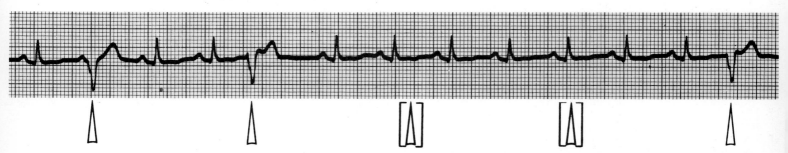

Figure 8–42. Apparent and concealed ventricular premature complexes in parasystole.

The markedly variable coupling intervals between parasystolic and normal beats favors the development of fusion beats, and these are quite common in parasystolic rhythms. The reason is the frequent fortuitous proximity of these two beats, favoring the partial penetration of the ventricles by both pacemakers simultaneously.

WIDE QRS COMPLEX BEATS

From this description of ectopic rhythms, it is evident that ventricular beats can simulate supraventricular beats with bundle branch block. In fact, the similarity poses a major problem in the interpretation of an ECG. Nevertheless, certain findings help to differentiate the origin of beats having wide QRS complexes.

1. **Duration.** Supraventricular beats with bundle branch block tend to be narrower than beats of ventricular origin because at least part of the propagating impulse travels in the normal intraventricular pathways. The entire ventricular mass is depolarized by the relatively slowly moving wave front from a ventricular pacemaker. As a rule, a QRS complex of 0.10 second or less is supraventricular; if 0.13 second or longer, it is probably ventricular. Either form of extrasystole is commonly found in the intermediary range.

2. **Configuration.** Supraventricular beats with wide QRS complexes tend to have more or less typical patterns of one form of bundle branch block. Ventricular beats, although they may resemble bundle branch block, tend to have a much greater distortion of the QRS complex (often referred to as bizarre).

Repolarization of ventricular beats generally undergoes much more drastic changes of sequence than do aberrantly conducted supraventricular beats. T waves of ventricular beats are often changed in direction and opposite to the principal QRS deflection and usually have a greater accentuated amplitude than normal beats.

3. **Retrograde A-V nodal conduction.** Impulses initiated at the A-V junction or low atrium expectantly depolarize the atria in a retrograde sequence. Impulses from the ventricles are usually blocked at the A-V node from entering the atria. Consequently, the presence of a P wave of altered contour following a wide QRS premature beat and associated with a change in the sinus pacemaker rate favors a supraventricular origin. In contrast, if a P wave that occurs after the ectopic wide QRS complex is not conducted to the ventricle and is unaltered in form, it is more likely a ventricular beat. This conclusion is enhanced if a compensatory pause follows the premature QRS complex.

4. **Fusion beats.** The finding of wide QRS complexes, some of which are narrower than the majority, suggests fusion beats involving both supraventricular and ventricular origins. The finding then identifies the wider QRS beat as ventricular in origin.

5. **Interference of the A-V node.** The impulse from a ventricular beat propagates into the A-V node so that the subsequent supraventricular wave front meets some degree of refractoriness. Of course, the nonconducted P wave following a VPC demonstrates absolute refractoriness of the A-V node. However, the conducted supraventricular beat that comes next may exhibit a prolonged PR interval, a sign of relative refractoriness. With an interpolated VPC, prolonged A-V conduction in the first complete cardiac cycle after the ectopic is quite common. Hence, the finding of delayed A-V conduction in the beat following a wide QRS complex beat suggests a ventricular origin.

Admittedly, differentiation of these forms of cardiac cycles is sometimes difficult because each criterion is quite limited when used alone. However, several criteria are often applicable and when used together usually allow a reasonably accurate interpretation. Even with such scrutiny, supraventricular complexes and VPCs are often not distinguishable, and electrophysiological studies with intracardiac recordings are necessary for precise identification.

Ventricular Tachycardia

The same automatic or reentrant mechanism that produces VPCs may cause repetitive beating. When three or more such beats occur consecutively, the term **ventricular tachycardia** is applied. The rate of this arrhythmia exceeds the natural rhythmicity of ventricular automatic tissue, which, as described in Ventricular Escape Rhythm is 20 to 60 per minute, depending on which portion of the ventricle contains the active pacemaker. As explained, these escape pacemakers become manifest only in conjunction with sinoatrial and A-V junctional bradycardia or arrest or with complete or high grades of intermittent A-V nodal block.

In the example in Figure 8–43, normal sinus rhythm is replaced by ventricular tachycardia. The patient was a 42-year-old woman who was convalescing from viral myocarditis. She had no symptoms at the time of this recording. Lead I is shown.

The sinus rhythm is interrupted by a solitary premature beat that begins during a P wave. The wide QRS complex (0.18 second), the opposing deflection of the QRS complex, and its failure to disturb the sinus rhythm all weigh in favor of its being of ventricular origin. Then after two sinus cycles, a similar beat appears to be followed by like beats that revert to sinus rhythm at the end of the strip. A ventricular rhythm is thus established. The dissocation between atrial and ventricular rhythms is evident by measurement with calipers and is confirmed by locating portions of P waves that exhibit no alteration of sinus cadence.

In effect, a ventricular pacemaker, at first producing a single premature beat, accelerates in excess of the sinus rate and takes over control of the ventricles. It encounters physiological ventricular-to-atrial block so that sinoatrial activity remains

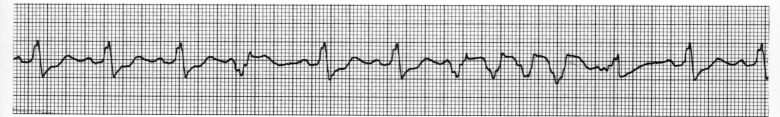

Figure 8–43. Sinus rhythm with single ventricular premature beat and subsequent rhythm control from a ventricular site.

undisturbed. Note that all ventricular complexes are similar. However, the rhythm is somewhat irregular, as is common for rhythms originating in the ventricles. Note also that the average rate is faster (170 per minute) than that of the sinus rate (80 per minute), which is the reason for the ventricular takeover.

Although included in the general category of ventricular tachycardia, such a rhythm of excitation that is less than 100 beats per minute is designated an **accelerated ventricular rhythm.** Ventricular tachycardia applies only to rates faster than this arbitrary speed. However, authorities differ in the precise cutoff between these two designations.

In the accelerated ventricular rhythm shown below, normal sinus rhythm is replaced by a rhythm consisting of

1. A-V dissociation.
2. Ventricular complexes that are changed in form or abnormally wide.
3. A ventricular pacemaker that is more rapid than the sinus pacemaker driving the ventricles, but less than 100.

In the second ventricular contraction, observe that the PR interval is shorter than in the sinus beats before it. The QRS complex of this beat is similar to those that follow without association with the sinus pacemaker. It is therefore presumed that this third sinus impulse is not conducted to the ventricles but rather that a late VPC has occurred, the first of a succession of ventricular beats appearing in a somewhat irregular cadence. There is no retrograde conduction, and atrial and ventricular rhythms are completely independent. This arrhythmia is a form of A-V dissociation produced by sustained excitation of a ventricular pacemaker. Because the rate is more rapid than is seen in ventricular escape rhythms (20 to 50 beats per minute), the rhythm represents a form of ventricular excitation.

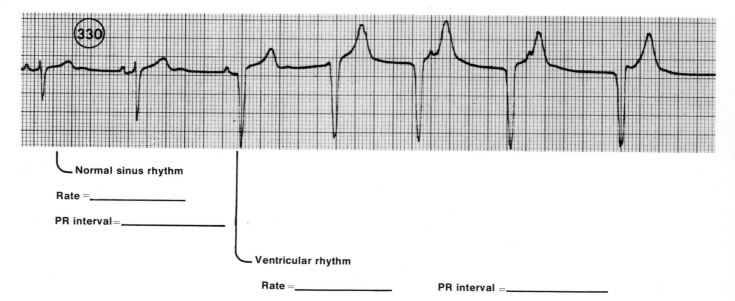

└ **Normal sinus rhythm**

Rate =_____

PR interval =_____

└ **Ventricular rhythm**

Rate =_____   **PR interval** =_____

Ventricular excitation was seen in an ECG obtained from a 52-year-old swimming coach who had symptoms suggestive of myocardial infarction. In the first of these two tracings, Figure 8–44A, a premature beat in which the QRS complex is widened and completely distorted appears, exhibiting a change in direction of the initial deflection.

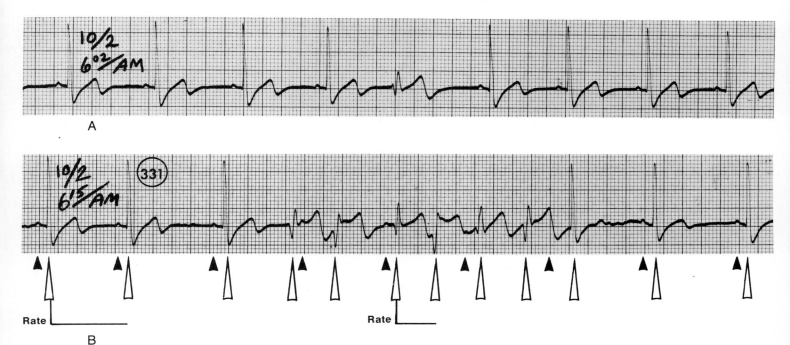

Figure 8–44. (A) Ventricular premature beat. (B) Ventricular premature beats—ventricular tachycardia.

On measuring out P waves, one would expect atrial depolarization to occur midway within the abnormal QRS complex (although none is visible). Subsequent atrial beats continue with no appreciable change in rhythmicity. Thus, this angle anomalous premature cycle has the typical features of a VPC.

A few minutes later, following the third sinus beat in Figure 8–44B, a premature beat with similar characteristics of the previously described ectopic beat is present. Five nearly identical beats then follow in rapid succession. During this paroxysm of tachycardia, independent atrial activity can be plotted throughout. Thereafter, sinus rhythm resumes.

On the tracing in Figure 8–44B, determine and compare the rates of the sinus and the ventricular rhythms. Is the ventricular rhythm regular or irregular? Does it begin with a premature beat (which may indicate a reentrant mechanism)?

Figure 8–45 demonstrates an episode of self-sustained ventricular activity recorded from a monitoring lead in a patient with suspected acute myocardial infarction. In addition to a mild sensation of midsternal chest discomfort extending to the neck, this patient experienced brief but frequent feelings of rapid palpitations.

During the run of ectopic beats, atrial activity can be measured out, and there is no alteration in cadence of the P waves. QRS complexes of the rapid rhythm are wide and abnormal in configuration. Also note that the small Q wave in the normal beats is absent in those of the arrhythmia. ST segments and T waves are also distorted and in a direction that opposes the main deflection of the associated QRS complexes. Furthermore, the ventricular rhythm in the paroxysm is irregular. These findings are typical of a ventricular rhythm. Because the rate averages about 100 beats per minute, it occurs

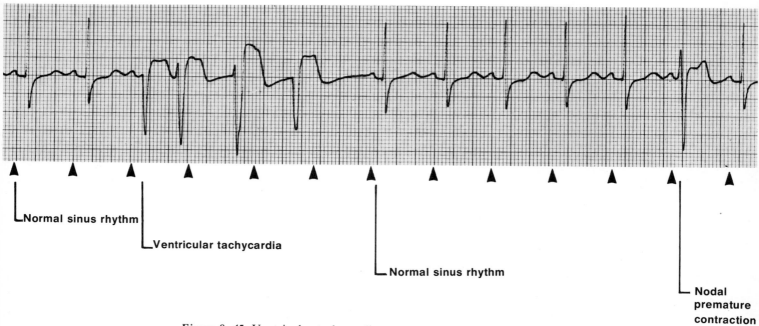

Figure 8–45. Ventricular tachycardia.

on the arbitrary border between an accelerated ventricular rhythm and ventricular tachycardia.

In test tracing 332 (taken from a Holter monitor), identify the sinus rhythm. Then observe the salient features of the ectopic rhythm: waveform configuration, QRS complex duration, rate, rhythmicity, concurrent atrial activity, and the mode of onset and offset of the arrhythmia.

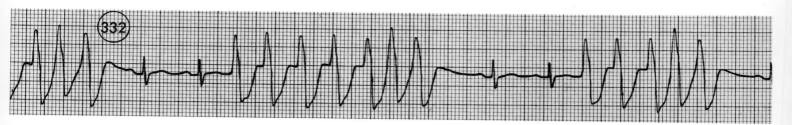

Determine the rates for the sinus and ventricular rhythms. Does the arrhythmia begin with a premature ectopic beat? Does it end with one? (An affirmative answer to both questions suggests that reentry is the underlying mechanism.) Is A-V dissociation present?

Atrial activity becomes more difficult to detect in dissociated rhythms as the ventricular rate increases. Only occasional P waves can be identified in the ECG in Figure 8–46.

At extremely rapid rates in ventricular tachycardia, atrial beats may be distinguished, and then only vaguely, by slight, rhythmically occurring disturbances on the baseline or on the waveforms. Such minor changes, in fact, may be the only clue for identifying the presence of A-V dissociation in wide QRS tachycardias. The ECG in Figure 8–47 presents such an example.

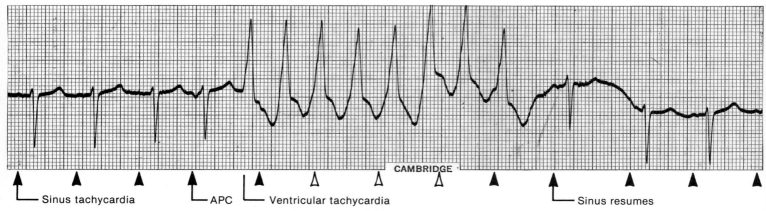

Sinus tachycardia   APC   Ventricular tachycardia   Sinus resumes

CAMBRIDGE

Figure 8-46. Rapid dissociated atrial and ventricular rhythms.

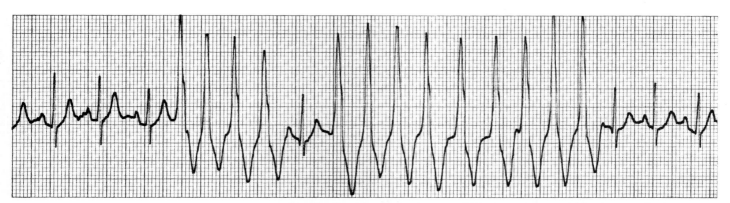

Figure 8-47. P waves in this dissociated rhythm are difficult to detect within the ventricular complexes. Minor variations in the baseline are the only markers of atrial activity.

The next group of ECGs illustrates transient periods of ventricular tachycardia.

1. Determine the basic rhythm and rate.
2. Mark isolated VPCs, if present.
3. Identify and bracket periods of ventricular tachycardia.
4. Using calipers, locate and mark P waves, if possible, through the periods of ventricular tachycardia.

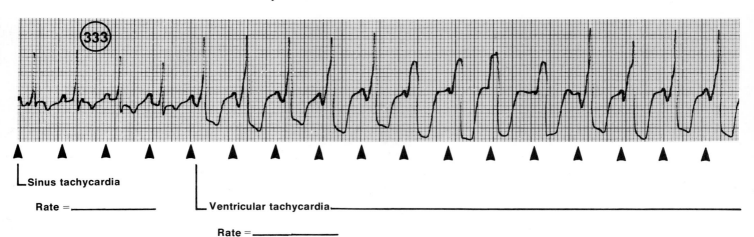

Sinus tachycardia

Rate =＿＿＿＿＿＿＿   Ventricular tachycardia＿＿＿＿＿＿＿＿＿＿＿＿＿＿＿＿＿＿＿＿＿

Rate =＿＿＿＿＿＿＿

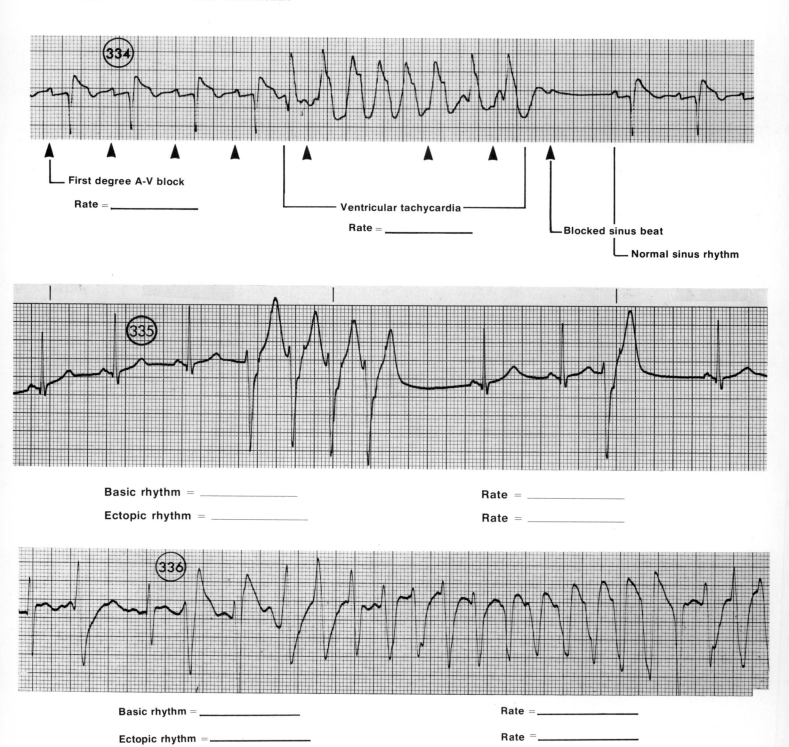

First degree A-V block

Rate = _____

Ventricular tachycardia

Rate = _____

Blocked sinus beat

Normal sinus rhythm

Basic rhythm = _____   Rate = _____

Ectopic rhythm = _____   Rate = _____

Basic rhythm = _____   Rate = _____

Ectopic rhythm = _____   Rate = _____

In strips 337 and 338, P waves seem to be visible in various places throughout the tracing, but these can be plotted out only roughly with calipers. The highly variable contour of the baseline is evidence of atrial activity out of phase with the ventricular rhythm. Measure out and mark P waves where possible.

At very rapid rates in ventricular tachycardia, the following features often appear:

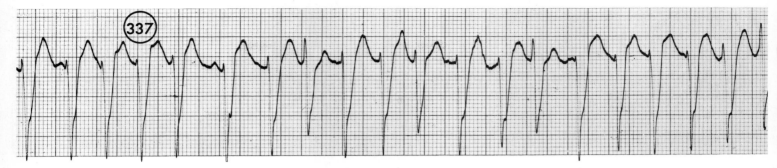

Ventricular tachycardia: Rate = _____

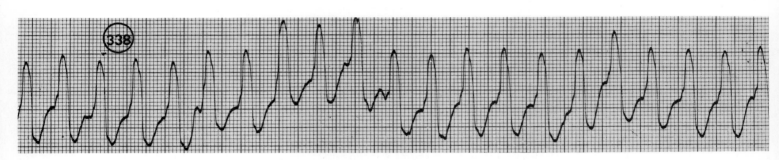

Ectopic rhythm_____   **Rate_____**

1. QRS complexes and T waves tend to vary from each other in contour and in amplitude. This is in part due to unidentifiable but superimposed atrial beats that are dissociated from the ventricular beats. In addition, the sequential events of depolarization and repolarization tend to be more variable from a ventricular focus than with normal electrical activation.

2. Ventricular pacemakers may be somewhat irregular.

3. QRS complexes merge directly with T waves, so that it becomes difficult or impossible to separate clearly the phases of depolarization and repolarization.

4. QRS complexes become broader and less well organized as the rate increases, owing to slower impulse transmission along conduction pathways. This property is an expression of relative refractoriness of individual conduction fibers.

Look for these features in tracings 339 and 340, examples of ventricular tachycardia at extremely rapid rates.

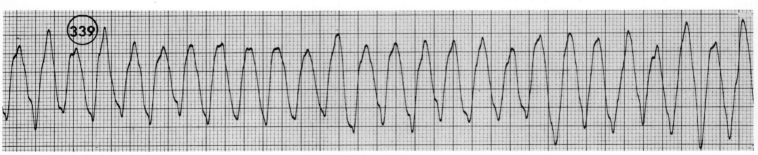

Rate_____   **Rhythm** *Regular* _____

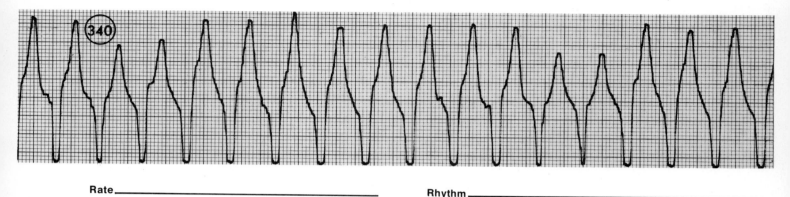

Ventricular tachycardia can produce cardiac contractions with such rapidity that the cardiac chambers do not have time to fill adequately during the intervals between contractions. This causes a diminution in the blood volume ejected with each contraction. Any gradation of low cardiac output may be associated with these arrhythmias, depending on the rate and the condition of the heart. The manifestations range from no symptoms or mild anxiety to lightheadedness or severe circulatory collapse and coma.

The clinical expression of ventricular tachycardia depends on the ventricular rate and the capacity for compensational adjustments by the myocardium and by the vascular system. For example, a person with impairment of myocardial contractile power or with drug-inhibited peripheral vasoconstriction is more affected by tachycardia at a given rate. In ventricular tachycardia, stroke volume is more compromised than in supraventricular tachycardias at the same rate because of the A-V dissociation (loss of atrial kick). The abnormal sequence of ventricular depolarization further limits the efficiency of myocardial contraction in ventricular arrhythmias.

Ventricular tachycardia may be recognized on physical examination by the rapid rate in combination with intermittent giant "a waves" (or cannon waves) in the jugular pulse. The explanation given for a giant "a waves" is the chance occurrence of some of the atrial beats just as the tricuspid valve has been snapped shut by the ventricular contraction. This venous pulse, of course, depends on the presence of A-V dissociation.

Anginal attacks may be precipitated by bouts of ventricular tachycardia in patients with coronary artery insufficiency. The ECG below was recorded in the emergency room on a man who had just collapsed. He was being examined for his complaint of persistent indigestion when he suddenly felt lightheaded and experienced air hunger with profound weakness. Blood pressure taken immediately was 50/?. Cardiac tones were distant, and the first heart sound varied in intensity from beat to beat. The ECG taken within minutes is shown in test strip 341.

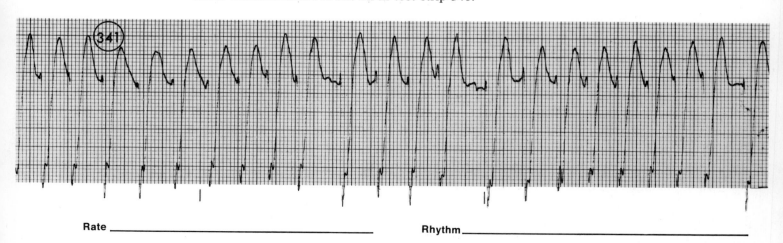

Describe the ECG as completely as possible. Explain the symptoms and clinical findings as they may relate to the arrhythmia.

Label tracings 342 to 346 completely; indicate atrial activity when possible.

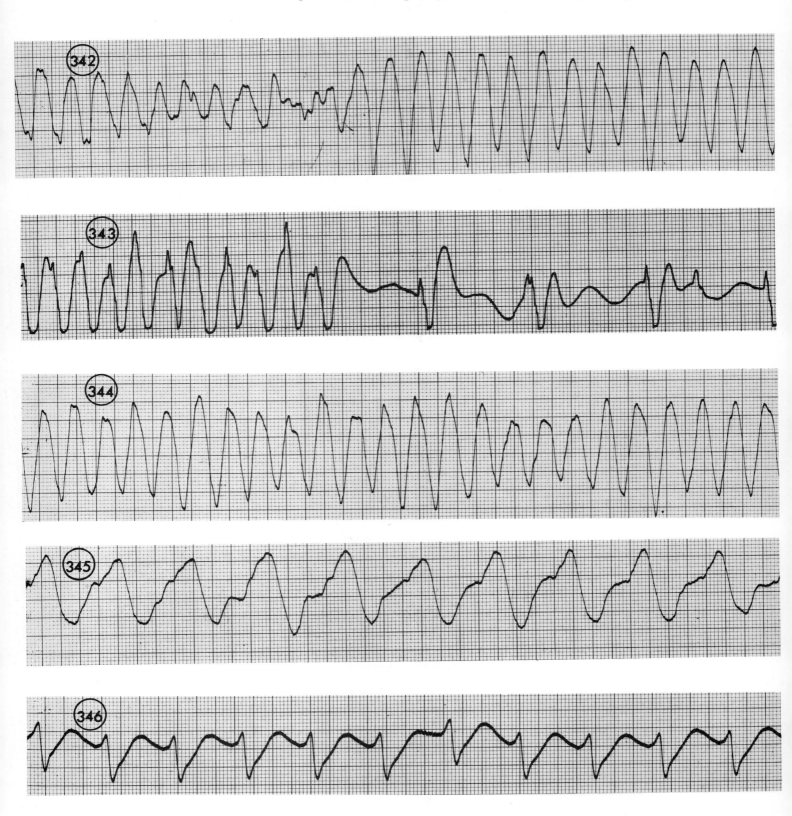

Almost certainly a sign of underlying heart disease, ventricular tachycardia is associated with myocardial ischemia in the majority of patients. It is especially common in acute myocardial infarction, when it is a harbinger of fatal arrhythmias, as we shall observe. Ventricular tachycardia is also a complication of other forms of congestive, hypertrophic, or inflammatory heart disease. It is sometimes found concomitantly with mitral valve prolapse and other types of valvular disease. Respiratory and metabolic disorders, most notoriously hypoxia and acidosis, predispose to ventricular tachycardia.

Those same drugs incriminated in VPCs are also causes of ventricular tachycardia. In general categories, the adrenergic agents are extremely important. Some individuals are inordinately sensitive to them, developing ventricular arrhythmias even with the minute amounts contained in such commonly used agents as the nonproprietary decongestants and stimulants.

Rarely, persons with paroxysmal ventricular tachycardia are found to have no underlying cardiac, pulmonary, or systemic disease. Although the attacks of tachycardia may result in hypotensive episodes, the condition is almost always self-limiting (after weeks, months, or even years) and rarely has life-endangering complications.

VULNERABLE PERIOD

As the ventricles recover from systole, they pass through a brief period during which a stimulus can initiate repetitive beats or wholly chaotic electrical activity. Known as the vulnerable period, this instant of instability occurs during a portion of the relative refractory period. On the ECG, the vulnerable period occurs just before or at the peak of the T wave, as shown schematically in Figure 8–48.

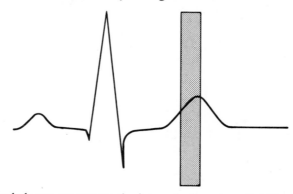

Figure 8–48. The shaded area represents the interval of superexcitability (vulnerable period).

The danger presented by the vulnerable period in some patients is that VPCs beginning during the vulnerable period of the preceding cardiac cycle may provoke ventricular tachycardia, flutter, or its more dire version, ventricular fibrillation. Such premature beats must necessarily have a very short coupling interval (i.e., a high degree of prematurity) to occur during the vulnerable period so that the initial deflection of the VPC is superimposed on the early portion of the T wave, a phenomenon referred to as **R-on-T.**

In the 1930s, the hazard of external electrical shock in production of fatal arrhythmias was studied in animals as it may apply to power-line workers. The special susceptibility of the heart to shock occurring near the peak of a T wave was identified. Since then, the mechanism and clinical relevance of the phenomenon have been extensively studied.

In brief, spontaneous VPCs posing the R-on-T relationship were originally thought to have a universally foreboding prognosis and to present one of the most reliable signs for predicting sudden cardiac death through arrhythmias. Yet some individuals present with frequent early VPCs and appear entirely immune to untoward effect. Information on this phenomenon does not yet allow for guidelines that may reliably distinguish these subtypes of responders.

Our current concept holds that stimulation during the vulnerable period of ventricular repolarization may result in multiple small reentrant circuits from a single premature beat. In turn, this leads to repetitive, self-perpetuating discharges at rapid rates, often resulting in total disorganization in the system for impulse formation and conduction.

Figure 8–49 illustrates the induction of ventricular tachycardia by this R-on-T mechanism. The incident was recorded with a Holter monitoring device on a 55-year-old woman who had been experiencing frequent episodes of weakness and syncope. Routine ECGs had failed to reveal any specific cardiac abnormality.

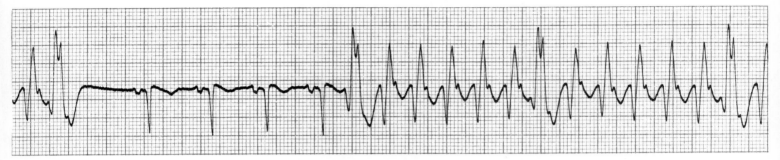

Figure 8–49. An episode of ventricular tachycardia is initiated by a ventricular premature beat occurring during the vulnerable period of the preceding beat.

The initial portion of the strip shows several QRS complexes with abnormal configurations. A short pause is interrupted by normal sinus rhythm that persists for only four cycles. During the recovery phase of the fourth cycle, a VPC occurs. This initiates a continuous run of ventricular complexes. During the period in which this patient was being monitored with the ambulatory equipment, she experienced repetitive runs of ventricular tachycardia lasting 6 to 12 seconds. All of the episodes were initiated with a VPC occurring during the recovery phase of a normal beat.

A heart that is free of structural disease appears to be resistant to the R-on-T phenomenon. For example, patients with ventricular parasystole or with malfunctioning electronic pacemakers unsynchronized to cardiac activity frequently receive depolarizing stimuli in the vulnerable period without incurring tachyarrhythmias. Epidemiological data also support the inference that persons with frequent and exceptionally early VPCs but without any other expression of heart disease are resistant to this electrophysiological phenomenon.

It is hearts affected by ischemic, inflammatory, or infiltrative disorders that are predisposed to untoward events from an R-on-T episode (Fig. 8–50). These conditions

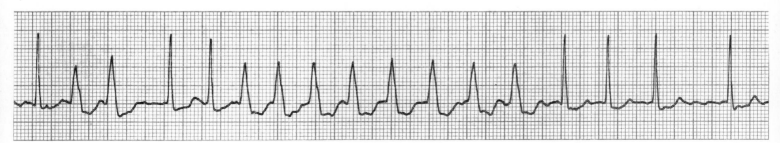

Figure 8–50. Ventricular premature beat with "R-on-T" relationship initiates a run of ventricular tachycardia.

evidently result in marked heterogeneity of electrophysiological properties in neighboring tissues, thus setting the stage for multiple reentrant events from a single stimulus. The VPC presenting with R-on-T in acute myocardial infarction is especially foreboding, a relationship that is even more prone to tachyarrhythmias if the infarction involves the anteroseptal wall and is complicated by a bundle branch block of either side.

Independent factors that also predispose to the risk of R-on-T induced arrhythmias are severe bradycardia and prolongation of myocardial repolarization. The latter condition, which is being recognized with increasing frequency, is described subsequently under The Long QT Interval.

DRUG THERAPY

Drugs that suppress impulse formation in the ventricles are used to control ventricular arrhythmias, whether of automatic or reentrant origin. Quinidine, procainamide (Pronestyl), and the beta-adrenergic blocking agents have been used extensively for this purpose.

These drugs of depression also have an effect on other functions of the heart. Sinus and atrial impulse formation are decreased, as is conduction time in the A-V node and in the Purkinje fibers. Myocardial contractile force may be reduced, and blood pressure lowered as well. All these actions must be considered to be dose-related, expected

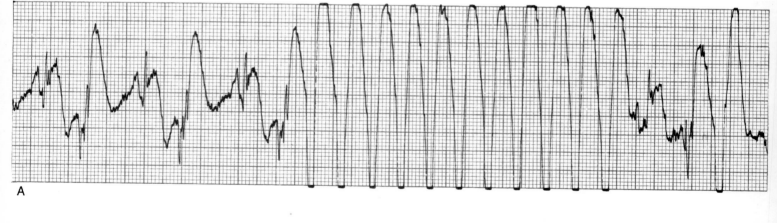

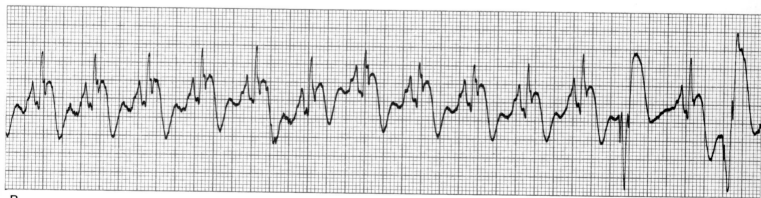

Figure 8–51. Treatment of ventricular tachycardia with lidocaine.

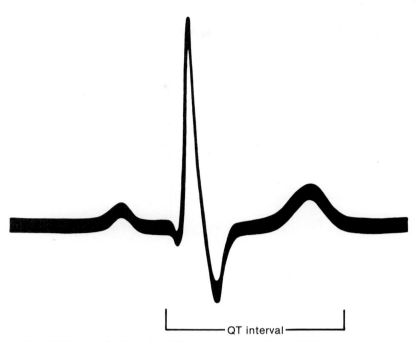

Figure 8–52. The QT interval. Measured from the onset of the QRS complex to the end of the T wave.

effects. Awareness of potential complications is critical in the use of the drugs. In addition, each of these agents can produce fairly common but unpredictable adverse reactions in other organ systems. A brief description of their numerous side effects is presented in Chapter 10.

Lidocaine (Xylocaine) is another agent having ventricular rhythm-suppressing properties. It has the advantage of having a highly selective action on the ventricles while producing little effect on the sinus node, atria, A-V node, and myocardium. Given by injection or infusion, it acts extremely rapidly, and its effects dissipate rapidly, thus offering a high degree of therapeutic control. Because of its effectiveness against VPCs and ventricular tachycardia and because of the relative freedom from other depressant actions on the heart, lidocaine has assumed paramount importance in critical care units.

For emergencies, undiluted lidocaine can be injected intravenously, and suppression of VPCs or ventricular tachycardia may occur within a few minutes. Once control is achieved, an infusion of the drug diluted in standard solutions is used to maintain a stable rhythm. Lidocaine, incidentally, has little effect on tachyarrhythmias of supraventricular origin.

To illustrate the use of lidocaine, the clinical series in Figure 8–51 is presented. The rhythm appeared suddenly in a 58-year-old man in the Coronary Care Unit. On the previous day, he had incurred a myocardial infarction that was complicated by heart failure; he was treated with digoxin and furosemide. Within 2 minutes after developing the arrhythmia, represented by tracing *A* in Figure 8–51, the patient was given 80 mg of lidocaine by intravenous injection. The transition to sinus rhythm (tracing *B*) occurred during the next minute, attesting to the speed of pharmacological action.

The following examples are continuous tracings from a 62-year-old teacher. They were obtained 1½ hours after admission to the Coronary Care Unit and demonstrate the effect of lidocaine on VPCs. The figures exhibit sinus rhythm with an intraventricular conduction defect and ventricular bigeminy.

Suppression of VPCs is evident within half a minute after the injection of lidocaine.

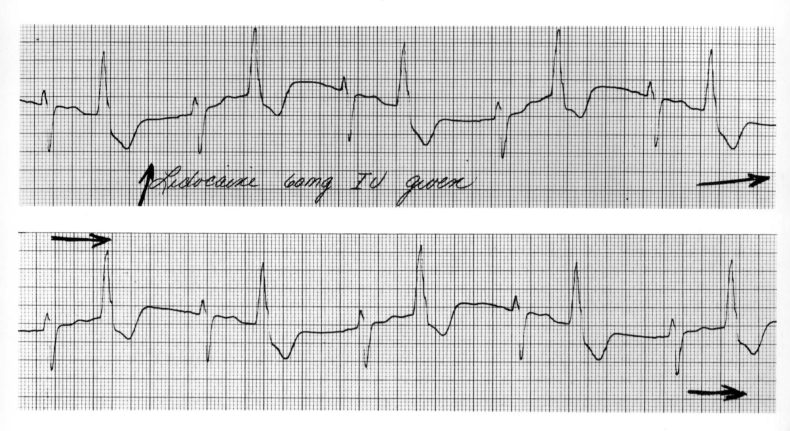

Lidocaine 60mg IV given

Suppression of VPCs is evident within half a minute after the injection of lidocaine.

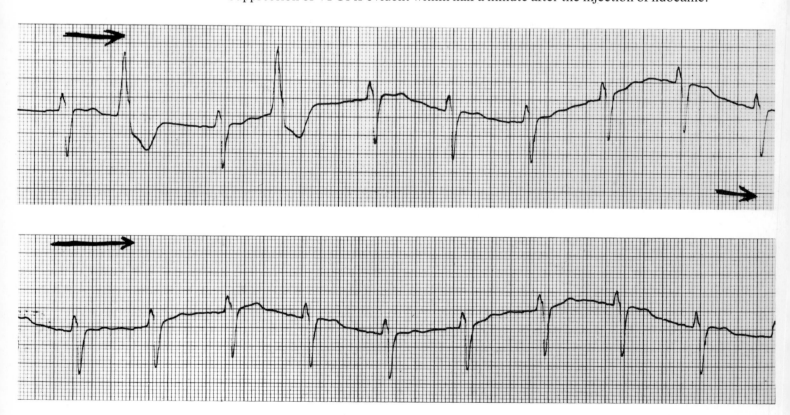

THE LONG QT INTERVAL

Prolongation of myocardial repolarization has already been referred to as predisposing to ventricular arrhythmias. This portion of the action potential is represented by the QT interval, measured from the beginning of the QRS complex to the end of the T wave, shown in Figure 8–52. Because only a relatively small fraction of this period is taken up by the QRS complex (depolarization), the QT interval reflects predominantly ventricular repolarization. Certain drugs, metabolic disorders, and constitutional susceptibility all may slow ventricular repolarization significantly, and in these conditions, the prolonged QT interval serves as an early warning sign for ventricular arrhythmias.

The QT interval is normally longer in bradycardias and shorter in tachycardias. The interval is usually less than 0.40 second, but it may be longer if the rate is very slow. Various formulas have been devised to adjust the interval according to rate to standardize the limits of normal. Such rules provide imprecise guidelines, but a QT interval longer than 0.45 second must be considered pathological regardless of heart rate and presumed to be an increased risk for the R-on-T phenomenon.

An exceptionally high incidence of recurrent ventricular tachycardias and sudden cardiac death has been discovered in some families in which a long QT interval is an inherited characteristic. Common among children of such families are episodes of syncope that may be caused by unrecognized arrhythmias.

A number of drugs increase the QT interval and predispose to the likelihood of R-on-T ventricular tachycardias. They include quinidine and, to a lesser extent, procainamide and disopyramide—paradoxically, drugs traditionally used to treat these arrhythmias. The phenothiazines and the tricyclic antidepressant agents also carry this liability in tachycardia-prone patients.

The long QT interval syndrome may be associated with certain metabolic disturbances such as hypokalemia and hypocalcemia and with extreme negative caloric imbalance as may be imposed by liquid protein diets. Powerful vagotonic stimulation (e.g., the Valsalva maneuver) also increases the QT interval momentarily and may be a triggering mechanism for ventricular tachycardia.

Some degree of successful management in persons with the long QT interval syndrome complicated by recurrent ventricular tachycardias has been accomplished with beta-adrenergic blocking drugs. Surgical interruption of the sympathetic innervation to the heart (by removal of the cervicothoracic or stellate ganglion) has proved useful in some individuals with drug-resistant arrhythmias.

TORSADES DE POINTES

A special form of ventricular tachycardia often associated with a prolonged QT interval is known as *torsades de pointes*. It is recognized by gradual beat-to-beat changes in configuration, amplitude, and cycle length of widened QRS complexes. The name refers to its electrocardiographic feature of appearing to twist around the isoelectric line. This undulating, polymorphic pattern is characteristically at a rapid rate (greater than 200 beats per minute). The tachycardia usually terminates spontaneously, and the clinical picture is typically one of recurring syncope of a seemingly benign nature. However, transition of the arrhythmia to ventricular fibrillation and sudden death is an ever present possibility.

The susceptibility to torsades de pointes is associated with severe slowing of myocardial repolarization. A QT interval greater than 0.5 seconds alerts the clinician to the threat of torsades.

Causes of torsades de pointes include all those that favor prolonging the QT interval. A congenital predisposition may be present. However, the condition is usually associated with drugs that have a strong dose-dependent tendency to retarding myocardial repolarization. Of all the drugs, quinidine is most notorious, although procainamide, disopyramide, mexilitine, and amiodarone are additional examples. Severe bradycardia associated with A-V conduction disorders is another important cause of the syndrome. Systemic conditions that may lead to torsades de pointes are hypokalemia, hypomagnesemia, alcoholism, hypothermia, and diffuse cerebral disturbances. These secondary causes of delayed repolarization commonly may precipitate episodes of ventricular tachycardia in patients who are already on drugs with a similar action. An example of a frequently offending combination resulting in torsades is hypokalemia induced by diuretic therapy in a patient taking quinidine.

Torsades de pointes was recorded in a 57-year-old man during treatment of acute myocardial infarction with the thrombolytic agent tissue plasminogen activator. His condition at the time of intravenous injection was stable except for tachycardia (Fig. 8–53A).

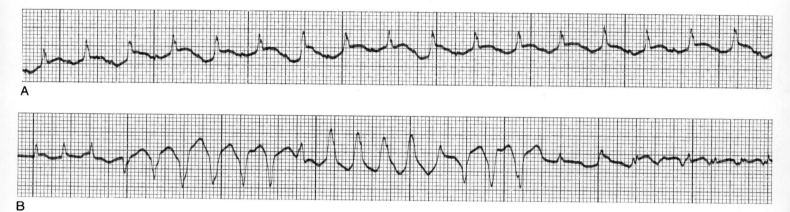

Figure 8–53. (*A*) Supraventricular tachycardia during the acute phase of a myocardial infarction. (*B*) Torsades de pointes develops during reperfusion in the same patient.

Atrial activity associated with consistent A-V conduction and narrow QRS complexes establishes the rhythm as supraventricular. Moments later, the tachycardia accelerated markedly (Fig. 8–53B).

In the initial portion of the tracing, atrial activity is indistinguishable. It was suddenly replaced by a wide QRS complex tachycardia having waveforms of alternating polarity.

This episode of torsades de pointes lasted only 4.2 seconds, and it did not induce symptoms. A chaotic supraventricular tachycardia follows. Several minutes later and without further therapy, the arrhythmia was replaced by sinus tachycardia.

Treatment of torsades de pointes requires special considerations because most standard drugs used to treat other forms of ventricular tachycardia prolong the QT interval and may be harmful. Torsades de pointes is preferentially treated with overdrive pacing—that is, the tachycardia is terminated by acceleration of heart rate with bursts of electronic impulses. Precordial electrocardioversion is also usually successful. Isoproterenol (which markedly shortens the QT interval) is generally the drug of choice (a clinical paradox considering that it may aggravate ordinary ventricular tachycardia). Trials with magnesium sulfate have demonstrated effectiveness in controlling torsades de pointes while exhibiting a high margin of safety. Drugs of depression that do not affect the QT interval appreciably (e.g., propranolol, phenytoin) are alternative therapeutic approaches. Of course, correction of the metabolic or pharmacological conditions leading to QT interval prolongation is imperative in effective control.

The patient whose rhythm is seen in Figure 8–54 was admitted to the telemetry

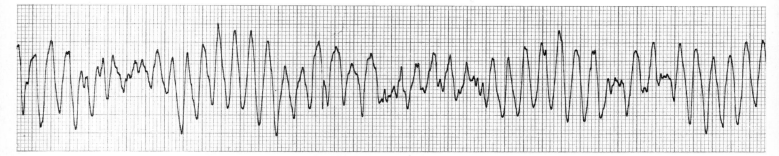

Figure 8–54. Torsades de pointes.

unit to investigate the cause of several near syncopal episodes. The nursing staff recorded three occurrences of torsades de pointes, which were treated with isoproterenol. The rhythm was eventually controlled with propranolol.

ELECTROCARDIOVERSION

Electric shock is frequently effective in converting ventricular tachycardia. This arrhythmia should be recognized immediately in the monitored patient and precordial shock applied when appropriate without any delay. When ventricular tachycardia arises from acute myocardial injury (not from drug toxicity), such prompt application is usually successful. However, the opportunity for conversion to a stable supraventricular rhythm diminishes rapidly with every moment's delay as the metabolic effects of circulatory failure accrue. When equipment for this procedure is not *immediately* available, a thump on the sternum with the closed fist occasionally induces conversion.

A helpful rule in deciding whether to use a drug or electrical means to treat ventricular tachycardia depends on the condition of the patient. If he or she remains alert and has at least a fair blood pressure or strong peripheral pulses, a fast-acting suppressor drug such as lidocaine can be given initially. If, instead, the patient becomes obtunded and has signs of circulatory failure, precordial shock is the better first approach.

The following sequential arrhythmias were treated with pharmacological and electrical agents. These strips represent selective tracings from a monitoring lead in the Coronary Care Unit. The patient is a 44-year-old construction laborer with a diagnosis of acute myocardial infarction.

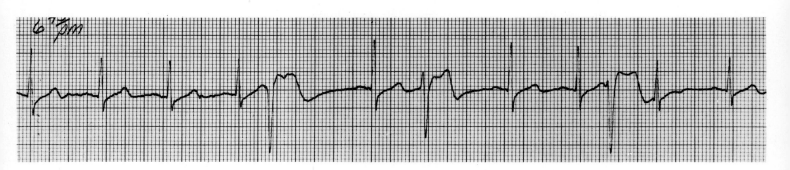

1. Moderately frequent uniform VPCs are present. These have a varying coupling interval, and two begin just after the peak of the T wave of the preceding beat.

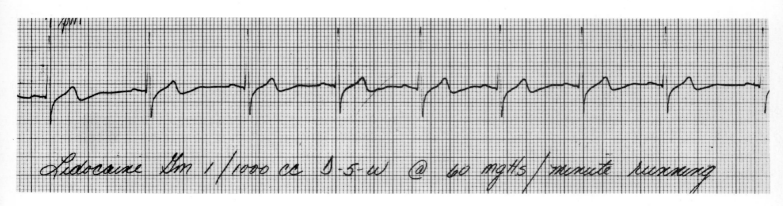

2. An infusion of lidocaine was started with satisfactory initial suppression of VPCs.

3. Suddenly VPCs recurred, some in pairs, also called couplets. Many continue to appear near the vulnerable period.

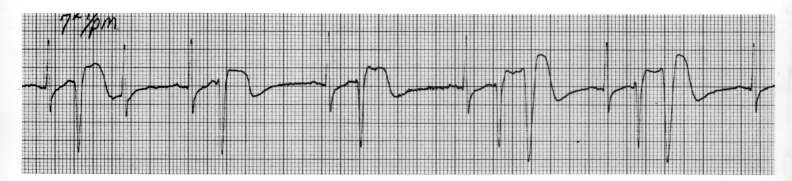

4. Before the rate of lidocaine infusion could be increased, a VPC occurring during the vulnerable period initiated ventricular tachycardia of approximately 250 per minute. The patient immediately became extremely restless, then began to have a generalized seizure.

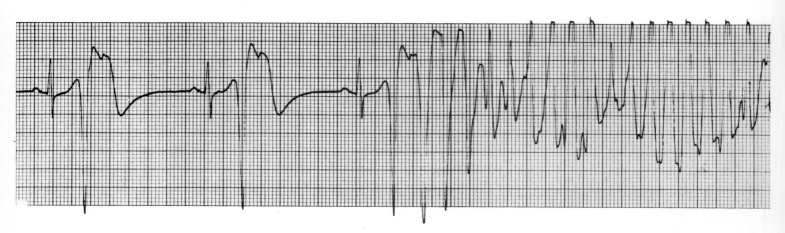

5. This tracing is continuous with the previous strip. The progressive waxing and waning of QRS amplitude, characteristic of torsades de pointes, is evident. The ar-

rhythmia at this rate can be properly called ventricular flutter. Slight changes found between the more definitive ventricular complexes may reflect P waves with A-V dissociation.

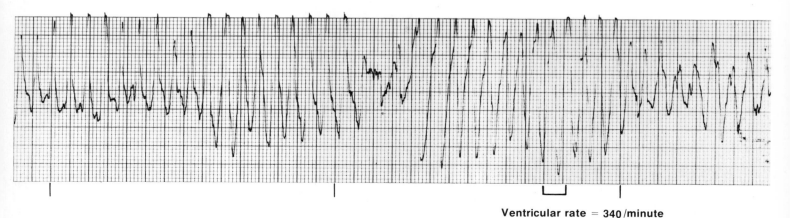

Ventricular rate = 340/minute

6. Convulsive movements were soon replaced by obtundation. Within a minute or two from onset of the tachycardia, 360 joules of direct current was applied to the anterior-lateral chest. Severe depression of ventricular activity then followed.

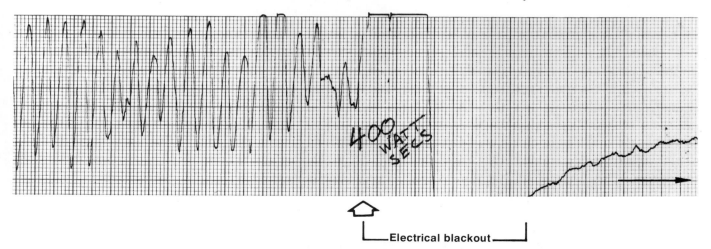

Electrical blackout

7. In these continuous rhythm sequences, notice the changes in rhythm. Observe the blocked sinus beats and multiform ventricular beats.

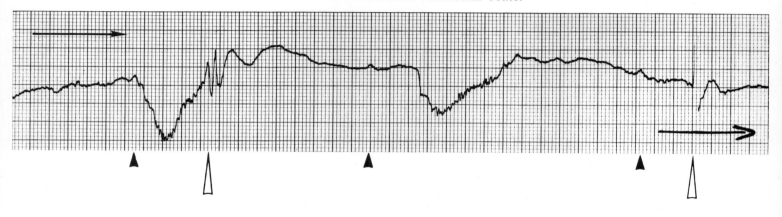

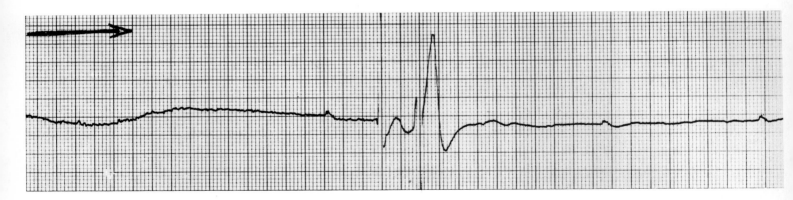

8. The period of extreme cardiac depression is now followed by a period of marked electrical instability. An A-V junctional or ventricular escape rhythm emerges with A-V dissociation. The gross baseline changes were caused by the patient's movement. However, distinct and rhythmic P wave activity can be distinguished throughout with calipers.

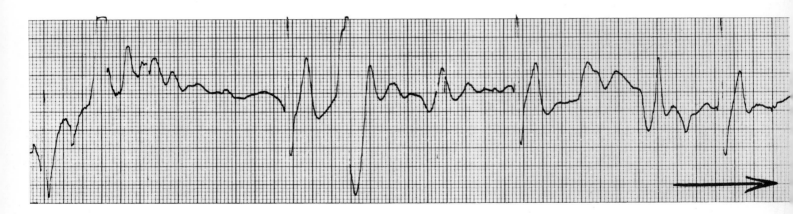

9. Moments later, A-V nodal conduction has been reestablished but severe depression is present (represented by 2:1 A-V block). In the later portion of the tracing, we find that second-degree A-V block is superseded by normal A-V conduction with normal PR intervals. A VPC is also identified, interrupting the normal sinus rhythm.

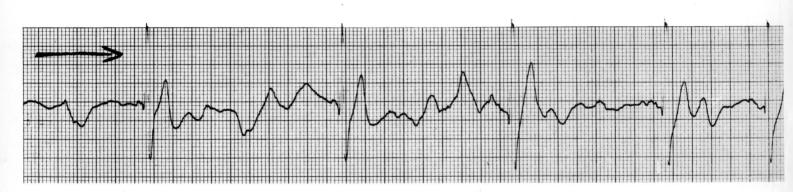

10. Effective cardiac contractions gradually returned (although frequent VPCs were present). The patient regained his full sensorium within a few minutes. Control of premature beats was thereafter controlled with beta blockers.

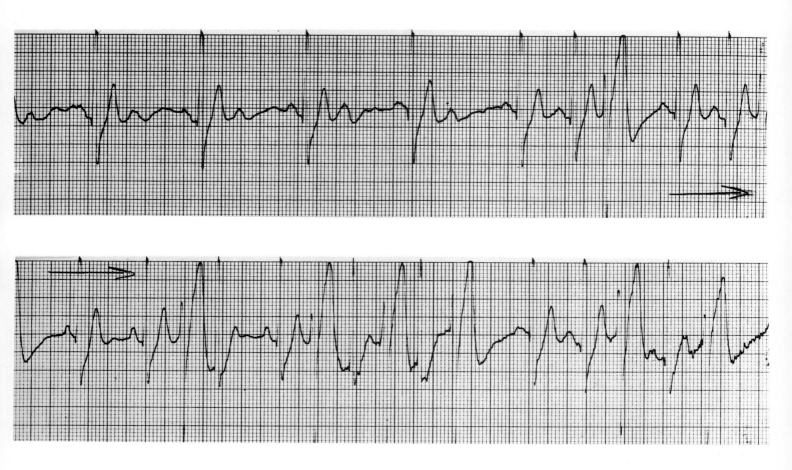

11. In subsequent days, VPCs became less frequent and appeared considerably later than the vulnerable period. The lidocaine concentration was gradually decreased; the drug was then discontinued altogether, with subsidence of all but occasional ectopic beats.

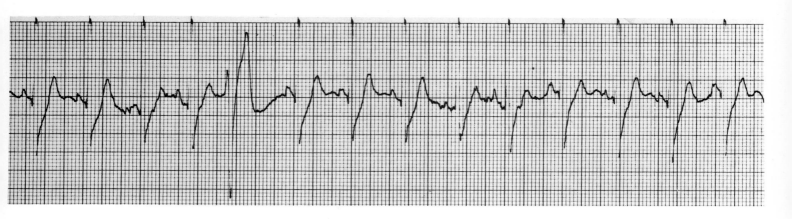

Ventricular Flutter

When ventricular activity causes an extremely rapid rate, the QRS complexes tend to merge with T waves, producing a continuous, wavy pattern with no clear separation between cardiac cycles. This pattern has been called **ventricular flutter** (Fig. 8–55).

The mechanism of ventricular flutter is similar to that of atrial flutter. However, in atrial flutter, the ventricles are protected to a degree against excessively frequent stimulation by physiological A-V block. In ventricular flutter, the ventricles contract so rapidly that there is inadequate time for chamber filling. Furthermore, the aberrant sequence of ventricular depolarization further compromises the effectiveness of myocardial contraction. Stroke ejection volume is inadequate, and circulatory failure ensues. Ventricular flutter differs from ventricular tachycardia only by its more rapid rate, causing continuous electrocardiographic oscillations. It is associated with profound cardiovascular collapse and loss of consciousness. Without definitive intervention, it is usually the immediate precursor of fatal ventricular fibrillation.

In the next test tracings (347 and 348), determine the ventricular rate. Do complexes vary in amplitude, duration, or configuration?

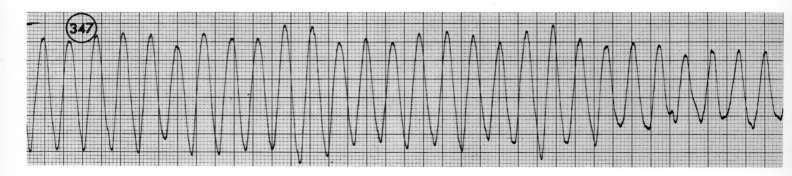

Rate = _____

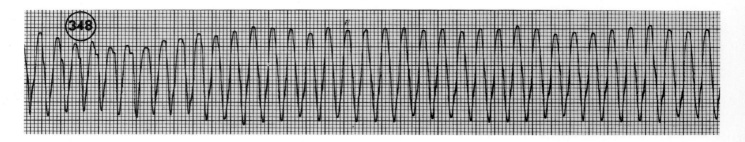

Rate = _____

Ventricular tachycardia and flutter may be complications of acute myocardial ischemia or infarction. Excessive adrenergic stimulation, such as caused by administration of catecholamine drugs or severe exercise, can produce these arrhythmias in already diseased hearts. They may also be manifestations of advanced toxicity due to digitalis. In each case, these disturbances of ventricular automaticity represent a more serious degree of excitation than VPCs. As with ventricular tachycardia, flutter can be initiated with a premature beat that occurs during the electrically unstable recovery period of the cardiac cycle.

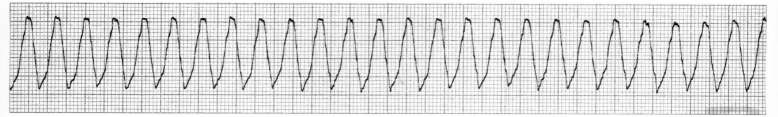

Figure 8–55. Ventricular flutter.

Figure 8–56 illustrates the induction of ventricular flutter by this R-on-T mechanism. The incident was recorded with a Holter monitoring device on a 61-year-old commuter with a history of myocardial insufficiency. The patient collapsed and died on a train. This tracing is the first electrocardiographically documented instance of sudden, unexpected death in the ambulatory population.

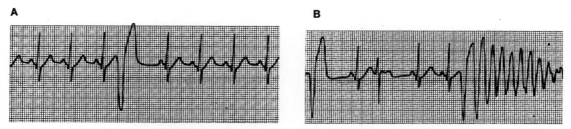

Figure 8–56. The R-on-T phenomenon as the provocative incident for ventricular flutter. (From Hinkle LE, Argyros DC, Hayes JC, et al: Role of early cycle ventricular premature contractions. Am J Cardiol 39:873, 1977.)

In tracing A, an isolated VPC occurs very early after a normal beat, its QRS complex interrupting the T wave at its expected peak. In tracing B, 3 minutes later, a similar beat occurs; it may even begin a bit earlier than the one described previously. There immediately follows a series of very rapid, wide QRS beats known as ventricular flutter. These beats soon deteriorate into the chaotic pattern of ventricular fibrillation, the transition between the two rhythms appearing at the end of this strip.

Ventricular Fibrillation

Sustained ventricular tachycardia and flutter lead inexorably to diminished myocardial performance and erratic electrical behavior. As circulatory failure from the tachycardia and progressive hypoxia affect the metabolism of the heart itself, QRS complexes become widened and more variable in contour. The next stage in the deteriorating function is **ventricular fibrillation.** Here, the impulses within the ventricles are formed and scattered too rapidly to propagate in an orderly sequence. Wave fronts overlap within the ventricular mass, and countless minute portions of the ventricles are in various states of depolarization and refractoriness. Consequently, the electrical activity of the ventricles is wholly chaotic, and no effective contraction occurs. If the heart could be viewed directly, one would see disjointed quivering of the ventricular surface instead of a vigorous, coordinated systole. Unlike atrial fibrillation, in ventricular fibrillation the primary pump of the heart is completely disabled and circulation stops.

Figure 8–57 demonstrates the electrocardiographic pattern of ventricular fibrillation. Note that no definitive complexes can be discerned.

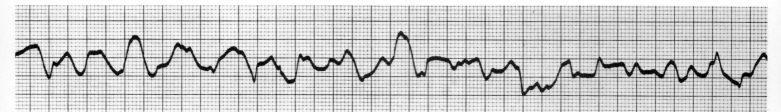

Figure 8–57. Ventricular fibrillation.

In the following examples, advanced electrical disorder of the ventricles is demonstrated. In some tracings, intermediary stages between ventricular tachycardia-flutter and fibrillation are present.

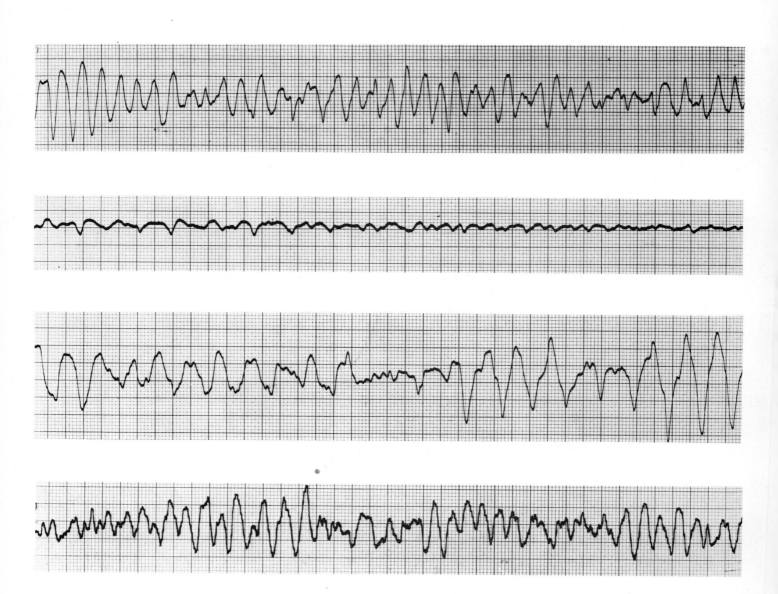

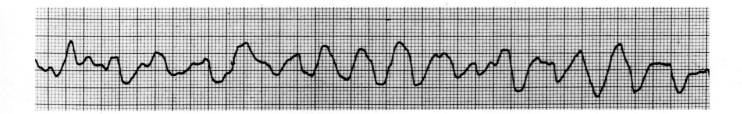

Electric shock treatment is often successful in restoring a high order of rhythm, providing that the prior condition of the heart was reasonably sound and that the procedure is administered within a minute or two after the appearance of ventricular fibrillation. A longer delay, particularly if cardiac compressions and assisted ventilations are not given or are ineffective, is associated with severe metabolic derangement, and the chances for rhythm conversion diminish rapidly with each passing minute. It is because of the rapid physiological deterioration that applying precordial shock within a minute or two after onset of ventricular fibrillation should be a goal of the Coronary Care Unit.

Within 10 to 15 seconds after the onset of ventricular fibrillation, seizure-like movement and loss of consciousness appear, attesting to the profound degree of circulatory arrest. Survival depends on prompt restoration of myocardial contractions. Conversion to an organized rhythm occasionally occurs spontaneously, but pharmacological or electrical measures generally are required. Cardiopulmonary resuscitation (CPR) is designed to maintain some degree of circulation until definitive therapy can be accomplished. Thus, CPR is intended to prevent the heart from deteriorating beyond the point at which rhythm conversion can be effective.

Electric shock treatment of ventricular fibrillation is demonstrated in the series in Figure 8–58. The patient was a 57-year-old police officer who complained of having chest pain for 2 hours before the first tracing. Acute myocardial infarction was documented on the standard ECG. The initial tracing shown here (Fig. 8–58A) was taken from a special monitoring lead after administration of morphine sulfate.

Two and a half hours later, the patient appeared comfortable and relaxed when the automatic alarm write-out system was suddenly activated. The patient simultaneously had clonic movements, lost consciousness, and became cyanotic and apneic. Electrical shock was given immediately. The tracings in Figure 8–58B and C show the results.

The rhythm recorded directly after the period of electrical shock and blackout is not identifiable. The QRS complexes are extremely prolonged, and atrial activity is obscure. With continuation into the second tracing, sinus rhythm is reestablished.

Because there are no distinct complexes in ventricular fibrillation, the electrocardioverting instrument cannot be synchronized with cardiac activity. Therefore, the automatic synchronizing control is ineffective. Instead, the operator must assure that the knob is turned to **defibrillate** (or the equivalent term as used by various manufacturers). This mode produces the discharge on activation of the switch; the instrument does not wait for a QRS complex spike, as it does in the synchronization mode. Inadvertently, using the latter in ventricular fibrillation (in which waveforms are poorly defined) may result in the failure of discharge.

When ventricular fibrillation appears suddenly even while the heart has been functioning adequately, the cause may be a premature beat during the vulnerable period. This sequence is common in acute myocardial infarction. It is known as **primary** ventricular fibrillation.

The following strips demonstrate the suddenness of the onset of primary ventricular fibrillation. The medical resident had placed additional precordial patches on a patient

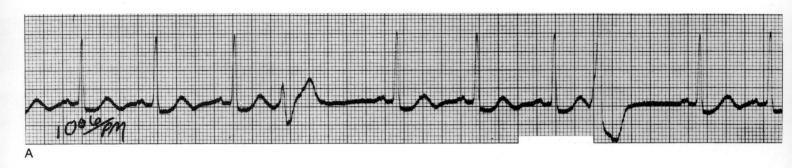

A

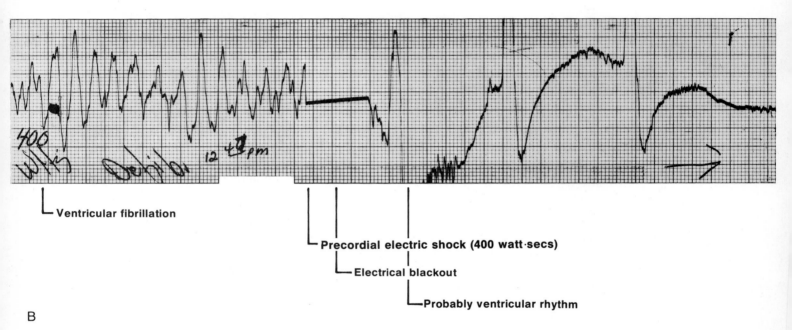

└ **Ventricular fibrillation**

└ **Precordial electric shock (400 watt·secs)**

└ **Electrical blackout**

└ **Probably ventricular rhythm**

B

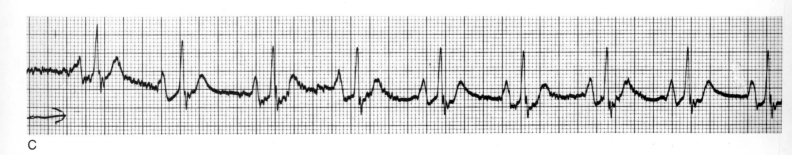

C

Figure 8–58. (*A*) Normal sinus rhythm with multiform premature contractions. (*B*) Electrical treatment of ventricular fibrillation. (*C*) Resumption of normal sinus rhythm.

to provide further information on the ectopics seen in strip 349. The second strip was recorded when the lead wire was removed from the V_1 electrode and reattached to an electrode in the V_2 position.

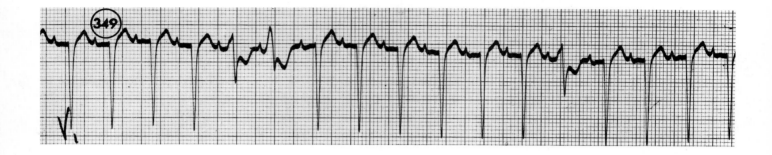

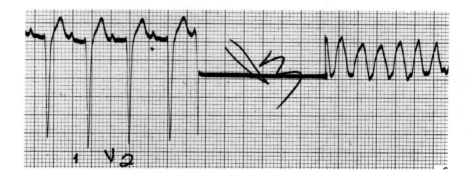

Ventricular fibrillation also occurs in the end stages of progressively deteriorating circulatory and metabolic function (as in shock and advanced myocardial failure). This form is referred to as **secondary** ventricular fibrillation. Resuscitation is much more difficult than in the primary form because of the superimposed metabolic disturbance of the body, as seen in the series in Figure 8–59.

The patient is a 48-year-old man admitted to the hospital because of gradually increasing dyspnea after an uncomplicated inferior myocardial infarction 7 months before. Furosemide, enalapril (an inhibitor of angiotensin-converting enzyme), and digoxin had been given in stepwise increments. In the emergency room, dyspnea at rest was evident, with signs of diffuse pulmonary edema. The ECG revealed a conduction defect that was of recent onset. Suddenly, the patient collapsed. The sequence in Figure 8–59 was recorded within the first 2 minutes.

Complete A-V block is present initially. The escape ventricular rhythm has an exceptionally wide QRS complex at a moderate and regular rate. An extremely premature beat interrupts the rhythm and initiates ventricular fibrillation alternating with ventricular flutter. Electrical defibrillation results in an extremely chaotic tracing, but the sharp deflections at a regular interval reveal a defined ventricular rhythm superimposed on gross movement artifact. The clear pattern of the original complete A-V block then emerges.

This patient was found to have global ischemic myocardial disease with advanced hypokinetic contractions. Susceptibility to ventricular fibrillation was presumably related to the progressing metabolic disturbance. The patient was referred for a cardiac transplant.

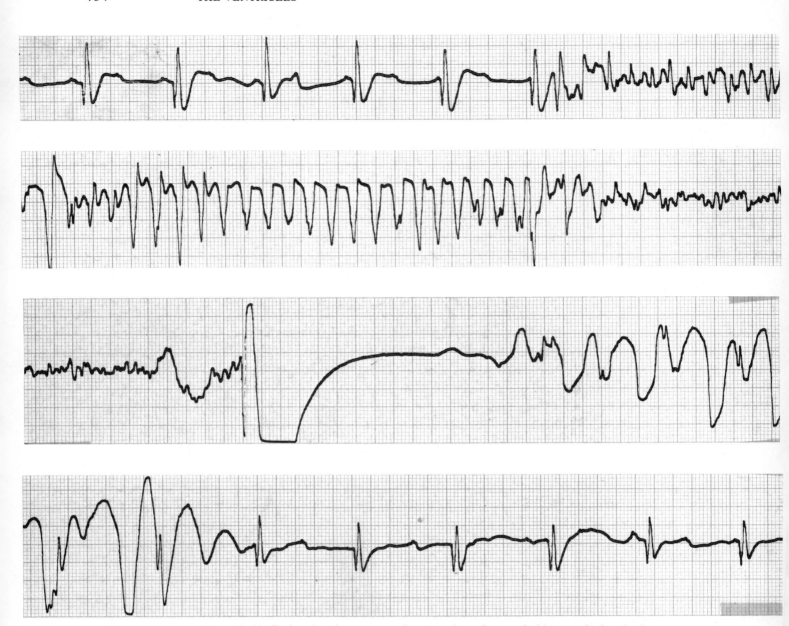

Figure 8–59. Series showing onset and conversion of an excitable ventricular rhythm.

VENTRICULAR TACHYARRHYTHMIAS

Coronary atherosclerosis is by far the preeminent underlying disease in ventricular fibrillation and the sudden cardiac death syndrome. In fact, the rhythms of ventricular excitation are the most important cause of death in the United States and in most other developed nations. In acute myocardial infarction, these fatal arrhythmias appear to arise at the periphery of the infarcted tissue, where viable cells are compromised by ischemia.

These observations underscore the importance of aggressive therapy in angina pectoris to lessen the frequency and duration of attacks and in myocardial infarction to limit the extent of injury. Furthermore, they provide a rationale for early recognition and treatment of VPCs when they complicate these conditions. Coronary Care Units were developed primarily to effect this goal.

Rhythm example number 350 is inserted here to illustrate the value of alert intervention in the management of acute myocardial infarction. The patient is a 58-year-old man in the Coronary Care Unit. On the previous day he sustained an acute anteroseptal wall infarction that was complicated by atrial fibrillation and treated with digoxin for ventricular rate control. Suddenly, without warning, the patient developed a wide QRS tachycardia associated with hypotension, air hunger, pallor, sweating, and panic reaction. The rhythm was interpreted as ventricular tachycardia and 80 mg of lidocaine was given intravenously. The tracing shown was recorded within 1 minute after injection. Prompt conversion was achieved in which atrial flutter became the superseding rhythm.

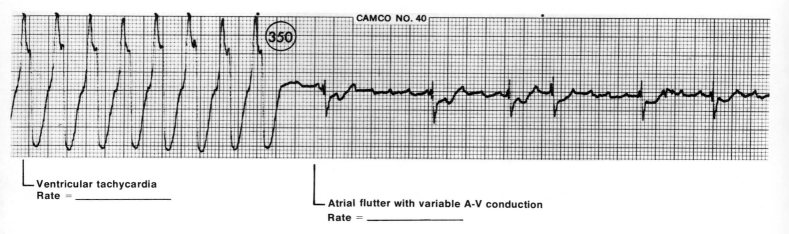

CAMCO NO. 40

350

Ventricular tachycardia
Rate = _____

Atrial flutter with variable A-V conduction
Rate = _____

VENTRICLE: IMPULSE FORMATION

Depression

Depression of impulse formation in the ventricles results in one of the three rhythm disturbances depicted in Figure 8–60.

Ventricular Bradycardia

The natural propensity of the unstimulated ventricles to beat at 20 to 50 times per minute may be severely depressed by metabolic or ischemic disease, resulting in **ventricular bradycardia.** Although this term is not often used in electrocardiography, it is appropriate and implies that supraventricular impulses are absent or not conducted and that impulse formation within the ventricles is depressed. The idioventricular rate is extremely slow, producing symptoms and signs of advanced cardiac output failure. The rhythm is usually irregular. General cardiac depression is frequently further reflected by markedly delayed ventricular depolarization with wide, varying QRS complexes. Diminished myocardial contractile force often accompanies the condition, further compromising cardiac output.

The patient whose ECG is shown in Figure 8–61 was transported to the emergency room of a small community hospital. The attendants reported that he was minimally responsive when found, and his wife stated that he had been having difficulty breathing for several hours and had experienced some chest pain and dizziness. The ventricular rate is irregular, with a rate ranging from 23 to 31. Between ventricular complexes, P waves can be identified at a rate in the low 30s.

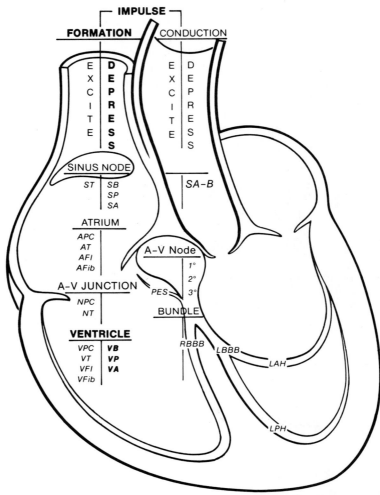

Figure 8-60. Depression of ventricular impulse formation. VB = ventricular bradycardia; VP = ventricular pause; VA = ventricular arrest.

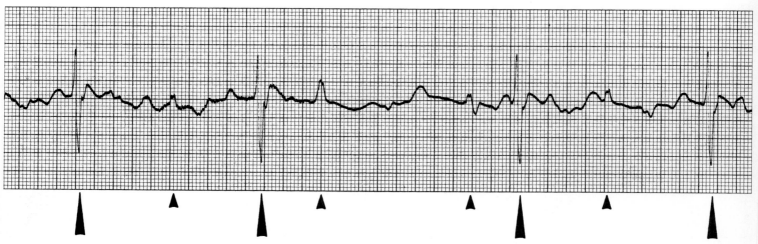

Figure 8-61. Ventricular bradycardia.

In test tracing 351, observe the character of QRS complexes (waveform, duration, and rhythmicity) and measure their rate.

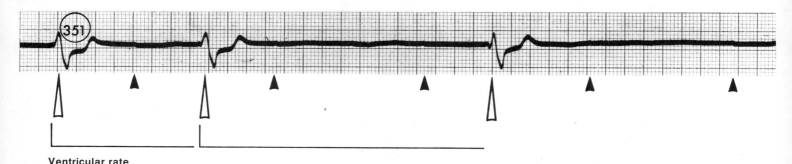

Ventricular rate

In treating ventricular bradycardia, vigorous and concerted measures are required to restore adequate cardiac output, including increasing the rate of the heartbeat and the effectiveness of myocardial contractility. A stimulatory agent such as isoproterenol may affect both, although such drugs increase the oxygen requirement of the heart. Improving contributing factors, such as hypoxia, acid-base imbalance, and major electrolyte excesses, deficiencies, or translocations is imperative. Indeed, these derangements are often the cause of myocardial depression, and specific therapy directed at other organ systems is the critical factor. In the most dire situations, CPR efforts may be essential to support the circulation until definitive therapeutic modalities are effective. A few illustrative examples will be presented.

In test strips 352 to 355, measure the rate and note the great variability in the cadence of impulse formation in the depressed ventricles. Also observe the extreme lengthening of ventricular depolarization in many instances, indicating marked depression of intraventricular conduction as well.

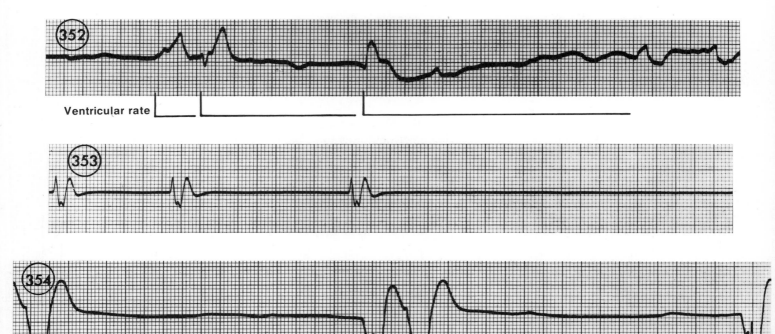

Ventricular rate

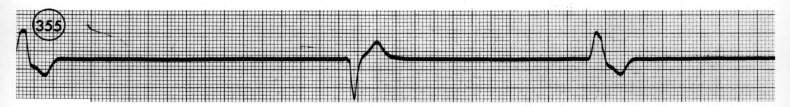

Progressive cardiac depression is evident in the following series of tracings taken on a 48-year-old man admitted to the Coronary Care Unit. The admission ECG indicated an acute myocardial infarction complicated by an atrial tachyarrhythmia, shown in test strips 356 and 357. During these recordings, the patient was alert and complained only of slight midanterior chest discomfort and nausea. Other than morphine for pain, he had been given no medication.

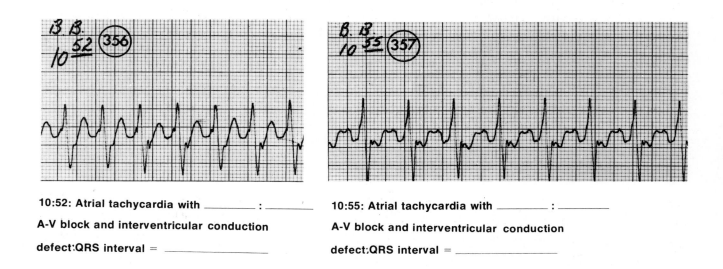

10:52: Atrial tachycardia with _____ : _____

A-V block and interventricular conduction

defect:QRS interval = _____

10:55: Atrial tachycardia with _____ : _____

A-V block and interventricular conduction

defect:QRS interval = _____

Within minutes, the patient experienced dyspnea and shortly thereafter lost consciousness. The following electrocardiographic samplings (tracings 358, 359, and 360) document the rapidly progressing deterioration of cardiac rhythm.

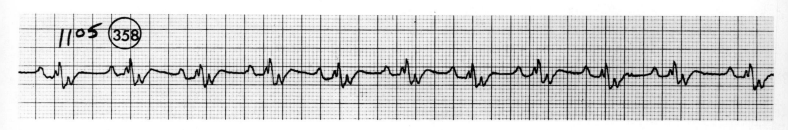

11:05: Normal sinus rhythm: Rate = _____

Further depression of conduction velocity: QRS interval = _____

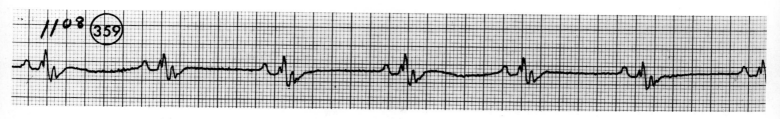

11:08: Sinus bradycardia: Rate = _____

Depression of sinus impulse formation

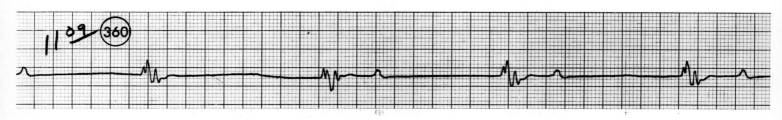

11:09: Sinus bradycardia: Rate = _____

Further depression of sinus impulse formation and depression of A-V conduction

producing complete A-V block and ventricular bradycardia: Rate = _____

Efforts at CPR were of no avail in a vigorous rescue attempt. The tracing below demonstrates the profound cardiac depression, recorded 6 minutes after the onset of collapse.

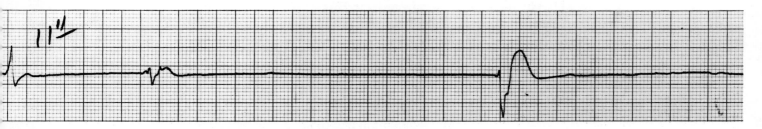

11:11 Depression of A-V junctional and ventricular pacemakers

Ventricular bradycardia with multifocal ventricular beats

In addition to continued CPR, digoxin was given intravenously and epinephrine by endotrachial tube. There was no evidence of cardiac recovery despite these measures, and within 15 minutes after onset the ECG revealed no spontaneous activity. A postmortem examination disclosed rupture of the left ventricular wall at the site of a large, infarcted area of recent origin.

Ventricular Pause

The rhythmicity of ventricular tachycardia may be interrupted by a momentary delay. This finding announces that myocardial depression is superimposed on myocardial irritability and is predictive of an unfavorable outcome.

Ventricular Arrest

When the ventricles fail to respond to intrinsic stimuli and do not maintain autonomous beating over a protracted period, the condition is designated ventricular arrest. No contractions occur, and without external circulatory support, permanent tissue damage occurs within a few minutes. Sudden transition from a tachycardia to ventricular arrest is shown in the tracing in Figure 8–62.

The following ventricular arrest sequence is from a 78-year-old woman with diffuse ischemic heart disease and refractory congestive heart failure. Progressive depression of ventricular impulse formation and conduction velocity is demonstrated in serial ECGs.

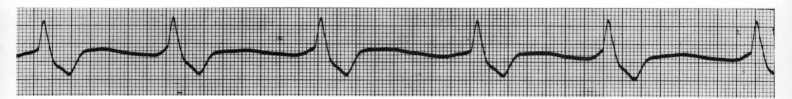

Ventricular rhythm: Rate = 40.

The rate, initially 28, slows to 20. Changes in ventricular depolarization appear with variation in QRS complex form (multiphasic beats) and further prolongation in QRS duration.

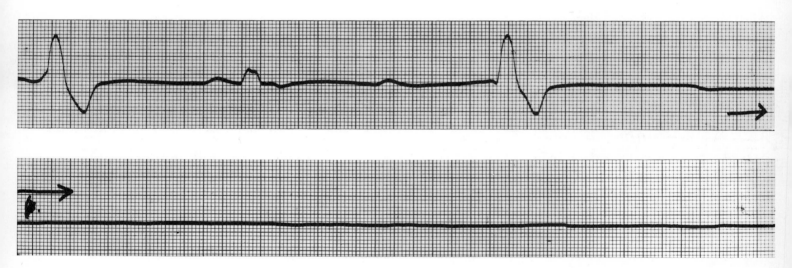

In continuous tracings, we observe severe ventricular bradycardia followed by total cessation of cardiac activity. The ECG becomes virtually a straight line. In this patient, immediate efforts at resuscitation failed to produce any cardiac response.

Ventricular arrest is highly resistant to rescue efforts, even when prompt, energetic, and well directed. External electroshock is ineffective. The heart sometimes responds to electronic impulses delivered through an intracardiac electrode, which, acting as an artificial pacemaker, drives the heart and affords a viable beat until other supportive measures can be instituted. Temporary external stimulation has also been accomplished in ventricular arrest using small, repetitive currents from the precordial paddles used for defibrillation.

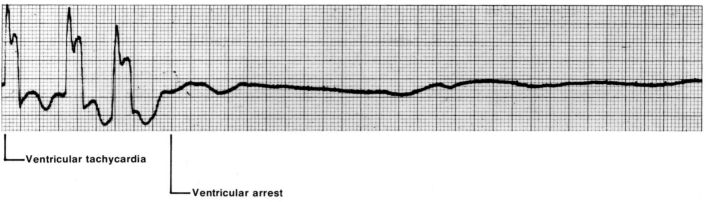

└─Ventricular tachycardia

└─Ventricular arrest

Figure 8–62. Cardiac arrest.

We have now proceeded through a discussion of all of the major forms of cardiac arrhythmias. The reader who has learned the basic principles, has observed carefully the illustrative points, and has practiced diligently with the test tracings should be able to interpret the wide range of rhythms that confront clinicians. Admittedly, rhythm abnormalities that are difficult to interpret appear frequently. Among arrhythmias most commonly vexing the electrocardiographer are those in which the QRS complex is prolonged and the question of origin arises. In the following section, detailed attention is given to this important challenge.

DIFFERENTIATION OF SUPRAVENTRICULAR RHYTHMS WITH ABERRANT VENTRICULAR CONDUCTION FROM VENTRICULAR RHYTHMS

The presence of QRS complexes of *less than 0.12 second* announces that ventricular depolarization has occurred through the ordinary conduction pathways. Such narrow complexes can therefore be assumed to be the result of impulses arising from a supraventricular source, specifically the sinus node, from specialized automatic foci in the atria, or from the A-V junctional tissues. In effect, rhythms associated with narrow QRS complexes rule out a ventricular origin.

A QRS complex of *longer than 0.12 second* may reflect the slowed ventricular depolarization characteristic of wave propagation from impulses arising in the ventricles themselves. What confounds these simplistic generalizations are those beats of supraventricular origin that, because of aberrant conduction in the ventricles, also produce wide QRS complexes. Differentiation of these beats from those of ventricular automatic foci can be very difficult. The distinction, however, must be made with the greatest accuracy attainable, for the diagnosis has a crucial bearing on major decisions regarding both prognosis and management.

A number of techniques may be enlisted to increase the certainty of correct diagnosis when the origin of a cardiac rhythm is in doubt. These include the following:

1. **Using multiple leads.** P waves, whose identification is so crucial for interpretation, may be poorly discernible on some leads. On the standard ECG, lead V_1 often provides the most clearly observed atrial activity, although no one lead should be relied on exclusively.

2. **Trying special leads.** With monitoring lead I, place the RA electrode over various sites of the right anterior chest, especially in the upper parasternal area. Alternatively,

with all the extremity leads attached as required for the standard ECG, the precordial electrode is used to explore the right chest, using the V lead mode.

    3. **Taking long tracings.** A break in the rhythm or a fortuitous time relationship between atria and ventricles (forming capture or fusion beats) can prove decisive in revealing the pacemaker site responsible for the QRS complexes. When they are infrequent, such events may be recorded only by taking a lengthy tracing.

    4. **Altering the rate of impulse formation or of A-V conduction.** Certain physical or pharmacological interventions may secure important advantages in diagnosing complex arrhythmias by changing the time relationship between atrial and ventricular activities. These techniques are discussed later under criterion 10.

    5. **Introducing special procedures.** The intraesophageal lead can be used to reveal atrial activity more clearly. The exploring electrode is threaded into the esophagus until the tip is positioned immediately adjacent to the atria. This technique can be applied with relative ease and safety (provided, of course, that electrical hazards are meticulously controlled).

    Similar information can be obtained from an intraatrial lead in which the exploring electrode is inserted into the right atrium by way of a peripheral vein. The His bundle electrogram is an extension of this technique, and it provides the definitive means for resolving the diagnosis of cardiac arrhythmias.

    In routine electrocardiography, the distinction between supraventricular beats with aberrant conduction and ventricular beats can usually be made with confidence by applying a battery of criteria. It cannot be overemphasized, however, that the proper use of these criteria requires sound understanding of the basic rhythm patterns and conduction defects, including the bundle branch blocks. The interpreter must become accustomed to meeting several criteria before arriving at a final diagnosis. At the same time, it must be acknowledged that even these criteria in consort have serious shortcomings. These limitations are frequently encountered in the Coronary Care Unit in the very patients for whom a precise diagnosis is so critical.

    The **major criteria** for differentiating supraventricular beats having aberrant ventricular conduction from ectopic ventricular beats are outlined below with illustrative examples.

1. Relationship Between Atrial Beats and Ventricular Beats

Determining if the atria beat in synchrony with the ventricles or if they beat independently of them is the single most important criterion to distinguish the two forms of rhythms associated with wide QRS complexes. This criterion, of course, depends on clear identification of atrial activity and is difficult with very rapid rates.

SYNCHRONOUS BEATING

Finding P waves that have a consistent and predictable time relationship to QRS complexes usually indicates that the dominant pacemaker is of supraventricular origin. The P waves may occur before each QRS complex or during or after each QRS complex (as occurs with A-V junctional pacemakers). P waves may outnumber QRS complexes in a consistent or inconsistent ratio (as in intermittent A-V block). The rule of synchrony applies to isolated escape or premature contractions as well as to sustained arrhythmias.

    From a patient with an acute myocardial infarction, the following tracing reveals a deep and abnormally wide Q deflection. The entire duration of the QRS complexes is prolonged. Atrial activity cannot be identified with certainty. The positive deflection just preceding each QRS complex may represent the T wave. However, there are few clues for the differentiation of ventricular tachycardia from supraventricular tachycardia with aberrant ventricular conduction.

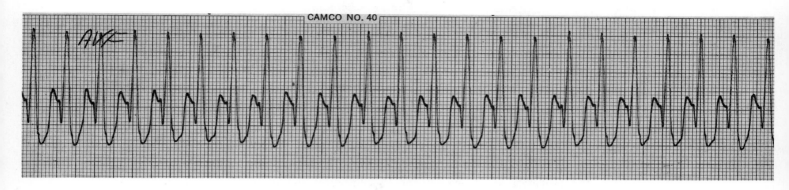

In this situation, it is helpful to look carefully at each beat, comparing corresponding points from beat to beat for any variation. Here, no appreciable changes in contour can be found, suggesting that there is no independent atrial activity (e.g., A-V dissociation). Unless atrial standstill is present (a rare condition), it is reasonable to assume that the tachycardia is of supraventricular origin.

Two *exceptions* to the above generalization are as follows:

1. In uncommon situations, an impulse generated in the ventricles is conducted in a retrograde direction to stimulate the atria.

2. A-V dissociation in which the atrial rate and the ventricular rate are, coincidentally, virtually the same. In such instances, the seemingly synchronous activity of atria and ventricles can be clarified at the bedside by deliberately altering the atrial rate or A-V conduction, as described later in criterion 10.

ASYNCHRONOUS BEATING

Identification of two independent rhythms—one controlling the atria and one the ventricles—establishes the presence of A-V dissociation and in most instances signifies the presence of a ventricular pacemaker. Such a relationship may be found in a premature beat in which the subsequent P wave is blocked; it may be noted in sustained arrhythmias of either a ventricular escape or an accelerated mechanism when an independent artrial rhythm is present.

An *exception* to the rule that A-V dissociation involves a ventricular pacemaker is in A-V junctional rhythms in which retrograde conduction to the atria is blocked. In this case, the nodal pacemaker dictates the ventricular beating and the atria are stimulated by a pacemaker proximal to the A-V node.

One must bear in mind that ventricular arrhythmias may arise in the proximal portion of the conduction system, anatomically close to the A-V junctional tissue. Consequently, it is expected that they often will behave similarly, including the tendency to exhibit retrograde conduction to the atria.

The following tracing demonstrates both supraventricular beats with aberrant conduction and ventricular beats, identified by close examination of the timing relationships of atrial and ventricular complexes.

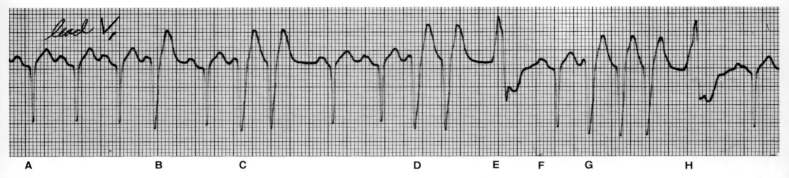

A, The basic rhythm is sinus tachycardia with a rate of 140 per minute.

B, A premature beat with a widened QRS interval occurs. This beat has the same initial contours as the conducted QRS complexes preceding it. The terminal portion of the beat, however, is slurred and is associated with alteration of the T wave. Thus, the premature beat appears to be of supraventricular origin, in which early ventricular depolarization takes place in the normal pathways but aberrant conduction occurs in the later phase of depolarization.

Because the P wave immediately preceding the premature beat is partially inscribed before the onset of the QRS complex, it can be assumed that the supraventricular premature beat is of nodal origin. Note that the P wave appearing after this beat does *not* exhibit any change in cadence from the dominant sinus rhythm. Therefore, it can also be assumed that there is no retrograde conduction.

C, Premature beats having the same characteristics as the previous one occur in tandem. Here again there is no disruption of the sinus rhythm, indicating absent retrograde conduction from the A-V junction pacemaker.

D, Reproduction of the paired nodal premature beats with aberrant conduction and retrograde block.

E, This beat also displays prolongation of the QRS duration, but it has a configuration that is entirely different from the ectopic beats previously described. In lead V_1, it is not typical of either right or left bundle branch block. The *initial* portion of the QRS complex is slurred, and there is no appreciable change in the cadence of the sinus beat following it. These findings favor a VPC.

F, Resumption of a sinus origin and conducted beat.

G, Recurrence of A-V junctional beats, this time as triplets, constituting A-V nodal tachycardia at an extremely rapid rate.

H, Beat of ventricular origin following the brief episode of nodal tachycardia.

This example illustrates both nodal and ventricular ectopic beats in a temporal association and depicts the electrical instability associated with extremely rapid rates.

2. QRS Complex Morphology

DIFFUSE INTRAVENTRICULAR CONDUCTION DEFECT

Prolonged QRS complexes that retain the same general configuration of previously normal beats suggest a diffuse abnormality of intraventricular conduction. Such changes may occur from cardiosuppressor drugs (quinidine, procainamide) or certain noncardiac drugs (emetine, used in treating amebiasis). Significant prolongation of the QRS complex with these agents is a sign of toxicity. Wide QRS complexes from diffuse intraventricular conduction disturbances also may be observed in severe hypoxia, in generalized myocardial diseases (ischemic, rheumatic, infectious from viral agents, and degenerative conditions), in ventricular aneurysms, in hypothermia, and in various electrolyte imbalances, most notably with severe hyperkalemia or hypercalcemia.

Severe hyperkalemia not only causes widening of the QRS complex but also reduction in the amplitudes of P waves. When this condition is advanced, a sinus rhythm may resemble a ventricular rhythm with atrial standstill. In the example in Figure 8–63, potassium excess produces a nearly terminal disorder of cardiac electrophysiology, but normal sinus rhythm persists. It illustrates a diffuse intraventricular conduction defect caused by a severe metabolic disturbance.

An 11-day-old boy was brought to the emergency room because of marked lethargy, rapid breathing, and emaciation. The mother remarked on his lack of voiding since discharge from the newborn nursery 6 days before. Because of the unexpectedly slow heart rate, an ECG was obtained; it revealed a sinus rhythm with markedly prolonged QRS complexes (Fig. 8–63A).

Because of the low-amplitude P waves and the extremely wide QRS complexes, one may mistake this rhythm for an accelerated ventricular rhythm. A cardiosuppressor drug, which might have been given to treat the latter arrhythmia, would certainly have had a detrimental action.

Blood was drawn for electrolytes and complete blood count. Moments later, the patient became apneic and had extremely distant heart sounds. Blood pressure was unobtainable. QRS complexes became progressively widened (Fig. 8–63B). After initiation of mouth-to-mouth ventilation, sodium bicarbonate was administered intrave-

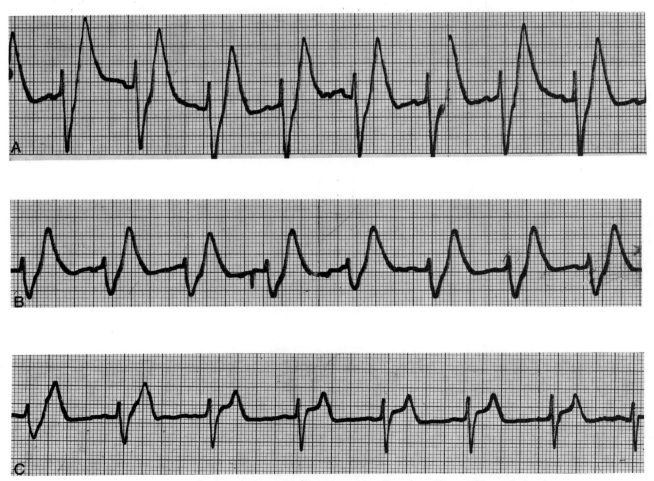

Figure 8–63. Series of electrocardiograms revealing the effects of hyperkalemia.

nously because of suspected uremic acidosis and hyperkalemia (suggested by tall and peaked T waves).

Prompt restoration of spontaneous breathing and normalization of the QRS complex ensued, as depicted below. Note the gradual narrowing of the QRS complex while it maintains the same general configuration. Sinus rhythm is evident here, endorsing the supraventricular nature of the wide QRS complex sequence (Fig. 8–63*C*).

Subsequently, laboratory examination revealed blood urea nitrogen of 215 mg/dl and a serum potassium concentration of 7.2 mEq/liter. Peritoneal dialysis was started soon after resuscitation. Congenital ureteral obstruction was eventually diagnosed, and the patient underwent successful surgical correction.

BUNDLE BRANCH BLOCK

When the pattern of ventricular depolarization is in the configuration of either right or left bundle branch block, the responsible pacemaker is most likely proximal to the bifurcation of the common bundle. Therefore, identification of a bundle branch block places the origin of the beat in a supraventricular focus. Unfortunately, impulses generated in either right or left ventricles can produce QRS complexes that closely resemble bundle branch blocks, and distinguishing between them requires using subtle and often not very reliable criteria.

RIGHT BUNDLE BRANCH BLOCK VERSUS LEFT VENTRICULAR BEATS. Both supraventricular beats with right bundle branch block and left ventricular beats are associated with a delay in the late portion of electrical systole in which the aberrantly conducted wave front moves toward the right. The essential difference between the two forms of beats is that those originating in the left ventricle distort the QRS complex early in its development as well, and consequently the initial portion of the QRS complex may be affected (Fig. 8–64).

Typically in lead I and in the monitoring lead, there is an abnormally wide S wave in right bundle branch block, but this is not longer than 0.04 second. The terminal prolongation in the left ventricular beats may be much longer and is of much greater variability in configuration. In addition, the Q wave in the left ventricular beats may be abnormally long.

From a different electrical perspective, the characteristic pattern of right bundle branch block in lead V_1 (small R, deep S, and tall and prolonged R') may also be present in the left ventricular beats. Usually, however, the initial R deflection is extended and eventually merges with R', intercepted only by a small S or no more than even a brief hesitation in the development of an entirely upright QRS complex.

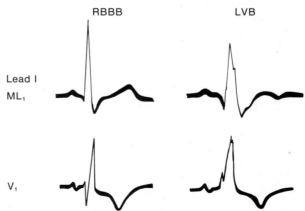

Figure 8–64. Characteristics differentiating right bundle branch block and left ventricular complexes.

LEFT BUNDLE BRANCH BLOCK VERSUS RIGHT VENTRICULAR BEATS.

Supraventricular beats with left bundle branch block depolarize the intraventricular septum in an abnormal direction (right to left) and create a wave front in the ventricular wall that moves predominantly from the right ventricle to the much thicker left ventricle. Consequently, the QRS duration is greatly prolonged. The QRS complex is directed almost entirely upward in lead I and in the monitoring lead; it is downward in lead V_1. The normal Q deflection in lead I and the monitoring lead is usually abolished, as is the normal small R deflection in lead V_1 (they may be present, but if so, are much smaller) (Fig. 8–65).

In beats arising from the right ventricle or intraventricular septum, the QRS complex pattern depends on the location of the pacemaker responsible (on the wall of the septum or the free wall of the ventricle), and thus the complex will be more variable. Nevertheless, the general character of the QRS complex tends to have the features stated above for left bundle branch block. Differentiation of the two forms may be assisted by the clues outlined below, although these criteria are far from infallible.

1. Right ventricular extrasystoles are relatively uncommon, whereas supraventricular beats with left bundle branch block are not.

2. On comparing the precordial leads of the standard ECG, the deepest QS deflection is usually found over the right precordial leads in left bundle branch block. In right ventricular beats, the deepest QRS deflection is usually over the left precordial leads.

3. In contradistinction to left bundle branch block, right ventricular beats often exhibit a prolonged Q deflection in lead I and in the monitoring lead and a prolonged R deflection in lead V_1.

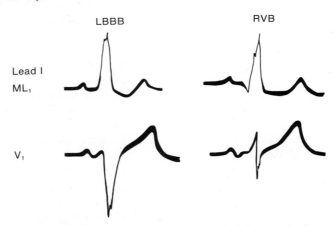

Figure 8–65. Configurations of left bundle branch block and right ventricular complexes.

In perspective, the recognition of a bundle branch block pattern is helpful in distinguishing between supraventricular beats with aberrant conduction and ventricular beats. It is crucial that the specialist in the critical care unit be thoroughly familiar with the bundle branch block pattern for the monitoring lead routinely used. At the same time, it must be appreciated that this means of distinguishing aberrantly conducted beats from ectopic beats is limited and that additional criteria should be enlisted in each diagnostic problem to minimize the chance of error.

One invaluable adjunct to diagnosis in sustained arrhythmias of uncertain origin is the review of tracings taken before development of the arrhythmia, searching for isolated beats with wide QRS complexes that resemble those now present and continuous. Since the earlier, single beats can usually be identified with confidence as to origin, similar beats observed during the sustained arrhythmia give reason to relate the two etiologically.

3. Post-Extrasystolic Pause

Keeping in mind the exceptions to the rule, the character of the interval following a premature beat can be helpful in differentiating supraventricular beats from ventricular beats. To review:

THE COMPENSATED PAUSE

Such a pause represents a delay in ventricular systole following a premature beat in which the dominant supraventricular rhythm continues after the extrasystole without a change in its established cadence. It is assumed that such premature beats are of ventricular origin because they cause a momentary refractoriness within the A-V nodal system to the natural oncoming supraventricular impulse. A blocked P wave can usually be found shortly after inscription of the premature QRS complex (unless the VPC is interpolated).

One exception to the compensatory pause rule is the occasional ventricular premature beat that is conducted in a retrograde direction through the A-V node to invade the atria and depolarize the sinus node. The result is a noncompensatory pause because the sinus node cycling is reset.

Another exception is the A-V junctional premature beat, which displays antegrade conduction to the ventricles but that blocks in retrograde propagation to the atria. In this instance, the supraventricular impulse produces a compensatory pause by the same mechanism as does a premature impulse arising in the ventricles. If the A-V junction beat is associated with prolonged intraventricular conduction and a wide QRS complex, it will be difficult if not impossible to distinguish it from an ectopic beat of ventricular origin.

THE NONCOMPENSATED PAUSE

Such a pause is produced by a premature beat that depolarizes the dominant sinus node pacemaker as well as the ventricles. Thus, the beat following the premature beat exhibits a change in its rhythmicity. This resetting of the sinus beat implies that the premature beat originated in a supraventricular focus (since most ventricular beats exhibit retrograde block).

Because the premature beat stimulates the sinus node prematurely, the subsequent sinus beat typically appears earlier in its cycling. The interpreter must, however, be alert to a variation in this generalization. The prematurely discharged sinus node sometimes hesitates in its refiring, and this delay can be quite substantial. It may even cause the sinus beat following a premature beat to appear late in the cycling pattern and, if appropriately timed, it may simulate a compensatory pause.

4. Regularity of Rhythm

The typical clock-like regularity of atrial and nodal escape rhythms and tachycardias is universally appreciated, as are the phasic variations of rate characteristic of sinus rhythms. Unfortunately, there is a generally accepted misconception that ventricular rhythms are distinctively irregular. In actuality, automatic firing in the common bundle and in the proximal Purkinje system tends to be quite regular. As pacemakers are activated farther distally in the Purkinje system, the rhythm generally becomes somewhat irregular as well as slower.

Grossly irregular rhythms are more characteristic of atrial fibrillation or atrial flutter with varying A-V block. When these rhythms are associated with very rapid ventricular rates, aberrant conduction is often present and the rhythms are mistaken for ventricular tachycardia.

In Figure 8–66, the grossly irregular rhythm at extremely rapid rates (at times about 275) suggests a supraventricular origin. This interpretation is supported by the finding of a premature beat exhibiting a narrow QRS complex (arrow) at the onset of each burst. It appears that a beat from the A-V junction has initiated a supraventricular tachycardia in which aberrant ventricular conduction occurs.

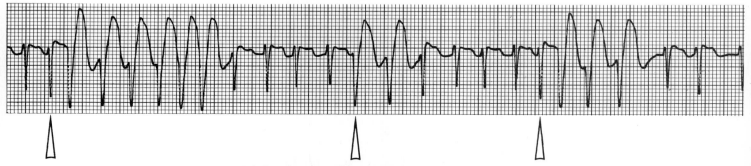

Figure 8–66. Brief paroxysms of a "wide QRS" tachycardia.

An extremely important form of irregular rhythm is the type with very wide QRS complexes at very rapid rates. These findings suggest atrial fibrillation with an accessory ventricular pathway, particularly when the rate is above 220 beats a minute. It is the form of ventricular preexcitation that presents normal early ventricular depolarization (no delta wave) before the onset of the tachycardia (see criterion 11, below).

5. Onset of a Tachycardia

The activity immediately preceding a tachycardia should be studied with special care, because the origin is often revealed. The presence of an atrial or nodal premature beat at the onset is strong evidence in favor of a supraventricular tachycardia. This diagnosis is further supported if subsequent QRS complexes become rapidly and progressively widened and deformed. In ventricular tachycardia, QRS complexes, by contrast, tend to be uniform in morphology and duration throughout, with the exception of torsades de pointes, already described.

The sinus tachycardia represented in Figure 8–67 is suddenly interrupted by a wide QRS tachycardia. There is no P wave at the onset to suggest a supraventricular tachycardia, but the changes in contour throughout the ectopic tachycardia probably reflect superimposed atrial activity (suggesting A-V dissocciation). The slight irregularity of the QRS complexes and the lack of progressive widening during the more rapid tachycardia favor the diagnosis of ventricular tachycardia.

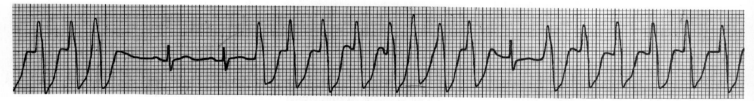

Figure 8–67. Ventricular tachycardia.

6. Captured Beat

A narrow QRS complex that interrupts a series of wide QRS complexes often indicates the presence of A-V dissociation. The intermittent captured beat represents ventricular depolarization along normal conduction pathways and an origin in a supraventricular pacemaker; the impulse from this pacemaker penetrates the A-V node to arrive at the common bundle just at a time when the ventricular conduction system is receptive to it. In other words, the His-Purkinje fibers, dominated by a ventricular pacemaker, respond to an occasional supraventricular impulse if that impulse reaches the system when enough time has elapsed from the previous beat to allow recovery from its refractory period. Thus, the intermittent and fortuitous captured beat provides evidence that the principal ventricular pacemaker is located in the ventricles themselves, and that an independent supraventricular pacemaker is simultaneously operant. This principle is illustrated in the ECG in Figure 8–68.

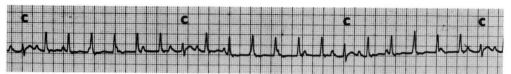

Figure 8–68. Rhythm strip showing ventricular tachycardia (rate 136 per minute) and occasional capture beats (C) with normal QRS complex. Note that the P wave of the capture beat (C) is conducted with a prolonged PR interval, indicating the presence of first-degree A-V block. (From Helfant RH [ed]: Bellet's Essentials of Cardiac Arrhythmias, 2nd ed. WB Saunders, Philadelphia, 1980, p. 148.)

7. Fusion Beat

The fusion beat is a variant of the captured beat and has the same implications when it appears amidst a group of QRS complexes of wide configuration. Such a beat (the first portion of which represents a supraventricular-initiated impulse and the remainder,

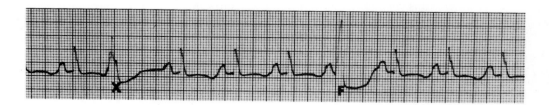

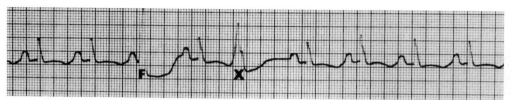

Figure 8–69. Continuous rhythm strip demonstrating ventricular premature beats (X) and fusion beats (F). Note that the QRS of the fusion beats is of intermediate contour between the sinus beat and the ventricular premature beat. (From Helfant RH [ed]: Bellet's Essentials of Cardiac Arrhythmias, 2nd ed. WB Saunders, Philadelphia, 1980, p. 141.)

a ventricular-originated impulse) reveals independent pacemaker activity. Hence, in a tachycardia with intermittent fusion beats, the presumption is that the basic rhythm is ventricular tachycardia. Fusion beats that reveal the identity of premature beats are demonstrated in the tracing in Figure 8–69.

8. The Ashman Phenomenon

Supraventricular beats that occur relatively soon after a slow cycle beat exhibit a tendency to aberrant ventricular conduction (Fig. 8–70). Known as the Ashman phenomenon, this feature is caused by the longer refractory period associated with slower rhythms. This characteristic is found in atrial fibrillation as well as in other forms of supraventricular rhythms.

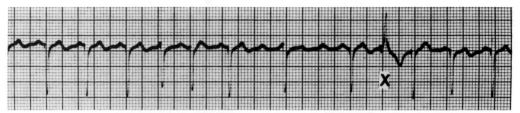

Figure 8–70. Aberrant conduction. Note that the aberrantly conducted beat (X) has a short coupling interval whereas the beat preceding it (which is normal in contour) follows a long pause. The aberrant beat has a right bundle branch block configuration. (From Helfant RH [ed]: Bellet's Essentials of Cardiac Arrhythmias, 2nd ed. WB Saunders, Philadelphia, 1980, p. 142.)

9. T Waves

Beats that have aberrant ventricular conduction have altered repolarization as well. However, the change in T waves associated with such beats is not generally as drastic as that observed in beats of ventricular origin. Ventricular beats usually exhibit T waves that are reversed in direction to the main QRS deflection. The T waves of ventricular beats also tend to be of greater amplitude than those found in supraventricular beats, even those with aberrant conduction.

In the example of bigeminal rhythm in Figure 8–71, the second beat of each pair (which is premature and has a wide QRS complex) has a blocked P wave at the interface between the QRS complex and the T wave. The configuration of this junction varies somewhat from beat to beat because of slight changes in sinus rate. The blocked but

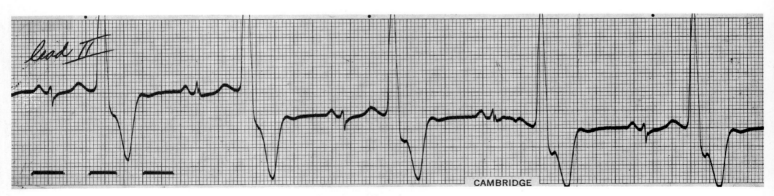

Figure 8–71. Reversal of T wave direction.

on-time P waves establish that atrial activity is not disturbed by the premature beat. This independent atrial and ventricular beating is evidence that the premature contractions originate from the ventricles. Reversal of T wave direction in comparison to the QRS deflection is evident in Figure 8–71. The fixed coupling interval between the sinus beats and the ventricular beats suggest that a reentrant mechanism of impulse conduction in the ventricles is responsible for the premature activation.

10. Rate Changes

In rhythms in which it cannot be readily determined if atrial and ventricular activity are dependent or independent, interventions that change the rate of either atria or ventricles can be extremely helpful in interpretation. Clinicians have various means of accomplishing such change at the bedside of cardiac-monitored patients.

VAGOTONIC MANEUVERS

In some tachycardias, the rate may be abruptly slowed with parasympathetic stimulation, such as carotid pressure, gag reflexes, and exposure of the face to cold water. This responsiveness strongly suggests that the tachycardia is of supraventricular origin, the slowing occurring either through suppression of the sinus, atrial, or A-V junctional pacemaker or through accentuation of physiological A-V block. In addition, the ventricular slowing may expose atrial activity, thus allowing a precise diagnosis from P wave tracking. Atrial flutter with aberrant conduction can often be diagnosed in this manner when the etiology is otherwise quite obscure. It must be emphasized that a lack of response to a vagotonic maneuver does *not* rule out a supraventricular mechanism for a tachycardia. This statement is particularly applicable to tachycardias associated with the ventricular preexcitation syndrome.

The value of vagotonic maneuvers is demonstrated in Figure 8–72.

In *A*, the rhythm is rapid and regular with Q waves of greater than 0.04 seconds, consistent with the diagnosis of anterolateral myocardial infarction. The QRS complex duration is 0.16 second. The baseline between QRS complexes and recognizable T waves varies slightly from beat to beat so that consistent atrial activity cannot be identified.

In *B*, the carotid pressure maneuver is performed as a diagnostic (and potentially therapeutic) trial. This intervention induces a sudden slowing of the ventricular rate and discloses the pattern of atrial fibrillation. The rhythm is complex, however, because a regular ventricular rate does *not* occur with atrial fibrillation unless the pacemaker driving the ventricles is electrically isolated from the atria (as in complete A-V block). Yet, the fact that the ventricular rate responded sharply to vagal stimulation is strong evidence that the pacemaker is located above the ventricles themselves. Thus, it is inferred that the ventricles were being paced by automatic tissue in the A-V junctional

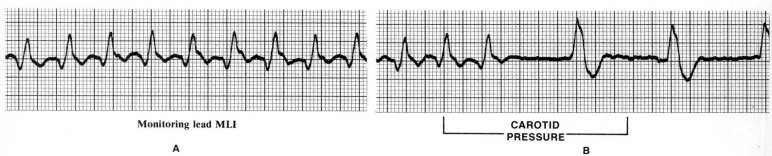

Monitoring lead MLI

CAROTID
PRESSURE

A   B

Figure 8–72. Effect of vagotonic activity on a tachyarrhythmia.

area and that complete A-V block was present. Interestingly, the rhythm that emerges after carotid stimulation has the typical configuration of left bundle branch block in the monitoring lead. It appears that increased vagal tone blocked a portion of the conduction pathways beyond the A-V junctional pacemaker.

A word of caution: Vagotonic maneuvers create a sudden and powerful imbalance of autonomic control, usually associated with a strong reactive stimulation of the sympathetic system. Ventricular premature beats rather frequently follow carotid pressure or comparable interventions. Admittedly rare complications, ventricular tachycardia and ventricular fibrillation have been reported after attempts to convert supraventricular tachycardias with these maneuvers. The messsage is obvious: When such techniques are used for differential diagnosis, proper precautions for coping with induced cardiac emergencies must be assured and should include an indwelling intravenous line, appropriate drugs, and resuscitation equipment.

PHARMACOLOGIC INTERVENTION

Edrophonium (Tensilon) can be used to achieve the same vagotonic reaction as the physical maneuvers mentioned previously. The ventricular rate will likely be slowed in supraventricular tachycardias owing to inhibition of the responsible pacemaker or to reduction in the frequency of impulses conducted across the A-V node. As with the vagotonic maneuvers, the tachycardia may also be converted to a sinus rhythm, thus resolving both the diagnosis and the clinical problem. Similarly, procainamide (Pronestyl) may reveal the mechanism of a supraventricular tachycardia. On the other hand, this drug also suppresses ectopic pacemakers in the ventricles so that simply slowing the ventricular rate does not imply a specific etiology. Incidentally, the use of lidocaine (Xylocaine) to distinguish tachycardias is not generally advisable. Although this agent is quite effective in abolishing ventricular automaticity, it may *enhance* A-V conduction. If the rhythm is of supraventricular origin with intermittent A-V block, the tachycardia may be seriously aggravated.

11. Preexcitation Syndrome

Because of important features of tachycardias associated with ventricular preexcitation and because of the increasing frequency of recognition of this disorder, the preexcitation syndrome deserves special mention. Differentiation of preexcitation tachycardia from ventricular tachycardia is often difficult because of the extremely rapid rates and the bizarre aberrancy often produced. The following clues may provide a key to the correct diagnosis of ventricular preexcitation syndrome with tachycardia:

1. The diagnosis of preexcitation syndrome has been established on ECGs predating the tachycardia.

2. Ventricular rates greater than 250 beats per minute, even briefly, strongly suggest a ventricular preexcitation mechanism with a supraventricular pacemaker.

3. Delta waves may be present during the tachycardia, but they are most often absent. The explanation is probably that the accessory pathway used during the normal rhythm becomes the retrograde pathway of the reentry circuit during the tachycardia. This frequent absence of a delta wave in tachycardias associated with the pre-excitation syndrome is not widely appreciated and has been responsible for their being treated as ventricular tachycardia. Fortuitously, lidocaine and electrocardioversion, the most commonly employed methods for treating ventricular tachycardia, are both highly successful in terminating supraventricular tachycardias in preexcitation. An exception is the use of lidocaine in atrial fibrillation in the presence of ventricular preexcitation as explained in criterion number 12.

4. Vagotonic stimuli are generally of no avail in converting supraventricular tachycardias associated with preexcitation. Enhanced vagal tone does not ordinarily affect the bypass tract to any substantial degree, although it may slow direct conduction in the A-V node.

12. Atrial Fibrillation

It is particularly difficult to differentiate the origin of broad QRS complexes in the presence of atrial fibrillation. However, identifying clues can often be found, as in the next two examples.

In this two-channel recording (Fig. 8–73), atrial fibrillation is associated with narrow QRS complexes (0.10 second), signifying that ventricular depolarizations proceed along the normal conduction system. One exception is noted in which an inordinately early QRS complex is prolonged (0.13 second). The initial portion of this waveform appears unchanged, but the terminal portion is aberrant, with its depolarizing wave front directed rightward (positive in lead V_1 and negative in lead V_5). Thus, a right bundle branch block pattern is recognized. It is concluded that conduction of this beat has occurred from an atrial impulse but that rate-related fatigue of the right bundle branch resulted in a block; the right ventricle was activated from a wave front proceeding aberrantly from the left ventricle.

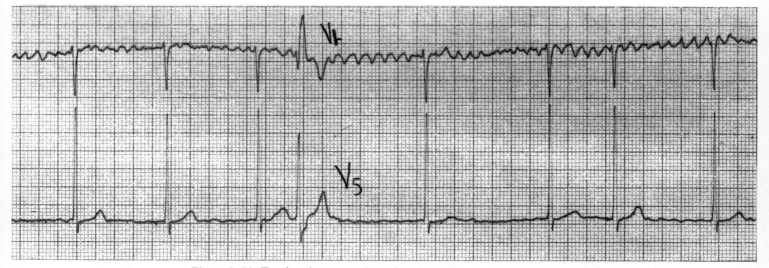

Figure 8–73. Tracing demonstrating wide QRS complexes in the presence of atrial fibrillation.

Atrial fibrillation is illustrated in Figure 8–74. In this tracing, all QRS complexes are markedly widened (0.17 second). Note also the perfect regularity of the ventricular rhythm, a response that would not be expected in uncomplicated atrial fibrillation. One must conclude that ventricular activity is independent of atrial activity, thus defining complete A-V dissociation. Because the ventricular rate is 70 per minute, it is considered an accelerated rhythm rather than escape rhythm. The pacemaker may be either from the A-V junctional tissue (with aberrant ventricular conduction) or from an automatic site within the ventricles. Considering that this tracing is from lead V_1, the downward initial portion of the QRS complexes is abnormal (normal left-to-right septal depolarization would cause an upright initial deflection). The terminal and major portion of these waveforms is directed leftward (away from the V_1 electrode). These findings suggest that the ectopic pacemaker is situated in the right ventricle (or the right side of the intraventricular septum). This recording is an illustration of digitalis toxicity in

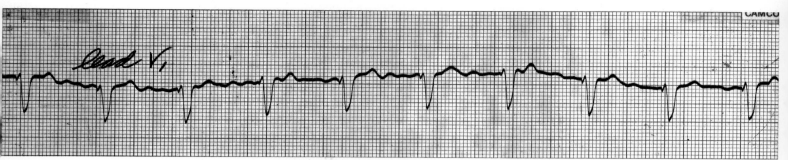

Figure 8–74. Wide QRS complexes in the presence of atrial fibrillation with complete A-V block.

which the A-V block and the accelerated ventricular pacemaker are functional manifestations. Both abnormalities disappeared on withholding the drug. Atrial fibrillation persisted, although the ventricular rate response became rapid.

SELF-EVALUATION: STAGE 3

Give a complete interpretation of the following electrocardiograms.

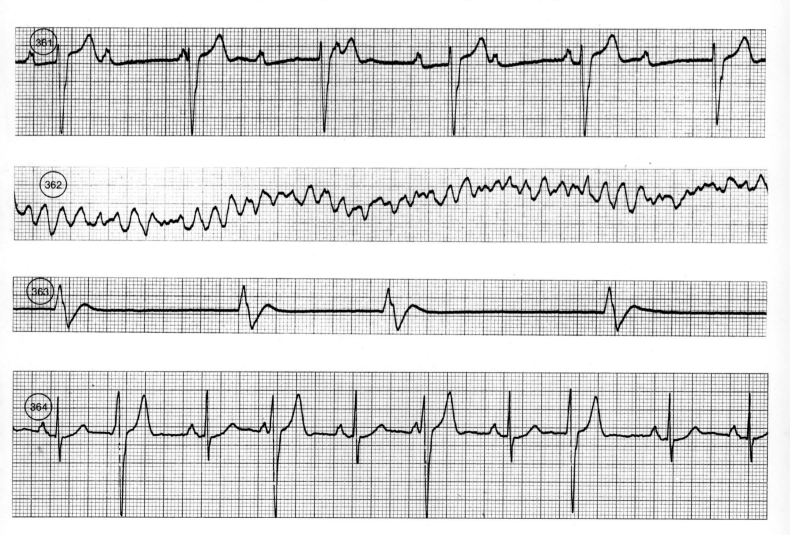

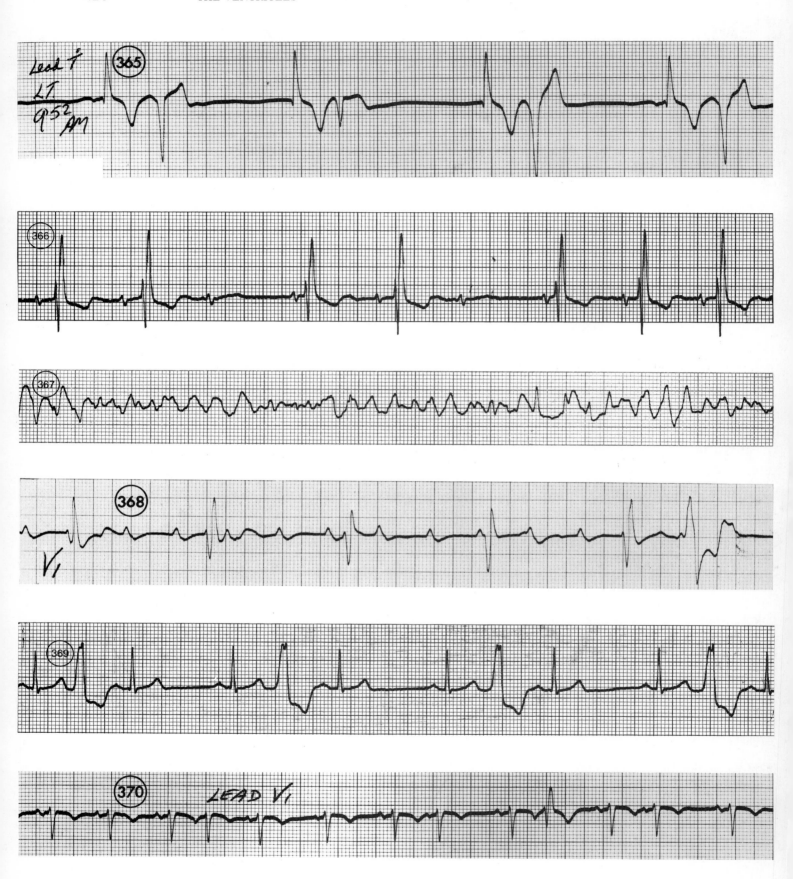

365 Lead 7 / LT / 9⁵² AM

366

367

368 V₁

369

370 LEAD V₁

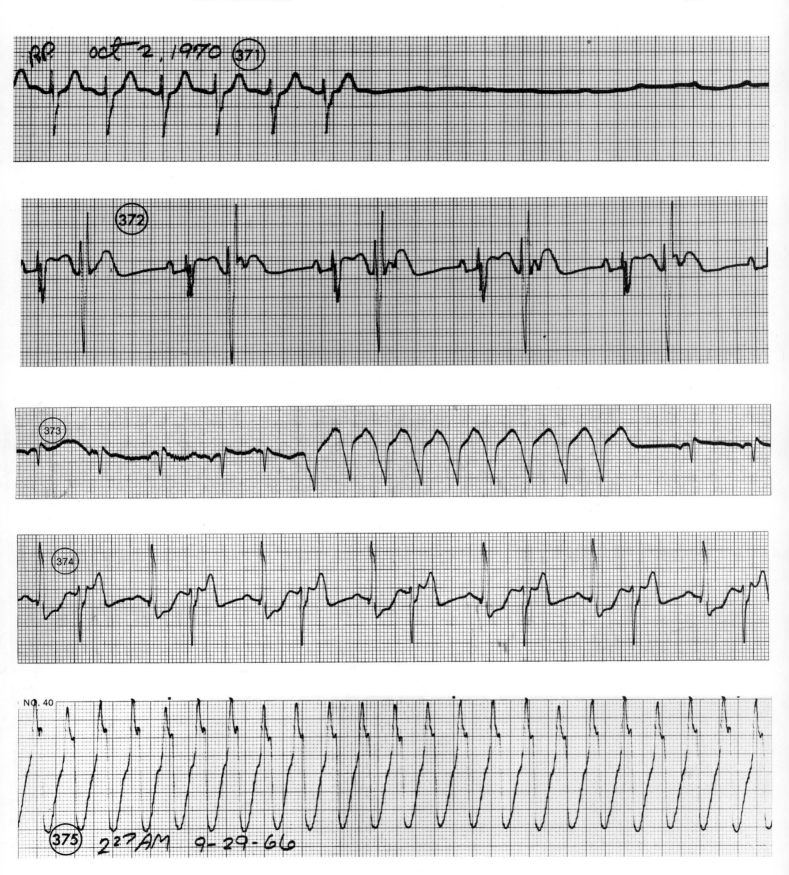

RP   oct 2, 1970   (371)

(372)

(373)

(374)

NO. 40

(375)   2²⁷AM   9-29-66

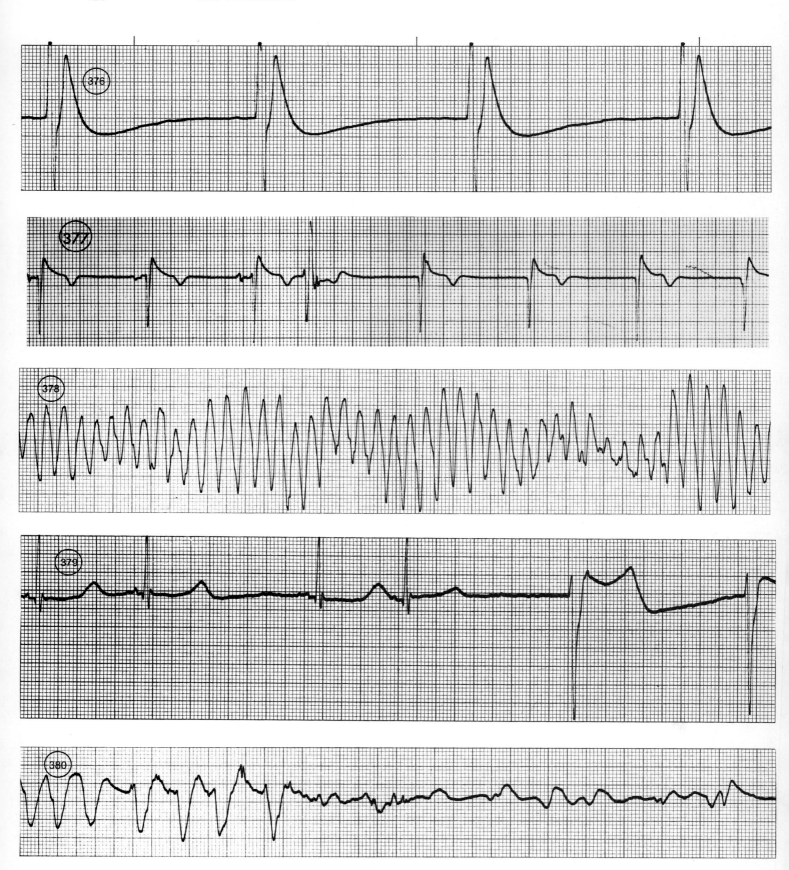

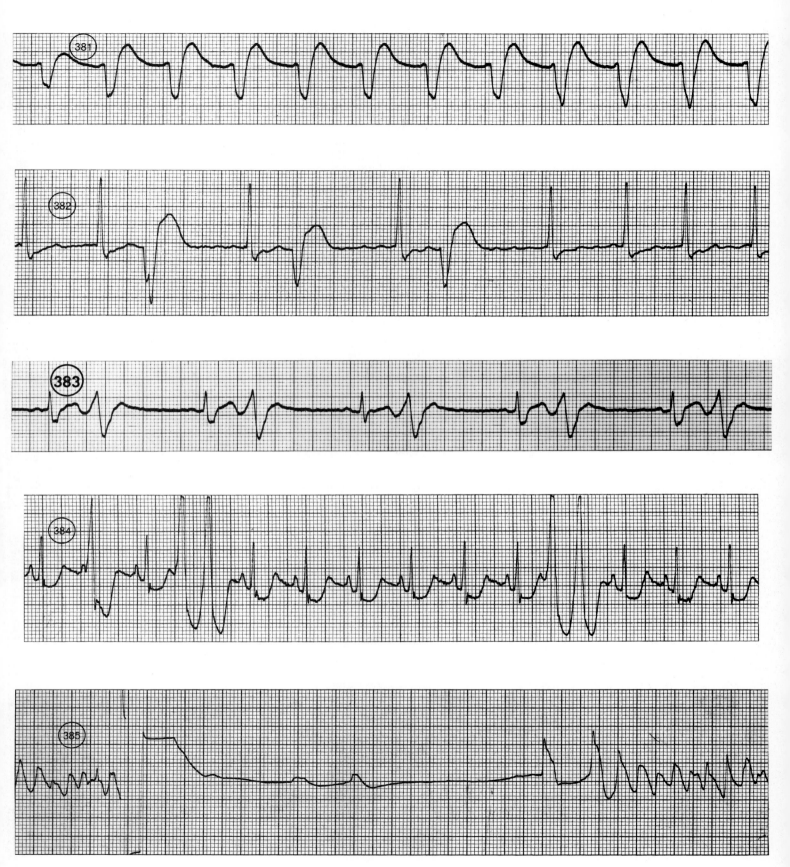

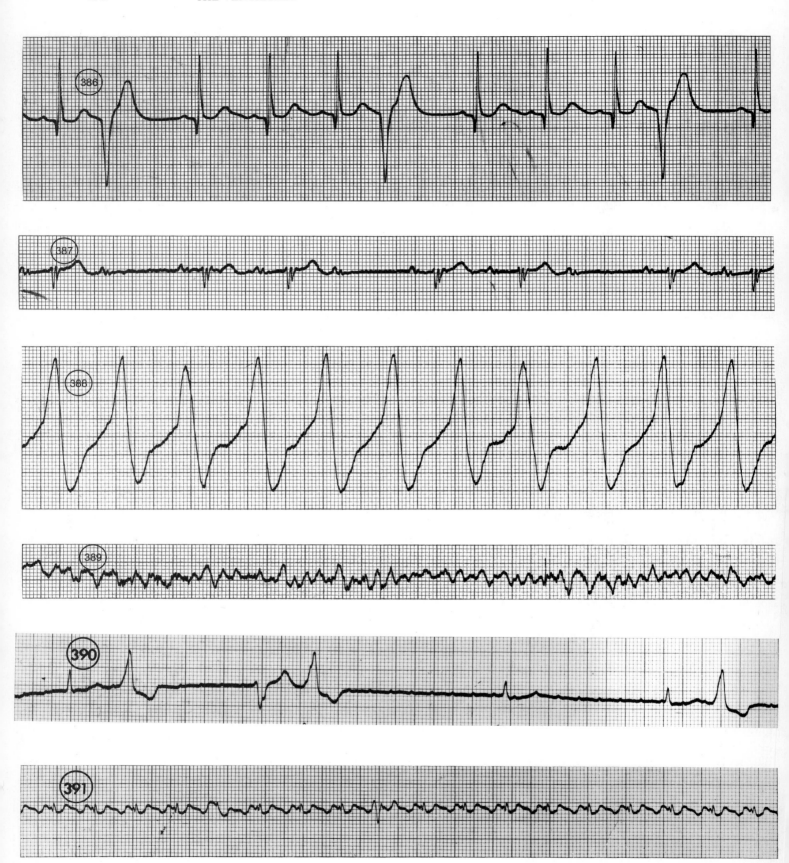

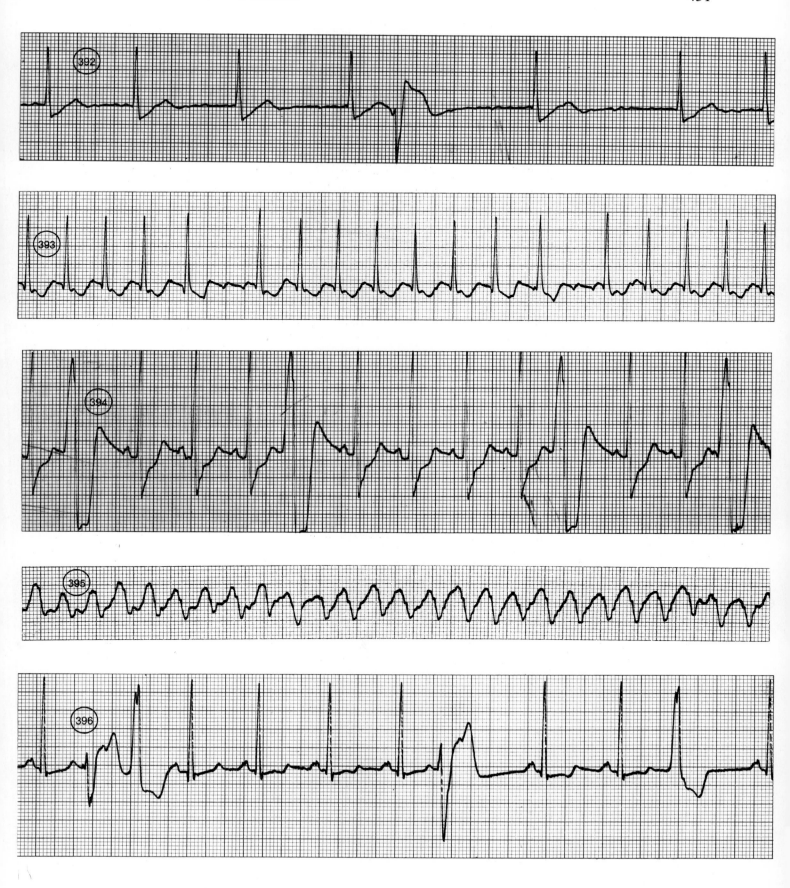

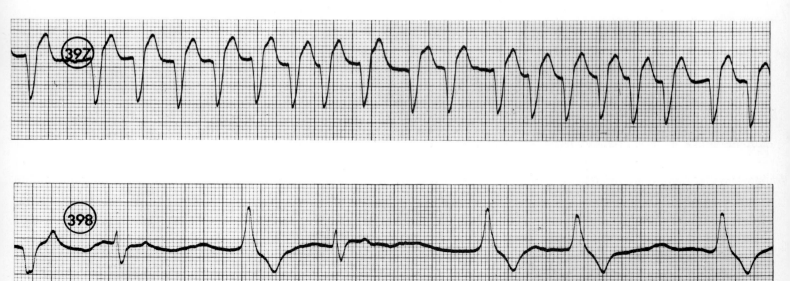

9 The Electronic Pacemaker

ELECTRONIC IMPULSE FORMATION
Excitation
ELECTRONIC PACEMAKER COMPONENTS
Energy Source
Conductor Lead
Electrode
ELECTRONIC PACEMAKER RHYTHM
METHODS OF APPLYING AN ELECTRONIC PACEMAKER
Transvenous Approach
Transthoracic Approach
External Approach
BRADYCARDIC INDICATIONS FOR THE ELECTRONIC PACEMAKER
Rhythms of Depressed Impulse Formation
Rhythms of Depressed Impulse Conduction
ASSESSING ELECTRONIC PACEMAKER CAPTURE
Pulse Generator
The Electrodes
Myocardial Response
ELECTRONIC PACEMAKER LEAD PATTERNS
THE ASYNCHRONOUS ELECTRONIC PACEMAKER
The Ventricular-Inhibited Electronic Pacemaker

ASSESSING ELECTRONIC PACEMAKER SENSING
Oversensing
Failure to Sense
Testing the Ventricular-Inhibited Pacemaker
THE ELECTRONIC PACEMAKER CODE
Chamber Paced
Chamber Sensed
Sensing Response
THE ATRIAL PACEMAKER
PHYSIOLOGICAL PACEMAKERS
The Atrial Synchronous Pacemaker
The Noncardiac Rate-Responsive Pacemaker
The Atrioventricular Sequential Pacemaker
The Universal Pacemaker
PACEMAKER-MEDIATED TACHYCARDIA
TACHYCARDIC INDICATIONS FOR THE ELECTRONIC PACEMAKER
The Atrial Overdrive Pacemaker
The Ventricular Overdrive Pacemaker
THE EXPANDED ELECTRONIC PACEMAKER CODE
AUTOMATIC IMPLANTABLE CARDIO-VERTER-DEFIBRILLATOR
SELF-EVALUATION: STAGE 4

Preceding chapters have presented the physiology of the heartbeat and the disorders of rhythm that result from abnormal formation and conduction of impulses. Attention is turned now to the use of electronic impulses provided to substitute for missing or blocked natural impulses, thereby protecting against excessive cardiac slowing. We will also see how the electronic pacemaker can be adapted to treat tachycardias by

433

interrupting their reentrant circuits. In the arrhythmia schematic and for labeling electrocardiograms (ECGs), we use a symbol representing a lightning bolt for the electronic impulse (Fig. 9–1). In fact, the brevity and the intensity of the impulse are appropriate in this analogy.

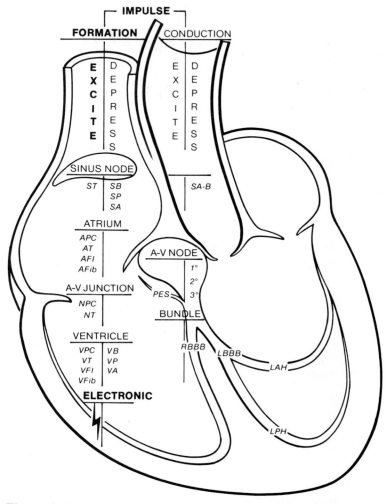

Figure 9–1. Electronic impulse formation. EPM = electronic pacemaker; ⚡ = symbol for electronic pacemaker impulse.

ELECTRONIC IMPULSE FORMATION

Excitation

Electrical impulses of small amperage are emitted at a rate set by an electronically controlled generator (or power unit). These impulses are conveyed along a connecting wire to an electrode that lies directly against the myocardial wall. The entire assemblage, known as an electronic pacemaker, represents one of the most revolutionary advances in modern cardiology.

Electronic impulses applied directly to the heart initiate a depolarizing wave front in the responsive myocardium. The wave front is propagated from the point of contact to the remaining portion of the cardiac chambers through contiguous myofibrils and specialized conducting fibers (Fig. 9–2) in the same manner that ectopic beats propagate from a single, natural focus of stimulation.

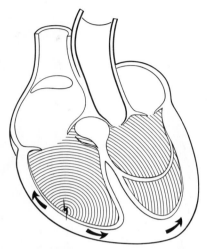

Figure 9–2. Wavefront propagation from an electronic pacemaker stimulus.

ELECTRONIC PACEMAKER COMPONENTS

To stimulate the myocardium, the electronic pacemaker must have the capability for both producing an electrical discharge and transmitting it to the heart. These functions are accomplished by a source of electrical energy and a conducting wire ending in an electrode tip.

Energy Source

The electronic pacemaker operates as a battery-powered unit. This power pack emits small electrical discharges at regular intervals and is therefore referred to as a pulse generator.

The **external** pulse generator is designed for temporary electronic pacing, primarily for initial support of critical bradycardias. As the name implies, the unit functions from outside the body and is usually connected to the heart by a conducting wire inserted through a venous channel. The unit is the size of a small transistor radio, and it operates by conventional dry-cell batteries. The external unit has dials for adjusting both power output and rate of discharges (Fig. 9–3).

Permanent pacemaker support requires the implanting of a pulse generator. Typically it is embedded through a small surgical incision in the subcutaneous tissue of the anterior chest wall just below the clavicle. The **internal** pulse generator is about the circumference of a stethoscope head. As with the external generator, it has the ability to be reprogrammed to alter its function.

Conductor Lead

Electrical transmission between the pulse generator and the heart is effected through a flexible metal wire having excellent electrical conducting properties. The wire or

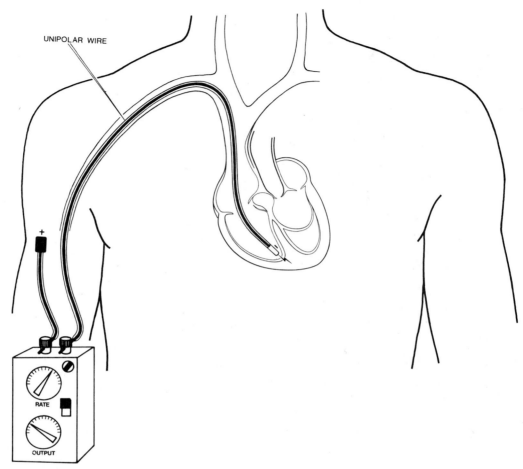

UNIPOLAR WIRE

RATE

OUTPUT

Figure 9–3. Endocardial electronic pacemaker with temporary external power pack.

leads must be electrically insulated (except at either end of the lead) so that the impulse is not dissipated into adjacent tissue.

Electrode

To stimulate the heart from a pulse generator, the impulse must be conveyed directly to the myocardial wall. The actual contact is made by a small electrode at the tip of the conducting wire as it emerges from the insulating layer. The electrode itself is broader than the wire (to protect against electrical injury to the myocardium from repeated stimulation and to lessen the risk of myocardial perforation). The venous electrode is constructed of exotic metals, usually platinum-iridium, which are not only highly conductive but also can be polished to such a fine degree as to deter the adhering of minute aggregates of platelets and other circulating particles. Wires inserted into the myocardium during surgery also have an insulated segment with exposed wire at the myocardial end as well as at the end available for attachment to the pulse generator.

Conducting wire-electrode systems may be either unipolar or bipolar. The **unipolar** design incorporates the cardiac electrode as the negative terminal of the electrical circuit with a second wire or the metallic shell of the implanted pulse generator serving as the positive electrode. In the **bipolar** system, there are actually two wires (some within the same insulating wrap), each ending in an electrode a short distance apart.

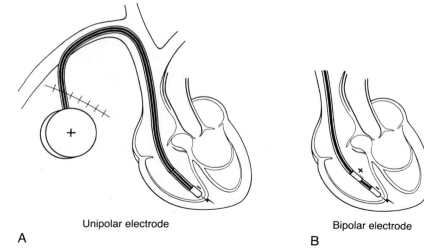

Figure 9-4. Depiction of unipolar (A) and bipolar (B) electrode systems.

The electrical circuit is completed by cardiac tissue and blood interposed between the two electrodes. These two systems are demonstrated in Figure 9-4.

ELECTRONIC PACEMAKER RHYTHM

The pulse generator emits an electrical signal that appears on the ECG as a sharp deflection with an extremely short duration and return to baseline. This inscription is purely an electrical phenomenon rather than electrophysiological (that is, a disturbance passing through living tissue). The artifact, which is too rapid to be mistaken for a physiological event, is commonly referred to as a **spike**. Electronic pacemaker spikes are identified at regular intervals in the rhythm strip in Figure 9-5.

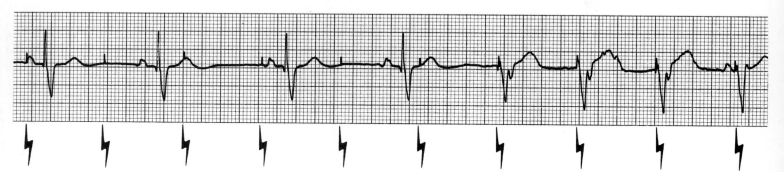

Figure 9-5. Electronic pacemaker spikes appearing at regular intervals.

To the left of the tracing, electronic pacemaker spikes appear in bold relief without any evidence of cardiac response (note spikes at regular intervals during sinus rhythm). Near the middle of the ECG, the electronic pacemaker spike is followed by a prominent deflection that represents the ventricular response. It is important to note that the depolarizing wave front begins *immediately* after the stimulating impulse. In addition, the resultant QRS complex is wide (usually greater than 0.14 second), caused by the relatively slow propagation of the wave front through contiguous myocardial fibers (similar to a spontaneous beat arising from the ventricles). An abnormal ST segment and T wave, of course, follow the wide QRS complex, representing altered repolarization after aberrant depolarization.

There follows a series of electronic pacemaker-QRS complexes, indicating that each electronic impulse stimulates the heart. The rate of this electronic rhythm is precisely regular (check with calipers), as is characteristic of basic pulse generator activity. On reviewing Figure 9–5, we have observed an electronic pacemaker rhythm that begins without any evident effect on the heart but later stimulates the ventricles consistently with each impulse. The early portion of the tracing familiarizes the reader with the visible electronic element; the latter portion combines it with the typical cardiac response. The pulse generator in this portion of the tracing is said to **capture** the ventricles.

The set of tracings in Figure 9–6 represents selected leads from a standard ECG and demonstrates an electronic pacemaker rhythm with complete ventricular capture. Each cardiac cycle is initiated by an electronic stimulus occurring at an exact rate of 74 per minute. Each pulse generator spike is seen as a sharp deflection, and the cardiac response follows it with no measurable delay. The amplitude and direction of the spike vary according to the lead in which the rhythm is recorded.

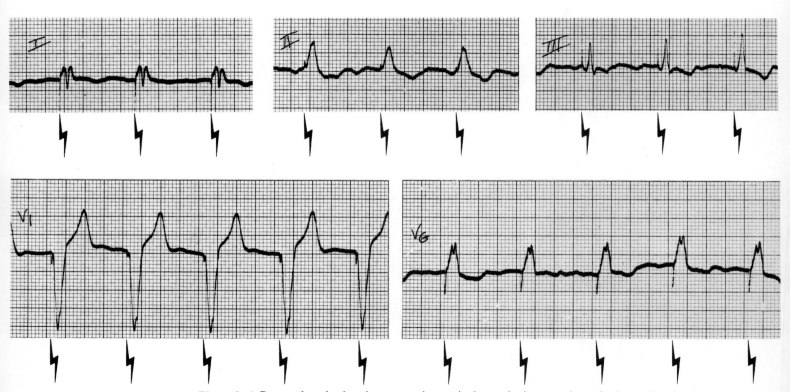

Figure 9–6. Pacemaker rhythm demonstrating typical ventricular complexes in the various leads.

This pacemaker is controlled by a pulse generator connected to a wire electrode inserted through a vein and passed into the apex of the right ventricle. The ensuing wave front moves upward from this point through the right ventricle, and it moves leftward, upward, and posteriorly through the left ventricular wall. Consequently, the direction of the QRS complex in each lead is predictable: Leads I, II, and V_6 are predominantly upright; lead V_1 is entirely downward. Lead III, having its positive electrode near the cardiac apex, has a QRS complex that is negative at first and strongly positive thereafter. Definitive P waves are not evident in any lead because the underlying supraventricular rhythm is atrial fibrillation.

Tracings 399 to 402 are examples of ventricular electronic pacemaker rhythms. Label each electronic artifact and observe the features of each cardiac response, the presence of a QRS complex and its duration, the ST segment T wave contours, and the basic supraventricular rhythm.

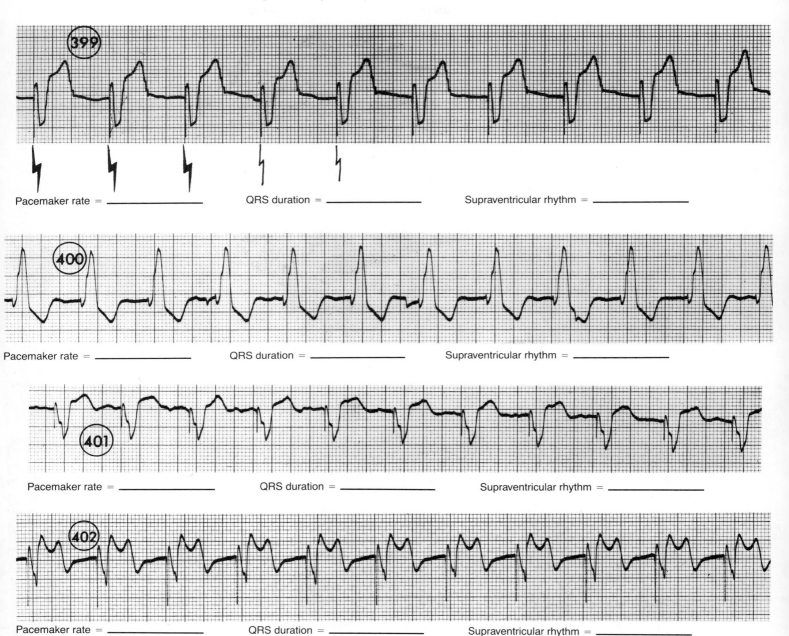

Pacemaker rate = _____   QRS duration = _____   Supraventricular rhythm = _____

Pacemaker rate = _____   QRS duration = _____   Supraventricular rhythm = _____

Pacemaker rate = _____   QRS duration = _____   Supraventricular rhythm = _____

Pacemaker rate = _____   QRS duration = _____   Supraventricular rhythm = _____

From the preceding exercises, it should be clear that the electronic ventricular pacemaker rhythm has the following electrocardiographic characteristics:

1. The rate has a clock-like regularity.

2. The electronic pacemaker deflection, or spike, is recognized by its extreme brevity.

3. The QRS complex begins immediately after the electronic pacemaker stimulus.

4. The QRS complex is markedly prolonged.

5. The QRS complex, the ST segment, and the T wave of electronically initiated ventricular beats exhibit the contours of anomalous wave front conduction.

6. The atrial rhythm, even if normal, may be entirely independent of the ventricular electronic pacemaker rhythm.

In the previous series of ECGs, every electronic pacemaker impulse has initiated a cardiac response. In each instance, we describe this relationship as **complete ventricular capture**. Electronic pacemakers may fail to capture the ventricle for one of a number of reasons, a subject for later discussion.

The next series of ECGs, tracings 403 to 405, again illustrate electronic pacemaker rhythms with complete ventricular capture. In each case, the electronic pacemaker was used to protect the heart against excessive slowing in complete A-V block. As you can expect in this arrhythmia, the artificial pacemaker stimulates the ventricles directly while the atrial rhythm continues independently without interference from the pulse generator system. In each of these examples, diagram the electronic pacemaker spike, determine its rate and rhythmicity, and interpret simultaneous supraventricular activity.

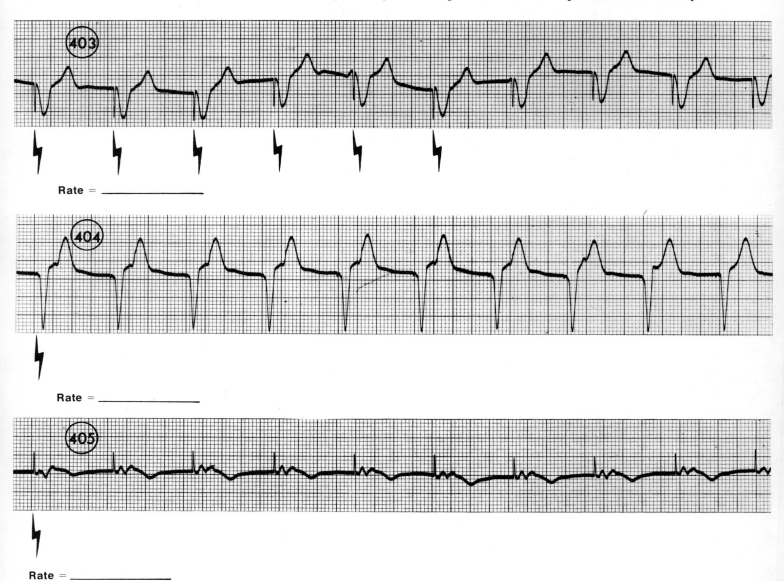

Rate = _____

Rate = _____

Rate = _____

Complete the symbols in tracings 404 and 405.

Because the electronic pacemaker is used to treat a variety of arrhythmias that involve depression of impulse formation and impulse conduction, attention should be given to the underlying arrhythmia in a descriptive interpretation. The next three tracings of ventricular pacemaker rhythms demonstrate variations in rhythm disturbance. In Figure 9–7, no atrial activity is visible. All cardiac activity appears directed by the artificial pacemaker. One can conclude that the natural rates of intrinsic pacemakers of the sinus node, atria, and the A-V junction are slower than the rate of the electronic pacemaker; in effect, atrial standstill is present.

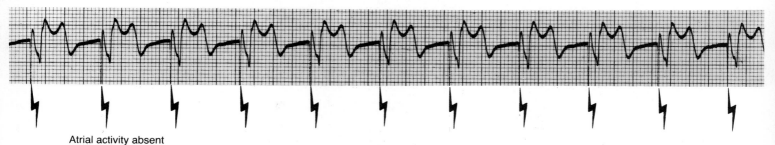

Atrial activity absent
Electronic pacemaker rhythm: Rate = 80

Figure 9–7. No atrial activity is discernible in this pacemaker-maintained rhythm.

In Figure 9–8, the pattern of atrial fibrillation is clearly evident. Nevertheless, the electronic pacemaker is initiating every heartbeat and at a regular rhythm, as in the previous tracing, and the ventricular complexes generated are singular in form. Here, one can conclude that A-V block prevents the atrial fibrillation impulses from entering the His-Purkinje system.

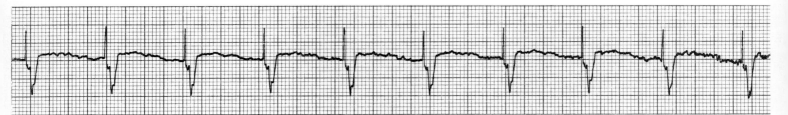

Figure 9–8. Electronic pacemaker-controlled ventricular rhythm at a rate of 71 beats per minute in the presence of atrial fibrillation.

In the example of complete A-V block in Figure 9–9, independent atrial and electronic pacemaker rhythms can be clearly discerned. Calipers are helpful in locating P waves.

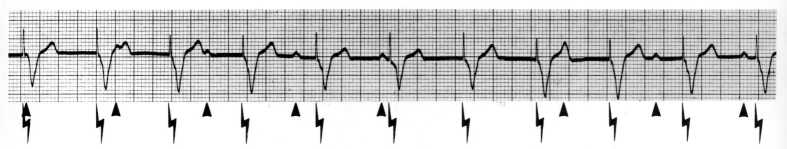

Figure 9–9. The ventricular rhythm is controlled by a regular electronic pacemaker stimulus. P waves do not result in normal QRS complexes even after delays as long as 0.56 second. An advanced degree of A-V block is present.

Mark the P waves and electronic pacemaker spikes in ECGs 406 and 407. What underlying arrhythmia is present?

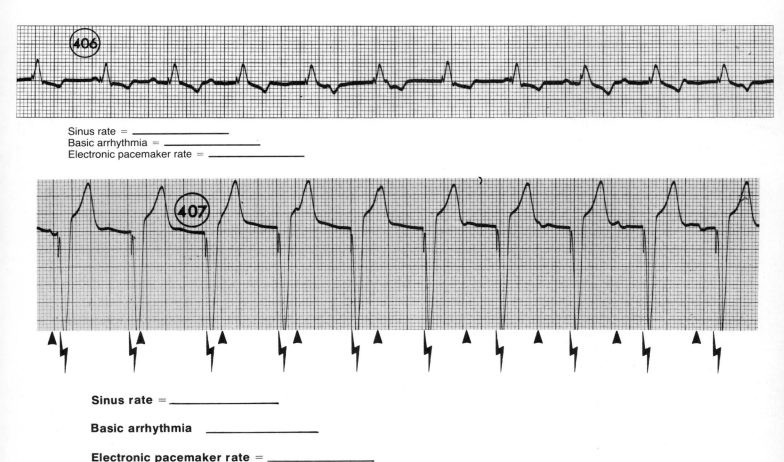

Sinus rate = _____
Basic arrhythmia = _____
Electronic pacemaker rate = _____

Sinus rate = _____

Basic arrhythmia _____

Electronic pacemaker rate = _____

METHODS OF APPLYING AN ELECTRONIC PACEMAKER

Transvenous Approach

The temporary electronic pacemaker previously described is inserted through a vein leading into the right cardiac chambers. This method is referred to as the transvenous approach (or **endocardial** system). Most electronic pacemakers installed for permanent use are also of this type. This approach is relatively nontraumatic and is easily performed under fluoroscopic observation. Once the wire-electrode system is in place, a permanent pulse generator can be inserted into a pocket underneath the skin, and the connecting wire then extends through a subcutaneous tunnel into the access vein. The entire system is thus completely internalized and protected against infection. Modern technology has miniaturized such implantable pulse generators to little larger than the head of a stethoscope (Fig. 9–10). Almost all permanent pacemakers are powered by lithium-iodide batteries, capable of functioning continuously for several years. For stabilizing electrode position, some connecting wires have **protuberances** (or **tines**) near the electrode, designed to lodge among the trabecular projections of the endocardial

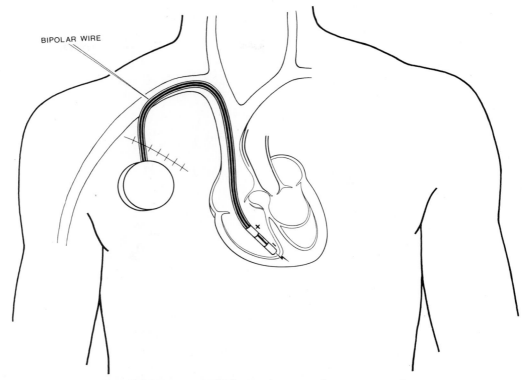

BIPOLAR WIRE

Figure 9–10. Endocardial (transvenous) electronic pacemaker, permanent.

wall. Other connecting wires incorporate an **active-fixation** feature in which the electrode can be screwed into the endocardial wall (Fig. 9–11).

Transthoracic Approach

By an alternative approach, the wire leads can be applied directly to the epicardial surface of the heart where the electrodes are sewn or screwed into the myocardial wall (Fig. 9–12). The pulse generator is also placed into a subcutaneous pocket. Although more secure than the transvenous, this **epicardial** system requires a thoracotomy. This

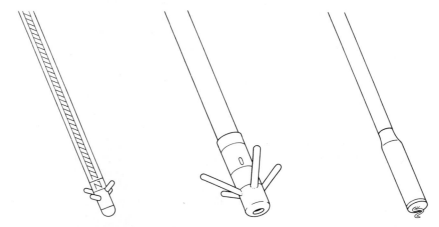

Figure 9–11. Endocardial electrode tips.

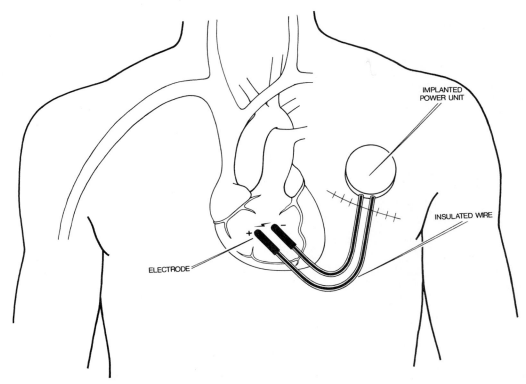

Figure 9–12. Epicardial electronic pacemaker.

method is the original technique used for inserting an electronic pacemaker, but it is seldom used now. The approach is indicated in those individuals in whom the risk of displacement of the endocardial electrode is predictably high. It can be used in individuals at increased risk for thromboembolism or with inadequate venous access. Transthoracic is also the approach of choice in most children.

Another form of the wire electrode is used for intervention in bradycardic emergencies. The system is packaged in a kit that includes an intracardiac needle for inserting the pacemaker electrode through the anterior thorax and a cable for attachment to an external power source. These intracardiac wires should be replaced as soon as possible, as their capability to stimulate cardiac response is often limited.

Specially developed wires can also be used as electrodes and are most often used for management of dysrhythmias experienced after open-heart surgery. These wires are supplied with a suture-type needle that is used to insert the wire through the cardiac tissue at the time of surgery. The wires then are brought through to the surface of the thorax, where they can be attached to a temporary power pack should the patient require pacemaker support.

External Approach

In extreme emergencies, electronic pacing may be applied entirely external to the chest. Bursts of electricity from surface electrodes are delivered with enough energy to propagate through the chest wall mass to the heart. The ECGs in Figure 9–13 were obtained from a 78-year-old man who experienced recurring syncopal attacks even with an implanted electronic pacemaker. Cardiac and respiratory arrest occurred suddenly during ambulance transport, and cardiac compression and ventilation were carried out. On arrival at the emergency department, the patient had no vital signs. The ECG revealed

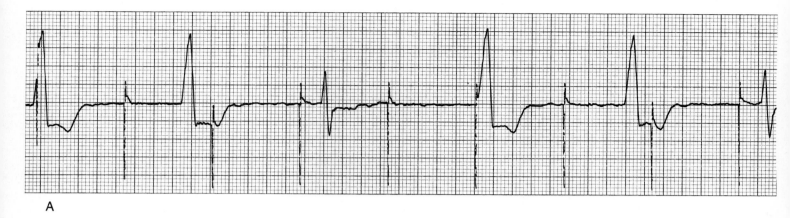

A

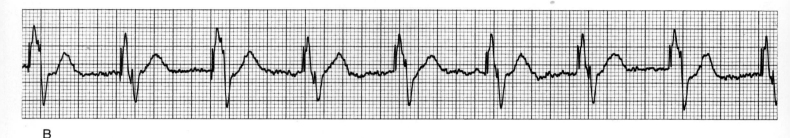

B

Figure 9–13. Failure of an implanted electronic pacemaker is treated in the emergency department with application of external electrodes and resultant electronic pacemaker rhythm.

idioventricular rhythm with two forms of complexes (strip A). It is evident that the electronic pacemaker is not stimulating the myocardium since spikes appear without QRS complexes. Treatment with bicarbonate, epinephrine, and continued cardiopulmonary resuscitation (CPR) produced no response. Thereafter, pacing was tried using anterior and posterior electrodes connected to an instrument having defibrillator/external electronic pacemaker capacities (strip B). Capture of the ventricles was immediately achieved, promptly followed by restoration of cardiac function and return of consciousness. Ultimately, a stable rhythm was obtained by repositioning the endocardial electrode of his permanent pacemaker.

BRADYCARDIC INDICATIONS FOR THE ELECTRONIC PACEMAKER

An electronic pacemaker serves to protect against symptomatic bradycardia from depressed impulse formation or conduction. An additional application of the electronic pacemaker is to terminate tachycardias by interrupting the reentrant mechanism (to be introduced later).

Rhythms of Depressed Impulse Formation

Patients who have excessively slow sinus rates (or sinus arrest) are subject to symptomatic bradycardia. This condition is often accompanied by dysfunction of the natural escape mechanisms, an inherent property of automatic fibers in the atria, the A-V junctional tissue, and the ventricles. Patients are thereby deprived of the normal back-up support system to protect the heart when the usually dominant pacemaker fails. In effect, an electronic pacemaker provides an artificial escape mechanism for these patients.

Figure 9–14 demonstrates severe sinus bradycardia with absence of natural escape beats. The electronic pacemaker controls the ventricular rhythm throughout.

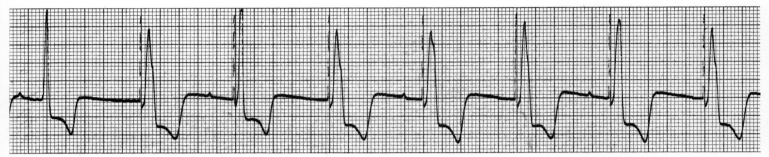

Figure 9–14. Severe sinus bradycardia (rate = 31) is the reason for insertion of this pacemaker.

Rhythms of Depressed Impulse Conduction

Severe impairment of impulse conduction through the A-V node makes the ventricles depend on escape automatic firing of fibers beyond the block. Such escape pacemakers in the distal A-V junctional tissue or in the ventricles are usually too slow (and often too erratic) to reliably support the circulatory demands for normal daily activity. The electronic pacemaker, stimulating the ventricles beyond the site of A-V block, safeguards the heart against symptomatic bradycardia and asystole. This application is shown in Figure 9–15.

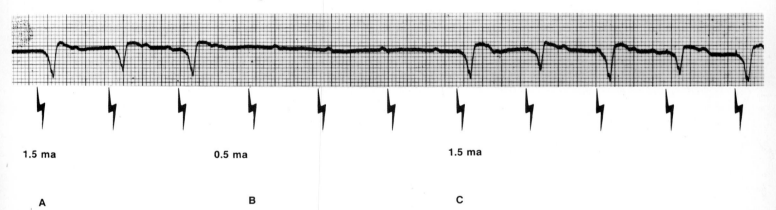

1.5 ma   0.5 ma   1.5 ma

A   B   C

Figure 9–15. The absence of ventricular conduction is observed when the electrical output from the ventricular pacemaker is reduced. At *A*, ventricular complexes are produced by an electronic pacemaker artifact. At *B*, loss of ventricular capture when the output from the generator is reduced exposes sinus rhythm with complete A-V block and ventricular arrest. On increasing the output, *C*, complete ventricular response is restored.

In Figure 9–16, sinus beats can be identified throughout without evidence of A-V conduction. The electronic pacemaker rhythm (producing QRS complexes) is regular, and all stimuli occur independently of the atrial rhythm. Thus, it functions with consistent ventricular capture in the presence of complete A-V block.

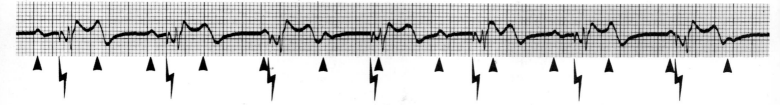

Figure 9–16. Sinus rhythm with complete A-V block; electronic pacemaker with complete ventricular capture.

Atrial flutter is recognized in Figure 9–17*A*, taken from a monitoring lead. There is no A-V conduction, as evidenced by variability of the relationship of atrial flutter waves and the QRS complexes (variable FR interval). In Figure 9–17*B*, the ventricles are stimulated by an electronic pacemaker at a rate of 71 beats per minute. The pacemaker was inserted as an urgent procedure when the patient developed complete A-V block with an idioventricular escape rate of only 20 to 30 beats per minute following administration of Inderal for severe hypertension.

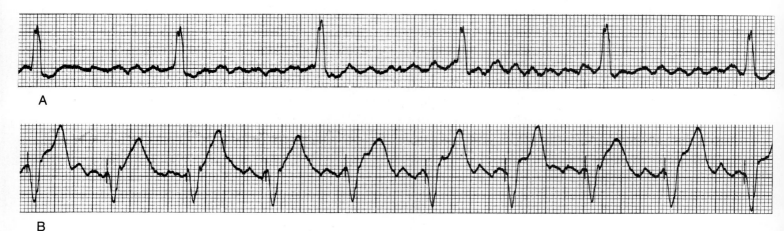

A

B

Figure 9–17. Pacemaker insertion to maintain a rhythm in the presence of depressed A-V conduction. Strip *A* shows the existence of atrial flutter with complete A-V block and ventricular activity at a rate of 40 beats per minute. Strip *B* was recorded in the same patient after insertion of a ventricular pacemaker.

Provide a complete descriptive interpretation of test tracings 408, 409, and 410. Include the electronic pacemaker and the underying atrial rhythm. Is A-V conduction present?

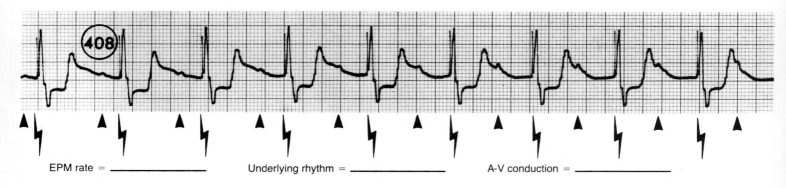

EPM rate = _____   Underlying rhythm = _____   A-V conduction = _____

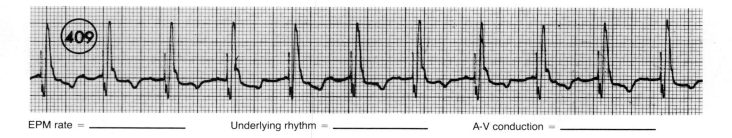

EPM rate = _____   Underlying rhythm = _____   A-V conduction = _____

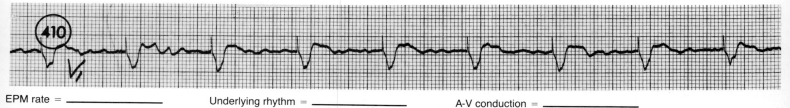

EPM rate = _____   Underlying rhythm = _____   A-V conduction = _____

ASSESSING ELECTRONIC PACEMAKER CAPTURE

Proper function of the electronic pacemaker depends on several distinct components: (1) sufficient energy output from the pulse generator with each impulse, (2) an intact wire-electrode system that completes an electrical circuit, and (3) responsiveness of the myocardium to the artificial stimulus. Failure of any one of these components results in loss of cardiac stimulation, termed **failure to capture**.

Pulse Generator

In test tracing 411, a temporary electronic pacemaker was inadvertently turned off. Interpret the rhythm before and after the event.

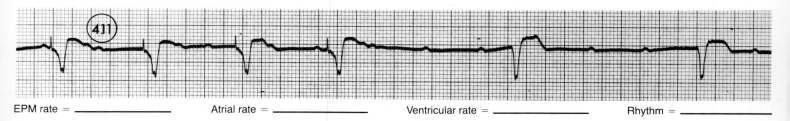

EPM rate = _____   Atrial rate = _____   Ventricular rate = _____   Rhythm = _____

Figure 9–18 demonstrates temporary electronic pacemaker failure in which the power output was deliberately reduced to below that required to provide ventricular

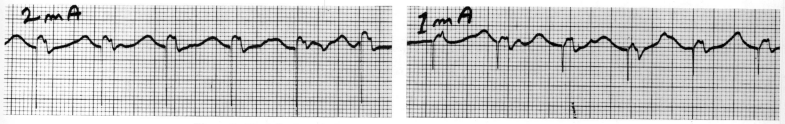

Figure 9–18. Adjustments in power output.

stimulation. This maneuver was performed to check the sensitivity of the pacemaker system and the placement of the electrode introduced through a subclavian vein. With the pulse generator set at an output of 1.0 milliampere, consistent ventricular stimulation is achieved. The tracing was recorded from the monitoring lead.

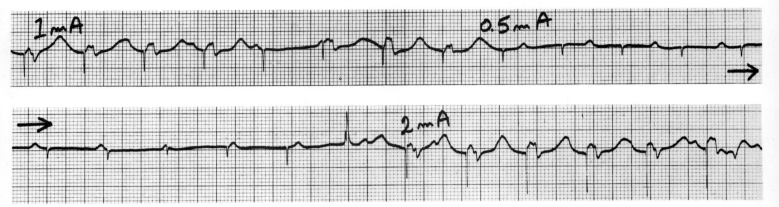

Figure 9–19. Loss of ventricular capture on reducing power output.

The setting is gradually reduced, and at 0.5 milliampere (Fig. 9–19) spikes are observed without QRS complexes following. P waves are present throughout the subsequent 6.8-second period of ventricular asystole, which is interrupted by a narrow QRS escape beat. This complex is probably of A-V junctional origin because it does not appear to be induced by an atrial beat. At this time, the power output is rapidly increased to 2.0 milliamperes and complete ventricular capture is restored. It is evident that a serious bradyarrhythmia would have resulted had the higher pulse generator output not been restored. Note that the electronic pacemaker spike varies in amplitude in proportion to the differences in energy emitted.

The term *milliampere* (mA), incidentally, is an expression of electrical power. The prefix *milli-* (one-thousandth) is used for convenience because of the relatively small amount of energy emitted by the electronic pacemaker.

Figure 9–20 was recorded 4 days after onset of an acute myocardial infarction. A temporary electronic pacemaker was introduced through the brachial vein to control severe bradycardia present on admission to the Coronary Care Unit. The tracing was made at the time the pulse generator was turned off to check the underlying rhythm, thereby assessing the need for a permanent pacemaker.

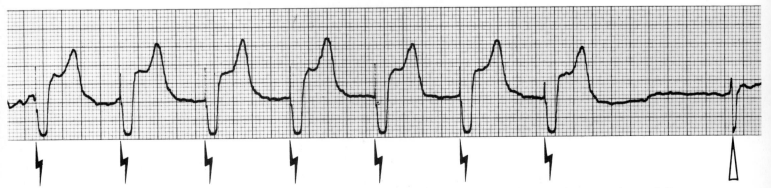

Figure 9–20. Identification of basic arrhythmia on cessation of electronic pacemaker activity.

After a pause of 2 seconds, a supraventricular beat occurs. During this pause, the pattern of atrial fibrillation is evident. The origin of the ventricular beat cannot be established in this tracing. It is a narrow QRS complex that could be conducted from the fibrillating atria or it could be an A-V junctional escape beat in the presence of complete A-V block. Continued recordings revealed QRS complexes of similar configuration and duration appearing irregularly at a rate averaging 60 per minute. This finding favored the diagnosis of atrial fibrillation with depressed (*but present*) ventricular conduction.

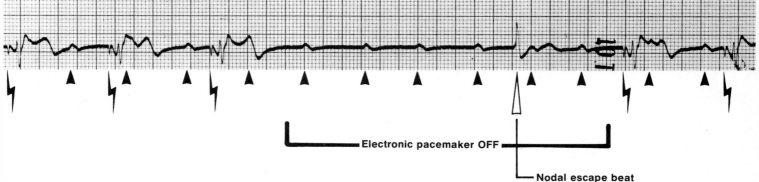

Electronic pacemaker OFF

Nodal escape beat

Figure 9–21. Sinus rhythm with complete A-V block; temporary cessation of pacemaker power.

At the beginning of Figure 9–21, an electronic pacemaker rhythm showing ventricular capture is evident. The temporary pacemaker unit was inserted to control the ventricular rhythm in complete A-V block. The pulse generator is turned off momentarily. Observe cessation of all electronic pacemaker spikes and ventricular activity until an A-V junctional escape beat appears after a 3-second asystolic period. Sinus activity continues without change. On turning the pulse generator back on, spikes reappear and ventricular capture is evident.

Failure of chamber capture with the intentional decrease in external pulse generator output to determine the threshold of myocardial sensitivity has already been studied (see Fig. 9–18). Eventually, even "permanent" electronic pacemakers lose the capacity to capture the ventricles as battery strength decays beyond a critical level. Battery life occasionally deteriorates prematurely. This problem is shown in the next example.

The ECG was obtained on routine monthly follow-up of an elderly patient who had long-standing complete A-V block and who was wholly dependent on electronic pacemaker support (Fig. 9–22). It was recorded from a telephone link using a sensing device placed over the patient's pulse generator. The signal was then transmitted to a central monitoring receiver. The pulse generator, powered by a lithium battery, was implanted one and a half years earlier.

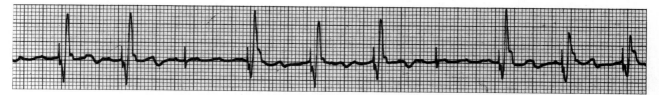

Figure 9–22. Intermittent ventricular capture by electronic pacemaker.

The basic rhythm is atrial flutter with complete A-V block and fixed-rate ventricular electronic pacing. Some electronic pulses produce a ventricular response; others do not. The patient was entirely asymptomatic. Prolonged observations revealed no instances when more than a single pulse failed to capture. Even so, this discovery led to prompt replacement of the pulse generator, which was connected to the original electrode wire. Complete capture was achieved with the new pacemaker. Ordinarily, a lithium battery provides adequate power for about 5 years.

Test tracing 412 reveals failing pacemaker capability in a permanent electronic pacemaker. Identify the noncapturing impulse, the electronic pacemaker and the basic cardiac rhythm.

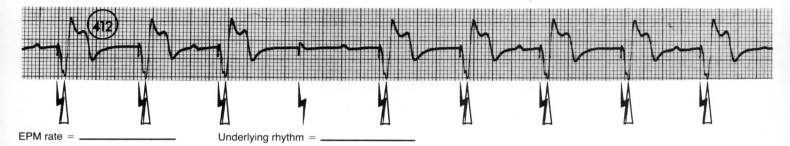

EPM rate = _____   Underlying rhythm = _____

Even the single missed stimulation, as demonstrated in the tracing above, is highly significant, because a reliable electronic pacemaker system performs its function of pacing with unbroken consistency. In this instance, this finding was the electrocardiographic evidence for excessive battery wear, and the implanted pulse generator was replaced before symptomatic bradycardia resulted.

A more advanced degree of power failure is exemplified in Figure 9–23. Here the paced beats evident at the beginning of the tracing suddenly stop while the electronic pacemaker spikes continue on without interruption. During this period, a sinus rhythm is evident but there is no conduction to (or response of) the ventricles, indicating complete A-V block. Finally, after a period of 5.6 seconds, a ventricular beat occurs. It is immediately preceded by an electronic pacemaker spike, and its configuration and duration are similar, *if not precisely identical,* to the earlier paced complexes. One could conclude that this beat represents a capture response (although it may be a fusion beat in which a portion of the QRS complex is produced by a simultaneous biological escape depolarization). There follows immediately afterward a noncapturing electronic pacemaker impulse and then a spontaneous beat with QRS configuration similar to that

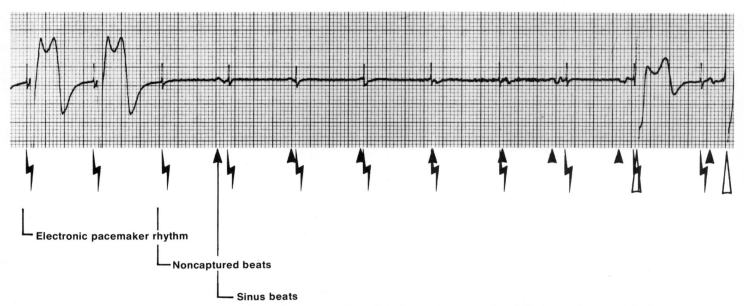

Electronic pacemaker rhythm

Noncaptured beats

Sinus beats

Figure 9–23. Asystole occurs when the electronic pacemaker fails to produce ventricular response for 5.6 seconds and the sinoatrial impulses fail to conduct to the ventricles.

of the previous ventricular beat, thus indicating an operative escape phenomenon. We conclude that this earlier beat is not the result of an electronic pacemaker stimulus.

The Electrodes

Connector leads are manufactured to withstand small degrees of flexion imposed by each heartbeat. Rarely, the wire fractures so that no impulse is conveyed from the pulse generator to the heart. This event results in complete absence of electrocardiographic spikes, and of course, the heart must revert to its natural rhythm. More commonly, the integrity of insulating material around the lead is compromised, and some of the electrical discharge is dissipated into the surrounding tissue. Total loss of electronic pacemaker function may occur with a defective insulating cover, simulating lead fracture. Alternatively, the signal may reach the electrode (producing a spike) but may be too weak to induce a response. The outcome, complete or intermittent failure to capture the ventricles, is similar to reduced power in the pulse generator itself.

Myocardial Response

Finally, the interface between the electrode of the connecting lead may impede conduction to the myocardium to such an extent that capture fails. Displacement of an endocardial lead tip is perhaps the most common cause. In addition, the tissue between the electrode and the myocardial wall may develop scar, thrombus, or infarction. Critically reduced sensitivity may also be caused by replacement of myofibrils by collagen, amyloid, or other infiltrating processes. Any of these problems may appear exactly as if energy discharge from the pulse generator itself is deficient and responsible for loss of cardiac stimulation.

To review, the presence of electronic impulses on the ECG without a resultant complex indicates that the entire pacemaker system is intact but that the magnitude of discharge to the myocardium is inadequate, whether it results from faulty pulse generator power, connector lead insulation defect, electrode placement, or myocardial responsiveness. A complete break of the connecting lead (or its attachment to either the pulse generator or the electrode tip) disrupts the entire system so that there is no evidence of spike on the ECG, and there is, of course, no capture of the cardiac chamber.

ELECTRONIC PACEMAKER LEAD PATTERNS

Transvenous pacing from the right ventricle produces a depolarizing waveform that spreads from the right to the left ventricle. Therefore, the waveform moves toward the positive pole of lead I, and the QRS complex is upright; it moves away from the positive electrode of lead V_1, and the QRS is downward, as shown in Figure 9–24.

Finding QRS complexes that are opposite to the expected direction (i.e., downward in lead I and upward in lead V_1) is in keeping with left ventricular pacing. This complication could occur with the transvenous pacemaker if the wire electrode penetrates deep into the coronary sinus or if it perforates the intraventricular septum. (Another explanation of a downward QRS complex in lead I is that the right arm/left arm leads have been interchanged.)

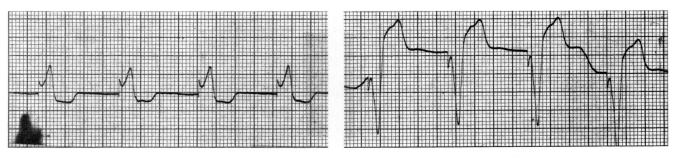

Lead I   Lead V₁

Figure 9–24. Typical patterns produced by an electronic pacemaker electrode located in the right ventricle.

THE ASYNCHRONOUS ELECTRONIC PACEMAKER

The properties of an electronic pacemaker system studied thus far are as follows:

1. It fires continuously at set intervals regardless of the spontaneous activity of the intrinsic cardiac pacemakers.

2. It fires at an absolutely unvarying rate as determined by a fixed setting.

From these examples, it is evident that the electronic pacemaker-stimulated ventricular rhythm functions independently of the inherent atrial rhythm as well as from ectopic beats originating in the ventricles. This, the most basic type of electronic pacemaker design, is known as the **fixed** or the **asynchronous** mode (referring to its lack of synchrony with the natural heartbeat).

This "single-minded" mode represents the earliest design of the electronic pacemakers, first used in humans in 1958. It is still a serviceable system for selected patients, specifically those with a natural heart rate less than about 60 beats per minute and without a tendency toward ectopic tachyarrhythmias. It is all the more fitting if the patient does not indulge in heavy physical activities (requiring a rapid heart rate) and does not have advanced myocardial insufficiency.

A disadvantage of the asynchronous electronic pacemaker is the potential for inducing tachycardia in the presence of additional impulse formation from spontaneous sources. For example, if ectopic ventricular beats occur or if the conduction system recovers from complete A-V block while an electronic pacemaker is operative, the ventricles respond to more than one pacemaker and a situation called **competitive**

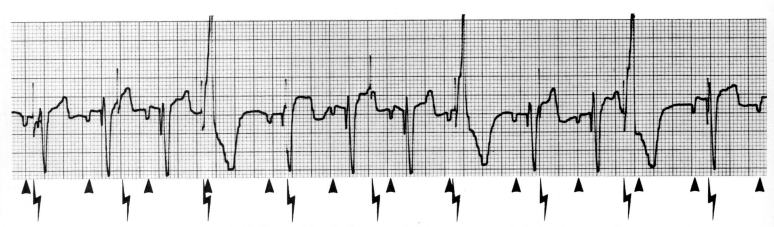

Figure 9–25. Competitive rhythm control between sinus and electronic pacemakers.

rhythms results. When such competition is sustained, serious tachyarrhythmias may result.

Note in strip 413 that an electronic pacemaker spike can be seen superimposed on the QRS of normally conducted beats. The electronic pacemaker continues to fire every 0.80 second despite the presence of sinus-initiated ventricular activity. Calculate the rate for the electronic pacemaker rhythm and the sinus node.

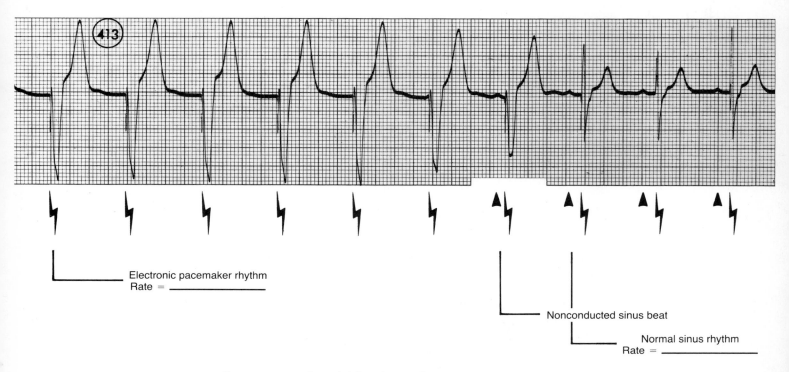

Electronic pacemaker rhythm
Rate = _____

Nonconducted sinus beat

Normal sinus rhythm
Rate = _____

Spontaneous sinus-initiated ventricular complexes in Figure 9–25 occur at a rate of 96 per minute. Despite this normal activity, the electronic pacemaker fires at a rate of 66 per minute. Note that the electronic pacemaker controls the fourth, eighth, and eleventh beats. If the P waves that occur simultaneously with the electronic pacemaker beats had been conducted, the heart rate would have been temporarily increased.

Figure 9–26 illustrates a failure of ventricular capture caused by faulty electrode position. The electronic pacemaker had been inserted during cardiac arrest, according to the Advanced Cardiac Life Support (ACLS) protocol of the American Heart Association. The initial portion of the tracing reveals electronic pacemaker spikes (without ventricular stimulation) occurring at a rate of 71 impulses per minute. Two spontaneous complexes that are independent of the electronic pacemaker rhythm and have a rate

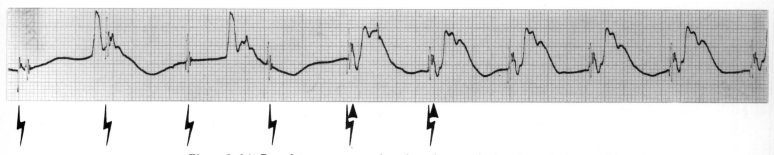

Figure 9–26. Complete capture results when the ventricular electrode is repositioned.

of 43 beats per minute then occur. During this period, the electronic pacemaker fires but fails to capture the ventricles. The transvenous wire electrode was readjusted, with resultant consistent stimulation of the ventricles, as seen in the last six cycles.

Although the asynchronous electronic pacemaker fires at the rate set with invariable consistency, the rate can be adjusted to best suit the needs of the individual patient. Of course, adjusting the external pulse generator in temporary pacemakers is easy. Also, in most models of implanted pacemakers, the rate can be easily adjusted using a radio-controlled device placed on the skin directly over the pulse generator. A set heart rate, although achieving adequate cardiac performance at rest, is sometimes too slow for ordinary activity. Elderly patients in particular, who have more limited myocardial reserve for exertional stress, are more dependent on acceleration of heart rate during physical effort. In patients with electronic pacemakers and slow fixed heart rates, increasing the rate (e.g., from 60 to 75) can improve cardiac output and thereby promote achievement of daily activities. Figure 9–27 illustrates this adjustment (from a rate in the 80s to a rate of 140 per minute) in a patient with complete A-V block and electronic pacemaker dependency.

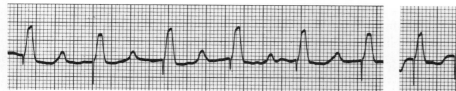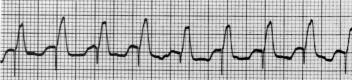

Electronic pacemaker rate = 83

EPM rate increased to 140 by manual control dial

Figure 9–27. Adjustment of rate.

Sometimes an electronic pacemaker is set to a faster rate to obliterate frequent premature beats. In this type of rate adjustment, the more rapid ventricular depolarization from the artificial pacemaker does not allow enough time for the development of ectopic beats from the ventricles.

Frequent ectopic beats, particularly those with a short coupling interval, may occur even with the faster settings of the pulse generator. In the asynchronous type of pacemaker, this activity may result in a very rapid heart rate, some beats from the electronic pacemaker and some from the automatic or reentrant focus (or foci). In sustained supraventricular or ventricular rhythms, the asynchronous pacemaker continues on, driving the heart even faster. An example of this situation is presented in Figure 9–28.

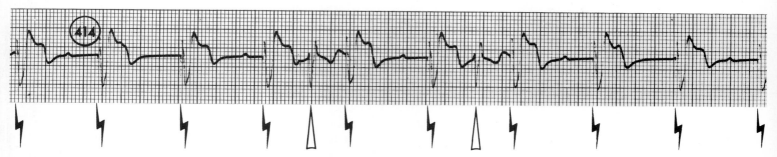

Lead V₁

Figure 9–28. Complete A-V block with an electronic pacemaker rhythm in the presence of spontaneous beats.

Complete A-V block is evident at the beginning of the tracing with an independent sinus rhythm. Spontaneous beats occur intermittently and momentarily double the cardiac rate. What is the origin of the spontaneous beats?

In addition to the resultant tachycardia from simultaneous electronic and intrinsic pacemakers, there is also the possibility of an artificial impulse firing just at the critical period of hyperexcitability in ventricular repolarization. Thus is created an R-on-T phenomenon with the potential for inducing sustained ventricular tachycardia as described in Chapter 8.

The liability of the asynchronous electronic pacemaker to produce tachycardias by combining electronic stimulation and normal beats has been overcome with the development of the inhibited mode pulse generator, which has the capability for stopping impulse emission when spontaneous beats occur.

The Ventricular-Inhibited Electronic Pacemaker

This next generation of electronic pacemakers incorporates a sensing wire-electrode lead. It picks up spontaneous electrical currents in the heart and conveys them to the pulse generator, thus informing the unit of every natural heartbeat. The pulse generator responds by shutting off its impulse emission; it then emits an impulse only after the lapse of a preset interval, as shown in Figure 9–29.

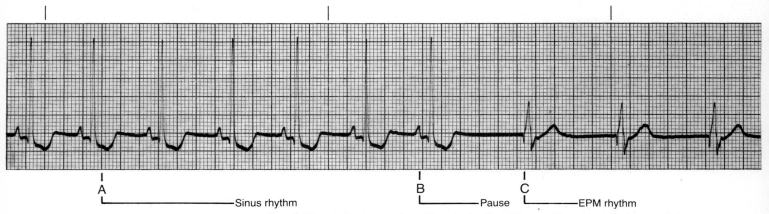

Figure 9–29. A sinus-initiated rhythm, *A*, is evident in the first 7 beats. Cessation of sinus activity, *B*, results in a 1.0-second period of asystole, which is terminated by the firing of the electronic pacemaker at *C*. The last three beats all exhibit characteristics of a ventricular pacemaker-induced complex.

Sustained inherent ventricular activity continuously inhibits the pulse generator output. On the other hand, the electronic pacemaker establishes a sustained rhythm at a constant rate if spontaneous beating remains suppressed. The interplay between spontaneous and **ventricular-inhibited** electronic-pacemaker rhythms is demonstrated in Figure 9–30.

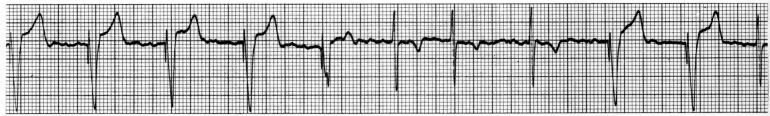

Figure 9–30. Cardiac control alternates between normal conduction from fibrillating atria and electronic pacemaker-produced activity.

In Figure 9–30, the basic rhythm is atrial fibrillation. The ventricular rhythm initially is electronically controlled at a rate of 73 beats per minute. A spontaneous irregular ventricular rhythm appears at a somewhat faster rate, presumably responding to impulses from the atria. However, after several beats, the inherent rhythm slows to a critical point at which the latent electronic pacemaker then takes over.

Figure 9–31 demonstrates how the electronic pacemaker serves as an artificial escape mechanism.

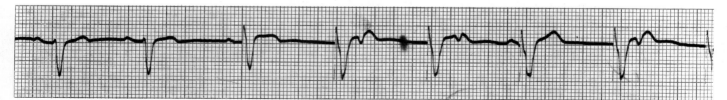

Figure 9–31. Slowing of the sinus rate to 57 beats per minute permits the electronic pacemaker to control the rhythm as an artificial escape mechanism.

The tracing begins with a sinus rhythm at the rate of 64 beats per minute. Slight slowing to 57 beats per minute occurs. However, before the atrial depolarization can be conducted to the ventricles, an electronic pulse that stimulates the ventricles appears. The electronic escape rhythm continues at the rate of 62 per minute. Thus, the inhibited electronic pacemaker becomes activated, preventing the heart from slowing beyond a set rate.

In another example of the escape pacemaker function (Fig. 9–32), the inhibited ventricular pacemaker turns on after every other sinus beat.

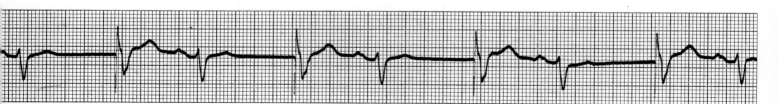

Figure 9–32. The artificial escape mechanism produced by the electronic pacemaker prevents the patient from having a critically slow sinus rate.

This electronic pacemaker bigeminy ensures that a rate no less than 58 beats per minute is maintained even in the presence of severe sinus bradycardia. Note that the escape interval (measured from the beginning of the conducted ventricular complex to the beginning of the electrical pulse) remains precisely constant at 1.02 seconds.

The capability of sensing an inherent beat and turning off the pulse generator discharge represents a great advantage over the fixed output of the original electronic pacemaker. In effect, this newer pacemaker acts as an artificial escape mechanism becoming operative on demand when the natural heart rate falls below a predetermined level. For this reason, it is referred to as the **demand mode** electronic pacemaker.

Appropriate function of an inhibited pacemaker includes two factors:

1. Capture of myocardial response when it fires.

2. Sensing of inherent activity, which results in inhibition of the electronic pacemaker firing mechanism.

ASSESSING ELECTRONIC PACEMAKER SENSING

In Figure 9–33, sinus rhythm is interrupted by a series of atrial premature complexes ending in a pause. This pause is terminated by an electronically stimulated beat acting as an escape pacemaker. Sinus rhythm is then resumed. Note that a P wave appears immediately before the electronic pacemaker spike, but it occurs too late to produce a ventricular complex.

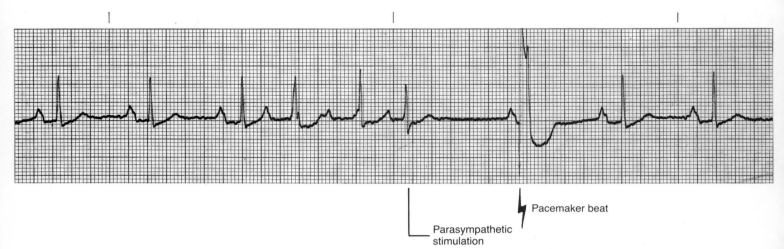

Parasympathetic stimulation

Pacemaker beat

Figure 9–33. Emergence of electronic pacemaker activity when the supraventricular firing rate is delayed after suppression of rapid atrial beats through parasympathetic stimulation.

The tracing in Figure 9–33 points out the standby pacemaker function of the ventricular-inhibited type. In this instance, it was prevented from firing by the more rapid (and thereby dominant) sinus node impulses. To test both the sensing function and the pacing function, slowing of the sinus rate was induced by carotid stimulation. Here, we have observed the intended purpose of the electronic pacemaker: to take over as pacemaker for the ventricles when the natural heart rate slows below a critical point. The maneuver demonstrated that the sensing device alerted the pulse generator of a delay in the natural rhythm. The pulse generator, in turn, fired a discharge at the proper interval, and that discharge resulted in the initiation of ventricular depolarization.

In another example of the ventricular-inhibited pacemaker, Figure 9–34 shows the interplay between natural and electronic pacing. After three normally conducted sinus beats, there is a pause of 1.00 second. This pause is terminated by a complex having

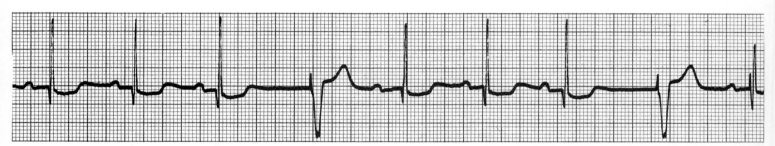

Figure 9–34. Proper function of a synchronous ventricular pacemaker. Initiation of pacemaker-induced beats is inhibited by the presence of normal sinus-ventricular complexes.

the pattern of ventricular origin. Thereafter, the sinus pacemaker regains control of the rhythm for three more cardiac cycles. Another pause of 1.00 second occurs and is interrupted by another ventricular complex. Note that both of these escape beats are preceded by a rapid deflection from baseline (a spike), identifying its electronic source. This electronic pacemaker has an intact sensing *and* pacing system that generates a stimulus when the patient's own sinus rate falls below a critical level, in this instance less than 60 beats per minute.

Another interaction between spontaneous and electronic pacemakers is illustrated in Figure 9–35. In lead V_1, an electronic pacemaker rhythm (A) is suddenly replaced by a sinus rhythm (B) in which ventricular depolarization is of the right bundle branch block pattern. Note that the rates of these two rhythms are very nearly the same. The sinus rhythm dominates until the sinus activity slows beyond a critical point (in this case, it slows to a very slight degree; measure the rates), and the electronic pacemaker once again activates its impulse formation mechanism. Measure the rate for the electronically produced rhythm.

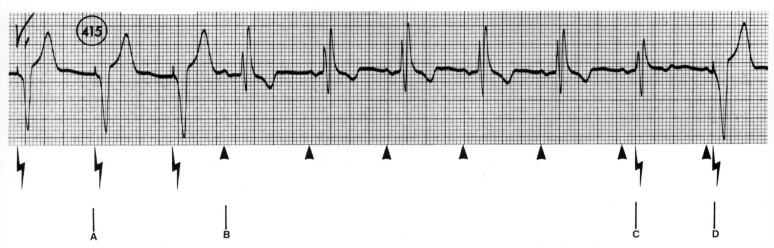

Figure 9–35. Spontaneous and electronic pacemaker rhythms as functions of rate. *A*, electronic pacemaker rhythm: Rate = _____. *B*, normal sinus rhythm with right bundle branch block. Carefully determine the rate of each cardiac cycle using the one-beat ruler. At *C*, an electronic pacemaker spike appears at the beginning of the QRS complex. However, the QRS form is similar to that of the sinus beats (right bundle branch block pattern). This is, therefore, also a sinus beat. The electronic impulse does not induce a response. At *D*, an electronic pacemaker spike with ventricular capture occurs.

Notice that an electronic pacemaker spike appears just before the next to last ventricular complex (*C*). However, the P wave preceding it and the right bundle branch block pattern of the QRS immediately following it identify this cardiac cycle as a sinus beat. Obviously, the electronic pacemaker stimulus did not result in a ventricular response. This finding does not represent a failure of capture of the electronic impulse because of a faulty pulse generator or a misplaced electrode. Rather, the spike was initiated after the ventricular conduction system had already been activated by the sinus beat, so that the ventricles could not respond to the electronic stimulus.

In tracing 416, an electronic pacemaker rhythm that is interrupted by frequent premature beats is evident. The recording is from the monitoring lead. The electronic pacemaker is a permanent ventricular-inhibited type inserted from the transvenous approach. What is the rate of the electronic pacemaker? Which ventricle is being paced electronically? From which ventricle do the premature beats probably arise? Does the sensor-pacer system exhibit normal turn-on and turn-off functions?

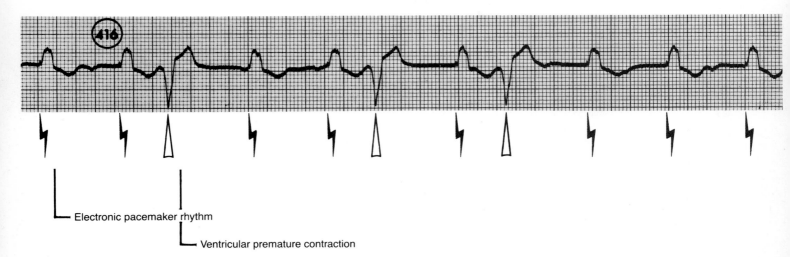

Electronic pacemaker rhythm

Ventricular premature contraction

The normal turn-on and turn-off function of the ventricular-inhibited electronic pacemaker is demonstrated in tracings 417 to 419. In each instance, the pacemaker had been inserted because of symptomatic bradycardia associated with sinus node dysfunction. Each ECG begins with the electronic pacemaker rhythm in which a dissociated sinus rhythm may be evident. As the sinus rate increases to above that of the electronic pacemaker, the sinus node impulse takes over ventricular pacing. At this point, the pulse generator lapses into the standby mode and electronic pacemaker spikes are no longer present. In each case, the sinus rate was accelerated by having the patient stand suddenly or perform mild exercise to check the electronic pacemaker sensing system.

In test tracings 417 to 419, identify the rate of the electronic pacemaker rhythm, the dissociated sinus rhythm (if present), and the character of the rhythm that takes over.

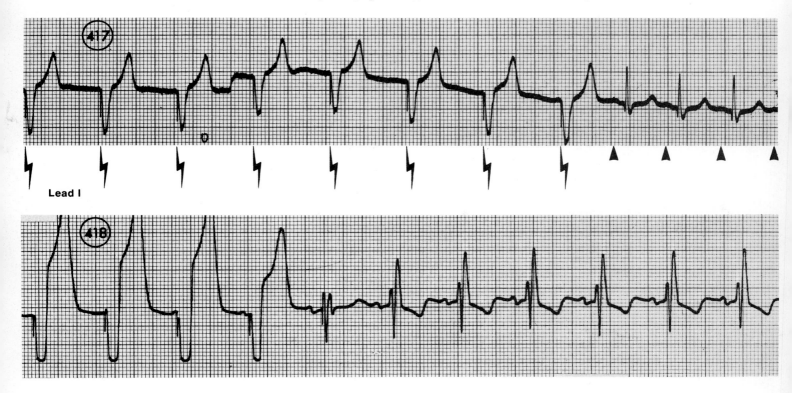

Lead I

Lead V₁

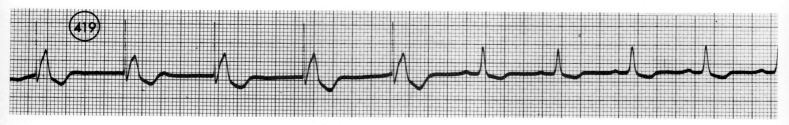

Monitoring lead

Note in the natural rhythms any features of the cardiac cycle that may be a clue to the identity of disorders affecting the impulse formation or impulse conduction systems.

Figure 9–36 begins with a sinus beat having a right bundle branch block pattern followed by an electronic pacemaker spike with ventricular capture and altered QRS complex and T wave. Then a normal sinus beat appears at a shorter interval than the previous sinus to electronic pacemaker interval, demonstrating a quickening of the sinus rate. The subsequent cycle also has a P wave and a similar QRS-T configuration. However, the QRS complex is preceded by a typical electronic pacemaker spike immediately at its onset. Here, one can assume that depolarization from the sinus impulse was too far advanced into the intraventricular conduction system for the electronic pacemaker discharge to produce an independent wave front. Two similar events are recorded later on in this tracing. This interaction between natural and artificial pacemaker results from the pulse generator being set at a very slightly slower rate than the predominant rate of the sinus pacemaker.

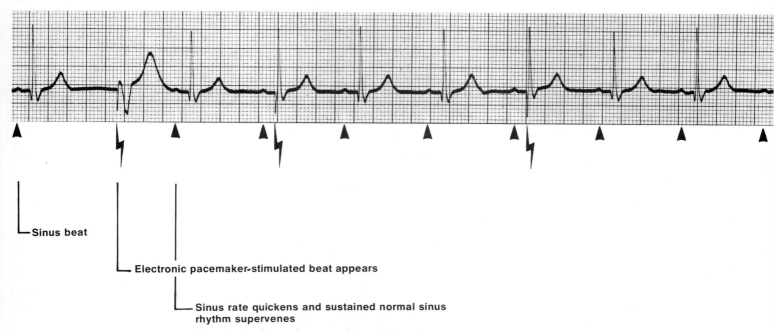

Sinus beat

Electronic pacemaker-stimulated beat appears

Sinus rate quickens and sustained normal sinus rhythm supervenes

Figure 9–36. Intermittent pacing activity of a ventricular inhibited electronic pacemaker.

An electronic pacemaker is sometimes adjusted to a faster rate to control frequent premature beats, as shown in Figure 9–37.

The upper tracing exhibits a sinus rhythm with complete A-V block, fixed-rate electronic pacing of the ventricles at 72 per minute, and multiform ventricular premature beats. The latter momentarily delay the electronic pacemaker, indicating that a sensor-inhibition system is present and functioning properly. Standard drugs for control of the ectopic beats were tried, but the patient tolerated them very poorly.

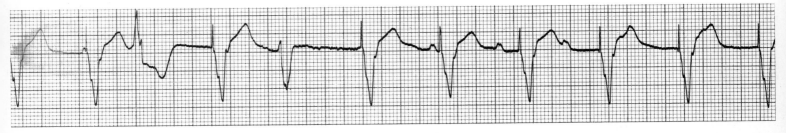

A

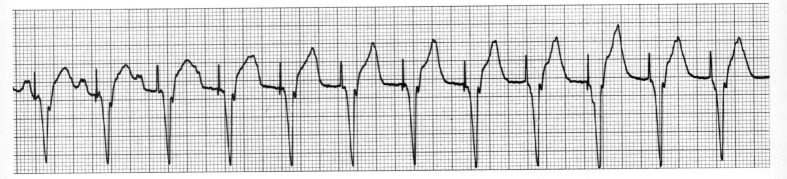

B

Figure 9–37. In strip *A*, the patient experiences ventricular ectopics when the electronic pacemaker is set at a rate of 70 beats per minute. Strip *B* illustrates elimination of ectopics by increasing the rate of the electronic pacemaker to 93 per minute.

The lower tracing reveals more rapid pacing at 93 per minute. Ventricular ectopic beats are no longer present. Presumably, the faster rate does not allow enough time for spontaneous generation of impulses from the ventricles. With this trial, a decision was made to keep the pacemaker at a more rapid rate.

Fusion beats—that is, complexes from two stimuli—are commonly observed in ventricular electronic pacemaker rhythms in the presence of a supraventricular rhythm with a functioning A-V node. The first three complexes of Figure 9–38 are formed by electronic stimuli. A nonstimulating P wave occurs before each of these complexes. Because the sinus rhythm is slightly faster than the electronic, the P wave emerges progressively sooner in each subsequent beat, eventually stimulating a portion of ven-

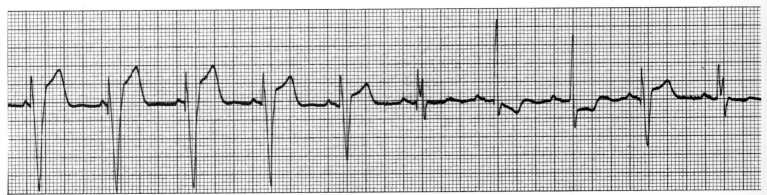

Figure 9–38. Note the fusion beats that occur during transition in ventricular control from supraventricular to electronic pacemaker impulse formation.

tricular depolarization. The eighth complex appears to be entirely of sinus origin, and preceding complexes represent transitional configurations of combined, or fused, sinus and electronic depolarization.

The marked depression of the ST segment was present in the admitting ECG before a temporary electronic pacemaker was inserted for protection against symptomatic sinus node dysfunction. Wholly electronically paced beats exhibit a markedly elevated ST segment. With the ninth beat, the sinus node rate slows slightly, and electronic pacemaker spikes begin to influence depolarization of the ventricles once again, resulting in more fusion beats.

Additional examples of fusion beats are presented to further illustrate this common phenomenon. Figure 9–39 begins with a normal sinus rhythm at a rate of 75 beats per minute. A minimal slowing of the sinus node rate starts with the fourth beat. This cycle exhibits a change in QRS configuration with an abrupt upward deviation and a slightly altered ST segment. With subsequent beats, the cause of these changes becomes more obvious as the rhythm converts to complete control by a ventricular pacemaker. The gradual change in configuration coincides with the gradual slowing in sinus rate, allowing more and more influence of the electronic pacemaker on the complex appearance until the final complex is under total control of the electronic pacemaker.

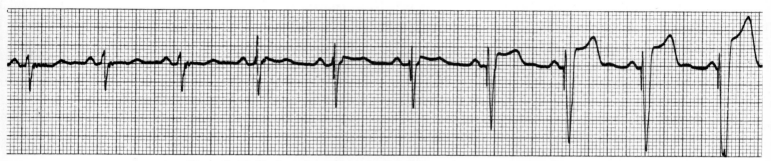

Figure 9–39. Fusion of supraventricular and ventricular initiated complexes occurs during transition from one controlling rhythm to another.

Figure 9–40 begins with a sinus rhythm with a prolonged PR interval. The reason for insertion of a pacemaker becomes evident following the third complex, when a P wave occurs without resulting ventricular activity. At this point, a QRS of ventricular origin occurs, preceded by a pacemaker spike. The seventh complex, which has a QRS with a supraventricular configuration, has a spike superimposed on the QRS. The pacemaker sensing system had already initiated an impulse, and simultaneously normal conduction occurred. This is not failure to sense, but rather coincidental firing of both the biological and electronic pacemakers, resulting in a fusion beat.

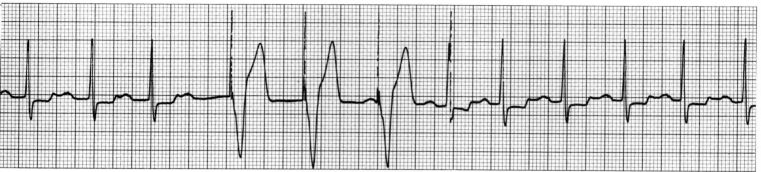

Figure 9–40. Normal sensing function despite superimposition of a pacemaker spike on a normal QRS complex.

The following examples depict normal turn-off function of the ventricular-inhibited pacemaker in response to ectopic beats. Figure 9–41 begins with typical electronic pacemaker spikes and subsequent wide QRS complexes at a rate of 72 per minute with 0.82-second intervals between each beat. The rhythm is interrupted by a premature beat, with a somewhat narrower complex. Immediately thereafter, the expected electronic pacemaker spike does not appear on time (check for 0.82-second interval). However, a spike does appear with an interval of 1.30 seconds from the preceding pacemaker beat, but 0.84 second from the ectopic beat. From this point on, the electronic pacemaker rhythm resumes its pacing function at the original rate with interruption by a second ventricular premature complex (VPC). Thus is shown properly functioning electronic pacing with intact sensing of ectopic beats resulting in a momentary cessation of pacing.

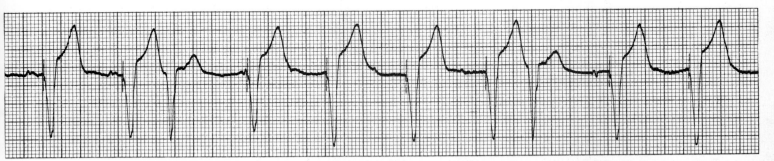

Figure 9–41. Appropriate inhibition of pacemaker activity when ventricular ectopic beats occur.

Clinicians often attempt to estimate the percentage of time during which the electronic pacemaker is operative. Strips presented here are actually too short to be representative. In this tracing (Fig. 9–41), it would appear that the electronic pacemaker is controlling the rhythm about 80% of the time.

A sinus beat begins the tracing in Figure 9–42, but a superimposed electronic pacemaker spike initiates a portion of the QRS depolarization. The electronic pacemaker rate is slightly faster than the sinus rate, so that subsequent fused beats become progressively more controlled by the electronic stimulus. The fourth and fifth complexes are entirely of electronic pacemaker origin. A VPC that inhibits electronic impulses then appears, and the sinus rhythm with ventricular control returns. An electronic stimulus can be seen in the QRS complex of the ninth beat, but it occurs too late to produce any response.

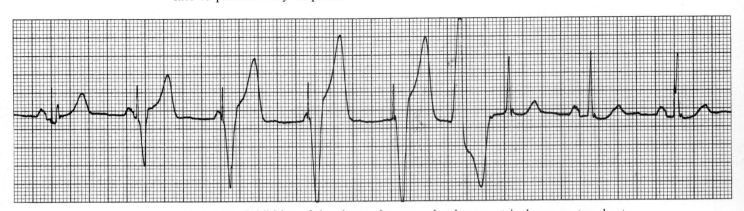

Figure 9–42. Inhibition of the electronic pacemaker by a ventricular premature beat.

A sinus delay following the second beat allows emergence of an impulse from the electronic pacemaker, and ventricular capture is evident (Fig. 9–43). Immediately

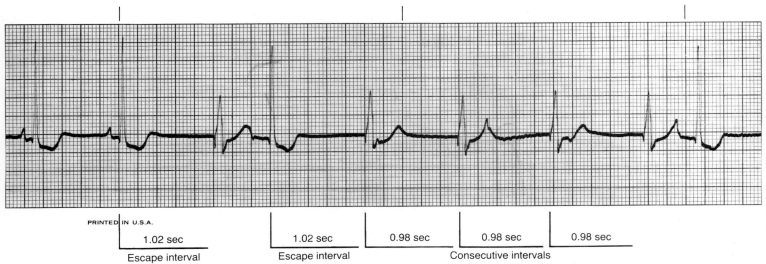

1.02 sec   1.02 sec   0.98 sec   0.98 sec   0.98 sec

Escape interval   Escape interval   Consecutive intervals

Figure 9–43. Inhibition of ventricular pacemaker by atrial premature activity.

thereafter there appears an atrial premature complex (APC) that momentarily inhibits the electronic pacemaker rhythm, measured at 62 beats per minute in the subsequent four beats.

Note that the interval from both the sinus beat and the APCs to the subsequent electronic pacemaker beats is longer than that between consecutive electronic pacemaker beats. This delay in the electronic pacemaker **escape interval** is a feature of some pacemakers and is known as **hysteresis.** The delay has been designed to prevent the demand electronic pacemaker from kicking in too early when the rate of the intrinsic rhythm slows naturally (as during sleep) while maintaining its capacity to beat at a more rapid rate when needed. In practical terms, hysteresis is advantageous only when a sinus rhythm is dominant or intermittent. A disadvantage of this feature is that it leads some interpreters to assume that the pulse generator is faulty. Thus, fewer electronic pacemakers are currently manufactured with the feature of hysteresis.

Oversensing

Extraneous events in the cardiac cycle or external stimuli may result in an unintended pacemaker turn-off referred to as **oversensing.** Oversensing occurs when the sensitivity of the inhibitor mechanism is set high enough to respond to incidental electrical phenomena. In addition to its normal inhibition when cardiac depolarizations are sensed, the electronic pacemaker may become quiescent in the presence of electronical activity of other cardiac events, as demonstrated in Figure 9–44.

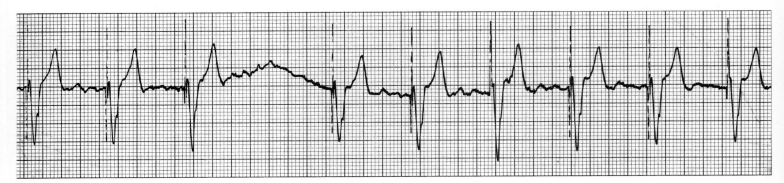

Figure 9–44. Inhibition of a ventricular demand pacemaker by movement of the baseline.

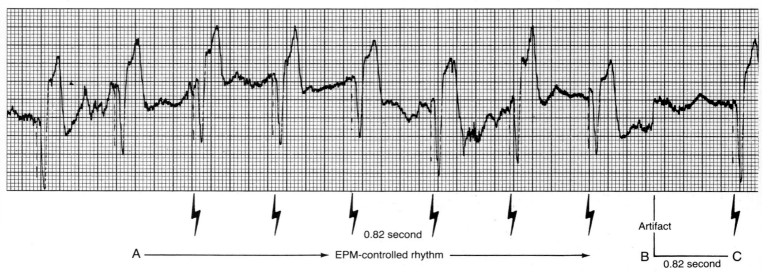

Figure 9–45. Electrical interference is obvious throughout the electronic pacemaker-controlled rhythm at the beginning of the strip, at *A*. The artifact at *B* is of sufficient amplitude to be sensed by the pacemaker, and the pacemaker is inhibited. At point *C*, a spike occurs at 0.82 second after the interference, indicating that the pacemaker timing interval was reset by the artifact.

A ventricular-inhibited pacemaker is observed pacing at a fixed rate with complete ventricular capture. The presence of atrial fibrillation without evident ventricular response indicates complete A-V block. A pause during which there is no spontaneous beat or electronic pulse occurs. It is likely that the wandering baseline produced enough of an electrical disturbance to be interpreted by the pulse generator's sensor as a spontaneous ventricular depolarization. The generator then follows a nondiscriminating response of inhibiting the pacing mechanism. After an interval of 1.48 seconds, pacing resumes at the previously established rate. This false sensing was corrected by using an external programmer to reduce the sensitivity of the unit. Of course, this change in sensitivity of the generator increases the risk of failure to detect ectopic ventricular activity.

Output of the demand mode electronic pacemaker can also be inhibited by extra-cardiac stimuli. For example, strenous physical exercise may place the demand electronic pacemaker into the quiescent mode. Generalized seizures or tremors, such as in severe Parkinson's disease, may produce strong enough myopotentials to shut off electronic pacing, even producing prolonged asystole in patients who are totally electronic pacemaker-dependent. Figure 9–45 illustrates such an event.

Electronic pacemaker inhibition from ordinary activity of skeletal muscle can gen-

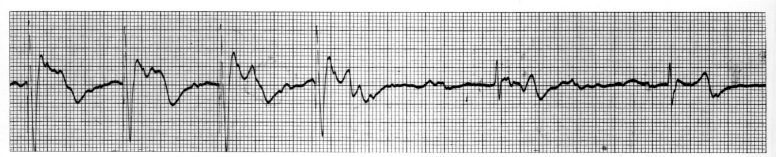

Figure 9–46. An escape rhythm (rate = 33) was exhibited in an airport employee when his ventricular pacemaker was turned off by equipment in the environment.

erally be ameliorated by adjusting the sensitivity of the pulse generator to increase the threshold for extraneous myopotentials.

Strong electromagnetic forces in the environment can result in demand pacemaker turn-off. This effect was discovered in a pacemaker-dependent airport worker who incurred repetitive episodes of syncope until it was realized that the episodes coincided with the rotations of a nearby powerful radar emitter (Fig. 9–46). Similar effects are produced by emissions from close contact with electrical generators, vehicular engines, and microwave ovens. Properly cautioned, patients need not fear interference from common household and workplace appliances.

The preceding strips have presented the complication of oversensing. Before continuing on to the opposite problem of failure to sense, the normal relationship of intrinsic and electronic pacemaker rhythms is again reviewed.

The interaction of a demand electronic pacemaker and intrinsic supraventricular rhythms is shown in Figure 9–47. The patient was a 63-year-old fisherman with a history of losing consciousness on several occasions, placing him in great jeopardy. Evidence of sinus node dysfunction was demonstrated by carotid stimulation and other parasympathetic stimulating maneuvers. The cardiac examination and ECG were otherwise unrevealing of any disorder. A ventricular-inhibited electronic pacemaker was implanted transvenously, and no further syncopal episodes occurred. Its protective function can be appreciated following the ectopic beat recorded here.

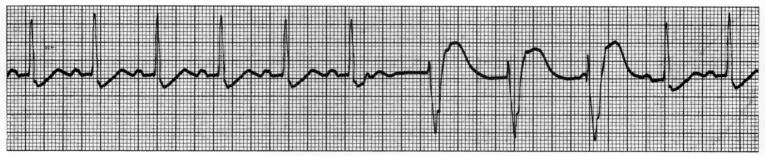

Figure 9–47. Ventricular pacemaker activity assumes control for three beats following a blocked premature atrial beat.

A premature atrial beat occurs and is blocked within the A-V conduction system (P wave with no ensuing QRS complex). After a pause of 0.84 second (hysteresis delay), the electronic pacemaker discharges for three consecutive beats at the preset rate of 72. Thereafter, the sinus node recovers from the shock of the atrial premature beat and resumes its usual control of the rhythm. Note that the sinus node pacemaker rate is more rapid than the electronic pacemaker.

Failure to Sense

As with failure to capture, presented earlier, **failure to sense** is a serious situation requiring immediate intervention. The following strips are used to illustrate lack of sensing and the resulting complications. In Figure 9–48, the electronic pacemaker spike occurs despite the presence of VPCs. The spike can be seen during the ST segment of the first ectopic beat and near the peak of the T in the second VPC. A review of the R-on-T phenomenon producing ventricular tachycardia as presented in Chapter 8 will identify the concern of this spike falling on the T wave.

Figure 9–49 shows the production of a short run of ventricular tachycardia resulting from the R-on-T phenomenon. In reviewing the strip, the electronic pacemaker spike can be seen superimposed on the first QRS, and it gradually moves farther behind the intrinsic QRS until it provokes ventricular tachycardia when it hits the vulnerable period

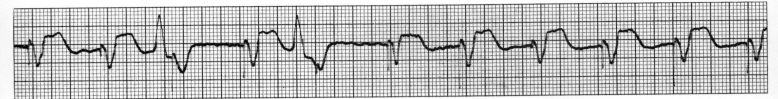

Figure 9–48. Spikes on the T wave indicate failure of the electronic pacemaker to sense inherent cardiac activity.

of the fifth cycle. At the end of the strip, an electronic pacemaker-controlled rhythm at a rate of 72 can be seen. This is the same rate for the electronic pacemaker activity throughout the strip, but in the initial segment the rhythm was controlled by the intrinsic pacemaker, which was firing at a rate of 75.

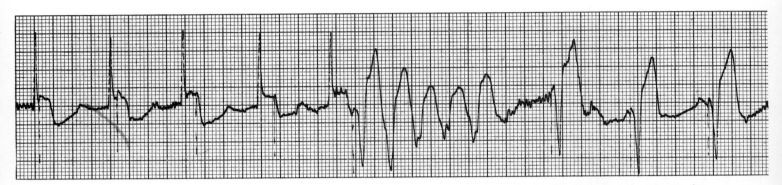

Figure 9–49. A short run of ventricular tachycardia occurs as the result of a nonsensing electronic pacemaker firing during the T wave of a normal cardiac cycle.

Testing the Ventricular-Inhibited Pacemaker

When a ventricular-inhibited electronic pacemaker is in place but a sustained spontaneous rhythm at a faster rate causes continuous suppression of electronic pacemaker firing, examination at the bedside or by ECG reveals no evidence of its proper sensing and pacing function. However, there are two simple methods to determine if both are operable. One method is to slow the intrinsic heart rate to less than that preset in the pulse generator. Sufficient slowing is often produced by deep breath holding, the Valsalva maneuver, or carotid pressure, as shown in Figure 9–50.

The sinus rhythm of 76 beats per minute slows abruptly with vagal stimulation from breath holding, and after an interval of 0.90 second, the electronic pacemaker begins firing at the rate of 60 beats per minute. Capture of the ventricles is evident with each discharge. On release of breath holding, the sinus rate accelerates and overtakes the electronic pacemaker rate. At this point, the electronic firing ceases altogether. This sequence confirms that the sensing mechanism and the pacing (firing and capturing) system of the electronic pacemaker are intact. Note the transition of rhythms designated by the arrow. Which pacemaker is driving the ventricles in this instance?

Another example of testing the demand electronic pacemaker sensing and firing systems during inhibition is presented in Figure 9–51. The initial rhythm is not easily discerned, but it is most likely atrial flutter (rather than atrial fibrillation) because of the regular ventricular rate. Marked prolongation of QRS duration is also noted. A

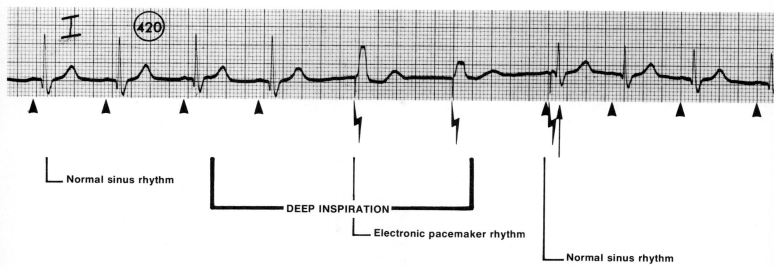

Figure 9–50. Appearance of an electronic pacemaker rhythm during slowing of the sinus rate.

deep breath evidently increases the degree of intermittent A-V block, producing enough of a pause to enlist an electronic pacemaker discharge. Capture of the ventricles is evident with a change in QRS-T morphology. The electronic pacemaker rhythm continues on at a rate somewhat slower than that of the earlier intrinsic rhythm.

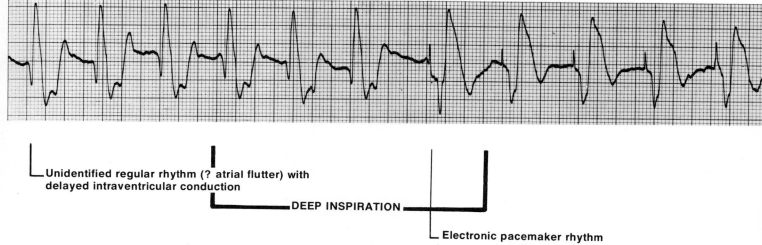

Figure 9–51. Testing of a demand pacemaker sensor system in the presence of spontaneous rhythm.

The second method of checking the quiescent ventricular-inhibited pacemaker is with the use of a magnet. When a magnet is placed directly over a subcutaneous pulse generator, the magnetic force activates a switch that breaks the circuit required for inhibition. Thus, the pacemaker is converted to the fixed (or asynchronous) mode, emitting discharges at the preset rate regardless of intrinsic cardiac activity. Electronic impulses appear immediately on application of the magnet amidst the spontaneous beats. Some electronic impulses may capture and some may not, depending on refractoriness at the time of the impulse. Their presence does demonstrate that the firing mechanism is functioning, as shown in Figure 9–52.

Atrial fibrillation is evident in test tracing 421, and the ventricular response rate, as expected, is irregular. When the ventricular rate slows beyond a critical point, an

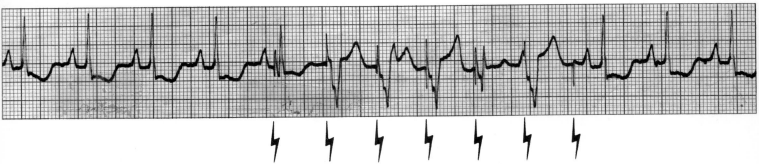

Figure 9–52. Electronic pacemaker spikes appear with application of a magnet over the generator.

electronic pacemaker spike appears. Locate all electronic pacemaker spikes. Are intervals between each R deflection of spontaneous beats and the next electronic pacemaker spike constant (i.e., the duration of the escape period)? When firing successive discharges, does the electronic pacemaker maintain a constant rate? Are the intervals between successive electronic pacemaker spikes different from the escape intervals? Do electronic pacemaker stimuli capture the ventricles?

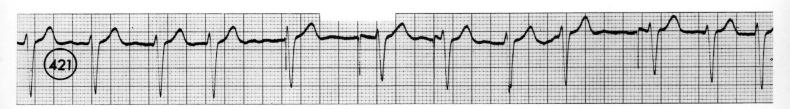

This tracing illustrates a well-functioning sensor system and impulse-generating mechanism, but the electronic pacemaker fails to stimulate the ventricles. An x-ray taken at this time revealed that the transvenous pacing wire had become dislodged from the apex of the right ventricle and that its tip now rested in the outflow track of the pulmonary artery. Complete capture of the ventricles was attained by repositioning the wire.

The next series of tracings illustrates many rhythm problems occurring within a relatively brief period. They were recorded from a 66-year-old man who received a permanent transvenous electronic pacemaker on the previous day. Write a complete rhythm interpretation for each tracing.

1. 8:15 AM: The following three continuous strips are from the standard ECG taken on the first postoperative day. Until this time, no defect in the pulse rate had been detected since implantation of the electronic pacemaker. During the recording, the patient developed a period of lightheadedness and apprehension.

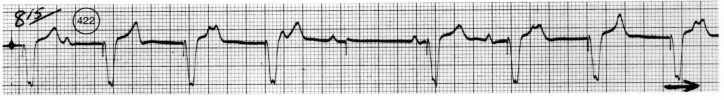

Interpretation _____

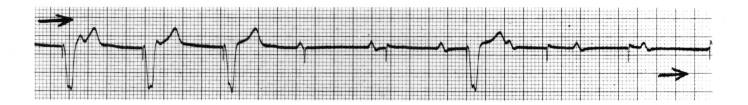

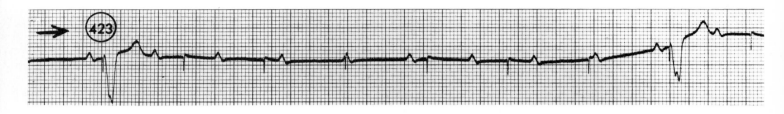

Interpretation _____

2. 8:27 AM: The patient no longer had symptoms when lying supine but experienced lightheadedness upon sitting up.

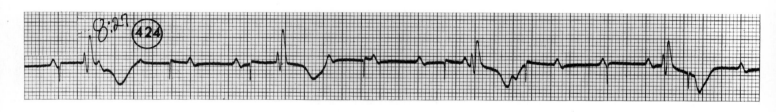

Interpretation _____

3. 8:33 AM: Isoproterenol infusion was started: 1 mg/1000 ml 5% D/W at 50 drops per minute.

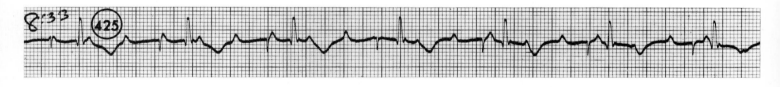

Interpretation _____

4. 8:47 AM: The patient can tolerate sitting upright without symptoms. However, he now complains of palpitations.

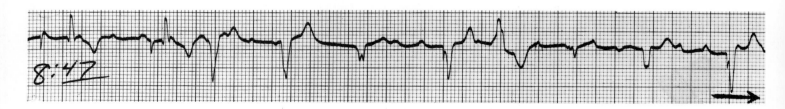

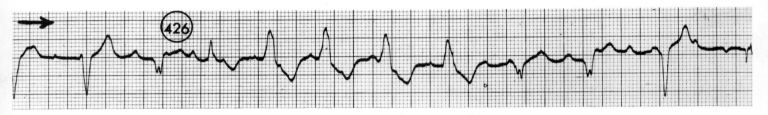

Interpretation _____

5. 8:49 AM: The isoproterenol infusion rate was reduced to 30 drops per minute.
6. 8:54 AM: Palpitations have disappeared.

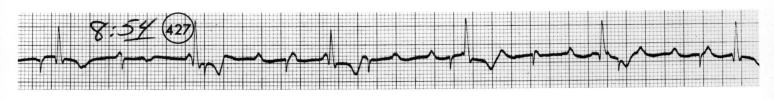

Interpretation _____

7. 9:15 AM: Monitoring leads were attached to the patient, and the recording was made by another instrument.

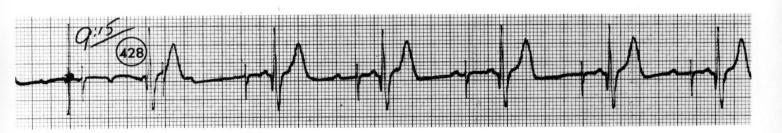

Interpretation _____

8. 9:45 AM: The patient was taken to the operating room with the intention of implanting an epicardial electronic pacemaker to replace the transvenous endocardial one. (This decision was made because of several previous episodes of pacemaker failure due to changing electrode position of the transvenous wire.) Tracing recorded at 9:58 AM.

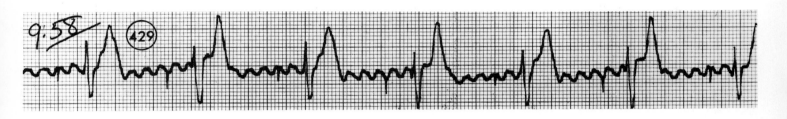

Interpretation _____

9. 10:05 AM: An endotracheal intubation was performed. Blood pressure was maintained.

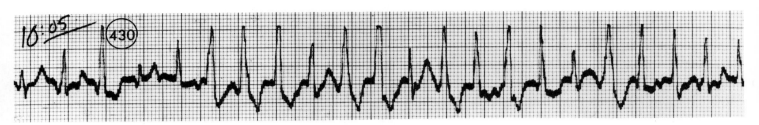

Interpretation_____

10. 10:06 AM: Isoproterenol infusion was stopped, one 1 minute later this tracing was recorded.

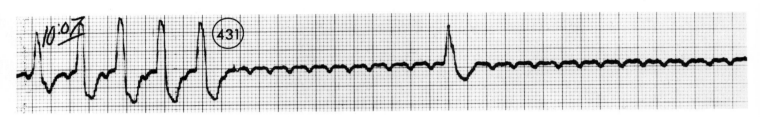

Interpretation_____

11. 10:08 AM: Ventricular beats were stimulated by a succession of fist blows to the chest by the surgeon. Meanwhile, isoproterenol infusion was restarted at 100 drops per minute momentarily, then slowed to 50 drops per minute when a spontaneous heartbeat reappeared.

12. 10:09 AM: Stable rhythm was maintained with isoproterenol infusion while the surgeon proceeded with the thoracotomy and epicardial electrode placement.

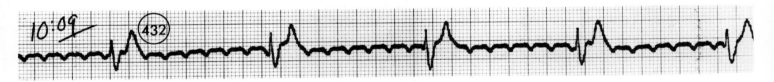

Interpretation_____

13. 10:45 AM: Wires from the epicardial electrodes were connected to the electronic pacemaker power unit. Technical problems then interfered with the electrocardiographic recording. Nevertheless, the desired information could be ascertained from this tracing.

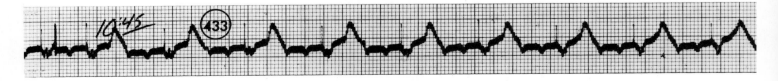

Interpretation_____

14. 10:47 AM: Isoproterenol infusion was discontinued.

15. 11:20 AM: The lead from the standard ECG taken in the recovery room is shown below. Thereafter the cardiac rhythm remained entirely stable.

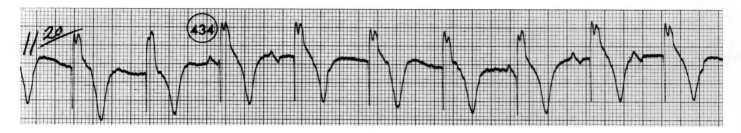

Interpretation

The episodes just illustrated reveal in dramatic fashion a sequence of complications with an electronic pacemaker and with a drug and how both modalities are used in conjunction until a difficult arrhythmia is controlled. Clearly apparent is the importance of establishing a secure transvenous position for the electronic pacemaker at the outset.

Rarely, the myocardium may fail to act as a minimally effective pump, resulting in a presentation of cardiac arrest, while the ECG reveals a fairly normal rhythm, rate, and wave forms. This paradox is known as **electromechanical dissociation.** In most instances, the rhythm deteriorates rapidly, and the patient cannot be resuscitated. An electronic pacemaker is inappropriate because the existing intrinsic electrical activity is unable to induce an effective contraction, indicating mechanical not electrical dysfunction. Rupture of the myocardium and massive infarction are the most common causes.

The term *fixed-rate* pacemaker may lead to some confusion. It refers to the electronic pacemaker design that emits impulses at a constant set rate regardless of the natural heart activity (see The Asynchronous Electronic Pacemaker). It differs, of course, from the demand (inhibited) electronic pacemaker, which has an impulse-forming mechanism that turns on or off in response to competing intrinsic cardiac rhythms. Even so, the demand pacemaker also fires at a *fixed rate* when it paces continuously.

Of the two types of electronic pacemakers, the demand mode (synchronous) is far more common. Although it is substantially more expensive than the fixed mode unit, the pulse-inhibiting feature offers a valuable protective advantage against excessively rapid rates from combined natural and electronic rhythms.

This potential for creating excessively rapid rates or ventricular dysrhythmias was the stimulus for converting from pacemakers that fired at a fixed rate to pacemakers that are inhibited by the patient's own complexes. However, the strip in Figure 9–53 illustrates that patients who have pacemakers without the sensing capability are occasionally admitted. This 87-year-old patient was admitted in April of 1989 for replacement of his 8-year-old pulse generator. The nurse who recorded the strip, presuming that the patient had an inhibited pacemaker, notified the physician of the failure to sense. The cardiologist acknowledged that the patient had an asynchronous fixed-rate ventricular pacemaker because the underlying rate at the time of initial implantation of the pacemaker 18 years before had been in the 20s, and no spontaneous complexes had been recorded since the insertion. The occurrence of frequent inherent beats lasted for less than 30 minutes, and no further biological complexes were seen during the remaining 24 hours of the patient's hospital stay. This tracing then does not demonstrate failure of the pacemaker to sense the patient's own rhythm, but rather it shows proper functioning of a noninhibited ventricular pacemaker.

It is sometimes possible to learn a great deal about electronic pacemaker function

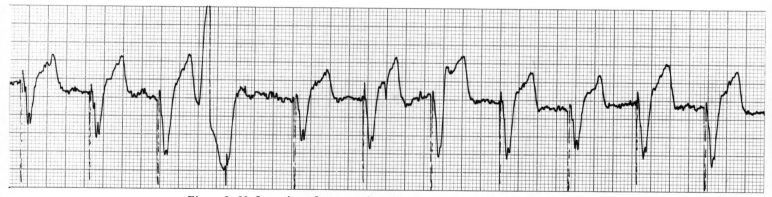

Figure 9–53. Insertion of an asynchronous pacemaker in the spring of 1989 produces a strip with apparent failure to sense.

and its interaction with the natural rhythm by detailed examination of a few beats. The next example provides this opportunity, serving as a review of electronic pacemaker interpretation. The patient was a 70-year-old diabetic man admitted with acute cholecystitis and suspected sepsis. Blood pressure is 95/50. A laparotomy was planned as soon as the patient's condition had been stabilized. A temporary bipolar electronic pacemaker was inserted on admission because of bradycardia (Fig. 9–54).

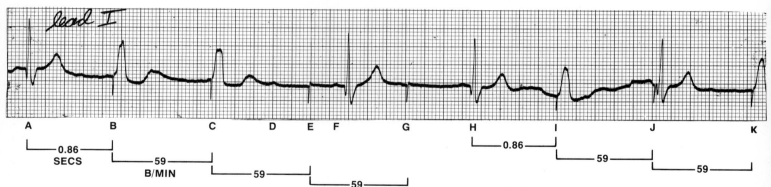

Figure 9–54. Malfunction of pacing and sensing in a transvenous ventricular inhibited electronic pacemaker.

The first beat (A) from lead I is of sinus origin, and it exhibits typical right bundle branch block. In the following beat, an electronic pacing spike is seen (B), initiating a ventricular depolarization having a left bundle branch block pattern. The escape interval between the R deflection of the first beat and the electronic pacemaker spike is 0.86 second. The next beat (C) is also an electronic pacemaker-stimulated cycle with left bundle branch block pattern, and the set pacing rate of the electronic pacemaker is observed to be 59 beats per minute.

A nonconducted P wave then occurs (D) followed by an electronic pacemaker spike (E) appearing at precisely the same rate as before. This time, however, the electronic impulse is not followed by a QRS complex, indicating a failure of pacer capture. A P wave then emerges (F), and this wave is conducted, again producing a ventricular depolarization with right bundle branch block. The electronic pacemaker spike occurring at G does *not* exhibit any delay from the preset rate of 59 beats per minute, as expected. This finding demonstrates that the sensing component has failed to respond to the spontaneous beat so that the pacing unit was not inhibited. Noncapture is also noted. However, after the next spontaneous beat (H), recognized as a sinus beat with right bundle branch block, an electronically induced beat with left bundle branch block pattern (I) is again observed at the previously established escape interval of 0.86 second. This cardiac cycle exhibits intact sensor and pacer functions of the power generator. Subsequently, an electronic pacemaker spike (J) occurs at the preset rate of 59 beats per minute, but it occurs *after* a spontaneous P wave. Because the form of the QRS complex that follows has a right bundle branch block configuration, it can be assumed that ventricular depolarization was initiated by the sinus impulse, the electronic pacemaker impulse occurring too late to stimulate the ventricles. The last cycle of the tracing (K) is clearly an electronically paced beat with left bundle branch block pattern. However, a defect in sensing is once again observed because the spontaneous R deflection did not induce any pause in the firing sequence of the electronic pacemaker.

Thus, from detailed examination of a few beats, a great deal can be learned of the functioning of an electronic pacemaker and its interaction with a natural rhythm. In this example, the problem of intermittent failure of pacing and sensing was corrected by a slight change in the position of the pacing lead. Mild hypotension was also improved by increasing the pacemaker rate to 70 beats per minute.

The following schema (Fig. 9–55) is used to review the process for assessing proper function of a ventricular-inhibited (demand) pacemaker. Evaluation can be simplified to the following steps:

1. Intrinsic complex present—spike absent   } proper sensing
2. Intrinsic complex absent—spike present   }
3. Spike present—ventricular complex present} proper capture

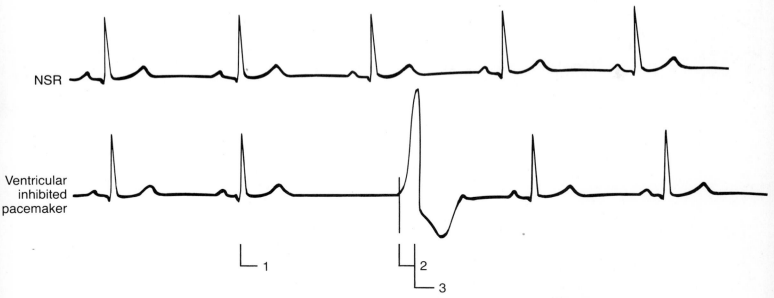

Figure 9–55. Schemata depicting normal function of a ventricular inhibited pacemaker.

THE ELECTRONIC PACEMAKER CODE

Before progressing to more complex models of electronic pacemakers, you will need to know the terminology applied to the various types of pacemakers. This terminology defines the functions according to a simple, standardized code system established by the Intersociety Commission on Heart Disease (ICHD): A Revised Code for Pacemaker Identification (Table 9–1). Before the code was adopted, descriptions of electronic

Table 9–1. ICHD PACEMAKER CODE (1981)

I Chamber paced	II Chamber sensed	III Response to sensing
V (ventricle)	V (ventricle)	I (inhibition)

Modified from data from Parsonnet V, Furman S, and Smyth NP: A revised code for pacemaker identification. Pacemaker Study Group. *Circulation* 64:60A–62A, 1981.

pacemakers became increasingly confusing and cumbersome as additional technological features were incorporated.

The electronic pacemaker code uses a series of letters representing the pacing mode and the cardiac chamber(s) involved in a specific pacemaker. Following is a description of the code as applied to the ventricular-inhibited, demand mode, pacemaker.

Chamber Paced

The first letter in the series always indicates the location of the pacing electrode. **V** specifies that the electronic pacemaker is pacing a ventricle. (An **A** would indicate atrial pacing, a mode to be presented later).

Chamber Sensed

The second letter signifies the presence of sensor function and indicates the chamber sensed. The electronic pacemaker just described is represented by a **V** in the second position because it incorporates a sensor in the ventricles.

Sensing Response

I, the third letter in the series, indicates that the electronic pulses will be inhibited by spontaneous depolarizations, such as premature beats. (An **I** in this space would indicate that the generator triggers a stimulus in response to sensing activity, a function to be explained later.)

According to this terminology, the demand mode system studied earlier is designated **VVI**. The letters designate that the electronic pacemaker

1. Paces the ventricles,
2. Senses spontaneous activity in the ventricle, and
3. Turns off pacing in response to sensed activity.

The VVI pacemaker represents the basic instrument used to prevent symptomatic bradycardias. It is most suitable for patients with advanced degrees of A-V block (intermittent or temporary) and for patients with sinus node dysfunction coupled with failure of reliable inherent escape rhythms. The method is restricting in the sense that pacing is performed at a constant rate (regardless of physical activity) and that the artificial pacemaker creates an A-V dissociation with loss of physiological synchrony of atrial and ventricular contractions. Thus, a ventricular pacemaker limits cardiac output because there is loss of atrial kick and its preset escape rate precludes an automatic adjustment to meet circulatory demands. Even so, this form of electronic pacemaker is usually quite satisfactory for those individuals who lead a sedentary life-style and who enjoy freedom from serious tachyarrhythmias.

In the accepted electronic pacemaker code, the letter **O** signifies that no function is present. The symbol can be used for any position of the series. For example, the fixed mode (asynchronous) pacemaker described originally in the chapter is designated **VOO** (ventricular pacing without the capability for sensing or inhibiting).

For sedentary patients, an electronic pacemaker that provides a ventricular escape rhythm may be adequate to prevent symptoms of excessive cardiac slowing. However, fixed ventricular pacing may limit more active, pacemaker-dependent patients. Because of failure of heart rate acceleration and lack of chamber sequencing, these individuals may experience fatigue, lightheadedness, or dyspnea even with slight exertion, limitations known as the **pacemaker syndrome.** Stepping up the ventricular pacemaker rate may overcome the symptoms but sometimes at the expense of producing disturbing palpitations at rest and accelerating battery decay.

THE ATRIAL PACEMAKER

In sinus node dysfunction, the pacemaker syndrome may be alleviated by placing the pacing lead in the atrium instead of in the ventricles. By this strategy, the atrial rate can be held above a set minimum; the atrial impulse passes through the A-V node and Purkinje conduction systems and thus preserves the normal sequence of atrial and ventricular contraction. By restoring atrial kick, cardiac output may be increased appreciably and lessen symptoms. An example of **atrial pacing** is seen in Figure 9–56. Note that the PR intervals are constant throughout, as normal A-V conduction is undisturbed.

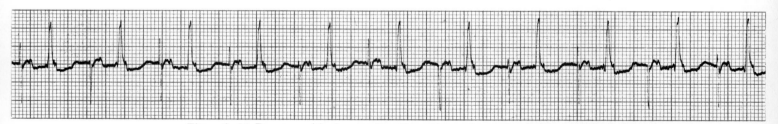

Figure 9–56. P waves with abnormal configuration and a prolonged PR interval follow electronic pacemaker spikes with a rate of 82 per minute.

Some atrial pacemakers incorporate a sensing lead to inhibit pulse generator firing when the sinus rate accelerates beyond the pacing rate or if atrial ectopic rhythms occur (Fig. 9–57). In effect, the VVI pacemaker is modified to an AAI, simply by the lead placement.

A problem often encountered with the AAI pacemaker is the inability to sense P waves because of their low amplitude. The pacemaker spikes in Figure 9–58 can be seen superimposed on the sinus P waves. The patient had the pacemaker inserted to prevent symptoms associated with severe sinus bradycardia, a side effect of his propranolol therapy. Increasing the sensitivity of the generator was unsuccessful.

The security of a lead in the atrium has been greatly enhanced by new designs of electrode tips. A major problem remains, however, because most patients with sinus node dysfunction have disease in other areas of excitable tissues, and many eventually develop A-V block. Of course, atrial pacing is absolutely dependent on an intact A-V conduction system.

Figure 9–59 demonstrates the problem that can evolve when the patient develops A-V block after insertion of an atrial pacemaker. The fourth and tenth atrial spikes produce a P wave that is not conducted. An atrial spike is superimposed on the ST segment of each of these escape beats. This electronic pacemaker impulse is also non-

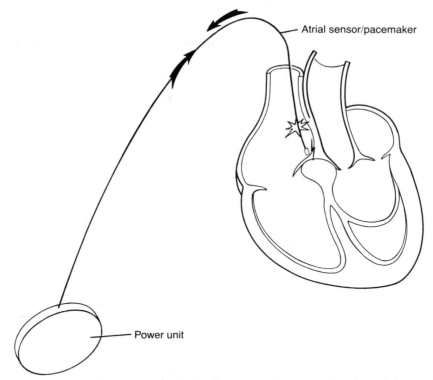

Figure 9–57. Schemata depicts lead placement in the atria. Note: In sketches of electronic pacemakers, the star is used to represent sensing function. The lightning symbol indicates pacing function.

conducted, not because of A-V block but because the ventricles have not yet repolarized after the escape depolarization.

The problem of the pacemaker syndrome in sinus node dysfunction and in A-V block is also addressed by new designs of electronic pacemakers. By restoring the functional advantages of normal cardiac dynamics in response to activity, exercise performance may be substantially improved. Admittedly, the **physiological** electronic pacemakers in current use have complex capabilities. The essential features of each of the major types are presented here with illustrative tracings.

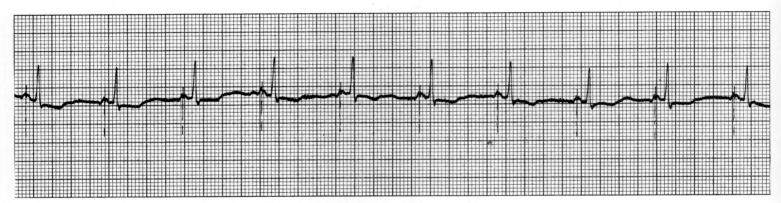

Figure 9–58. Failure of sensing of an atrial pacemaker.

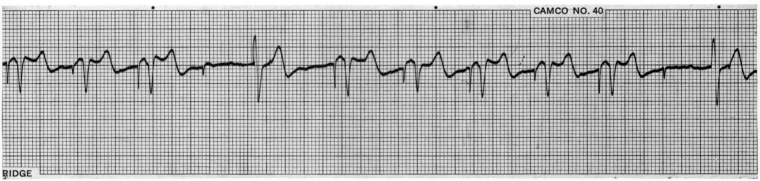

Figure 9–59. Atrial pacemaking in the presence of complete A-V block.

PHYSIOLOGICAL PACEMAKERS

To provide a more physiological action of the heart, particularly during times of increased work load, two fundamental approaches of bioengineering have been taken:

 1. Rate-responsive pacing. The pulse generator paces at varying rates in response to the natural heart rate, which is in turn a function of the degree of physical work.

 2. Atrioventricular sequential pacing. The pulse generator is capable of maintaining the normal sequential relationship between atrial and ventricular contractions.

The Atrial Synchronous Pacemaker

To begin, a relatively simple mode of electronic pacing is described to familiarize the reader with certain principles. In A-V block, the sinus node apparatus and atrial conducting system may be intact so that the atria beat at a rate governed by venous return and hemodynamic pressure in the right atrium. (These are the most important mechanisms by which the sinus node responds to changes in work load.) In the atrial synchronous electronic pacemaker, the sinus rhythm is sensed and transmitted to the pulse generator and this rate determines the rate of ventricular pacing using the following components (Fig. 9–60).

- A **sensor lead** in the right atrium informs the pulse generator of natural atrial depolarizations.
- The **pulse generator** senses each intraatrial interval, converts it to rate, and after an appropriate delay (an artificial PR interval) responds by firing.
- The **pacing lead** is placed in the right ventricle. Through it ventricular pacing is coupled to each atrial depolarization.

By this design, the sinus pacemaker triggers the ventricular pacemaker, and these events are separated by a delay that is equivalent to the PR interval. Thus, the normal heart rate changes associated with everyday activity are maintained even in the presence of complete A-V block. The electronic pacemaker, in effect, serves as an artificial A-V node. This feature is demonstrated in Figure 9–61.

 Caliper measurements reveal a slight variation in electronic pacemaker spike intervals. At the same time, PR intervals remain constant. Thus is demonstrated a variable atrial rate with a constant artificial interval from the natural P wave to the electronic stimulation. Because this duration is not a natural one, it is referred to as the **PV interval** (time between onset of P wave to appearance of the electronic pacemaker spike). Note the variable PP rate and consistent PV interval in the schema that follows (Fig. 9–62).

 The rate-responsive electronic pacemaker is appropriate for patients who have

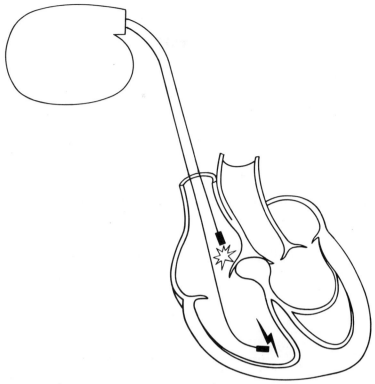

Figure 9–60. Synchronous mode electronic pacemaker.

complete A-V block and have reasonable acceleration of sinus rate on increased effort. For example, some individuals with pacemaker-dependent forms of AV nodal disease have entered athletic competition using this mode. It is also useful for patients who have global myocardial disease and who cannot enlist an appreciable increase in contractility (and stroke volume) for relatively low-level tasks, such as climbing stairs and carrying groceries. This function is illustrated in the tracing in Figure 9–63, which was obtained from a 76-year-old man. The patient had a demand ventricular pacemaker implanted 4 years before, but it was replaced by a rate-responsive pacemaker because of excessive fatigue on walking.

Of course, the coupling of ventricular stimulation to atrial depolarization restores the natural synchrony of atrial and ventricular contractions, and the properly timed

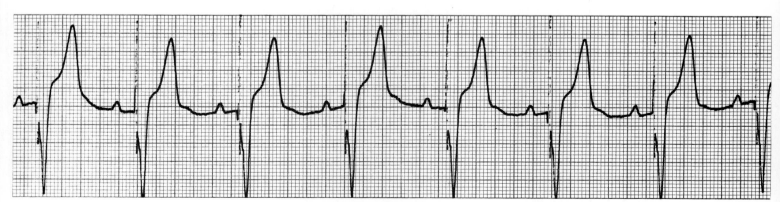

Figure 9–61. Activation of the ventricles by a P wave synchronous electronic pacemaker.

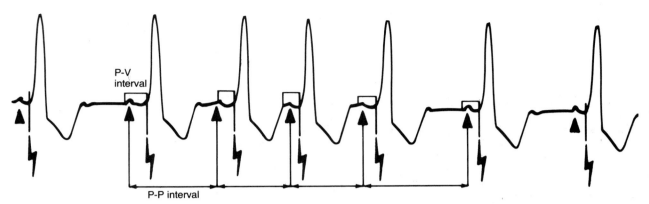

Figure 9–62. Schemata of atrial responsive pacemaker depicts variance in P-P intervals but stable P-V interval.

artificial PR interval is a critical factor in this relationship. Thus, rate augmentation with exercise and atrioventricular synchrony are combined in the atrial synchronous pacemaker to more effectively eliminate symptoms associated with the pacemaker syndrome.

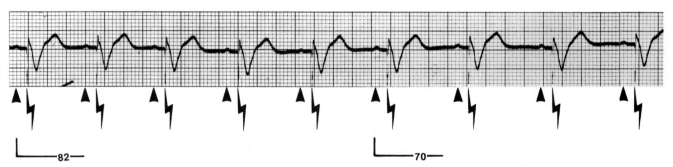

Figure 9–63. Sinus rhythm with synchronized ventricular electronic pacemaker response.

Certain features of the atrial synchronous pacemaker are integrated into the pulse generator circuit to protect against spontaneous cardiac activity of a deleterious nature. For example, a **lower rate limit** for atrial depolarization is programmed. Should the sinoatrial rate fall below this level, the electronic pacemaker converts to fixed-rate ventricular pacing (Fig. 9–64).

The sinus rate in the rhythm in Figure 9–64 varies between 69 and 74. At the faster rate, the ventricular pacemaker fires after an interval of 0.32 second. As the rate begins to slow with the seventh cycle, the pacemaker converts to a VVI mode at a rate of 72 per minute (sinus rate is 69 per minute).

Five other conditions in which an atrial synchronous pacemaker would convert to a ventricular pacemaker are as follows:

1. Displacement of the atrial sensing electrode.
2. Fracture of the atrial sensing lead.
3. Break in the integrity of insulation in the atrial sensing lead.
4. Malfunction of the pulse generator (including critical reduction in battery strength).
5. Development of sinoatrial arrest.

The atrial synchronous pacemaker also has an **upper rate limit** for atrial sensing. Various models have different established limits and may be programmed, usually to just above the maximum rate anticipated for the patient's usual activity. When the limit is exceeded, the pulse generator steps down the atrial signals by losing its 1:1 con-

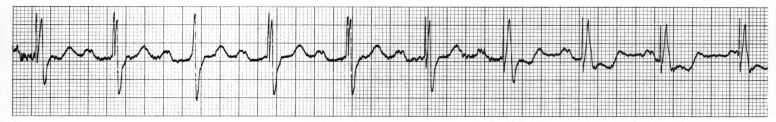

Figure 9–64. Conversion of an atrial synchronous pacemaker to a fixed-rate ventricular pace-maker.

duction and providing an artificial, intermittent A-V block. In some pacemakers, this is a 2:1 A-V block (Fig. 9–65).

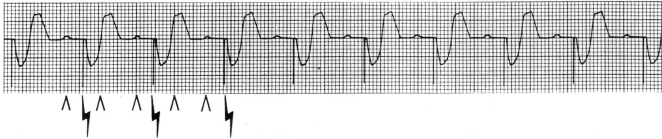

Figure 9–65. Rapid atrial activity results in production of 2:1 block. (Courtesy of Dell Dinicola of Medtronic, Inc.)

In other models of atrial synchronous pacemakers, a Wenckebach type of periodic block occurs (Fig. 9–66).

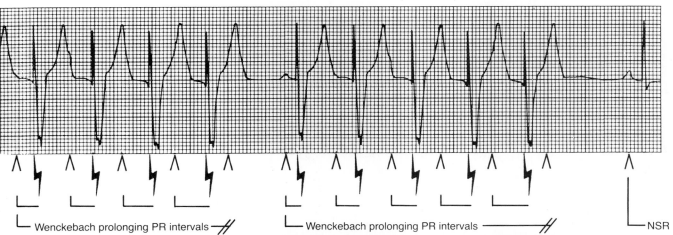

Wenckebach prolonging PR intervals —//—   Wenckebach prolonging PR intervals ————//—   NSR

Figure 9–66. Conversion of typical pacemaker function to Wenckebach block when atrial rate becomes excessive. (Courtesy of Dell Dinicola of Medtronic, Inc.)

Most rate-responsive electronic pacemakers also have a sensing lead in the ventricles. It is included to further protect the heart against spontaneous ventricular activity. In this way, the pulse generator functions in the ventricular inhibited mode, described earlier.

Figure 9–67*A* is an ECG that demonstrates a rate-responsive ventricular pacemaker; it was obtained from a 32-year-old man with mitral valve prolapse and two episodes of syncope while playing tennis. In the electrophysiology laboratory, resting

first-degree A-V block progressed to complete A-V block under provocation of a vagotonic drug. A variable-rate ventricular pacemaker was chosen because of the patient's
desire to continue vigorous sports.

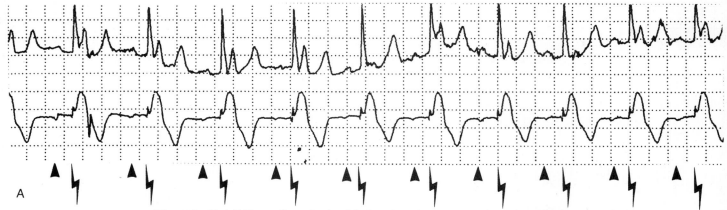

Figure 9–67. (*A*) Recording obtained from a young man with a rate-responsive electronic pacemaker.

A simultaneous two-channel recording is shown. (In this tracing, the grid was
printed with a matrix dot system at the same time that the ECG was recorded. Note
that 0.04-second markings are eliminated.) Atrial tracking is evident in which sinus rate
variations associated with respiration dictate the ventricular pacing rate. (Use calipers
to detect the slight changes in rate.)

An ECG was then obtained immediately after the patient completed climbing 15
steps (Fig. 9–67*B*).

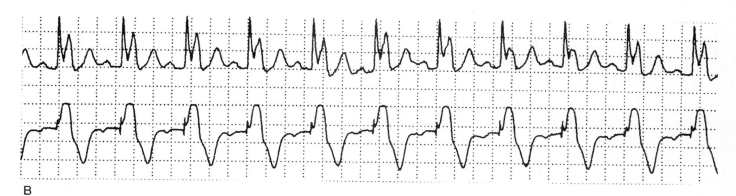

Figure 9–67. (*B*) After exercise, the electronic pacemaker rate has increased in response to the
increase in sinus firing.

Sinus rate has increased as a natural response to exercise. The electronically paced
ventricular rate increases correspondingly, and atrioventricular sequential contractions
are preserved. The patient is shown here to maintain atrioventricular synchronous
activity while accelerating the heart rate to support physical exertion. He did return
to vigorous athletics, with excellent tolerance. Figure 9–67*C* demonstrates that even
such complex electronic pacemakers incorporate protection against spontaneous and
competing rhythms.

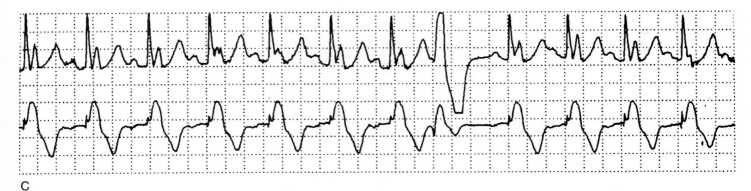

C

Figure 9–67. (*C*) A ventricular premature complex has resulted in inhibition of ventricular stimulation by the pacemaker.

The paced ventricles continue to respond to atrial drive as slight rate variations can be measured. However, momentary suspension of ventricular pacing occurs when a premature beat is sensed. The event indicates the presence of ventricular sensing/inhibitory function.

The features of the two-lead atrial synchronous pacemaker are designated VDD according to standard terminology:

First letter: V = pacing occurs in the ventricles.

Second letter: D = atrial and ventricular sensing is present, the D representing dual or double chamber.

Third letter: D = inhibition of the pacemaker can occur in both ventricular and atrial chambers when ectopic activity is sensed, and ventricular activity is stimulated in response to atrial activity. Thus a dual (D) function of inhibition and stimulation are present.

The letter **I** in the third position indicates that the electronic pacemaker output is inhibited when it senses spontaneous depolarization. The letter **T**, indicating that the atria trigger the ventricles, can be substituted in the third position if the inhibition function is not included.

A fourth letter, **P**, is also given for additional functions that can be adjusted by external programmers. Such adjustments may include that of rate, power of output, and sensitivity. A fifth letter may be included to indicate the function of tachycardia control (to be described later). However, these last two letters are customarily omitted in ordinary clinical reference.

The Noncardiac Rate-Responsive Pacemaker

In persons with diffuse cardiac disease, the unreliability of the sinus node and the tendency toward supraventricular tachycardias have limited the usefulness of the VDI pacemaker. Consequently, further technological improvements are sought to circumvent the unpredictability of the sinoatrial pacing by monitoring work load more directly. These efforts have taken several different directions. Ventricular pacemakers may be triggered by changes in blood pH, body temperature, oxygen level in the subcutaneous tissue, respiratory frequency, QT interval, and mechanical vibrations. All these factors vary to a more or less predictable degree with exercise.

MOTION-RESPONSIVE PACEMAKER

Most interest in the development of extracardiac variables to govern cardiac rate centers on the use of the whole body's natural resonance to physical activities. Currently available is an electronic pacemaker (manufactured under the name Activitrax) with rate-responsive capability using this principle to reflect the degree of effort expended. Its pulse generator contains a piezoelectric crystal that detects small mechanical vibrations from ordinary physical activity. When the vibrations are above threshold amplitude, a voltage signal is transmitted to the pacing unit. The pacing unit, in turn, responds at a rate that reflects the frequency as well as the strength of the signal received (Fig. 9–68).

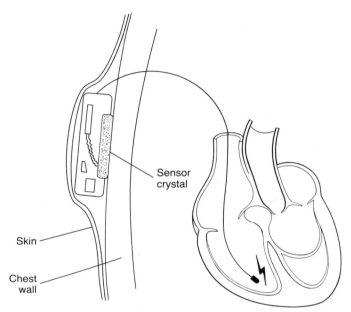

Sensor
crystal

Skin

Chest
wall

Figure 9–68. Motion-responsive pacemaker. A sensor on the inner side of the pulse generator responds to body motion. A pacemaker lead stimulates a chamber at a rate determined by the extent of body motion. Either atrial or ventricular leads may be used.

The motion-sensitive crystal within the pulse generator acts as an artificial sinus node, using external pressure waves from body movement rather than hemodynamic changes to match heart rate to the level of physical activity. This variable-rate system requires only a single lead for pacing. In persons with sinus node dysfunction but with reliable A-V conduction, the pacing lead can be placed into the atria, thereby maintaining normal atrioventricular synchronization.

For rate-responsive pacing in patients with A-V block, a single-chamber system requires a ventricular lead. The pulse generator drives the ventricles at varying rates in response to signals from body movement. This system establishes an A-V dissociation (in the absence of retrograde conduction to the atria) and thus loses atrioventricular synchrony. In the tracing in Figure 9–69, changes in paced ventricular rate can best be appreciated using calipers.

Rhythm strip A in Figure 9–69 was recorded while the patient, recovering from a myocardial infarction, was at rest. Very slight changes in rate can be detected (73 to 75 per minute). During a cardiac rehabilitation walk (strip B), the patient's rate increased to the high 80s. The increased activity is responsible for the increased rate of the pacemaker: all ventricular events are controlled by the pacemaker.

Figure 9–70 illustrates a typical clinical application of a rate-responsive ventricular pacemaker. Mr. A.K., 74 years old, was admitted to the telemetry unit with a history

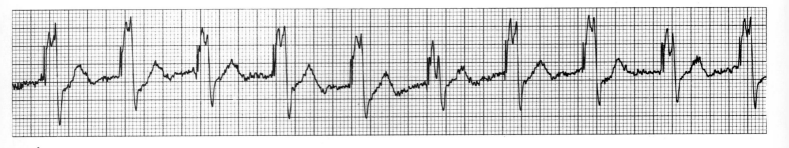

A

B

Figure 9–69. Body motion-responsive ventricular pacemaker showing rate change with activity.

of periods of lightheadedness and two syncopal episodes. His admission pattern (strip *A*) revealed complete A-V block with a ventricular rate of 29.

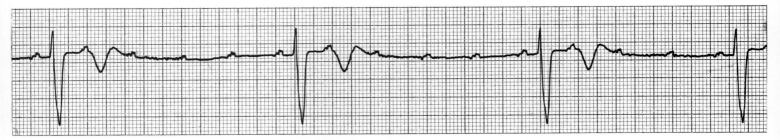

A

Figure 9–70. (*A*) Admission strip reveals complete A-V block.

A VVI pacemaker with a rate of 70 was inserted within hours of admission (strip *B*). He continued to experience symptoms of low cardiac output after discharge and subsequently was readmitted for insertion of a ventricular rate-responsive pacemaker.

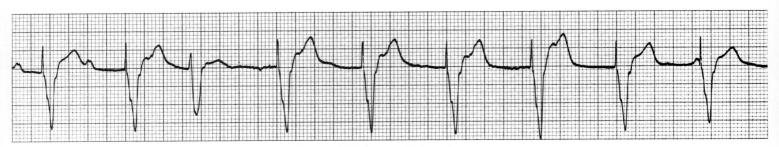

B

Figure 9–70. (*B*) A VVI pacemaker was inserted.

Strip *C* shows the typical pattern when Mr. A.K. was active. Nonconducted atrial activity can be identified throughout the strip.

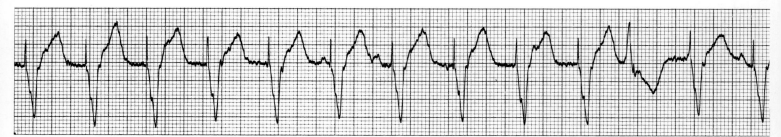

C

Figure 9–70. (*C*) Symptoms of decreased cardiac output continued, and the patient was readmitted for insertion of a rate-responsive electronic pacemaker.

A rate-responsive pacemaker may incorporate an inhibitory function so that spontaneous depolarizations turn off pacemaker firing momentarily, as shown in Figure 9–70*C*. A premature ventricular beat is followed by a pause. Subsequently, the electronic escape mechanism in which the pause is 0.75 second from the preceding spontaneous beat is evident. This system is another form of VVI pacing.

Four parameters on the motion-responsive pacemaker can be adjusted by an external radio transmitter:

1. The basic rate is set between 60 and 80 beats per minute, establishing the rate at which the pacemaker functions at minimum physical effort.

2. The upper limit for pacemaker firing is programmed from 100 to 150 beats per minute so that pacing does not accelerate excessively regardless of the degree of physical effort. This feature is particularly useful for patients who are subject to angina with very rapid heart rates.

3. Threshold amplitude for body motion can be adjusted to respond to effort levels that are mild (such as walking) up to vigorous (such as jogging). Thus, the sensitivity for triggering is individualized according to anticipated activity and for filtering extraneous signals (tremor, seizures, vehicular motion).

4. Rate can be adjusted to provide a pacing frequency for any given rate of voltage signals. Ideally, optimal ventricular rate is programmed for each level of physical exertion. It must be emphasized that the pacing rate of the motion-responsive pacemaker remains fairly constant at any given level of physical activity.

The Atrioventricular Sequential Pacemaker

When the sinus pacemaker is not reliable in patients with complete A-V block, the atrial synchronous pacemaker is ineffective. Abandoning the feature of rate responsiveness, an alternative strategy for these patients is the atrioventricular (A-V) sequential pacemaker depicted in Figure 9–71. By producing a properly timed contraction of the atria before each ventricular contraction, this method augments ventricular filling and has an appreciable effect on stroke volume. In this way, the benefit of atrial kick is preserved to compensate for loss of rate responsiveness during effort. Pacing wires in *both* an atrium and a ventricle restore the natural sequence of atrial and ventricular contractions.

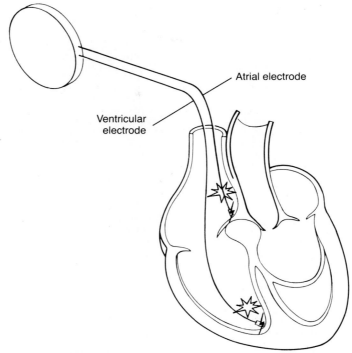

Figure 9–71. A-V sequential pacemaker.

The A-V sequential pacemaker rhythm is depicted schematically in Figure 9–72.

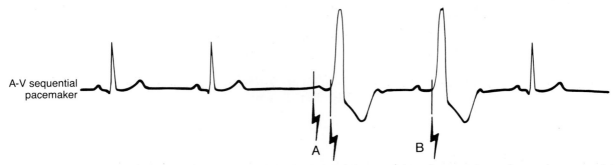

A-V sequential
pacemaker

Figure 9–72. Schemata of an A-V sequential pacemaker demonstrates electronic pacemaker stimulation of both the atrium and ventricle (A), as well as ventricular stimulation in response to a biologic P wave (B).

The pulse generator drives both atrial and ventricular chambers while maintaining a short delay between impulses. The delay serves as an artificial A-V node, simulating the natural PR interval and facilitating ventricular filling. The duration of this A-V interval (an artificial PR) may be preset by the manufacturer or externally programmed after insertion of the pulse generator. A tracing demonstrating A-V sequential pacing is presented in Figure 9–73.

An atrial pacemaker spike is followed by a poorly defined P wave (as is commonly observed in atrial pacing). After an interval of 0.20 second, another pacemaker spike produces a ventricular depolarization. Note that the atrial pacemaker is precisely reg-

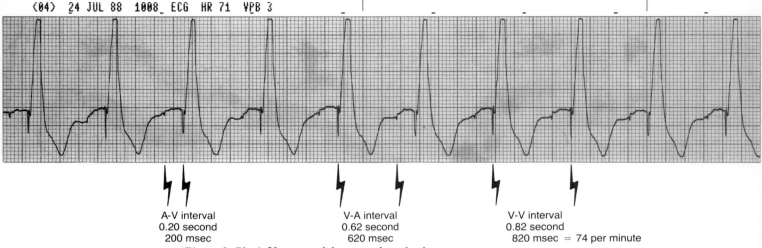

〈04〉 24 JUL 88 1008_ ECG HR 71 VPB 3

A-V interval	V-A interval	V-V interval
0.20 second	0.62 second	0.82 second
200 msec	620 msec	820 msec = 74 per minute

Figure 9–73. A-V sequential pacemaker rhythm.

ular at 74 pulses per minute and that the A-V intervals are uniform. The V-A interval (from ventricular spike to subsequent atrial spike) is 0.62 second. For convenience in expressing such small intervals, it has become common for electrocardiographers to use milliseconds (msec). Accordingly, the A-V interval here is 200 msec and the V-A interval is 620 msec. The interval from one ventricular spike to the next (termed the V-V interval) is another way of representing rate and should be equal to the combined A-V and V-A intervals (620 msec plus 200 msec = 820 msec = 74 per minute).

A-V sequential pacing is of benefit even at rest to the patient who, because of severely restrictive myocardial reserve, is unable to use increased stroke volume to overcome an inappropriately slow natural sinoatrial rate. Studies on A-V sequential pacing demonstrate an increase in cardiac index of about 20% in most patients when compared with fixed-rate pacing of the ventricles. (Cardiac index is a measure of cardiac output adjusted to the body surface area).

The patient in the ECGs in Figure 9–74 had been experiencing vision disturbances and dizzy spells with activity. Initial monitoring revealed only sinus rhythm (Fig. 9–74A).

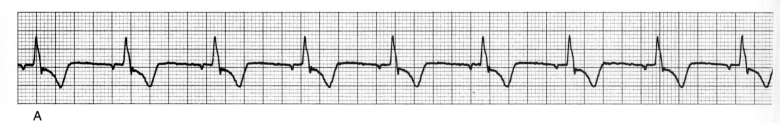

A

Figure 9–74. (A) Sinus rhythm was recorded on admission to the telemetry unit.

However, vagal maneuvers produced severe sinus node and A-V node dysfunction, resulting in rates that dropped into the 50s. A VVI pacemaker was inserted and was programmed to fire when the ventricular rate dropped below 75 (Fig. 9–74B).

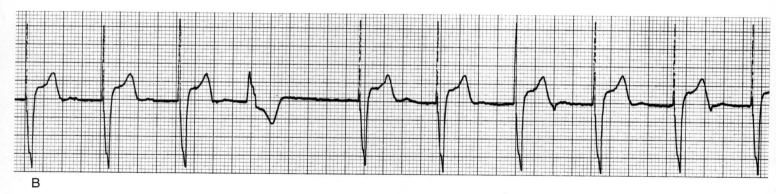

Figure 9–74. (*B*) Rhythm strip obtained after insertion of a VVI pacemaker.

Despite the presence of the ventricular-inhibited electronic pacemaker, the patient continued to experience lightheadedness. This problem was alleviated by insertion of an A-V sequential pacemaker set at precisely the same rate as his previous VVI pacemaker (Fig. 9–74*C*).

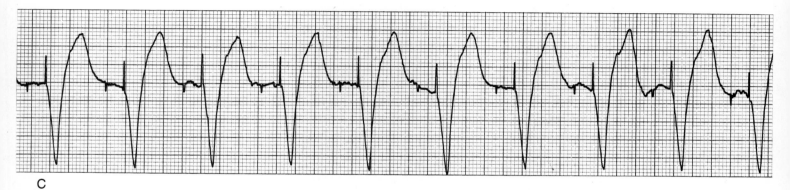

Figure 9–74. (*C*) Symptoms of reduced cardiac output were ultimately eliminated when an A-V sequential pacemaker was substituted for a VVI pacemaker.

A 62-year-old woman complained of increasing difficulty in performing household activities. Sinus bradycardia was the only notable finding on the initial evaluation. An ambulatory monitor documented her cardiac rhythm during 23½ hours. The tracing in Figure 9–75*A* was quite typical of the resting rhythm. (The two leads were recorded simultaneously with chest electrodes in positions that most closely resemble leads I and V₁.)

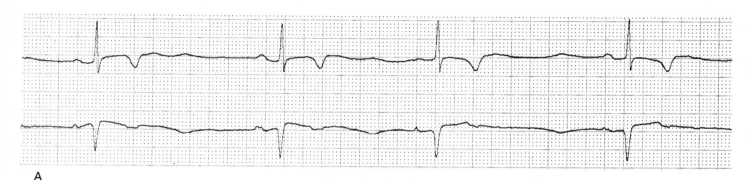

Figure 9–75. (*A*) Resting rhythm of a patient unable to perform normal household activities.

The sinus rate of 35 beats per minute at rest accelerated only slightly in response to walking and other ordinary exertions, never increasing beyond 55 per minute. In addition, frequent nonsustained tachycardias appeared unrelated to activity (Fig. 9–75B).

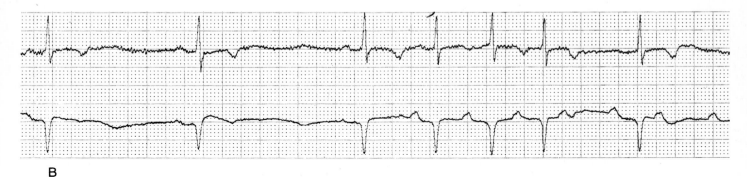

B

Figure 9–75. (*B*) Tachycardia unrelated to exertion.

A series of four atrial beats interrupts the sinus rhythm. The usefulness of simultaneous leads is clearly demonstrated here, where the P waves of the atrial beats in Figure 9–75A are obscured within the T waves of the preceding beats but are clearly evident in Figure 9–75B. Also note that the atrial arrhythmia exhibits Wenckebach periodicity (gradually lengthening P waves), with the tachycardia ending at the blocked atrial beat.

This example illustrates the bradycardia-tachycardia syndrome often associated with sinus node dysfunction. The patient was referred for electronic pacemaker implantation.

Because this patient was very active, an A-V sequential pacemaker was selected to optimize her effort tolerance (Fig. 9–75C).

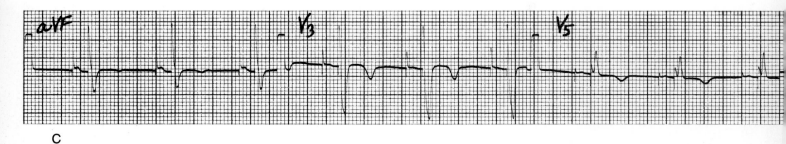

C

Figure 9–75. (*C*) Insertion of an A-V sequential pacemaker for bradycardia-tachycardia syndrome permits resumption of normal activity.

Note than an electronic impulse precedes each P wave, indicating programmed stimulation of the atrial rhythm. After 0.17 second, each impulse is followed by another electronic impulse, which in turn precedes a ventricular complex. Thus, an artificial PR interval in which stimulated atrial and ventricular depolarization occur at a favorable (or synchronized) timing is created. With this intervention, the patient was able to resume vigorous activities without undue fatigue.

Most A-V sequential pacing systems have sensing-inhibition components to protect against competition with ectopic beats. The most commonly used design has this function only in the ventricles. It is classified as the DVI system (**D** for dual-chamber pacing, **V** for ventricular sensing, and **I** for ventricular inhibiting). Figure 9–76 provides an

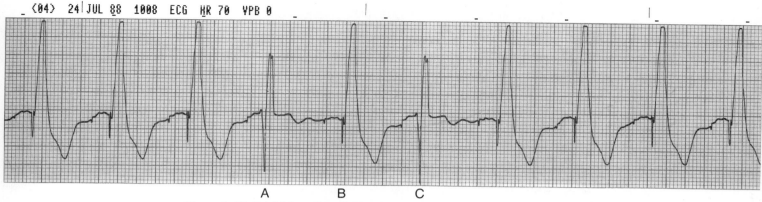

Figure 9–76. Inhibition of an A-V sequential pacemaker after a ventricular premature complex.

example of the A-V sequential pacemaker with inhibition of pacing following ventricular ectopy.

A-V sequential pacing controls the rhythm initially. At point A, a premature wide QRS complex appears 0.15 second after an atrial stimulus. The anticipated ventricular spike does not follow but is inhibited by the premature ectopic depolarization. A complete A-V sequential paced beat then resumes at B, followed by another premature ventricular beat at C, with inhibition of a ventricular pulse. Thereafter, an A-V sequential paced rhythm resumes.

Timing intervals must be analyzed very carefully to verify that both electronic and biological complexes are sensed properly and that inhibition and pacing occur appropriately. In the tracing in Figure 9–76, the atria are paced at a rate of 73 pulses per minute (the A-A interval is 0.81 second) with an A-V interval of 0.19 second. In the A-V sequential rhythm, the duration between the ventricular pulse and subsequent atrial pulse (V-A interval) is consistently 0.61 second. After the ectopic beat, however, atrial pacing occurs after an interval of 0.68 second (R-A interval). This slight delay is an inherent part of the pulse generator mechanism.

The DVI pacemaker is highly serviceable for most patients with complete A-V block. However, the absence of atrial sensing may result in competition with natural sinus and atrial beats. Spontaneous development of atrial tachycardia or fibrillation negates the advantage of A-V sequential pacing because the atrial pacemaker simply adds to the already overstimulated atria. In the presence of complete A-V bock, the ventricles, of course, are protected from these tachyarrhythmias.

The **committed** A-V sequential pacemaker is obligated to ventricular firing after each atrial stimulus as shown in Figure 9–77. In this pacemaker example, the patient is primarily in an A-V sequential rhythm. The activity of the committed electronic pacemaker can be determined by closely examining spike locations. Two functions of all A-V pacemakers are demonstrated at the ends of the strip. The first two beats exhibit normal function of ventricular pacemaker control in response to sinoatrial activity. The P-V interval is 0.19 second. The last cycles on the strip show complete cardiac control by the pacemaker, with atrial and ventricular spikes separated by an A-V interval of 0.20 second (200 msec). Beats 3, 4, 5, 9, and 10 are intrinsic beats. Close examination of the ninth beat reveals an atrial spike at the expected V-A interval of 440 msec. The QRS, however, does not resemble the other ventricular complexes induced by the pacemaker, and is not preceded by a spike. Rather, a spike occurs at an A-V interval of 200 msec at the top of the QRS. The presence of this spike at the prescribed time after the atrial spike is evidence that the A-V sequential pacemaker is a committed pacemaker. It can be appreciated by looking at this strip that if the PVC had occurred slightly earlier, the ventricular spike would have occurred near the vulnerable period

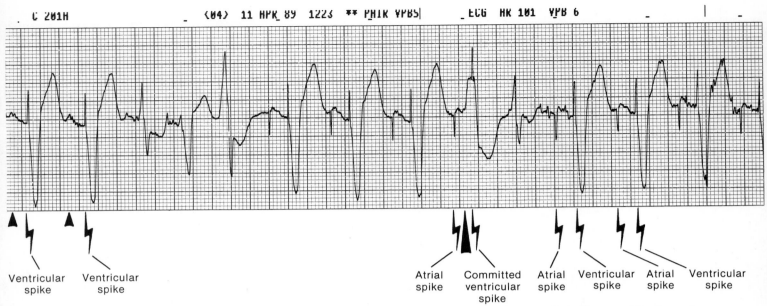

Figure 9–77. Ventricular pseudofusion beats reflect combined depolarization resulting from simultaneous supraventricular and electronic pacemaker stimuli.

of the intrinsic complex with the potential of initiating ventricular tachycardia. The patient's other biologic complexes show no evidence of pacemaker activity. This can be verified by searching for spikes at expected intervals. There are no atrial spikes at V-A intervals of 440 msec, nor any ventricular spikes at P-V intervals of 200 msec.

In some instances of atrial fibrillation developing shortly after implantation of a DVI pacemaker, it is suspected that the pacemaker may have been responsible. Furthermore, induction of ventricular tachycardia has been observed in the committed pulse generator when the ventricular electronic impulse occurred during the vulnerable period of a spontaneous ventricular beat. To address the potential hazards of obligatory ventricular firing after each atrial depolarization (whether electronic or sinoatrial in origin), two mechanisms (safety window firing and the noncommitted mode) have been developed.

In Figure 9–78, the characteristics of the **safety window** feature can be identified. The typical A-V sequence of electronic pacemaker activity can be seen in the majority of beats. However, beats 3 and 8 possess altered appearances. The atrial spike can be clearly delineated by measuring the V-A intervals. A notch is present within the QRS complexes of beats 3 and 8. In each case, this artifact is equidistant from the preceding atrial spike (120 msec). This compares with the normal firing during A-V sequential pacing of 180 msec. The generator, having sensed the intrinsic QRS, initiated a ventricular spike at an interval shorter than the normal firing interval. The early firing of the ventricular pulse prevents occurrence of an electrical discharge during the vulnerable repolarization phase of these two cardiac cycles. This safety window timing is usually an A-V interval of 110 to 120 msec. Two other beats possess configurations that differ from the typical A-V sequentially produced patterns. Beat 4 is probably a supraventricular complex (note the change in the QRS and T wave appearance). Complex 10 is a combination of the spontaneous ventricular beat and the A-V sequentially initiated ventricular complexes (compare the duration and appearance of the QRS and T wave configurations). The characteristic of this beat is similar to fusion beats produced when VPCs and supraventricular beats are superimposed and is thus referred to as a **pseudofusion** beat.

The pulse generator of some models of DVI pacemakers has the capability to sense

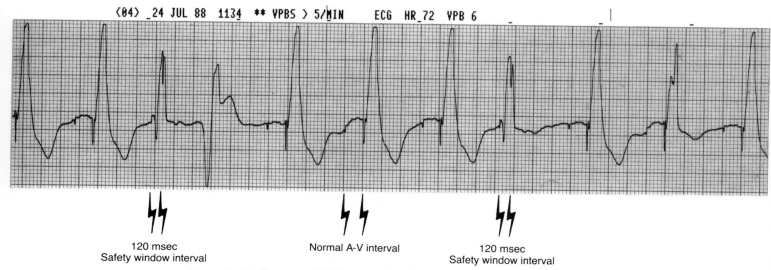

<04> _24 JUL 88 1134 ** VPBS > 5/MIN   ECG HR_72 VPB 6

120 msec
Safety window interval

Normal A-V interval

120 msec
Safety window interval

Figure 9–78. Committed DVI pacemaker demonstrating the safety window feature.

ventricular activity *during* the electronic PR interval (more properly called the A-V interval). Should a ventricular ectopic beat occur during this period, the firing is inhibited.

This **noncommitted mode** of pacemaker can be examined in Figure 9–79. The strip begins with complete control of the rhythm by the A-V sequential pacemaker. The fourth beat has both an atrial and a ventricular spike. However, the QRS complex and T wave have altered configurations. The fifth beat has an atrial spike (V-A interval is normal), which is followed by a QRS of supraventricular configuration. This atrial spike is *not* followed by a ventricular spike at any expected interval (normal A-V sequential interval or safety window interval). This noncommitted DVI feature can be seen again in the last beat of the strip. Reexamining the fourth cycle, we can now identify it as a pseudofusion beat.

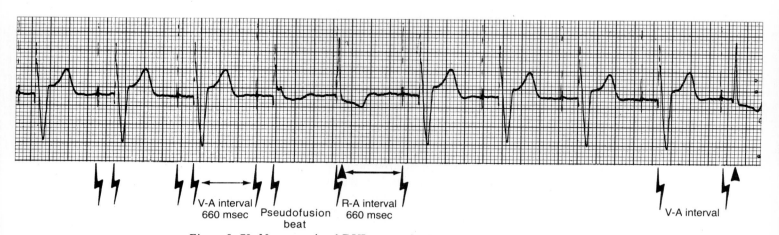

V-A interval
660 msec   Pseudofusion   R-A interval
                 beat   660 msec

V-A interval

Figure 9–79. Noncommitted DVI pacemaker.

The A-V sequential pacemaker is typically used for the treatment of bradyarrhythmias. In Figure 9–80, however, an A-V sequential pacemaker was used to eliminate ectopic ventricular beats. The patient was admitted for episodes of lightheadedness and blurred vision. It was suspected that the A-V sequential pacemaker that had been inserted the previous year was malfunctioning. The admission rhythm strip (Fig. 9–80A) reveals appropriate DVI pacemaker activity and the presence of runs of ventricular

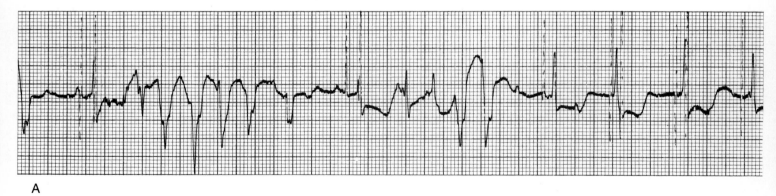

A

Figure 9–80. (*A*) Episodes of ventricular tachycardia occur between A-V sequential pacemaker activity.

tachycardia—the true cause of the presenting symptoms. Treatment with usual antiarrhythmics was attempted, but the patient experienced many adverse reactions.

The rate of the A-V sequential pacemaker was increased from 88 to 106 per minute, and the ventricular tachyarrhythmia was eliminated (Fig. 9–80*B*).

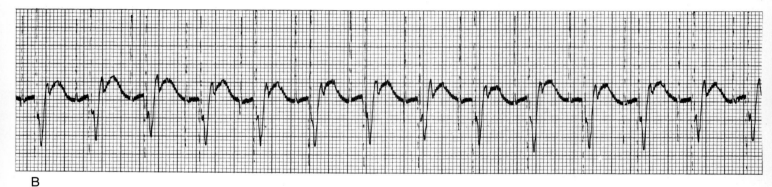

B

Figure 9–80. (*B*) Elimination of ventricular tachycardia when the rate of the A-V sequential pacemaker is increased to over 100 per minute.

The DVI pacemaker is satisfactory in most patients with complete A-V block and sinus node dysfunction because the A-V block protects the ventricles if supraventricular tachyarrhythmias or atrial fibrillation develops. However, the absence of atrial sensing results in competition with supraventricular rhythms, reducing the hemodynamic benefit of synchronous pacing. Furthermore, atrial pacing competing with ectopic beating may be responsible for initiating atrial fibrillation in some patients, eliminating A-V synchrony altogether. To solve this problem, the function of atrial sensing-inhibition has been added to the dual-chamber pacemaker, to be described next.

The Universal Pacemaker

The most comprehensive version of the electronic pacemakers is the universal (or fully automated) system. It combines the functions of rate responsiveness and A-V sequential pacing along with various inhibitory safeguards and programming capabilities already described (Fig. 9–81).

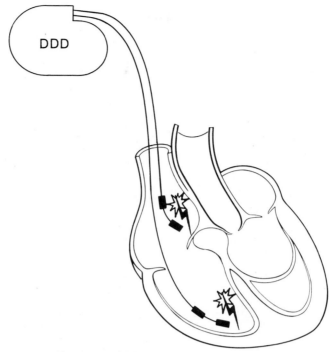

Figure 9–81. The universal (DDD) pacemaker.

Specifically, the universal pacemaker performs the following functions:

- It *paces* dual chambers to maintain sequential contractions of atria and ventricles in complete A-V block. In the absence of an acceptable spontaneous sinoatrial rhythm, it reverts to the function of an **A-V sequential pacemaker.**
- It *senses* spontaneous atrial depolarizations, triggering ventricular pacing. When a sinus rhythm is present and its rate falls within an acceptable range, this rate-responsive feature behaves precisely like the **atrial synchronous pacemaker.** It enables a natural sinoatrial rhythm to govern heart rate even in complete A-V block.
- It *inhibits* atrial and ventricular pacing in response to sensed premature atrial and ventricular depolarizations. In atrial flutter or fibrillation with complete A-V block, it functions as a VVI pacemaker.

The universal pacemaker is designated the DDD system, referring to its dual-chamber pacing, sensing, and inhibitory-triggering capabilities. It provides the most physiological electronic pacing available to match exertional demand in the compromised myocardium.

The following series demonstrates the use of a complex electronic pacemaker and many of its special features.

The tracing in Figure 9–82A was recorded by a paramedic at the home of a semiconscious 50-year-old man who had collapsed without warning. Blood pressure could not be obtained, although peripheral pulses were detectable. History revealed minor episodes of lightheadedness during the previous several weeks.

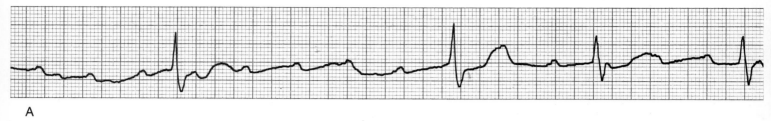

A

Figure 9–82. (*A*) Field monitor strip obtained by paramedics on a semiconscious 50-year-old man.

Using telemetry and radio instructions, the paramedic injected 0.6 mg of atropine. The tracing in Figure 9–82*B* was recorded 2 minutes later.

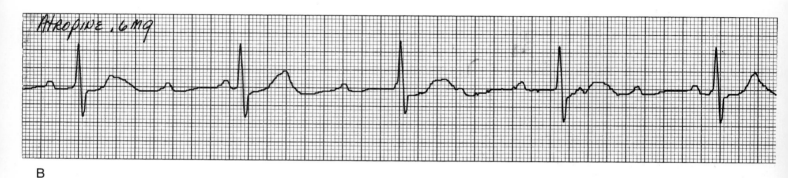

B

Figure 9–82. (*B*) Rhythm following administration of atropine.

Consciousness and blood pressure improved only slightly, and an infusion of isoproterenol at 10 µg per minute was administered, achieving return of normal mentation and a blood pressure of 100/50. The tracing in Figure 9–82*C* was obtained, and stable vital functions were maintained throughout transport to the hospital.

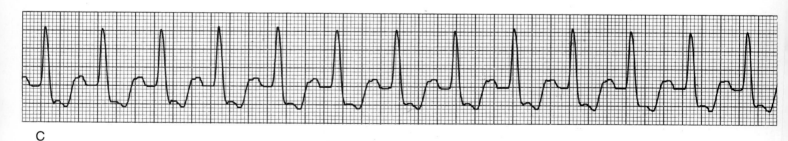

C

Figure 9–82. (*C*) Isoproterenol infusion provided cardiovascular support throughout transport to the hospital.

Intermittent complete A-V block was documented during the last episode of syncope, and a thorough workup revealed sinus node dysfunction but no evidence of myocardial ischemia. Because the patient was a high school coach in a physically demanding role, the universal pacemaker was chosen for optimum cardiac function. With the patient at rest, the feature of dual pacing is shown in Figure 9–82*D*.

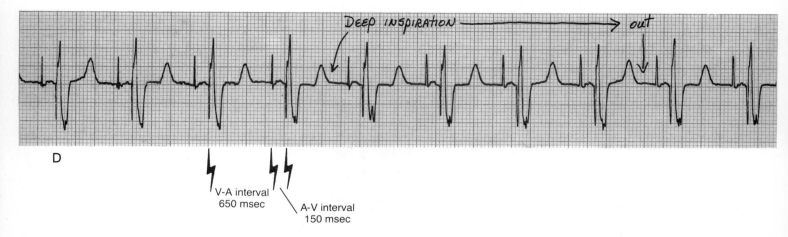

Figure 9–82. (*D*) The A-V sequential mode of the DDD controls the rhythm throughout this monitor strip.

The precise regularity of atrial pacing, even during a respiratory maneuver, is in keeping with an A-V sequential pacemaker rhythm. The somewhat indistinct contour of the P wave is typical of atrial pacing. In each cardiac cycle, a ventricular spike follows the atrial spike after an interval of 150 msec (0.15 second), an artificial A-V interval preset by the manufacturer. Functioning in the A-V sequential mode, the pacemaker provides complete atrial and complete ventricular capture.

The DDD pacemaker responds to spontaneous atrial depolarizations by turning off atrial pacing. This function is demonstrated in the tracing in Figure 9–82*E*, in which A-V sequential pacing is replaced by atrial synchronous ventricular pacing when the native atrial rate exceeds 76 beats/minute.

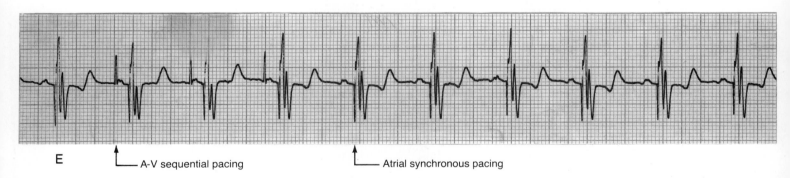

Figure 9–82. (*E*) DDD pacemaker exhibiting A-V sequential and atrial synchronous modes.

The capability of the DDD pacemaker to support increased physical activity by responding to an accelerated sinoatrial rate is shown in Figure 9–82*F*, recorded immediately after the patient climbed a flight of stairs. The heart rate has increased to 110 beats per minute, observed at the beginning of the tracing. Atrial pacemaker spikes are not seen because the natural sinus pacemaker is dictating the atrial rate (i.e., atrial pacing by the pulse generator is inhibited by the spontaneous atrial rhythm). Ventricular pacing is governed by the sinus rate. Thus, an atrial synchronous rhythm is maintained to support the higher demands of physical exertion.

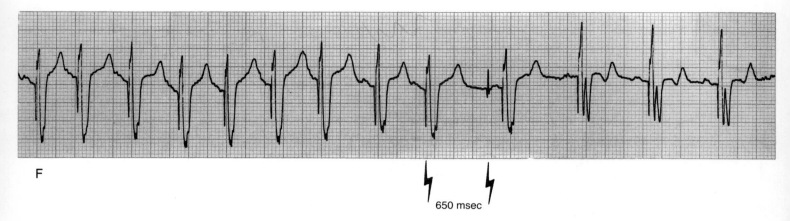

F

650 msec

Figure 9–82. (*F*) Changes in sinus rate result in the DDD pacemaker alternating between atrial synchronous and A-V sequential modes.

As the sinus rate slows after exercise, natural P waves emerge and become visible. The rate continues to slow until, after an interval of 650 msec following a ventricular pacemaker stimulus, atrial pacing recommences. This sequence demonstrates the protection afforded by the universal pacemaker against excessive slowing while preserving the advantage of A-V sequential function.

For review of the functions of the universal pacemaker and for learning some additional features, tracings of a 41-year-old fire fighter are presented (Fig. 9–83). He had experienced giddiness and weakness on heavy effort for 2 or 3 weeks. On a detailed examination, the only abnormality detected was severe first-degree A-V block with a PR interval of 0.36 second. Electrophysiological studies were then performed, and rapid atrial pacing induced transient complete A-V block, presumably caused by fatigue within the A-V nodal system. The idioventricular rate of 40 to 50 observed in this period would account for insufficient cardiac output to support strenuous activity. Recent history of a tick bite with a large red lesion in the axilla suggested the possibility of Lyme disease; a high serum titer confirmed the diagnosis. Lyme disease is occasionally complicated by cardiac conduction disturbances as a late manifestation.

An electronic pacemaker was indicated, and the DDD type was selected because of its physiological advantages in active patients. The series in Figure 9–83 was obtained on a routine pacemaker checkup 1 year after the acute illness. During this time he was free of symptoms.

In Figure 9–83A, pacing of the ventricles responds to a changing sinus rate associated with respiratory function. Atrial tracking is clearly evident as the rate accel-

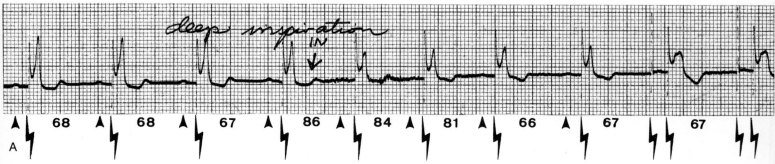

deep inspiration

A   68   68   67   86   84   81   66   67   67

Figure 9–83. (*A*) DDD pacemaker response to a rate change induced by deep inspiration.

erates from 68 to 84 cycles per minute. The subsequently rate slows to 66 per minute on continued breath holding (a vagotonic effect), and the pulse generator switches to dual-chamber pacing. The rate of A-V sequential pacing is fixed at 67 pulses per minute.

In Figure 9–83B, the rate of atrial synchronous pacing slows below a critical level, here induced by vagal stimulation.

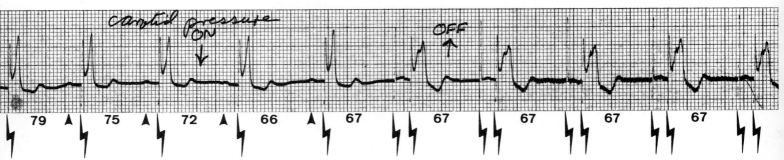

Figure 9–83. (*B*) Vagal stimulation results in assumption of control of both atria and ventricles by the electronic pacemaker when sinus rate slows.

With sinus slowing to the critical point of 66 beats per minute, atrial pacing begins. An A-V sequential rhythm again replaces the atrial synchronous rhythm. Note that the atria in the A-V sequential mode are now paced at a fixed rate. This test establishes the *lower rate limit* at which the pulse generator will allow either chamber to function. The A-V interval is consistently 0.16 second.

In Figure 9–83C, a premature beat interrupts this rhythm, illustrating the inhibitory function.

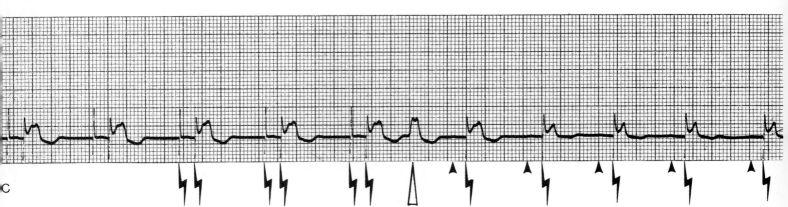

Figure 9–83. (*C*) Interruption of DDD rhythm by a ventricular premature complex.

During A-V sequential pacing, a ventricular premature beat occurs. Both atrial and ventricular firing are inhibited momentarily. A pause following the premature beat allows recovery of the natural atrial pacemaker, and a spontaneous impulse is generated. With this change, atrial synchronous pacing is restored, and the rate is slightly more rapid.

Atrial sensing pacemakers also have an upper rate limit to protect against supraventricular tachycardias. To test the *upper rate limit* of this pacemaker, the heart rate was increased by exercise (Fig. 9–83D). After the patient ran in place for 1 minute, his heart rate accelerated to 109 beats per minute, and atrial pacing was inhibited (shown on the left). Appropriate atrial tracking is demonstrated as the pulse generator has assumed the atrial synchronous mode. After the patient ran for 2 more minutes, the atrial rate increased to 143 (on the right). At this work load, the upper limit for atrial rate has been exceeded, and the pulse generator automatically goes into the ventricular inhibitory mode. The A-V conduction system is proved to function normally as each atrial beat leads to a ventricular stimulation. Note that the A-V interval has increased during exercise from 0.17 to 0.20 second. Although this increase is small, it is an abnormal response to exercise. Little is known about the long-term cardiac effects of Lyme disease, but in this instance a mild disturbance of A-V conduction has persisted despite full recovery otherwise.

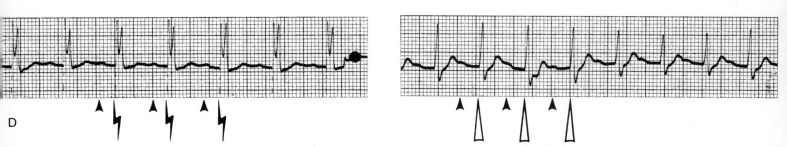

Figure 9–83. (*D*) Tracings reveal DDD function with increasing heart rates during exercise.

After exercise, the heart rate gradually slows, and the rate at which atrial synchronous pacing kicks in can be determined (Fig. 9–83*E*). Here the upper rate limit for atrial tracking-ventricular pacing is shown to be 124 beats per minute. Note that the rate of the paced rhythm is slightly more rapid than the previous natural rhythm and that the pulse-generated A-V interval is slightly shorter than the natural one.

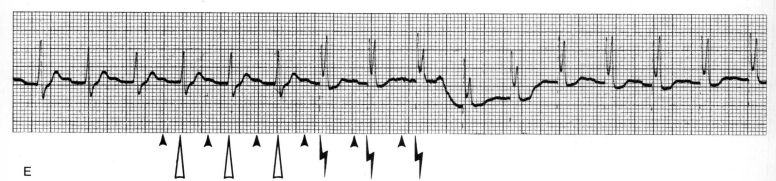

Figure 9–83. (*E*) Resumption of atrial synchronous mode as the heart rate slows after exercise.

Function of the universal pacemaker can be further checked using a magnet placed over the pulse generator. As in the electronic pacemakers described earlier, the magnet turns off inhibitory function, forcing both chambers into the pacing mode. In Figure 9–83*F*, atrial synchronous pacing is replaced by the A-V sequential mode when atrial sensing is inhibited by the magnet. The capability for atrial pacing is demonstrated. The *magnet rate* is 93 pulses per minute. Manufacturers set a specific rate at which each pacemaker will respond under magnet control.

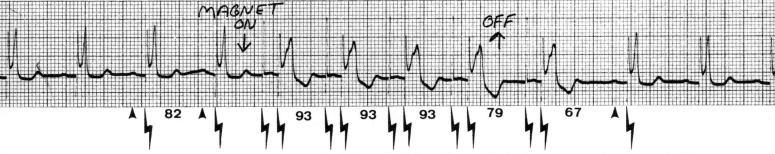

Figure 9–83. (*F*) Magnet inhibition of atrial sensing results in the generator changing to the A-V sequential mode.

The magnet-induced rate can be forced even when the pulse generator is already in the A-V sequential mode, as shown in Figure 9–83*G*. On application of the magnet, the A-V sequential rate increases abruptly from 67 to 93 pulses per minute. Although there is no change in the pacing function except for rate, this maneuver provides a sensitive and reliable index of battery life. As the battery decays, the magnet rate decreases. Consequently, plotting this rate on periodic checkups is a valuable way of detecting impending battery failure.

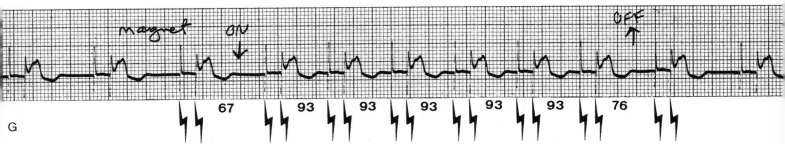

G

Figure 9–83. (*G*) Magnet application during A-V sequential pacing causes an increase in the rate of impulse formation by the generator.

The series of tracings in Figure 9–84 demonstrates how the universal pacemaker protects against tachycardia and against bradycardia while also providing a physiologically favorable interaction between atria and ventricles. The patient was a 71-year-old woman who had angina and was treated for frequent presyncopal symptoms. For many years, she also experienced brief but disabling bouts of rapid palpitations for paroxysmal reentrant tachycardia associated with an intranodal dual-pathway mechanism. Symptoms of lightheadedness and palpitations completely disappeared after insertion of a permanent DDD pulse generator. Six weeks later, she underwent special testing to evaluate the various pacemaker functions. Short lead strips are presented in Figure 9–84*A*, revealing a sinus rhythm with synchronous electronic ventricular pacing.

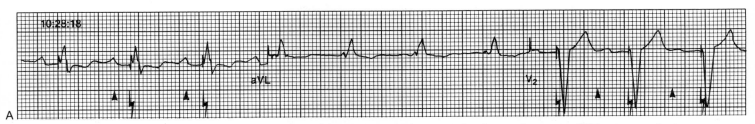

A

Figure 9–84. (*A*) A DDD pacemaker responds appropriately to a sinus rate of 90 beats per minute.

These tracings exhibit a constant P-V interval (from the onset of the P wave to the electronic spike) even as the rate varies slightly, signifying that atrial synchronous pacing is present. The constant P-V interval of 0.22 second (220 msec) indicates a consistent relationship of atrial and ventricular activation.

To evaluate the safeguard functions of the pulse generator against tachycardias, upper rate limit activity was observed during monitored exercise. The patient walked on a treadmill at 2.0 miles per hour at a grade of 3.5%. After 2 minutes of exercise, the sinus rate increased to 130 beats per minute (Fig. 9–84B).

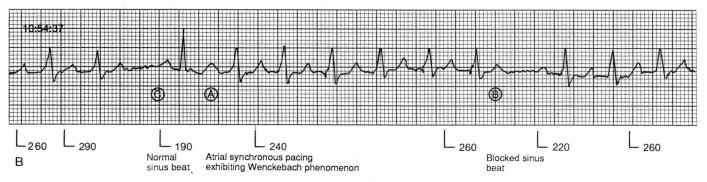

Figure 9–84. (B) The Wenckebach function of the DDD pacemaker replaces the 1:1 conduction when the sinus rate exceeds the upper rate limit of 120 beats per minute (see the text for details of the strip).

Going first to the middle portion of the tracing (A), atrial synchronous pacing is identified. Note that the P-V interval gradually lengthens in consecutive beats until a blocked sinus beat occurs (B). Thereafter, atrial synchronous pacing is resumed, and progressive PV lengthening recurs. The classical form of second-degree A-V block with Wenckebach periodicity is recognized; here, the block is a desired and programmed function of the pulse generator in response to supraventricular rates above a preset rate. This intermittent blocking slows the ventricular rate response to excessively rapid supraventricular beats. In this case, the ventricular rate (based on a whole minute count) was 116 beats per minute.

A variation of the rhythm is seen at the beginning of the tracing. The blocked sinus beat in the Wenckebach cycle is followed by a sinus beat (C) with normal A-V conduction (0.19 second). It results in a narrow ventricular complex with normal intraventricular conduction.

This cycle exhibits several features that require explanation. The appearance of the normal cardiac complex (intrinsic P wave, PR interval, and QRS appearance) reveals appropriate sensing and inhibition by the electronic pacemaker in the presence of atrial and ventricular function. The PR interval is shortened to 0.19 second, and the ventricles are no longer driven by the electronic pacemaker. The pulse generator remains on standby for both atrial and ventricular pacing. From this observation, we conclude that the pulse generator has been programmed to provide an escape ventricular impulse when the delay after an atrial depolarization exceeds at least 0.19 second.

On continued treadmill walking for an additional minute at the same speed and incline settings, the sinus rate has increased to 140 beats per minute (Fig. 9–84C). Atrial synchronous-ventricular pacing persists, but the A-V block has increased to a ratio of 3:2, again with Wenckebach periodicity. Consequently, the ventricular rate is only 93 beats per minute at a time of increased physical exertion.

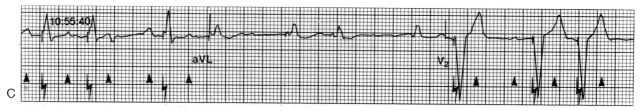

Figure 9–84. (*C*) At an atrial rate of 140 beats per minute, a Wenckebach ratio of 3:2 develops.

The treadmill walking continues for another half minute, and the test is stopped due to fatigue. Pacemaker activity reverts to a 1:1 conduction as the sinus rate slows below the preset upper rate limit setting of 125 beats per minute in response to the termination of exercise (Fig. 9–84*D*).

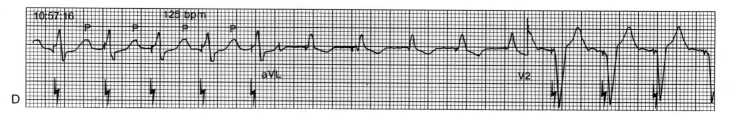

Figure 9–84. (*D*) During the recovery phase of the stress test, 1:1 conduction is again attained as the sinus rate drops to 120 beats per minute.

A 68-year-old woman who had experienced episodes of paroxysmal atrial tachycardia for many years developed A-V block after a small infarction. Her cardiologist prescribed a universal pacemaker to correct her heart block and prevent recurrent tachycardia. The tracings in Figure 9–85 were recorded during her routine stress test to determine pacemaker function 6 weeks after insertion.

In Figure 9–85*A*, the patient reached a heart rate of 120 beats per minute and continued in 1:1 atrioventricular synchrony. The P-V interval measured 280 msec. She was tolerating the exercise well, and her blood pressure was 130/80.

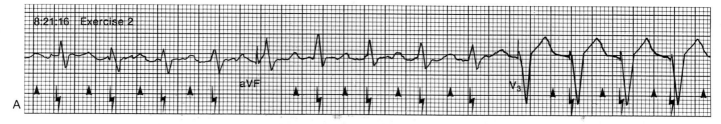

Figure 9–85. (*A*) A universal pacemaker maintains a 1:1 ratio when atrial rate is less than the programmed upper rate limit.

One minute later, when her sinus rate exceeded the programmed upper limit of 125 beats per minute, the pacemaker initiated supraventricular blocking with a 2:1 ratio, and the ventricular rate decreased. In Figure 9–85*B*, the sinus rate of 146 can be seen, with a ventricular rate of 73.

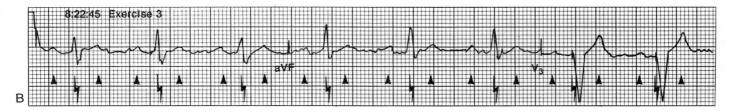

Figure 9–85. (*B*) An atrial rate of 146 results in 2:1 block by this universal pacemaker.

The upper rate limit characteristics of the electronic pacemaker have been documented in this evaluation. This mechanism is important for protecting against paroxysmal tachycardias. The second-degree A-V block phenomenon is a *normal* function of the programmed pacer and should not be considered a malfunction. However, this A-V block mechanism restricts the normal acceleration of ventricular rate response to physical effort. In this instance, it resulted in an inappropriately reduced rate because an increased heart rate is the preeminent variable for supporting increased work load. At this time, the stress test was terminated because the patient's blood pressure dropped to 108/70 and she felt weak. In this case, the patient led a sedentary life, and the limitation of exercise-induced bradycardia rarely interfered with her ordinary activity. Should a patient experience symptoms of decreased output during physically stressful activities, the universal pacemaker can be reprogrammed so that the 2:1 block mechanism will be initiated at a higher rate limit.

A review of additional pacemaker acronyms is appropriate at this time. Normal biological cycle intervals, such as P-P interval, R-R interval, and PR interval, have been used in previous chapters. To interpret complex pacemaker rhythms, another group of acronyms has evolved. A few such letter symbols are described here.

V-V: Interval between consecutive ventricular paced complexes (artificial R-R interval) as seen with totally ventricular pacemaker-controlled rhythms.

A-V: Interval between pacemaker-initiated atrial complex and subsequent related pacemaker-initiated ventricular complex (artificial PR interval).

V-A: Interval from ventricular pacemaker-initiated complex to following pacemaker-initiated atrial complex.

R-V: Interval between any biological QRS (sinus or ectopic origin) and subsequent ventricular pacemaker-induced complex (VVI pacemaker pattern).

R-A: Interval between biological QRS and subsequent atrial pacemaker-induced complex.

A-R: Interval between atrial pacemaker-induced complex and the subsequent biologically produced ventricular complex (requires intact A-V node).

P-V: Interval from onset of P to subsequent ventricular electronic pacemaker spike.

If antegrade conduction through the A-V node occurs and if the ventricular sensor detects a spontaneous depolarization during the artificial A-V interval, ventricular pacing will be inhibited. In effect, the fully automatic pacemaker can be entirely quiescent in the presence of an atrial rhythm of moderate rate which conducts to the ventricles.

The ventricular sensor will also function by inhibiting stimulation should spontaneous ventricular beating occur, identical to the function of the ventricular demand pacemaker. Ectopic ventricular beats inhibit atrial stimulation as well. After a VPC, the atrial pacing rhythm is reset, as in Figure 9–86. The R-A following the VPC and the V-A intervals are both 620 msec.

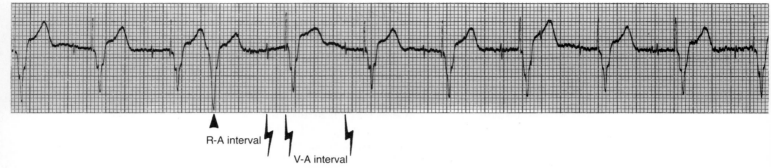

R-A interval

V-A interval

Figure 9–86. The atrial rhythm is reset after a ventricular premature complex.

PACEMAKER-MEDIATED TACHYCARDIA

One liability of the atrial sensing lead is its potential for acting as an artificial accessory pathway, setting the stage for a reentrant circuit in which the pacemaker itself is a component of the circuit. In this complication of the DDD pacemaker, a retrograde impulse passes from the ventricles through the A-V node to the atria. The impulse stimulates the atria, enters the atrial sensing lead, and then passes to the pulse generator. This event triggers a ventricular impulse. Fortuitously timed, the entire circuit may be repeated in the classic reentrant pattern, establishing a sustained supraventricular tachycardia with the atrial sensing lead, the pulse generator and the ventricular pacing lead serving as the descending limb of the circuit. An example of pacemaker-mediated tachycardia is presented in Figure 9–87.

The ventricles are being paced at the upper rate at which the pulse generator is programmed. Rapid pacing is sustained because each ventricular depolarization is conducted to the atria, initiating an atrial depolarization. This event (which occurs after the programmed atrial refractory period) is sensed by the pulse generator, and it responds by firing a ventricular impulse after the programmed A-V interval. The cycle recurs and is repetitious throughout the tracing.

Pacemaker-mediated tachycardias often subside spontaneously as the retrograde conduction pathway fatigues. However, intervention is sometimes necessary.

Because the atrial sensing lead is an integral component of the reentrant circuit, interruption of its function terminates a pacemaker-mediated tachycardia. An easy and effective means of identifying and treating this arrhythmia is with a magnet placed over the pulse generator. The magnet breaks an electrical connection necessary for impulse sensing in both the atria and the ventricles. The electronic pacemaker is forced into the DOO mode, and the tachycardia stops abruptly. Of course, the tachycardia can recur once the magnet is removed. VPCs are the most common precipitating event of pacemaker-mediated tachycardias.

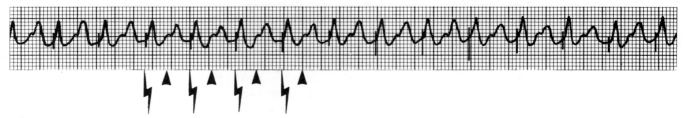

Figure 9–87. Pacemaker-mediated tachycardia.

Most individuals with A-V node dysfunction retain the capability for retrograde conduction, which is present in about one-fourth of those with complete A-V block. Consequently, most DDD pacemakers are designed to protect against the reentrant phenomenon by having an adjustable refractory period for atrial sensing. Pacemaker-mediated tachycardias can usually be prevented by programming this refractory period to extend beyond the interval required for completing a reentrant circuit.

Prevention of pacemaker-mediated tachycardias may also be achieved by depressing retrograde conduction with drugs, such as digitalis, verapamil or beta-adrenergic blocking agents. As a last resort for recurring tachycardias, the function of atrial sensing can be eliminated, converting the DDD pacemaker to the DVI (A-V sequential) or the VVI mode.

To emphasize one last point, pacemaker-*mediated* tachycardias are basically different from pacemaker-*induced* tachycardias. In the latter instance, an electronic impulse initiates a tachycardia by striking the action potential during its vulnerable period of repolarization, a mechanism described earlier under complications of electrical shock in Chapter 4, in the section entitled Electrocardioversion. Once the tachycardia is operant, the electronic pacemaker is no longer part of the circuit. There is no evidence for DDD pacemaker stimulation, because the ectopic tachycardia places it into the inhibited mode in both chambers.

A composite of basic types of electronic pacemakers is shown to highlight their different features (Fig. 9–88).

NORMAL SINUS RHYTHM. Normal sinus rhythm (NSR) is shown for reference.

ATRIAL-INHIBITED PACEMAKER. After a pause in the sinus rhythm, an electronic pulse occurs, driving the atria. This mechanism requires a sensor-inhibitor system in an atrium. The pacemaker preserves the normal sequence of atrioventricular contraction. It is used to control sinus node dysfunction, but only when A-V nodal conduction is intact.

VENTRICULAR-INHIBITED PACEMAKER. A pause in the sinus rhythm is interrupted by an electronic pulse, which produces a ventricular depolarization. A sensor-inhibitor system serves to prevent excessive ventricular slowing, even in complete A-V block. Ventricular pacing is asynchronous with atrial activity.

A-V SEQUENTIAL PACEMAKER. Slowing of the natural sinus rate turns on atrial pacing, and ventricular pacing follows after an appropriate interval. As the sinus rate becomes faster, atrial sensing once again turns off atrial pacing, but the interval exceeds the programmed quiescient period of the ventricles, and a ventricular escape pulse is emitted. This pacemaker preserves the physiological advantage of coordinated chamber contractions. Sensor-inhibitor pacemaker systems are required in both an atrium and a ventricle.

ATRIAL RESPONSIVE PACEMAKER. The ventricles alone are paced, but the rate at which they are paced is governed by the atrial rate. This pacemaker incorporates an atrial sensor and a preset A-V interval. It provides a mechanism by which appropriate cardiac acceleration can occur during periods of exertion, even in the presence of complete A-V block, while maintaining synchronous contractions of atria and ventricles. It depends on a normally functioning sinoatrial pacemaker.

UNIVERSAL PACEMAKER. This device combines the features of the atrial-responsive pacemaker and the A-V sequential pacemaker.

The electronic pacemakers described thus far have been used to protect against the bradycardia attendant to depression of impulse formation and/or impulse conduction. The newer designs improve cardiac function by approximating heart rate to match the degree of physical exertion or by maintaining the physiological advantage of atrioventricular sequential contractions. More complicated pacemakers combine both features. One further application of the electronic pacemaker is for the treatment of paroxysmal tachycardia by the function of overdrive pacing.

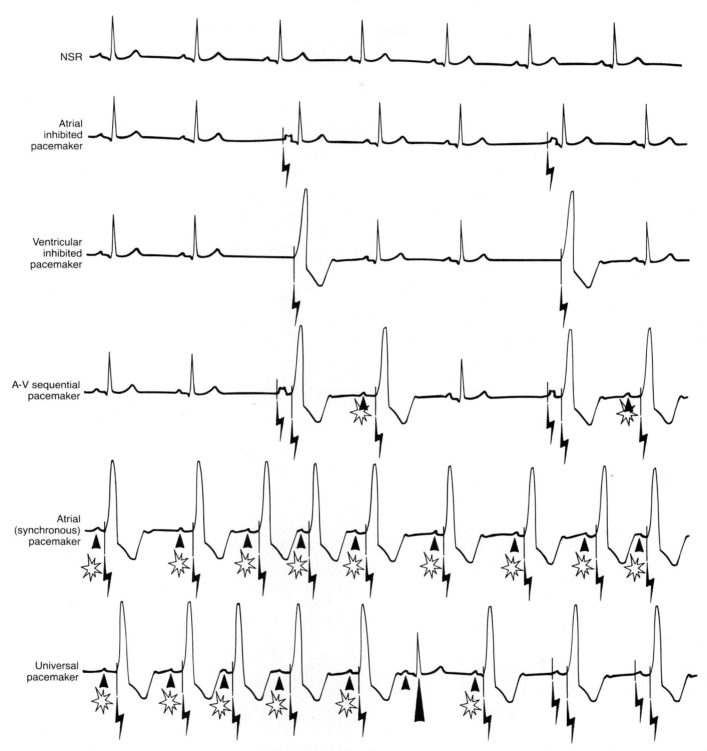

Figure 9–88. Schematic summary of types of electronic pacemakers. (▲ = spontaneous atrial complex; ✳ = sensed atrial complex; ⌇ = electronic pacing [atrial or ventricular])

TACHYCARDIC INDICATIONS FOR THE ELECTRONIC PACEMAKER

The Atrial Overdrive Pacemaker

Reentrant tachycardias depend on a reverberating electrical impulse in a closed loop of conducting tissue. If a series of electronic impulses are imposed into the circuit at a rate *faster* than the ectopic rate, the electronic stimuli supervene as pacemaker for the chamber(s), and the reentrant mechanism is suppressed. If the rapid electronic impulse suddenly stops, the reentrant circuit is no longer operative, thus allowing for resumption of control by the sinus pacemaker. By this strategy, **overdrive** pacing with a short burst of rapid impulses from a pulse generator is used to terminate ectopic tachycardias.

An example of atrial overdrive pacing is presented. It was used to treat recurring paroxysmal tachycardias developing in a patient who was in intensive care and had respiratory failure as a result of pneumonitis complicating advanced, chronic bronchitis. The arrhythmia (Fig. 9–89A) may have been provoked by intensive administration of adrenergic bronchodilators.

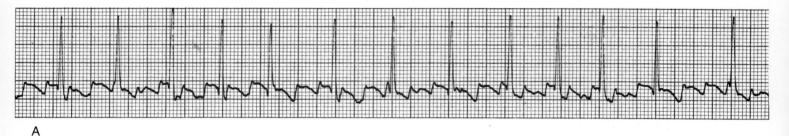

A

Figure 9–89. (A) Atrial flutter with variable conduction resulting in ventricular rates ranging from 130 to 75 beats per minute.

To manage any recurrences, a wire electrode was passed into the right atrium through the external jugular vein and attached to a battery-powered pulse generator with overdrive pacing capability. Moments after the appearance of another episode of tachycardia, the nurse activated the pulse generator unit. A burst of electronic impulses is evident, followed by sudden turn-off. The ensuing rhythm demonstrates absence of the ectopic rhythm and takeover by the normal pacemaker (Fig. 9–89B).

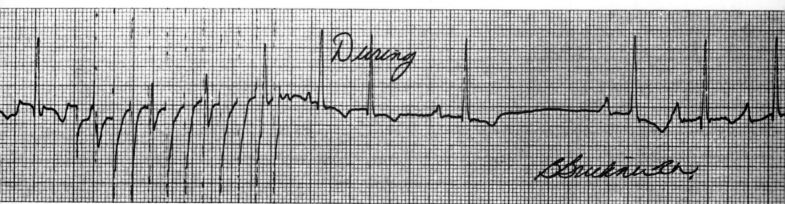

B

Figure 9–89. (B) Atrial overdrive pacing at a rate of 350 stimuli per minute converts atrial flutter to a sinus rhythm.

Atrial flutter with a ventricular rate of 100 per minute was observed at the beginning of the recording. A succession of electronic impulses suddenly occur at a rate of 350 per minute. Most of these impulses appear to capture the atria and some result in depolarizations of the ventricles. Immediately after the burst of 12 stimuli, a sinus rhythm supervenes at an irregular rate and with a PR interval of 0.29 second. Rapid intracardiac electronic pacing was used to interrupt a supraventricular tachycardia.

Temporary atrial overdrive pacing usually converts the rhythm within 3 to 4 seconds. The examples in Figure 9–90 show an unsuccessful attempt to override atrial tachycardia. The 56-year-old patient had had coronary artery bypass surgery 4 days previously and had been having increasingly more frequent atrial premature beats before developing tachycardia with an atrial rate of approximately 300 per minute (Fig. 9–90A).

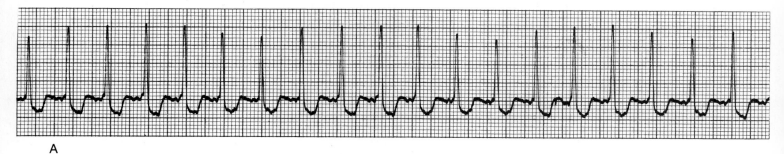

A

Figure 9–90. (*A*) Atrial tachycardia with a ventricular response rate of 150 beats per minute.

The nurse in the intensive care unit attached the external atrial generator to the existing wires placed during surgery. Following standard protocol, the pacemaker was activated at a rate of 350 per minute. When this overdrive rate was unsuccessful, the rate was increased to 650 per minute, the amperage was increased to 5 milliamperes, and the pacemaker was activated for a period of more than 5 seconds (Fig. 9–90B).

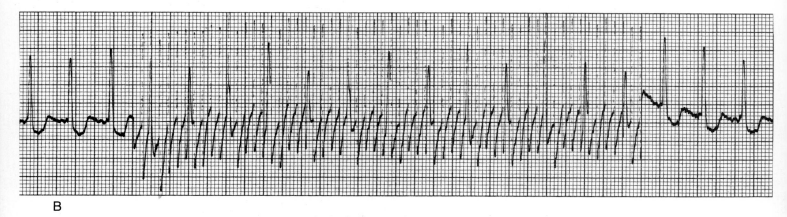

B

Figure 9–90. (*B*) Application of atrial overdrive pacemaking for 5 to 6 seconds.

The surgeon suggested that further attempts would probably also be unsuccessful because of the length of time since placement of the wires and resultant poor conduction from the wire to the surrounding myocardium. Conversion subsequently was effected with verapamil.

Because the atrial overdrive pulse generator fires at extremely rapid rates (some pulse up to 800 beats per minute), it is imperative that the temporary pulse generator never be attached inadvertently to the ventricular pacing lead. Rapid rates for atrial pacing are not hazardous to ventricular function because the ventricles are protected by the limited conduction capacity of the A-V node (just as in atrial flutter and fibrillation). On the other hand, such rapid pacing directly into a ventricular lead would be perilous.

Permanent overdrive pacemakers are now available for persons with a high risk of paroxysmal tachyarrhythmias, particularly for those who have extremely rapid supraventricular tachycardias that have proved resistant to drug therapy and who are not candidates for surgical interruption of a bypass tract. The implantable pulse generator can be activated by the patient, using a radio transmitter over the unit on first recognizing the symptoms of tachycardia. The battery-operated transmitter is activated manually for approximately 1 second.

Other forms of atrial overdrive pacemakers are automatic responders. With an atrial sensing lead, the pulse generator is activated when atrial depolarizations exceed a preset rate that turns on the rapid firing sequence in the electronic pacemaker. After a burst of several stimuli (usually three to six), it turns off. If the technique is successful, the spontaneous tachycardia is aborted.

The Ventricular Overdrive Pacemaker

Using the same principle, automatic overdrive pacing can be adapted for treatment of recurrent ventricular tachycardias. A sensing lead in the ventricle triggers a burst of impulses into a ventricular pacing lead when the natural rate is above the established upper limit.

Because overdrive pacing in the ventricles has the potential for inducing ventricular fibrillation, this method for control of recurring ventricular tachycardias has more limited application than in supraventricular tachycardias. Alternative methods such as electrocardioversion are preferred.

THE EXPANDED ELECTRONIC PACEMAKER CODE

To keep up with development of these more complex electronic pacemakers, the identification code system established by the ICHD has been modified. In 1987, the North American Society of Pacing and Electrophysiology (NASPE) and the British Pacing and Electrophysiology Group (BPEG) proposed changes in the code to embrace these advances.* For example, a letter in the **fifth** position refers to the **antitachycardia** mode. Here, the letter **P** indicates that the pacemaker is capable of overdrive *pacing*. An **S** in this position signifies that an electrical *shock* (greater than 1 millijoule) is discharged when a tachyarrhythmia occurs as described below.

The duration and intensity of the burst of overdriving impulses can be adjusted in some units by an external transmitter device, adjustments that are indicated by a letter in the **fourth** position. According to the recent coding system, **P** in this position states that rate and/or output can be *programmed*. The letter **M** indicates that *multiple* functions can be reset. The letter **C** denotes that the power generator has an output that can be communicated by telemetry. The complete pacemaker code is shown in Table 9–2.

---

* Bernstein AD, Camm AJ, Fletcher RD, et al. The NASPE/BPEG generic pacemaker code for anti-bradyarrhythmia and adaptive-rate pacing and antitachyarrhythmia devices. PACE 10:794–799, 1987.

Table 9–2. NBG PACEMAKER CODE (1987)

Code Positions				
I *Chamber* *Paced*	*II* *Chamber* *Sensed*	*III* *Response to* *Sensing*	*IV* *Programmable* *Functions*	*V* *Antitachyarrhythmia* *Functions*
V, ventricle	V, ventricle	T, triggers pacing	P, programmable rate and/or output	P, overdrive pacing
A, atrium	A, atrium	I, inhibits pacing	M, multiprogrammability of rate, output, sensitivity, etc.	S, shock
D, double	D, double	D, triggers and inhibits pacing	C, communicating functions (telemetry)	O, none
O, none	O, none	O, none	R, rate modulation O, none	

(Modified from Bernstein AD, Camm AJ, Fletcher RD, et al. The NASPE/BPEG generic pacemaker code for antibradyarrhythmia and adoptive-rate pacing and antitachyarrhythmia devices. PACE 10: 794–799, 1987.)

AUTOMATIC IMPLANTABLE CARDIOVERTER-DEFIBRILLATOR

One further technological step is the automatic antitachycardia device used for recurring ventricular tachycardia-fibrillation. The pulse generator (which is about the size of a cigarette pack) is inserted in a pouch formed within the abdominal wall (Fig. 9–91). It is connected to patch electrodes placed on the epicardial surfaces of the right

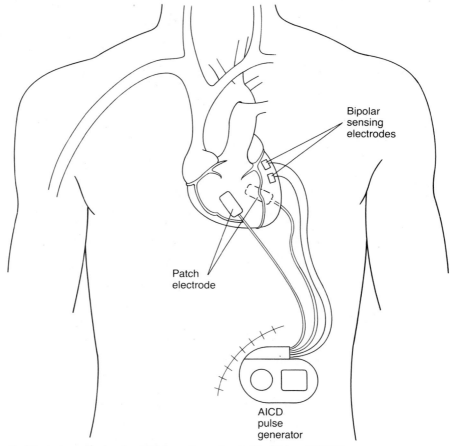

Bipolar
sensing
electrodes

Patch
electrode

AICD
pulse
generator

Figure 9–91. Automatic implantable cardioverter-defibrillator (AICD).

and the left ventricles for dispersing the electrical charge. Sensing electrodes are placed on the epicardial wall to monitor ventricular activity. (Alternatively, endocardial sensing leads may be used.)

On sensing excessive rate or the loss of organized ventricular complexes, the automatic implantable cardioverter-defibrillator (AICD) discharges within a programmed time, usually within 20 seconds. The energy of initial discharge is about 25 joules. Repeated shocks, usually set at somewhat higher levels of energy, may be given if the pulse generator does not recognize the return of distinct ventricular complexes.

Because internal electrical shock is delivered directly to the myocardium, the amount of amperage is relatively small compared with that required for external defibrillation. Nevertheless, it is strong enough for the patient to be aware of an uncomfortable jolt in the chest. Even so, it is desirable that the implanted unit recognize the arrhythmia and provide a shock before the patient has collapsed.

Electrophysiological studies were performed on a 55-year-old woman with recurring episodes of ventricular tachycardia of unknown cause. Fainting occurred with several of these events, and the condition proved resistant to drug therapy. An internal cardiac defibrillator was implanted, and at the end of this procedure ventricular tachycardia appeared. In the tracings in Figure 9–92, which are reduced in size, each set records three simultaneous external limb leads. Paper speed is 50 mm per second, giving a spread-out appearance of the waveforms and doubling of intervals; the sinus rate is 96. In Figure 9–92A, normal sinus rhythm is replaced by a ventricular rhythm.

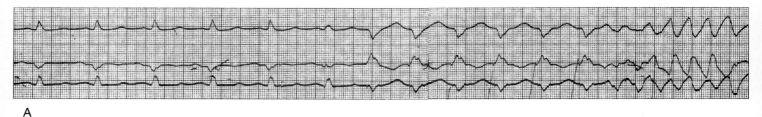

A

Figure 9–92. (*A*) An electrophysiological laboratory tracing shows onset of a ventricular rhythm (paper speed is 50 mm per second).

At 14 seconds from the onset of ventricular tachycardia, an electric shock is delivered automatically (Fig. 9–92B).

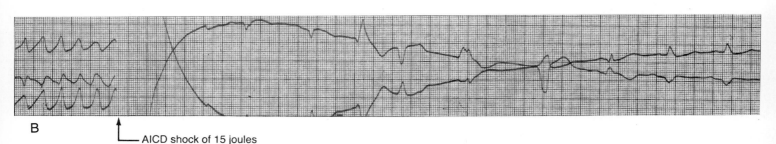

B

└─ AICD shock of 15 joules

Figure 9–92. (*B*) A 15-joule shock is delivered by an AICD.

A continuous tracing from this point demonstrates the electrical blackout, then a brief period of idioventricular activity and within seconds restoration of a sinus rhythm. Syncope with injury from a fall or cerebral ischemia was no longer a constant threat, and the patient eventually learned to tolerate the occasional jolts.

Progress in refining electronic devices is occurring very rapidly. Many types of pacemakers are now available to meet patients' individual needs. The more complicated arrhythmias can be managed with pacemakers having various combinations of functions. The introduction of systems that match heart rate to physical activity and synchronize chamber activity has provided important steps toward restoring the normal physiological action of the heart. Programmable units add another dimension of benefit, instructing the pulse generator on changing rate and intensity of impulse emissions, sensitivity for sensing, upper and lower rate limits for pacing, atrial refractory period, and atrioventricular sequencing. Under development are external units capable of transmitting information from the pulse generator, such as actual pacing and sensing levels, frequency of ectopic beats and A-V conduction, battery strength, impedance of leads, and memory of activity over extended periods. The automatic cardioverter-defibrillator units are continuing to be refined to enhance their efficiency. Certainly, bioengineering will continue its remarkable advances in electronic development while moving toward simplification of these complex devices for clinicians and patients.

SELF-EVALUATION: STAGE 4

Each of the following electrocardiograms demonstrates compound rhythms, and two or more statements are required. Give complete interpretations.

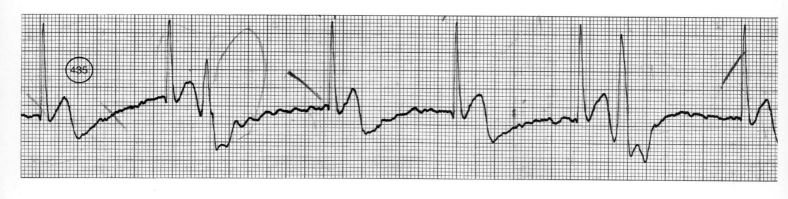

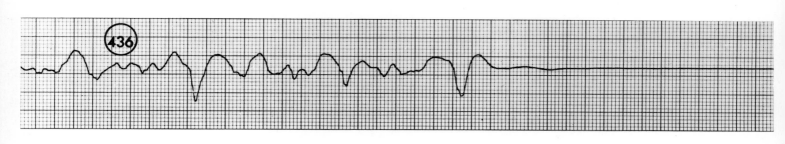

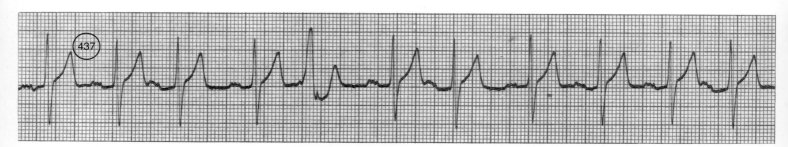

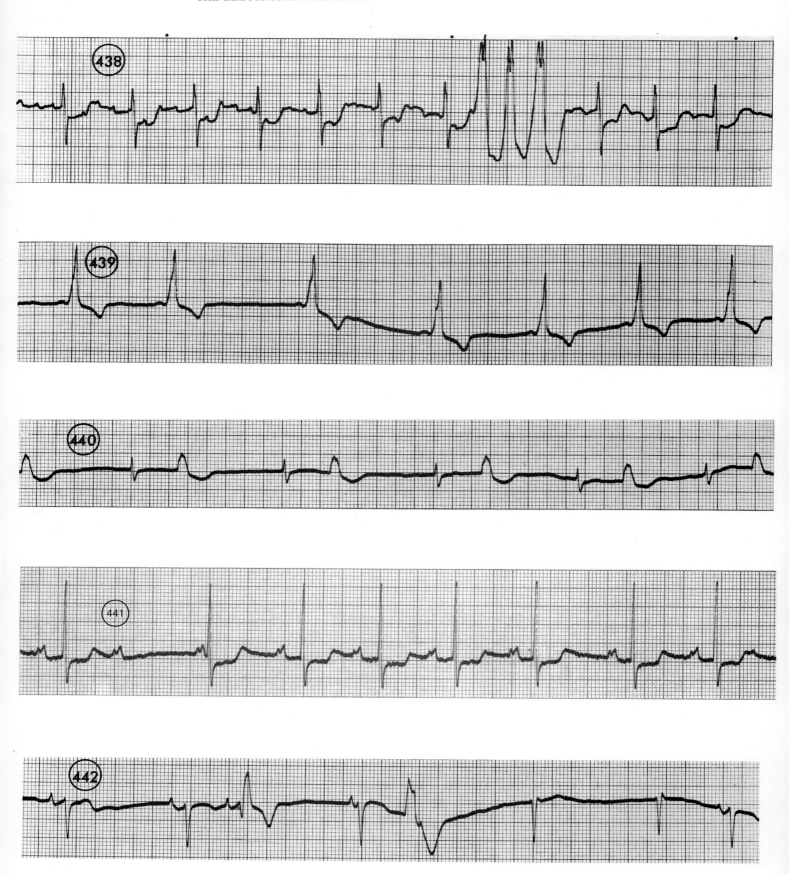

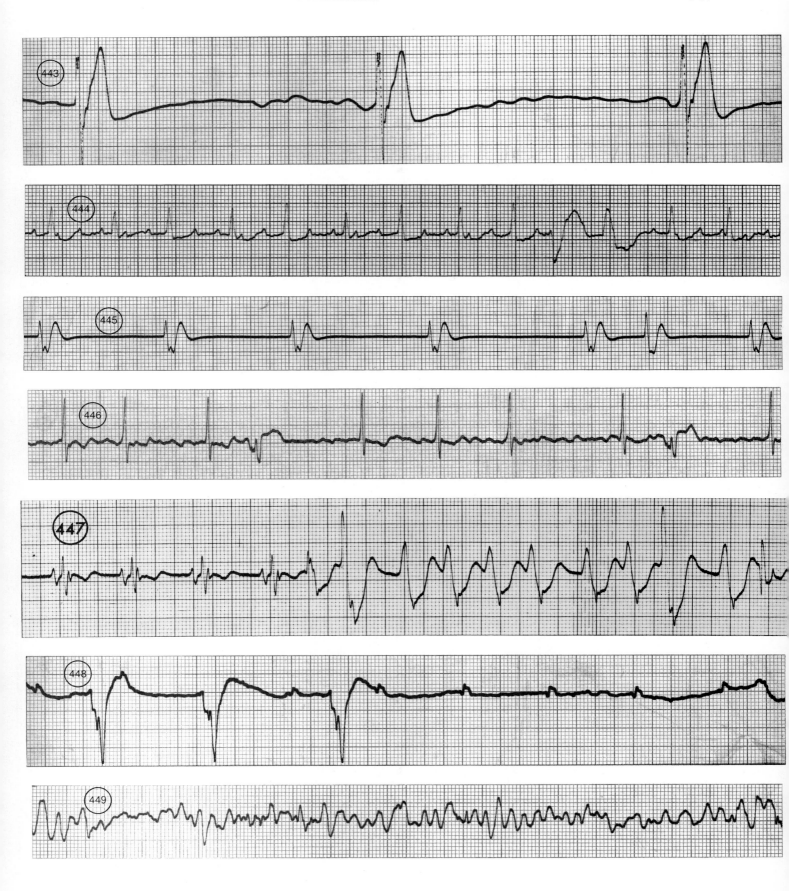

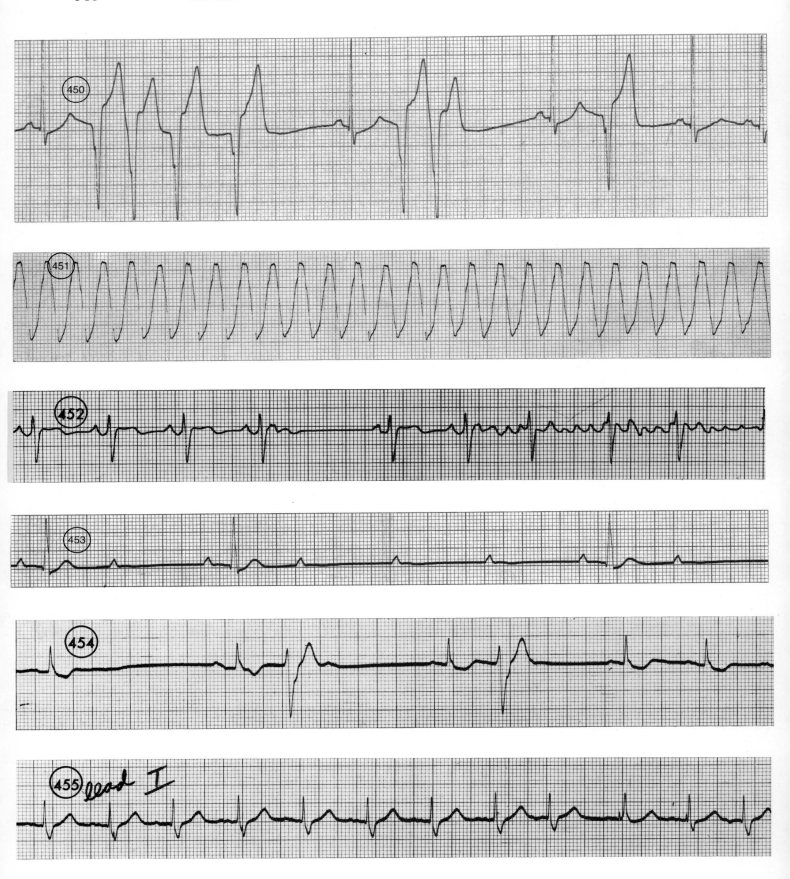

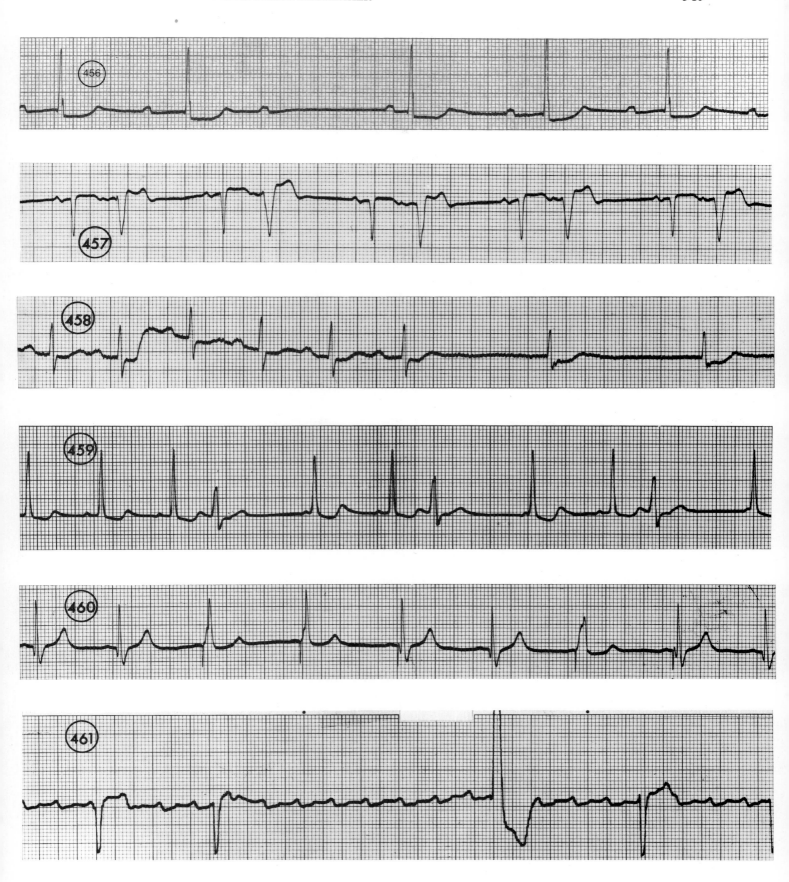

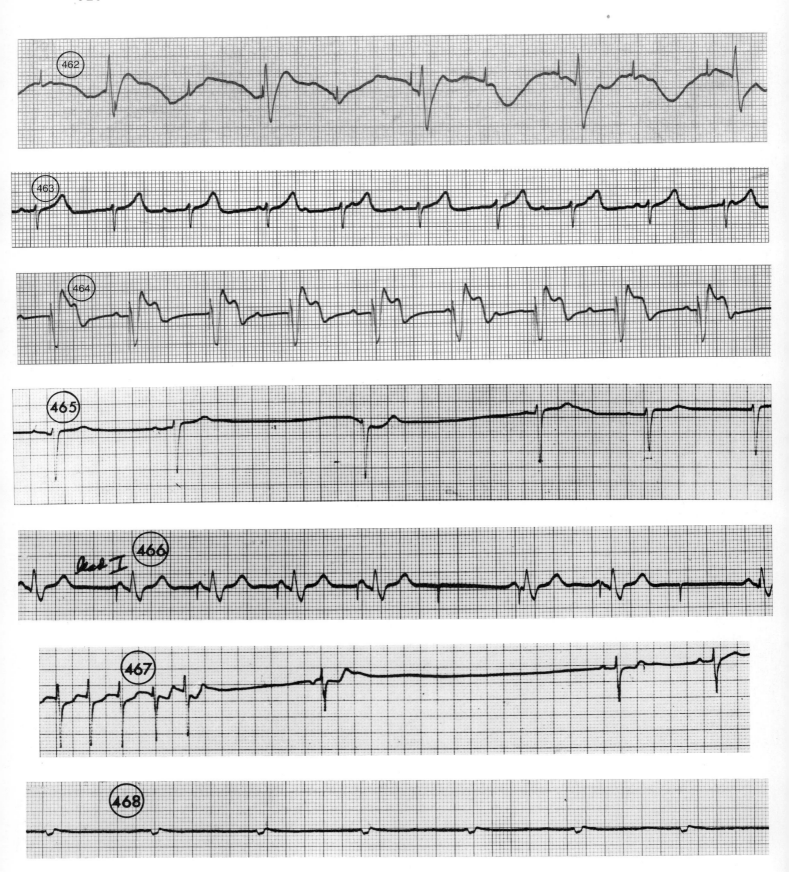

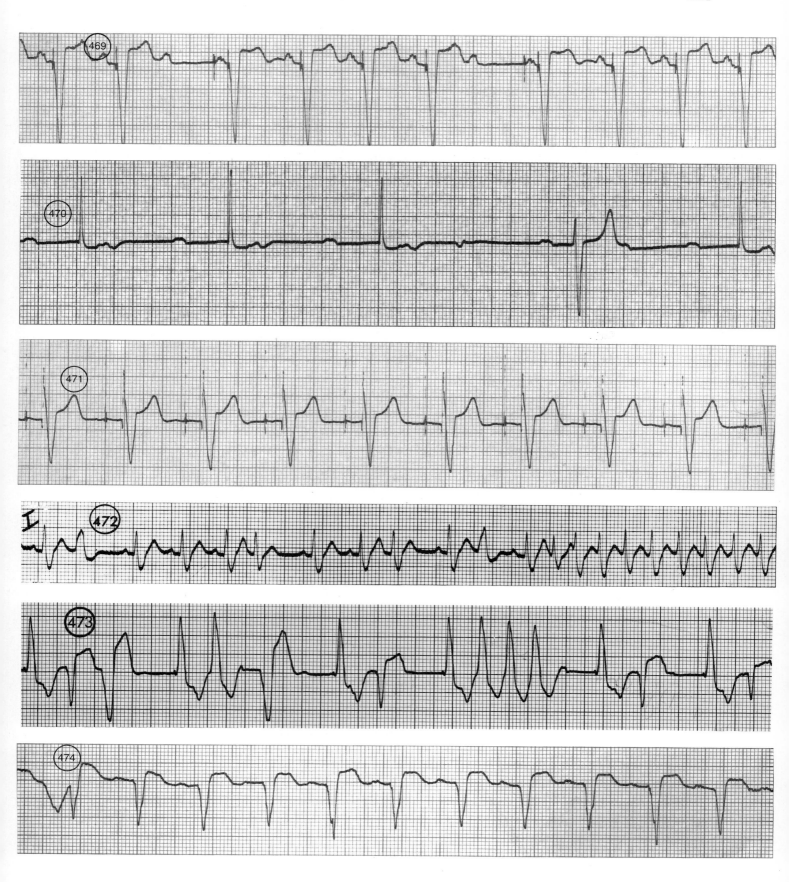

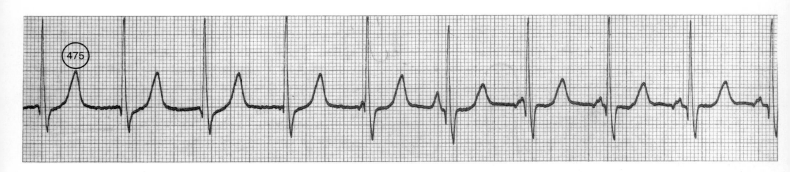

10 The Cardiac Drugs

DRUGS OF EXCITATION
Sympathetic Nervous System: Stimulation
Parasympathetic Nervous System: Inhibition
DRUGS OF DEPRESSION
Sympathetic Nervous System: Inhibition
Parasympathetic Nervous System: Stimulation
Drugs that Affect the Cell Membrane

DIGITALIS
Myocardium
Vasomotor Tone
Electrophysiology
Digoxin
GENERAL PRECAUTIONS WHEN ADMINISTERING CARDIAC DRUGS

This chapter outlines the actions of drugs commonly used in the Coronary Care Unit (CCU). Emphasis is on the conceptual framework for learning their effects on impulse formation and conduction. The chapter is also intended as a reference to the more important pharmacological features—both cardiac and extracardiac, both beneficial and adverse. This chapter is not meant to serve as a comprehensive text on pharmacology, nor does it indicate the choice of drugs for specific arrhythmias or the full range of their side effects. Special considerations for pediatric and pregnant patients are not covered.

Drugs used for treating disorders of the cardiac rhythm act either by enhancing or by inhibiting a specific component of the action potential. Many of them affect more than one component, resulting in complex changes in impulse formation and conduction. Some of the dual- or multiple-action drugs even have opposing effects on the action potential and therefore often alter cardiac function in unpredictable ways. In addition, they may directly affect the dynamics of myocardial contraction. Many of the cardiac drugs also modify peripheral vascular tone, then indirectly affecting cardiac function. Clinicians are becoming increasingly aware of a substantial incidence of **proarrhythmia** effect—that is, the exacerbation of arrhythmias by agents used to protect against them. Virtually all of the drugs used for treatment of arrhythmias have important effects on noncardiac organ systems.

This presentation of the cardiac drugs is arranged according to their predominant action, as summarized in the following outline:

A. Drugs of excitation: used for treatment of rhythms of depression
   1. Drugs that affect the autonomic nervous system
      a. **Adrenergic** (stimulators of sympathetic tone)
      b. **Anticholinergic** (inhibitors of parasympathetic tone)
B. Drugs of depression: used for treatment of rhythms of excitation

1. Drugs that affect the autonomic nervous system
   a. **Antiadrenergic** (inhibitors of sympathetic tone)
   b. **Cholinergic** (stimulators of parasympathetic tone)
2. Drugs that affect the cell membrane
   a. Block sodium channels
   b. Block beta-adrenergic receptors
   c. Prolong repolarization
   d. Block calcium channels

C. Digitalis: considered in a separate class because of its complex actions on the electrophysiology of the heart

Drugs are introduced by their generic names (with their brand names, when available, in parentheses). Thereafter, the drugs are referred to only by their generic names.

DRUGS OF EXCITATION

Sympathetic Nervous System: Stimulation

The **adrenergic agents** accelerate the rate of impulse formation and impulse conduction throughout the heart. They are used to treat bradycardias caused by depression of impulse formation or conduction. This group of drugs, known as **catecholamines**, includes isoproterenol, norepinephrine, epinephrine, dopamine, and dobutamine.

Actions. The catecholamines have the following actions:

- They bind to specific receptor sites on the membrane of excitable cells to activate adenylate cyclase, an essential mediator in the energy-consuming processes of cellular work. They compete with the natural sympathetic neurotransmitters, norepinephrine and epinephrine.
- They act indirectly on automatic and conducting fibers by augmenting sympathetic tone.

IMPULSE FORMATION

- They increase the rate (or slope) of spontaneous depolarization (Phase 4) of the action potential. Thus, automatic tissues accelerate their rate of firing.
- The sinus rate increases. Enhanced impulse formation in ectopic foci may result in premature beats and sustained rhythms from the atria, A-V junction, or ventricles.

IMPULSE CONDUCTION

- They increase the amplitude and maximum rate of depolarization after stimulation (Phase 0) of the action potential. Faster propagation of impulses occurs in conducting fibers in the sinoatrial, atrial, A-V nodal, and Purkinje systems.

MYOCARDIUM

- They increase performance of the myofibrils by
  1. Shortening the duration of systole.
  2. Strengthening the force of contraction.

This increased work, however, exacts a cost by markedly increasing oxygen demand by the myofibrils.

VASCULATURE

- They constrict or dilate blood vessels in various vascular beds. Although the catecholamines act similarly on impulse formation and conduction in the heart and on the myocardium, they differ markedly in their effect on peripheral vascular control.

EXTRACARDIOVASCULAR

- They relax smooth muscles in the bronchi.
- They inhibit secretions by the glands.

Adrenergic drugs may be either excitatory or inhibitory, depending on the specific receptors stimulated. In the cell membrane, **adrenergic receptors** that are involved in cardioacceleration and in myocardial enhancement are referred to as **beta receptors**. Because there are also beta receptors in other organs, those of the heart are further identified as **beta₁** receptors. Beta₂ receptors mediate relaxation of vascular, bronchial, intestinal, uterine, and urinary bladder tone.

Alpha-adrenergic receptors mediate vasoconstriction and contraction of the iris and the sphincters of the intestinal tract and urinary bladder.

Because the drug isoproterenol has pure beta-adrenergic actions, it serves as a standard of reference for these responses and is, accordingly, described first.

THE CATECHOLAMINE DRUGS

ISOPROTERENOL (ISUPREL). Isoproterenol is a synthetic drug with potent cardiac properties. It is used to accelerate heart rate and impulse conduction when a minimal effect on peripheral vascular tone is desirable.

Actions. Isoproterenol has the following actions:

- It stimulates impulse formation and impulse conduction in specialized cardiac tissues.
- It augments myocardial contractile force.
- It produces generalized **vasodilation** (skin, skeletal muscles, and splanchnic bed). This action is slight because the receptors promoting vasodilation are relatively weak compared with the opposing constricting muscles. Consequently, the reduction in peripheral arterial resistance and the decline in blood pressure resulting from isoproterenol are modest.

Isoproterenol serves as a temporary expedient in emergency bradycardias because of the following actions:

- It accelerates impulse formation in symptomatic sinus bradycardia.
- It increases impulse conduction velocity in advanced degrees of sinoatrial or A-V nodal block.
- It stimulates escape pacemaker activity in complete A-V block.

Isoproterenol has also been used to "unload" the heart in circulatory shock by reducing excessive vasoconstriction and promoting better perfusion of peripheral tissues. Expanding intravascular space with fluid volume expanders is a critical adjunctive measure. Dilation of the bronchial tree may afford an additional benefit. However, newer, direct-acting vasodilating agents have largely replaced isoproterenol for the treatment of shock. For bradycardic emergencies in the hospital setting, clinicians usually prefer the temporary electronic pacemaker.

Side Effects. Isoproterenol has limited use in the CCU for the treatment of bradycardias for the following reasons:

- It increases oxygen required by the myocardium.
- It generates ectopic beats. Ventricular ectopic beats are particularly likely when the automatic fibers are already unstable, as is common in acute myocardial ischemia, hypoxia, thyrotoxicosis, and with certain anesthetics (especially halothane).
- It causes central nervous system excitation.

- It produces atony of the bowel through inhibition of smooth muscle of the gastrointestinal tract.

NOREPINEPHRINE (LEVOPHED). Norepinephrine is used in the treatment of hypotensive shock to raise blood pressure through generalized vasoconstriction and enhanced myocardial contractions.

Actions. Norepinephrine is the natural neurotransmitter in sympathetic terminals throughout the body. It has the following actions:

- Beta-adrenergic (stimulatory) actions on automatic and conductile fibers and on the myocardium (like isoproterenol).
- Alpha-adrenergic action on both arterial and venous beds (in sharp contrast to isoproterenol), providing a powerful **vasoconstrictor** effect on the skin, skeletal muscle, kidneys, liver, and intestinal tract. Exceptions are the vascular systems of the brain and heart, which normally lack responsive vasoconstrictive receptors for adrenergic agents. (In persons with a predisposition, however, spasm of a coronary artery may be precipitated by norepinephrine stimulation.)
- Vasoconstriction, in conjunction with increased heart rate and myocardial contractile force, sharply raises blood pressure. Paradoxically, the strong, generalized vasoconstriction can induce a secondary parasympathetic reaction of such great magnitude as to cause marked bradycardia from excessive vagal tone (vasovagal reaction).

Side Effects. So intense is the vasoconstrictive action of norepinephrine that prolonged use of the drug may produce any of the following conditions:

- Ischemia of splanchnic organs or digits. (Arterial occlusive disease predisposes to such complications.)
- Harmful effects on various organs, including the heart, if administration is prolonged. Lysosomes are released from organelles in underperfused cells (especially in the splanchnic organs, where vasoconstriction is greatest). Of most concern, these digestive enzymes are deleterious to myocardial function.
- Skin necrosis from vasospastic ischemia if extravasation of infused norepinephrine occurs.
- Other cardiac and central nervous system effects similar to those produced by isoproterenol.

Alternative approaches that spare the more vital organs from vasoconstrictive forces have been adapted because of a better understanding of shock and the development of newer drugs to treat it. Nevertheless, norepinephrine remains the most potent of the pressor agents now available.

EPINEPHRINE (*ADRENALINE, British Terminology*). Epinephrine is produced exclusively in the adrenal gland by incorporating a methyl group into the norepinephrine molecule.

Actions. Epinephrine behaves similarly to isoproterenol and norepinephrine in respect to cardiac automaticity, conductivity, and contractility. It has mixed actions on the peripheral vasculature:

- Dilation of blood vessels of the skeletal muscles.
- Constriction of the vasculature of the skin, mucous membranes, and splanchnic beds.

Consequently, the overall effect of epinephrine on blood pressure is much less predictable than with the other agents. At high blood levels, epinephrine constricts the vessels of skeletal muscles, as well. Therefore, when large doses are administered, the drug behaves very much like norepinephrine.

- It stimulates the breakdown of glycogen, elevating blood sugar in defense of maintaining normal glucose levels. (The common symptoms of hypoglycemia—blanching, sweating, trembling, hyperexcitability, and tachycardia—are the result of epinephrine released from the adrenal gland in response to a rapid decrease in blood sugar.)
- It inhibits histamine release from mast cells. In this action, epinephrine plays a critical role in reducing the reactions of acute hypersensitivity.

Epinephrine is used to

- Stimulate the heart in cardiac arrest by intravenous injection.
- Control bleeding in surgery through vasoconstriction by combining it with a locally injected anesthetic agent.
- Treat anaphylactic reactions by suppressing histamine release from mast cells. Epinephrine also relaxes smooth muscles in the larynx and the bronchial tree, major targets of profound hypersensitivity reactions.

Side Effects. Potential reactions from epinephrine include any of the side effects listed for isoproterenol and for norepinephrine. At high doses, the drug has a strong, diffuse vasoconstricting action. In addition, it elevates blood sugar, causes mental excitation, and may elevate blood pressure to dangerous levels.

DOPAMINE HYDROCHLORIDE (INTROPIN). Dopamine is the immediate chemical precursor in the natural production of norepinephrine. It is a crucial neurotransmitter within the central nervous system. Depletion of dopamine in brain tissue is characteristic of certain advanced neurodegenerative states, such as Parkinson's disease.

Actions. Administration of dopamine has the following effects on the cardiovascular system:

- It triggers the release of norepinephrine from peripheral neuronal terminals. The action, therefore, parallels that of norepinephrine itself, having *both* alpha- (vasoconstrictor) and beta-adrenergic (myocardial) actions. This dual role is advantageous when a central pressor agent (positive inotropic) must be combined with a peripheral pressor effect.
- It dilates the renal vasculature through specific receptors in the kidneys. These receptors are uniquely responsive to dopamine. As a result, renal blood flow is augmented, with a subsequent increase in glomerular filtration rate and sodium excretion. This protective action on renal function gives dopamine a preferential value over norepinephrine in the treatment of hypotensive shock. Excessive doses, however, result in deleterious constriction of the renal vasculature.

As with norepinephrine, the direct accelerating effect of dopamine on impulse formation is neutralized in part by the reflex vagotonic stimulation from diffuse vasoconstriction.

DOBUTAMINE (DOBUTREX). Dobutamine is a synthetic catecholamine acting similarly to dopamine but having the following important distinguishing features:

- A more potent effect on myocardial contractility.
- A relative weak effect in accelerating sinus node function.
- A slight constricting action on peripheral vasculature.

Both left ventricular preload (left atrial pressure) and afterload (mean systemic arterial pressure) are reduced. Thus, dobutamine may improve contractility with comparatively less increase in oxygen demand than other adrenergic agents. Furthermore, dobutamine appears less likely to induce tachyarrhythmias. These properties provide advantages for treating myocardial insufficiency in myocardial infarction and immediately after cardiac surgery. The drug does not produce vasodilation in the renal bed and in this respect is not comparable to dopamine.

Dobutamine is the preferred vasopressor agent in acute left ventricular failure when the systolic blood pressure is normal or only slightly reduced. Alternatively, dopamine is used in cardiogenic shock when the blood pressure is severely depressed. An additional agent, such as nitroprusside or nitroglycerin, may be given to reduce pulmonary congestion in this form of hypotension.

Parasympathetic Nervous System: Inhibition

Drugs that suppress the frequency of parasympathetic impulses cause a shift in autonomic forces favoring a stronger sympathetic tone. Such agents are termed **anticholinergic** because they compete with the receptors for acetylcholine at the parasympathetic neuronal terminals. All drugs that act predominantly through this mechanism have similar effects on parasympathetic function of the heart, smooth muscles, and exocrine organs. Atropine is considered here as a prototype for this class of many agents.

ATROPINE. Atropine accelerates impulse formation in the normal sinus node and impulse conduction in the A-V node and is used in bradycardic emergencies involving these systems.

Actions. Atropine inhibits vagal nerve function. Thus normal parasympathetic tone, which is so important in regulating impulse formation in the sinus node and impulse conduction in the A-V node, is eliminated. The result is the absence of the cardiodecelerating effects of carotid pressure, emotionally induced vasovagal reactions, and other vagotonic reflexes.

Atropine may enhance **impulse conduction** in bradycardias caused by

- Sinoatrial block.
- Diffuse depression of atrial conduction.
- Second-degree A-V block, particularly of type I (Wenckebach periodicity). Atropine may decrease the PR interval in first-degree A-V block.
- Complete A-V block. Restoration of A-V conduction may result—wholly or partially—providing that the conduction disturbance is located in the A-V node itself. More distal conduction blocks are not corrected by atropine, because parasympathetic innervation does not extend into the His-Purkinje system.

Myocardial contraction is not directly affected by atropine and its congeners.

Peripheral vasomotor tone responds only slightly to atropine at usual clinical doses. The skin is an exception, however, with vasodilation causing a flush accompanied by dryness (inhibition of sweating). These are typical findings with high doses.

Large doses of atropine occasionally produce emergence of latent pacemakers in the A-V junctional tissues, which have a more rapid, parasympathetic-free rate than does the sinus node, resulting in nodal tachycardia.

Because atropine has no major effect on the peripheral vasculature (except at very high doses) and does not enhance cardiac excitability, it has distinct advantages over the adrenergic drugs in bradycardic emergencies.

Indications. Atropine is useful in severe bradycardia to promote more rapid **impulse formation** by the following mechanisms:

- It accelerates the sinus rate in sinus node depression.
- It promotes atrial and A-V junctional escape pacemakers in sinus arrest.
- It releases or accelerates automatic activity in the nodal-Hisian fibers when a

conduction defect in complete A-V block is proximal to these pacemakers. In complete A-V block caused by a distal lesion, atropine is unlikely to affect an idioventricular pacemaker because few, if any, vagal fibers are distributed to the ventricles.

Side Effects. Paradoxically, atropine in small doses (or as an early response to a higher dose) causes transient *slowing* of the sinus rate owing to direct stimulation of vagal tone in the central nervous system. For this reason, atropine given intravenously should be administered rapidly and in sufficient amounts. In addition, atropine may cause hypotension by central depression of vasomotor tone at very high doses. Otherwise, the drug is remarkably free of untoward effects on the cardiovascular system.

Noncardiovascular effects of atropine include the following:

- Depression of the exocrine functions (salivary glands, bronchial mucosa, and sweat glands).
- Inhibition of motor tone of visceral organs, frequently causing distention of the gastrointestinal tract and urinary bladder.
- Dilation of the pupils, causing excessive intraocular pressure in persons with closed-angle glaucoma.
- Cerebral hyperexcitability at high doses, followed by depression with increasing levels of toxicity.

DRUGS OF DEPRESSION

Rhythms of excitation are treated by agents that suppress impulse formation or conduction. They are referred to as **antiarrhythmic** drugs. Some of them act on the autonomic nervous system by blocking adrenergic activity or by increasing parasympathetic (vagal) tone. Others act directly on the cell wall, inhibiting ion transport that is crucial for depolarization and repolarization. Although many of the commonly used drugs affect the action potential in more than one way, the prevailing system for classifying these drugs is based on their dominant action.

Sympathetic Nervous System: Inhibition

DRUGS THAT DEPRESS THE CENTRAL NERVOUS SYSTEM

Recurring premature beats and tachycardias commonly occur during periods of high emotional tension in susceptible persons. These arrhythmias can often be lessened or eliminated by drugs that inhibit sympathetic activity in the central nervous system. The **tranquilizers** may thus serve as adjunctive (and sometimes primary) agents for treating rhythms of excitation when adrenergic stimulation plays a strong role. Examples of drugs that have proved useful in selected patients with frequent symptoms of supraventricular or ventricular tachycardia are alprazolam (Xanax), chlordiazepoxide (Librium), and diazepam (T-Quil, Valium).

Some of the antihypertensive drugs suppress sympathetic activity in regions of the brain responsible for maintaining peripheral vasopressor tone and cardioacceleration. Clonidine (Catapres) and methyldopa (Aldomet) are examples. These agents may be chosen preferentially for treating high blood pressure in patients who also have arrhythmias associated with high adrenergic tone.

DRUGS THAT BLOCK ADRENERGIC RECEPTORS

Control of rhythms of excitation may be achieved by inhibiting sympathetic stimulation at the cardiac receptor site for impulse formation and conduction. These sites are defined as the **beta-adrenergic receptors**. A large number of drugs in this category, of which propranolol is the prototype, are now available to clinicians. In the most widely accepted and current system of classification, they are designated Class II drugs. To adhere to this system, they are discussed later.

Parasympathetic Nervous System: Stimulation

DRUGS THAT ENHANCE VAGAL TONE

Parasympathetic activity counters adrenergic activity at impulse formation and conduction sites within the sinus node, atrium, and A-V node. Drugs that stimulate parasympathetic tone act similarly to carotid pressure and other vagotonic maneuvers. They may be effective in terminating supraventricular tachycardias.

EDROPHONIUM (ENLON, TENSILON). Edrophonium inactivates acetylcholinesterase, the enzyme responsible for hydrolyzing acetylcholine. Acetylcholine, the natural neurotransmitter of terminal parasympathetic fibers, accumulates under influence of this drug, greatly enhancing parasympathetic tone. In a normal heart, the augmented vagal tone results in slowing of sinus node function and prolongation of A-V conduction.

Edrophonium is often successful in converting atrial and A-V junctional tachycardias to sinus rhythm through strong vagal stimulation. Before continuing, it should be pointed out that this drug has been largely superseded by new drugs (namely, the calcium channel blocking agents) for treating supraventricular tachycardias. Edrophonium is currently used as a diagnostic test for myasthenia gravis (a disease of immunologically deficient receptors for acetylcholine at motor terminals) and to reverse the paralyzing action of curare-like drugs (which compete with acetylcholine on the receptor).

Although side effects of edrophonium have greatly limited its use, edrophonium remains a highly effective antiarrhythmic agent for intravenous administration. Its drawbacks are the constellation of symptoms from universal cholinergic stimulation: a flush, sweating, tearing, abdominal cramps, nausea and vomiting, headache, muscle fasciculations, and (in susceptible persons) bronchospasm. Sudden and dangerous degrees of bradycardia have sometimes been precipitated.

Edrophonium injected intravenously attains its full effect within a minute; its action is virtually dissipated within 10 minutes. Consequently, the drug has been used only in emergency situations.

Drugs used to enhance intestinal peristalsis or urinary bladder tone have parasympathetic-stimulating properties. Bethanechol (Myotonachol, Urecholine), an acetylcholine-like drug, may precipitate severe bradycardia when given to persons with sinus node dysfunction or A-V conduction defects.

Drugs That Affect the Cell Membrane

Attention now shifts to those drugs that affect cardiac rhythm principally by their action on the transport of ions through the cell membrane. The action potentials of fibers that form or conduct impulses is thereby altered. The site (or sites) and magnitude of alterations determine the antiarrhythmic properties of the individual drugs.

CLASS I: DRUGS THAT BLOCK SODIUM CHANNELS

Drugs that block sodium channels are bound to receptors in the fast channel of the cell membrane, predominantly those that affect **sodium transport**, and thus retard its inflow at the onset of depolarization. The results are as follows:

- Slowing of the upstroke (Phase 0) of the action potential.
- Reduced amplitude of the overshoot (Phase 1).

Potassium shifts are affected as well as sodium, and the overall effect may be responsible for prolonging the process of repolarization (Phase 3). The refractory period is thereby lengthened, and, in turn, excitability of the cell membrane and spontaneous depolarization (Phase 4) are decreased. Because of these properties, the terms **membrane stabilization** and **local anesthetic** are applied. Because disturbances in body potassium levels alter the intensity of the Class I drug effects, hyperkalemia and hypokalemia should be corrected before their administration.

The result of fast-channel inhibition is suppression of **automatic impulse formation**, which is most pronounced in the Purkinje fibers and in the myofibrils of the atria and the ventricles. The sodium channel blockers are used most effectively to control tachycardias of enhanced automaticity. They also increase the threshold for induction of ventricular fibrillation.

In addition, the sodium channel blockers are often successful in treating **reentrant tachycardias** of both atrial and ventricular types. The mechanism is probably by prolonging the effective refractory period in myofibrils and in Purkinje cells, thus obliterating unidirectional conduction within one limb of the reentrant circuit.

The sodium channel blockers have negligible effect on **sinus node** impulse formation (which is principally dependent on slow calcium channels). However, they may seriously intensify sinoatrial depression when sinus node dysfunction is already established. Sinoatrial block is especially susceptible to the depressive action of these agents. Sinus arrest and atrial standstill are expressions of their toxicity.

One can appreciate that suppression of automaticity carries the liability of impairing potential **escape pacemakers** should A-V block develop. Indeed, high degrees of A-V block are a contraindication for the sodium channel blockers (unless supported by electronic pacemaker back-up).

The sodium channel blocking agents depress **impulse conduction** in the atria, the A-V node, the Purkinje fibers, and the ventricles. The effect on A-V nodal conduction is most prominent during the HV interval. The drugs can be used to advantage to slow the ventricular rate in supraventricular tachycardias, including atrial fibrillation. In patients with disturbances of conduction, they carry the potential hazard of further impairing A-V and intraventricular impulse transmission.

The differences among the various sodium channel blocking agents depend on their relative potencies on various components of the action potential in special cardiac tissues—sinus node, atria, His-Purkinje fibers, accessory bundles, and ventricular myofibrils.

CLASS IA: DRUGS THAT PROLONG REPOLARIZATION

The Class IA drugs (quinidine, procainamide, and disopyramide) are the most extensively studied and prescribed of the antiarrhythmic agents. They have both direct and indirect actions on automatic fibers.

Direct Actions. The Class IA drugs have the following direct actions:

- They lower the transmembrane potential of the resting fiber.
- They decrease the slope of spontaneous depolarization (Phase 4).

Indirect Actions. Class IA drugs block acetylcholine at vagal nerve endings. This inhibition of parasympathetic tone (atropine-like effect) tends to counter the direct action on the cell membrane.

The net result of the dual and opposing actions of Class IA drugs depends on whichever influence dominates. At rest, a modest acceleration of sinus node rate and increase in conduction velocity in the A-V node usually occurs (dominant antiparasympathetic effect).

Innervation of the ventricles by parasympathetic fibers is probably negligible. This lack of counterbalancing forces is one factor accounting for the notable efficacy of Class IA drugs in suppressing ventricular tachyarrhythmias.

In **ventricular preexcitation**, the sodium channel blockers are quite unpredictable. When effective, they induce a unidirectional block in one limb of the reentrant circuit.

Paradoxically, the Class IA drugs commonly accelerate the ventricular rate response in **atrial flutter and fibrillation** by their atropine-like action. Rarely, the ventricles can respond with alarming acceleration of rate. In addition, the drugs can further increase the ventricular rate by reducing the frequency of impulse bombardment on the A-V node (lessening concealed conduction) and thereby increasing A-V nodal conduction.

Vasodilation by the Class IA drugs further complicates the response of impulse formation. Reduction of systemic blood pressure induces a counteracting alpha-adrenergic reaction of the sympathetic nervous system with resultant excitation in sinus rate and A-V conduction. In hypotensive shock, when cardiac output is strongly supported by adrenergic vasoconstrictor forces, the sodium channel blockers may further lower blood pressure.

The Class IA drugs do not ordinarily affect the **electrocardiogram** (ECG) except for minor changes in rate and PR interval. Some lengthening of the QRS complex and QT interval may occur and is dose related. At toxic levels, the drugs cause marked widening of the QRS complex, and this finding is an important warning sign for the electrocardiographer.

At usual clinical doses, the Class IA drugs have a negligible effect on the normal **myocardium**. However, their depressing action on the myofibrils is exaggerated in myocardial disease. Consequently, these agents always have the potential for worsening myocardial failure.

The more prominent characteristics of the individual Class IA drugs are summarized in the paragraphs that follow.

QUINIDINE. Used clinically for more than half a century and extensively studied, quinidine remains the standard agent for suppressing atrial and ventricular arrhythmias. Relatively short lived by hepatic metabolism, the drug usually must be taken four times a day. However, sustained-release formulations may lessen this requirement somewhat.

Side Effects. Quinidine induces distressing side effects in a third of recipients:

- Gastrointestinal symptoms (nausea and diarrhea are the predominant side effects). To protect against these reactions, quinidine is prepared as gluconate and polygalacturonate compounds.
- Vagolytic reactions causing symptoms from reduced salivation, pupillary fixation, intestinal peristalsis, urinary bladder tone, and sweating.
- Cutaneous hypersensitivity reactions (usually urticarial rash) are fairly common.
- Febrile reactions, thrombocytopenia, and bronchospastic or hypotensive crises are unusual but more serious problems.
- **Cinchonism** is a syndrome peculiar to quinidine and includes headache, tinnitus, visual and auditory disorders, and—at very high doses—delirium.
- Ventricular tachycardia with syncope. Torsades de pointes is the most characteristic form. Most susceptible are persons with a preexisting prolonged QT

interval. Although other drugs in this class also possess this liability, it is most pronounced with quinidine.

PROCAINAMIDE (PROCAN, PRONESTYL). Markedly different from quinidine in chemical structure, procainamide has remarkably similar antiarrhythmic properties. However, the route of excretion and side effects contrast strikingly.

Procainamide is eliminated principally by the kidneys. Dosage must be reduced in renal insufficiency, a particular caution in elderly patients. With a somewhat shorter plasma half-life than quinidine, procainamide requires oral administration at 3- to 6-hour intervals initially, then adjusted according to response and tolerance.

As with quinidine, procainamide may aggravate sinus node dysfunction, conduction abnormalities, and myocardial insufficiency. In contrast to quinidine, procainamide has minimal effects on autonomic fibers.

Side Effects. Certain complications of procainamide may appear early in administration:

- Depression or confusion can occur, although mental alterations are unusual.
- Gastrointestinal symptoms may appear but are much less prominent than with quinidine.
- Suppression of polymorphonuclear leukocytes, resulting in bacterial infection.
- Drug-induced fever.
- Vasculitis, Raynaud's phenomenon, and angioedema.

Another complication that tends to occur with long-term administration is a *lupus-like hypersensitivity reaction.* It may be associated with antibodies that develop against the patient's own cell nuclei. The syndrome is characterized by inflammatory changes in joints, serous membranes (pleura, pericardial, and peritoneal), fever, hepatomegaly, and splenomegaly. It is reversible on discontinuing procainamide. The syndrome occurs to some degree in nearly a third of patients taking the drug over several months.

DISOPYRAMIDE (NORPACE). Disopyramide is used principally to suppress ventricular tachyarrhythmias, most specifically ventricular premature beats and paroxysmal ventricular tachycardia. It is less successful in treating sustained ventricular tachycardia and tachyarrhythmias associated with digitalis toxicity. Although disopyramide may be effective in converting atrial tachyarrhythmias and for subsequently maintaining a sinus rhythm, the drug is not officially recommended for this purpose.

Disopyramide differs from quinidine in having a stronger tendency to increase refractoriness in the atria and the ventricles and little effect on A-V nodal and His-Purkinje fibers (where quinidine exerts its dominant action). Disopyramide may depress conduction in accessory pathways. Ordinarily, the drug produces no appreciable changes in PR interval and QRS complex and QT interval, although significant prolongation may occur in susceptible patients.

As with procainamide, the kidneys are the major excretory organs for the drug, and renal insufficiency dictates reduced doses.

Because of the strong vagolytic action of disopyramide, the ventricular rate in atrial flutter and fibrillation may accelerate excessively. Digitalis started beforehand protects against this possibility.

Side Effects. Disopyramide is relatively well tolerated by most patients. However, some potential problems deserve attention:

- Depression of myocardial contractility. This effect appears to be more prominent than with quinidine or procainamide. Therefore, the drug must be given with redoubled vigilance in patients with myocardial insufficiency.
- Atropine-like effect. Dry mouth, decreased sweating, pupillary dilation and loss of accommodation, constipation, and urinary retention are commonly experienced.

These symptoms from the vagolytic response are usually much more prominent than with quinidine. (A slow-release preparation of the cholinergic agent pyridostigmine has proved helpful in lessening the symptoms of disopyramide while not interfering with its antiarrhythmic properties.)

CLASS IB: DRUGS THAT SHORTEN REPOLARIZATION

The major action of the Class IB drugs (lidocaine, mexiletine, tocainide, and phenytoin) is to shorten repolarization, particularly in the Purkinje fibers. They are used with special efficacy in the treatment of ventricular tachyarrhythmias.

Actions. The Class IB drugs act directly on the cell membrane in the following mechanisms:

- They markedly accelerate the flow of potassium ions from the cell during repolarization. By this mechanism, shortening Phase 3 of the action potential is their major actions.
- They enhance the extrusion of sodium from the cell during Phase 2 of the action potential.
- They depress Phase 0 depolarization. This effect is relatively small.
- They decrease the slope of Phase 4 depolarization, thus suppressing automaticity.
- They raise the threshold for stimulation of the resting membrane, thereby reducing excitability.
- They eliminate the reverberating circuit in reentrant tachycardias by improving conduction in one limb or by inducing bidirectional block in one.

In general, the Class IB drugs are considered safer for control of ventricular tachyarrhythmias than those of Class IA, tending to be less proarrhythmic and to cause less myocardial depression.

LIDOCAINE (XYLOCAINE). Lidocaine is the principle agent used in the CCU to control ventricular tachyarrhythmias. It is highly effective and has a wide margin of safety. Parenteral administration is required.

Lidocaine is used to suppress ventricular premature beats and ventricular tachycardia. It also increases the threshold at which ventricular fibrillation is induced by electrical stimulation. Advantages of lidocaine include its **minimal effect** in

- Depressing impulse conduction in the Purkinje fibers.
- Depressing myocardial contractility.
- Reducing peripheral vasculature tone.
- Altering autonomic control.

Lidocaine has no appreciable effect on automaticity of the sinus node or atrial fibers or on impulse conduction in the A-V node. Consequently, lidocaine is ineffective in the treatment of atrial tachyarrhythmias.

The only electrocardiographic change noted is a minor reduction in QT interval owing to shortening of the refractory period in the His-Purkinje system. Ordinarily, the QRS complex is not prolonged.

Administration. Lidocaine is destroyed in the digestive tract; therefore, parenteral administration is necessary.

- Intravenous infusion is required or, in emergencies, undiluted intravenous injection. For out-of-hospital emergencies, the intramuscular route affords a practical expedient.
- Loading doses are given initially to saturate protein receptor sites in plasma.

- Maintenance doses are then established by infusion of the drug, appropriately diluted, to provide a continuous therapeutic effect without toxicity. Because of its short duration of action, lidocaine can be administered with a high degree of control by adjusting the infusion rate according to rhythm response.

Side Effects. Although lidocaine is remarkably free of untoward effects, they do occur and can be serious. The heart is seldom adversely affected, although this safety is less certain when there are underlying abnormalities:

- Further compromise of myocardial contraction can occur in patients with congestive heart failure.
- Complete A-V block may appear when A-V nodal disease is already present.
- The rate of the ventricular response to atrial flutter or fibrillation may increase because of the decreased refractory period of Purkinje fibers.

The preeminent complication of lidocaine, however, affects the central nervous system with increasing levels of toxicity by causing

- Paresthesias (especially around the mouth) or alteration in mood.
- Muscle twitching, reduced hearing, dizziness, and disorders of mentation with agitation and confusion. These signs and symptoms simulate those of hypoxia.
- Generalized seizures.

These problems generally subside promptly on discontinuing the drug because of the rapid dissipation of lidocaine effect. When hepatic insufficiency is present, however, metabolism is impaired; toxicity occurs at smaller doses and lasts longer.

ORAL/PARENTERAL AGENTS

Tocainide and **mexiletine** are similar to lidocaine in chemical structure and pharmacological effect. However, they differ by having the advantage of escaping first-pass degradation in the liver and of being absorbed effectively when taken by mouth. They are, in effect, oral versions of lidocaine, although both drugs can be given parenterally. These two Class IB drugs are described together because of their strongly similar properties and clinical indications.

Compared with lidocaine, the efficacy of tocainide and mexiletine is considered modest, particularly for life-threatening ventricular tachyarrhythmias. They are given principally for suppression of ventricular premature complexes; they are generally not as successful as lidocaine in controlling sustained ventricular tachycardias. Efficacy may be improved by combining either drug with another antiarrhythmic agent.

Actions. Mexiletine and tocainide have the following actions:

- They shorten the duration of the action potential in Purkinje fibers in greater proportion than the effective refractory period.
- They do not prolong the QT interval and are considered safe in patients with ventricular tachycardia associated with torsades de pointes.
- They have minimal negative inotropic properties and can be given with relative safety to patients with myocardial insufficiency.
- They are readily absorbed from the alimentary canal. They have a slower rate of elimination (principally in the liver) than do quinidine and procainamide; therefore, doses need be given only two or three times daily.

MEXILETINE (MEXITIL). Mexiletine appears to be even more effective than lidocaine in suppressing arrhythmias of increased automaticity in the Purkinje fibers. However, the drug has a greater tendency to impair impulse conduction in the His-Purkinje system, a prospect enhanced by hypoxia, hyperkalemia, or ischemia. Downward adjustment of dose is required for patients with hepatic or renal insufficiency.

Side Effects. The principal side effects of mexiletine are as follows:

- Gastrointestinal (nausea, anorexia, heartburn). Gastric symptoms are usually minimal if the drug is taken at mealtime.
- Neurological (diplopia, tremor, fatigue, and headache).
- Exaggeration of sinus node dysfunction and A-V nodal conduction defects when these conditions preexist.

TOCAINIDE (TONOCARD). In some patients with accessory pathways, tocainide has proved more effective than lidocaine for treating reentrant ventricular tachyarrhythmias.

Side Effects. Tocainide may produce the following problems:

- Gastrointestinal. Nausea, vomiting, and abdominal cramps are common, most notably in aged patients. Doses are best taken with meals to reduce gastrointestinal symptoms.
- Neurological. Paresthesias, vertigo, and tremor are associated with overdose, paralleling those side effects in lidocaine toxicity.
- Pulmonary. Fibrosis of the lungs can occur with long-term administration; therefore, periodic chest x-rays and pulmonary function studies are indicated.
- Suppression of bone marrow, which may involve red blood cells, leukocytes, or platelet production. Because of this hazard, the drug is reserved for treatment of ventricular tachyarrhythmias of a life-threatening nature.

Investigators have reported that arrhythmia control with combined tocainide and quinidine can be achieved while permitting lower doses and better toleration of each drug than with either drug used alone.

PHENYTOIN (DILANTIN). The antiepileptic drug phenytoin is also useful for treatment of ventricular tachyarrhythmias. It is less effective in suppressing supraventricular tachyarrhythmias, including atrial flutter and fibrillation. However, phenytoin is especially efficacious in tachycardias of either atrial or ventricular origin when associated with **digitalis toxicity.** Indeed, this condition provides the most distinctive advantages for phenytoin.

Actions. Phenytoin has the following actions:

- It counteracts the direct enhancement of automaticity by digitalis.
- It accelerates A-V nodal conduction, thus opposing the depressing action of digitalis in this tissue.
- It inhibits the hypothalamic center for sympathetic tone (reducing endogenous adrenergic stimulation).

Although phenytoin does not appreciably affect the sinus node, it may restore normal sinus function in sinus standstill or sinoatrial block if induced by digitalis. The drug may improve A-V conduction when it is impaired by digitalis and other drugs of depression. On the other hand, phenytoin may be hazardous in complete A-V block because it suppresses escape pacemakers. In atrial flutter and atrial fibrillation, phenytoin can increase the ventricular rate response.

Side Effects. Side effects of phenytoin are principally those of central nervous system disturbances:

- Labyrinthine dysfunction (with ataxia, vertigo, and nausea) and somnolence.
- Behavioral disorders often become evident as high blood levels are approached.

With chronic administration, gingival hyperplasia, hirsutism, and megaloblastic anemia are common complications.

Phenytoin has no effect on the autonomic nervous system except by its central suppressing action on sympathetic tone. At high blood levels, phenytoin may cause diffuse vasodilation that may be sufficient to produce hypotension, especially when given rapidly. Respiratory arrest is another potential complication of rapid intravenous injection.

CLASS IC: DRUGS THAT DEPRESS DEPOLARIZATION

Drugs of Class IC (flecainide, encainide, lorcainide, and propafenone) block the fast sodium channels and exert their major action on Phase 0 of the action potential. These newer drugs have proved most effective in controlling ventricular tachyarrhythmias. They appear promising for treating atrial tachyarrhythmias as well, although supporting clinical data are not as well established.

Actions. The Class IC drugs have the following actions:

- They markedly decrease the rate of depolarization (Phase 0) and the overshoot (Phase I) in atrial, Purkinje, and ventricular fibers.
- They inhibit impulse conduction (most notably in the His-Purkinje system).

In contrast to drugs of the IA and IB classes, they have but minor effect on any portion of repolarization, including the duration of the refractory period (Phase 3).

All of the Class IC drugs have but minor depressing effect on normal sinus activity, A-V conduction, and myocardial contractile force. However, the drugs may exacerbate underlying sinus node dysfunction, A-V conduction disturbances, and myocardial insufficiency. The Class IC drugs may appreciably lengthen the PR interval. Widening of the QRS complex also can be expected even in the therapeutic dosage range, but excessive prolongation is a warning of overdose.

Class IC drugs are well absorbed in the digestive tract and are therefore useful for oral administration.

FLECAINIDE (TAMBOCOR). Flecainide compares favorably with quinidine and disopyramide in its suppression of chronic ventricular arrhythmias, particularly in the more complex forms. Although clinical experience with flecainide for suppression of supraventricular tachycardias is very limited, it appears to be effective in some patients. In atrial fibrillation of recent onset, the drug is at least as successful as quinidine in restoring sinus rhythm. Flecainide may be the drug of choice for treating tachycardias involving accessory bundles. It is not effective in converting atrial flutter or atrial reentrant tachycardias to sinus rhythm.

Administration. Flecainide has a relatively long action (plasma elimination half-life of about 20 hours), permitting dosing only twice (and sometimes once) a day by mouth. The prolonged duration before steady state is reached dictates that at least 4 days should elapse after a given dose before incremental adjustments are made. It is poorly bound by plasma proteins, thus minimizing one source of drug interaction and other variables of dose regulation. Plasma concentrations closely reflect the pharmacological activity. A smooth transition from intravenous lidocaine to oral flecainide can be made in closely monitored patients in a CCU.

The principal route of clearance is the kidneys. Smaller doses are required in both myocardial and renal insufficiency. Although a small portion of the drug is excreted by the liver, the dose must also be reduced in patients with hepatic failure.

Side Effects. Potential cardiac complications from flecainide are as follows:

- Myocardial insufficiency precipitated or aggravated in susceptible persons because of the negative inotropic action.
- Proarrhythmia effect, increasing the duration or complexities of tachyarrhythmias. Because of these potential problems, flecainide is usually reserved for ventricular tachyarrhythmias refractory to other drugs. At the same time, it is acknowledged that a proarrhythmia effect is most likely in patients with the most severe forms of ventricular tachycardias.

- Sinus node depression.
- Conduction defects. A modest increase in the PR interval and in the duration of QRS can be expected. Excessive prolongation of either is a distinct sign of toxicity. A-V block of any severity or bundle branch block may develop.

Preexisting sinus node dysfunction or conduction defects of the A-V node or multifascicular branch block dictate against the use of flecainide without back-up electronic pacing.

Wide QRS complex tachycardias induced by exercise have been reported in which flecainide had a culpable role.

Noncardiac side effects of flecainide include the following:

- Autonomic dysfunctions (lightheadedness, blurred vision, and dry mouth).
- Gastrointestinal (nausea and diarrhea or constipation).
- Neurological (tremor, incoordination, paresthesias, mental disturbances, headache, and fatigue).
- Hepatic dysfunction.

Flecainide is reserved for patients with life-threatening ventricular arrhythmias, such as sustained ventricular tachycardia. These limitations were recommended following a clinical investigation initiated by the National Heart, Lung, and Blood Institute on efforts to suppress asymptomatic ventricular arrhythmias in patients who had suffered myocardial infarction. In multicenter trials, this drug was associated with a higher rate of mortality and nonfatal cardiac arrest in the study group than in the control subjects.

ENCAINIDE (ENKAID). Encainide is most successful in suppressing ventricular ectopy, including symptomatic and potentially lethal ventricular tachycardia. In addition, encainide may be effective in suppressing supraventricular tachycardias, especially those of A-V junctional origin and those associated with accessory pathways and ventricular preexcitation. In practice, encainide is often highly effective when these various tachyarrhythmias prove resistant to conventional drug regimens.

Actions. Encainide has the following actions:

- It strongly inhibits the conductance of ions across the cardiac cell membrane. This effect is most prominent in the AV nodal and Purkinje fibers. Its effect on the action potential curve is reflected in the ECG by lengthening of the PR interval and the QRS complex. These changes, however, do not correlate well in predicting drug efficacy or toxicity.
- It prolongs the refractory period of accessory pathway fibers more than those in neighboring normal pathways, accounting for its efficacy in ventricular preexcitation tachycardias.
- It has a relatively minor effect on the refractory period of excitable fibers, and no appreciable lengthening of the QT interval occurs.
- It increases the threshold for electronic pacemaker stimulation.
- It slightly depresses myocardial contractility when given intravenously. The drug is usually well tolerated in patients with left ventricular dysfunction.

Encainide has no anticholinergic effect.

Side Effects. Encainide is generally well tolerated, but it may affect the heart adversely by any of the following mechanisms:

- Accentuation of sinus node dysfunction.
- Exacerbation of arrhythmias. These occur fairly commonly in an electrically unstable ventricle.
- Adverse effects on hemodynamics. Detectable reduction of myocardial contractility and systemic blood pressure are seldom encountered.

- Accentuation of various degrees of A-V nodal block and block of multiple fascicles. Electronic pacemaker back-up is indicated in vulnerable patients.

Side effects in other systems are relatively uncommon and include the following:

- Headache, visual disturbances, dizziness, insomnia, tremor, and fatigue.
- Nausea, taste perversion, and constipation.
- Hepatic injury.
- Hyperglycemia.

Like flecainide, encainide was found in a multicenter trial conducted by the National Heart, Lung, and Blood Institute to impose an increased risk of mortality and nonfatal cardiac arrest in postmyocardial infarction patients. The drug is not recommended for patients with ventricular arrhythmias unless they are life threatening.

Administration. Encainide is metabolized in the liver to two longer-acting and more potent compounds. Together, these agents provide plasma levels that attain an antiarrhythmic effect with interval dosing of 8 hours. Because of the cumulative effect of bioactive metabolites, protracted use of encainide may eventually lead to cardiac depression. Dose reduction should be considered if the PR interval or QRS complex lengthens excessively. Liver disease reduces the efficacy of encainide. It is slowly excreted by the kidneys, and doses must be decreased in patients with advanced renal insufficiency.

PROPAFENONE (RYTHMOL). Propafenone is distinctive among the Class IC agents. In addition to its potent membrane-stabilizing effect, it also has a weak blocking action on beta-adrenergic receptors and slow calcium channels. These latter properties may enhance the primary arrhythmia-suppressing mechanism and play a deciding role in some arrhythmias that are resistant to other Class IC drugs.

Propafenone has high efficacy in controlling ventricular premature beats and recurrent ventricular tachycardia. However, the drug is officially approved for use only in patients with sustained tachycardia or in whom ventricular fibrillation has been documented (consistent with the restriction of the other Class IC drugs, encainide and flecainide). Propafenone may be even more efficacious in the treatment of supraventricular tachycardias, particularly those involving accessory pathways and the A-V node. It is often effective in preventing recurrent episodes of atrial fibrillation. Nevertheless, sanction for its use in supraventricular arrhythmias awaits further experience regarding safety.

Actions. Propafenone has the following actions:

- It markedly depresses sodium influx during depolarization.
- It slows conduction velocity mostly in fibers of the atria and A-V node. The PR interval lengthens and can be followed as a guide to dosage. Preexisting conduction defects in the sinoatrial or A-V nodes will likely worsen.
- It inhibits conduction in the ventricles and prolongs the duration of the QRS complex. Bundle branch block may be accentuated.
- It exerts a minor effect on the refractory period, shortening that of the Purkinje fibers while lengthening that of the ventricular myofibrils. This differential response may explain the high efficacy of propafenone in terminating sustained ventricular tachyarrhythmias. There is no appreciable increase in the QT interval.
- It suppresses conduction in accessory pathways. The intravenous form of propafenone is especially effective for terminating supraventricular tachycardias associated with ventricular preexcitation. The drug tends to block retrograde conduction in the accessory pathway, differing in this way from the beta-adrenergic and calcium channel blocking agents, which usually affect antegrade conduction within the reentrant circuit.

- It inhibits ventricular automaticity from digitalis toxicity and from myocardial ischemia.

Administration. In general, propafenone is well tolerated by most patients on long-term therapy, although cardiac dysfunction can be aggravated and extracardiac symptoms are fairly frequent. It is well absorbed when administered by mouth, although hepatic metabolism is extremely variable among patients. The serum half-life averages 6 hours but ranges from 2 to 32 hours. Genetically determined ''slow metabolizers'' are more vulnerable to side effects. Therefore, therapy must be guided by serial arrhythmia and electrocardiographic surveillance. Steady-state serum levels of propafenone can usually be attained after several days at 8- to 12-hour doses. It is recommended that the daily dose should not be raised in less than 3 days.

Side Effects. Propafenone has the following potential adverse effects on the heart:

- It may induce bradycardia in persons with sinus node or A-V node dysfunction.
- It intensifies conduction defects, as previously mentioned.
- It reduces myocardial contractility. This adversity is slight, however, and most patients with congestive failure tolerate the drug. The negative inotropic effect of propafenone is most prominent in acute myocardial injury, however, as encountered in acute ischemia or during open-heart surgery.
- It is potentially proarrhythmic, causing sustained and complex ventricular tachycardia. This complication is more likely in persons in whom the arrhythmia was present before treatment and in those with very low cardiac ejection fractions.

Noncardiac side effects of propafenone are common but mild:

- Blurred vision.
- Nausea, metallic or bitter taste, and constipation.
- Ataxia, headache, and tremor.
- Hepatic and hematological disturbances, rarely.
- Exacerbation of asthma (probably due to the beta-adrenergic blocking effect).

Dual therapy with propafenone and quinidine or procainamide has proved successful for complex ventricular arrhythmias. This strategy allows giving a lower and more likely tolerated dose of propafenone than does using this agent by itself. One precautionary note: quinidine has been shown to potentiate the action of propafenone by interfering with its hepatic breakdown.

Drug interactions also include the tendency of propafenone to increase the activity of a given dose of digoxin, warfarin, and metoprolol.

CLASS II: DRUGS THAT BLOCK BETA-ADRENERGIC RECEPTORS

The beta-adrenergic blocking agents compete with norepinephrine and other sympathetic neurotransmitters at the neuronal terminal. Beta-adrenergic blocking drugs have found wide utility in suppressing rhythms of excitation associated with excess sympathetic tone. In addition, they are used to lessen the work of the heart in angina pectoris and to reduce systemic arterial hypertension (through slower heart rate and reduced myocardial contractile force).

The place of the adrenergic blocking agents as inhibitors of sympathetic autonomic activity has been explained in Chapter 3 under Examples of Sinus Bradycardia, using propranolol as a prototype. In effect, these agents act *indirectly* at the cell membrane by counteracting adrenergic neutrotransmitters, the natural accelerators of membrane depolarization.

Adrenergic Actions. The beta-adrenergic blocking drugs affect the heart at several physiological sites:

IMPULSE FORMATION

- They inhibit sympathetic stimulation of the sinus node, thus blunting adrenergic acceleration of Phase 4 depolarization. This action has its most prominent effect in the normal heart. Sinus rate slows at rest, and acceleration during periods of enhanced sympathetic stimulation is blunted (such as during exercise, emotional excitation, hypoglycemic reactions, and hypotensive episodes).

    Although the beta-adrenergic blockers do not have a direct depressing action on the sinus node (independent of inhibiting sympathetic tone), they may severely depress the sinus rate in sinus node dysfunction.

- They inhibit other **automatic foci** under sympathetic control. Consequently, these drugs are useful in suppressing premature beats and sustained arrhythmias in the atria and ventricles when associated with enhanced sensitivity to sympathetic stimulation or in states associated with augmented catecholamine-mediated excitability, such as with physical effort, emotional stress, caffeine consumption, and postural hypotension. In such instances, the beta-adrenergic blockers may be remarkably effective, even in small doses.

- They act on central sympathetic centers as well as cardiac neuronal terminals to counteract tachyarrhythmias caused by digitalis. This interrelationship provides a favorable role for the beta-adrenergic blockers in controlling digitalis toxicity.

- They often prevent ventricular tachycardias in the long QT interval syndrome. No other class of antiarrhythmic drug seems to be as generally useful.

In organic heart disease (particularly ischemia), control of ventricular arrhythmias with beta-adrenergic blocking agents may require large doses, and antiarrhythmic effect may actually be by *direct* cellular depression of the myofibril or Purkinje fiber (see Nonadrenergic Actions, below).

IMPULSE CONDUCTION

- They cause an increase in the effective refractory period of fibers in the **A-V node**. This action provides the basis for reducing ventricular rate in response to atrial flutter and fibrillation, one of the most important indications of beta blockade. In normal sinus rhythm, the PR interval usually lengthens (reflected by a longer AH interval with no appreciable change in the HV interval). The beta-adrenergic blocking drugs may cause further progression of A-V block (this complication is compounded by their inhibiting adrenergic-sensitive escape pacemakers).

The increase in A-V nodal refractoriness may interrupt the circuit of bypass reentrant tachycardias. The combination of a beta-adrenergic blocker (to increase refractoriness in the A-V nodal fibers) and a Class IA drug (such as quinidine to increase refractoriness in accessory fibers) provides a powerful action to prevent or convert drug-resistant A-V bypass tachycardias.

VASOMOTOR

- They inhibit the vasodilatory (beta-adrenergic) receptors of sympathetic innervation to vascular smooth muscles. The vasoconstrictor (alpha-adrenergic) receptors are left unopposed. The result is increased peripheral vascular resistance and decreased blood flow to all but the cerebral vascular bed.

MYOCARDIUM

- They have negligible effect on normal atrial or ventricular myofibrils. On the other hand, the beta-adrenergic blocking agents tend to aggravate the decompensated myocardium, which depends on increased adrenergic tone to support contractility. By canceling cardiac sympathetic tone, increasing peripheral vascular resistance, and expanding intravascular volume (through reduced renal blood flow and retention of sodium), these drugs tend to worsen congestive heart failure. Beta-adrenergic blockade also reduces the capacity for heavy exercise, normally associated with strong sympathetic support for maximum myocardial contraction.

- They reduce oxygen consumption by the myocardium during effort. Patients with angina benefit by the lowering of heart rate, myocardial stimulation, and systolic pressure.

OTHER ORGAN SYSTEMS

Drugs producing beta-adrenergic blockade have important actions outside of the cardiovascular system:

- They increase airway resistance by decreasing the caliber of bronchi and bronchioles. Bronchospasm can be precipitated in patients with asthma.
- They inhibit the breakdown of carbohydrate and fat, thus complicating the management of diabetes mellitus. In addition, the sympathetic reflexes that protect against hypoglycemia through epinephrine-mediated release of glycogen are blunted. Beta-adrenergic blockade also suppresses the symptoms of epinephrine stimulation (tachycardia, sweating, tremor), which alert insulin-treated patients to hypoglycemic reactions.
- They inhibit the release of renin from the juxtaglomerular cells of the kidney. Renin initiates the angiotensin cascade for powerful vasopressor actions. The drugs are highly effective in lowering blood pressure of patients with hypertension of the high plasma renin activity type.

Nonadrenergic Actions. The beta-adrenergic blocking agents also act directly on the cell membrane through mechanisms mediated independently of the sympathetic nervous system:

- They slow the outward potassium flow during Phase 4 depolarization (similar to the Class IB drugs).
- They inhibit sodium influx during depolarization.
- They depress myocardial contractility.
- They reduce calcium channel transport.

These actions are referred to as the **quinidine-like** or **anesthetic effect**. It must be emphasized that these direct effects on ion transport through the cellular membrane are clinically apparent only at very high doses. However, the beta-adrenergic drugs may exert a subtle and unrecognizable effect on the cell membrane at ordinary blood levels, which could explain distinguishing features among them.

Administration. Hepatic metabolism of the beta-adrenergic blocking drugs is extremely variable; therefore, dosage must be adjusted according to response. The resting sinus rate serves as a convenient and generally reliable indication of the degree of adrenergic blockade. Comparable intravenous doses are much smaller than doses by mouth because of strong hepatic extraction with the latter route.

A **withdrawal syndrome** may occur when these drugs are discontinued. Chronic beta-adrenergic blockade renders the receptors hypersensitive to exogenous catecholamines. Patients who suddenly stop taking the drug after prolonged use are susceptible to developing marked sympathetic reactions (similar to paroxysms in pheochromocytoma) from the exaggerated response to endogenous catecholamines. Increased anginal symptoms and incidence of myocardial infarction have been reported during the withdrawal period. Consequently, gradual tapering of the drug is always recommended.

Side Effects. All of the beta-adrenergic blocking agents may cause functional disturbances:

- Gastrointestinal (nausea, constipation, and diarrhea).
- Neurological (easy fatigability, mental depression, insomnia, and intense dreams).

- Vascular (cold skin, nasal congestion, precipitation or aggravation of coronary arterial spasm, intermittent claudication, intestinal angina, Raynaud's syndrome, and digital ischemia).

NONCARDIOSELECTIVE BETA-ADRENERGIC BLOCKING AGENTS

All of the drugs that block beta-adrenergic receptors affect the heart and the release of renin, a reaction mediated through the beta$_1$ receptors. Certain drugs of this group also affect vascular tone, the bronchi, and glycogenolysis. These are referred to as **nonselective** beta-adrenergic blockers, which act at the beta$_2$ receptors. They include propranolol, nadolol, timolol, labetalol, and pindolol.

PROPRANOLOL (INDERAL). Among the many beta-adrenergic blocking agents currently available, propranolol has been the longest used and the most extensively studied. Having a fairly brief action, propranolol must be given several times a day to maintain steady-state blood levels. However, a recently introduced slow-release form permits less frequent administration.

The quinidine-like effect of propranolol has a synergistic action with adrenergic blockade in suppressing arrhythmias, even at ordinary doses. Thus, it is proposed that propranolol may have an advantage over several of the other nonselective agents that do not share this behavior on cell membranes.

On ingestion, a portion of propranolol is at first bound to proteins in the liver. The degree of binding is highly variable, causing marked differences in the effective dose among individuals.

NADOLOL (CORGARD). The most important difference from propranolol is the much longer action of nadolol. This property usually allows effective oral therapy for treatment of hypertension or angina by once-daily administration.

The major route of excretion is by the kidneys; therefore, lower dosages are appropriate for patients with renal insufficiency.

TIMOLOL (BLOCADREN). Although much more potent than propranolol, timolol has similar adrenergic-blocking properties and patterns of metabolism. Major attention was called to this drug in the Norwegian Multicenter Study Group because of its protective effect in long-term administration following myocardial infarction.

Timolol applied as eye drops constricts the pupil and ciliary body by blocking adrenergic receptors, reducing intraocular pressure in persons with chronic glaucoma. Enough can be absorbed systemically to aggravate bradycardia, A-V block, and myocardial decompensation in susceptible persons.

LABETALOL (NORMODYNE, TRANDATE). Labetalol combines the features of beta-adrenergic blockade with alpha$_1$-receptor blockade. Thus, cardiac dynamics as well as normal vasomotor tone are reduced. In clinical practice, the drug provides a potent lowering of blood pressure, and it has found most utility in the treatment of hypertension. Both oral preparations for long-term management and intravenous solutions for hypertensive emergencies are available.

Reflex and exercise-induced tachycardias are less common than with pure alpha$_1$-adrenergic blockers. Fatigue, depression, cold extremities, and impotence are less likely than with the simpler beta-adrenergic blockers.

Symptoms from postural hypotension may be prominent with labetalol, and standing blood pressures are indicated for assessment of ambulatory management. Following intravenous labetalol, the patient should remain supine for several hours.

In addition to the usual adverse effects of beta-adrenergic blockade—gastrointestinal, central nervous system, and autonomic symptoms—antinuclear antibody formation and vasculitis have been described, as in reactions to procainamide. Hepatocellular injury from the drug rarely occurs and is usually reversible on discontinuing.

Labetalol is metabolized and excreted both by the liver and kidneys. Twice-daily administration is generally required.

PINDOLOL (VISKEN). Although it is comparably potent in respect to adrenergic blockade, pindolol causes less cardiac slowing and less myocardial depressive effect *at rest* than does propranolol. In effect, these properties suggest that stimulation of sympathetic tone may occur, a property known as **intrinsic sympathomimetic activity**. To some degree, it counteracts the dominant blocking effect on adrenergic receptors. The clinical implication is a greater tolerance to pindolol by patients with bradycardia, myocardial insufficiency, or occlusive arterial disease. Additionally, the withdrawal reaction from pindolol is purported to be less severe than from propranolol.

The half-life of pindolol, like propranolol, is relatively short, usually requiring oral dosage two or three times a day. About half of the drug is metabolized and excreted as conjugated metabolites.

CARDIOSELECTIVE BETA-ADRENERGIC BLOCKING AGENTS
Drugs classified as cardioselective (atenolol, esmolol, metoprolol, and acebutolol) are comparable to the nonselective ones already described in respect to their inhibition of adrenergic receptors in the heart and in the renin-producing juxtaglomerular cells (beta$_1$ receptors). However, they have a relatively weak action on other adrenergic systems (beta$_2$ receptors). These distinctions between cardioselective and nonselective drugs are relative, however; all produce universal beta-adrenergic blockade at high blood levels.

In general, the cardioselective agents are better tolerated than the nonselective ones in patients with asthma, insulin-dependent diabetes, or peripheral arterial disease. They also suppress renin, are relatively free of side effects, and are notably effective in some forms of hypertension.

Cardioselective drugs are relatively lipid insoluble, are not metabolized by the liver, are poorly absorbed by the brain, and are excreted by the kidneys. Compared with the nonselective agents, plasma levels attained are generally more stable and have a more prolonged effect. Mental changes appear to be less prominent than with the noncardioselective drugs.

ATENOLOL (TENORMIN). In acute myocardial infarction, atenolol given intravenously appears to offer protection against extension of injury (judged by enzyme release and preservation of initial QRS contour) and against ventricular arrhythmias. Taken orally, it is also effective in suppressing both chronic benign and complex ventricular arrhythmias.

The antiarrhythmic effect persists for about 7 hours after intravenous infusion. Because atenolol has a longer half-life than metoprolol by oral administration, once-daily therapy is usually satisfactory for continuous adrenergic blockade.

METOPROLOL (LOPRESSOR). Because of its relatively short action, it is usually necessary to give metoprolol orally in divided daily doses. The drug can be administered intravenously in small incremental doses, the usual regimen in acute myocardial infarction.

ACEBUTOLOL (SECTRAL). This cardioselective agent also has moderate intrinsic sympathomimetic activity (see Pindolol). Used principally as a once-a-day dose for hypertension with minimal slowing of heart rate, acebutolol has special advantages in patients with bradycardia, bronchitis or emphysema, Raynaud's disease, or cold extremities. It is poorly absorbed into the cerebrospinal fluid and so has a minimal effect on the central nervous system. This property is especially advantageous for the elderly, who are more sensitive to the mental depression action of this class of drugs.

ESMOLOL (BREVIBLOC). This beta-adrenergic blocker is notable for its extremely rapid onset and brief duration of action. By intravenous administration, it provides an effective and easily adaptable agent for tachycardic emergencies. It is approved for use in supraventricular tachycardias. Although conversion to a sinus rhythm in atrial flutter and atrial fibrillation is unlikely, a significant slowing of ventricular response can usually be attained.

The beta$_1$ cardioselectivity of esmolol provides an advantage for patients with mild bronchospastic disorders. However, the higher doses sometimes necessary to control tachycardias are more likely to block beta$_2$ receptors and negate this advantage.

Administration. Available only in a form for intravenous use, esmolol is diluted in a saline or dextrose solution (not a bicarbonate diluent). After injection, it reaches a peak effect within 5 minutes. The pharmacologic half-life is reached within 10 minutes. There is no appreciable clinical effect after 1 hour.

Following an appropriate loading dose given by bolus injection over one minute, a steady state pharmacologic effect is maintained by continuous intravenous infusion. Should there be an insufficient slowing of the heart rate in the absence of untoward effects, the loading dose can be repeated after 5 minutes and followed, if indicated, by an increased maintenance dose.

Catabolism of esmolol is principally by the red blood cells. Consequently, it is safe even without dose adjustment when hepatic or renal function is reduced (unless severe).

Side Effects. Excessive reduction of blood pressure is the most common adverse effect of esmolol. Frequent blood pressure monitoring (preferably by intraarterial measurement) is mandatory. Symptoms from increased airway resistance or myocardial insufficiency are occasionally induced. Rarely, patients may experience neurological or gastrointestinal symptoms. Skin reactions at the site of the infusion dictate a change to another location, preferably through a centrally placed infusion line.

CLASS III: DRUGS THAT PROLONG REPOLARIZATION

The major actions of the Class III agents—bretylium, amiodarone, and adenosine—produce marked prolongation of the refractory period of selective cardiac fibers. These agents have extremely potent antiarrhythmic properties. Unlike the Class IA drugs, they have little effect on depolarization.

BRETYLIUM TOSYLATE (BRETYLOL). Bretylium counters reentrant mechanisms by prolonging repolarization. It is used in emergencies to control drug-resistant ventricular tachycardias and to treat ventricular fibrillation.

Action. Bretylium has the following actions:

- It markedly prolongs repolarization, an action reflected in lengthening of the QT interval. This mechanism decreases the differences between refractory periods in adjacent fibers within the Purkinje network and the ventricles, where impulse reentry is most likely. In acute myocardial infarction, bretylium may exert its major effect on the zone between normal and injured tissues.
- It stimulates automaticity. However, this effect is minor in the sinus node and the His-Purkinje fibers. Automatic firing may occur briefly after injection, probably caused by the release of norepinephrine. Once bretylium has accumulated in the endings of adrenergic neurons, it inhibits the norepinephrine release.

Bretylium can be dramatically effective in suppressing ventricular tachyarrhythmias that have proved refractory to more conventional agents. Ventricular fibrillation sometimes terminates after administration of bretylium, even when other drugs and electrical countershock have failed. The electrophysiological basis for these actions is not well understood. Because conversion of ventricular fibrillation occurs immediately but the antiarrhythmic effect does not reach maximum in ventricular tachycardia for up to 2 hours, different mechanisms may be operant.

Bretylium has little effect on impulse conduction. There is no impairment of the force of myocardial contraction, and hemodynamic parameters usually undergo no significant alterations.

Administration. Bretylium is available only for intravenous infusion or intramuscular injection. Its use is restricted to life-threatening ventricular arrhythmias.

Side Effects. Hypotension from impaired sympathetic reflexes is the most important adverse reaction to bretylium. On the other hand, sympathetic stimulation with initial therapy may cause transient ventricular ectopy, aggravation of hypertension, and enhanced digitalis effect with potential for toxicity.

AMIODARONE (CORDARONE). Amiodarone has a potent effect against recurrent supraventricular and ventricular tachycardias, even when standard drugs have been unsuccessful. Its effectiveness applies to the spectrum of cardiac etiologies: ischemia, congenital defects, myocarditis, and cardiomyopathy. The drug is singularly distinctive for its long duration of action, measured in weeks.

Amiodarone is highly effective in long-term suppression of arrhythmias in patients with the following disorders:

- Hypertrophic cardiomyopathy with recurrent ventricular tachycardia, a cause of exceptionally high risk for sudden death.
- Paroxysmal tachycardias associated with ventricular preexcitation.
- Atrial fibrillation, slowing the ventricular rate response or converting it to sinus rhythm even when electrocardioversion and other drugs have failed.
- Post myocardial infarction with complex ventricular arrhythmias.

Actions. Amiodarone has several distinguishing features:

- It markedly prolongs the refractory period of atrial, ventricular, and His-Purkinje tissue. PR, QRS, and QT intervals typically are prolonged; significant lengthening of the QT interval is an important clinical marker of amiodarone effect. Alterations in the T wave and increased U wave amplitude may occur as well.
- It blocks alpha- and beta-adrenergic receptors as well as calcium channel receptors.
- It reduces the rate of Phase 4 decrement in automatic cells. Amiodarone has minor effects on depolarization.
- Amiodarone increases the threshold for ventricular fibrillation.
- It decreases the force of myocardial contraction when given by intravenous injection. However, it has minimal effect on the myocardium with chronic oral administration.
- It dilates vascular smooth muscle, although slightly. Coronary and peripheral arterial resistance is reduced somewhat, tending to compensate for the negative inotropic effect.
- It acts during an extraordinarily long period, which may extend to several weeks.

Administration. There are three pharmacokinetic phases of amiodarone and its major active metabolite, desethylamiodarone:

1. Circulatory system distribution, which occurs rapidly, with drug eliminated from plasma within a few days.

2. Tissue loading of the various organ tissues, requiring several days. Elimination is relatively slow.

3. Adipose tissue fixation, taking several months. On discontinuing the drug, 1 to 3 months is required for complete elimination.

All three compartments must be saturated before a steady state is attained. Because amiodarone is so slowly absorbed, metabolized, and eliminated (chiefly by the liver), several days or weeks are often required before the full clinical effect of chronic administration is evident. Furthermore, there is a wide variation in individual sensitivity, its action is unpredictable, and it has serious potential side effects. Daily loading doses are usually recommended, with step-down to maintenance doses prescribed within 1 or 2 weeks. In practice, an effective and safe dose must be determined by individual trial and only with fastidious clinical and laboratory monitoring. During the dose loading period, it is prudent to monitor the durations of PR, QRS, and QT intervals daily.

Although the drug may be effective in treating atrial fibrillation and paroxysmal supraventricular tachycardia) with or without accessory bypass tracts), amiodarone is approved only for treatment of ventricular tachycardias that are life-threatening and then only after they have proved refractory to conventional agents.

Amiodarone may be combined with more conventional agents, generally with good compatibility.

Side Effects. The majority of persons taking amiodarone develop some adverse manifestations, but these are usually minor and tolerable. However, dangerous toxic reactions are possible and dictate that the smallest effective dose be used for maintenance therapy.

The major toxic effects of amiodarone are as follows:

- Pulmonary fibrosis. Pulmonary infiltrate and alveolitis may be intermediary reactions and are reversible. Periodic chest x-ray, diffusion capacity studies, lung scan, or a combination of these is essential for follow-up.
- Neurological disorders (including peripheral sensory and motor neuropathies, incoordination, tremor, and fatigability).
- Rarely, fulminant hepatitis occurs.

More common but generally less serious side effects of amiodarone are as follows:

- Sleep disturbances, probably the most common unpleasant reaction.
- Photosensitivity, which may be severe. A rash with a golden brown discoloration sometimes occurs in sun-exposed areas.
- Ocular discomfort and visual disturbances from precipitation of the drug in the corneas.
- Interference with thyroid metabolism and laboratory testing because of a high drug iodine content. Either hyper- or hypothyroidism may rarely result.
- Aberrations of liver enzymes are common. Sometimes bilirubin and alkaline phosphatase levels are elevated in a pattern suggesting biliary obstruction.

Although amiodarone has a low incidence of cardiac toxicity, it can aggravate or precipitate the following conditions:

- Sinus node dysfunction.
- Congestive myocardial failure.
- Ventricular tachycardia (with a tendency toward torsades de pointes).

ADENOSINE (ADENOCARD). Adenosine has recently been released for the emergency treatment of supraventricular tachycardia. Although the drug has not yet been placed in an official classification, it is included here because of similarities in action to the Class III agents.

Acting principally to delay conduction in the A-V node, adenosine is noteworthy for its extremely rapid action and high degree of success in treating supraventricular tachycardias. Adenosine, by prolonging the refractory period of A-V nodal fibers, is especially effective for suppressing reentrant tachycardias with an accessory (Wolff-Parkinson-White) or intranodal tract.

Adenosine is a natural substance (composed of a purine derivative and a sugar) that is found in nucleic acids and in high-energy phosphate bonds (e.g., ATP). Given as an intravenous bolus, it has a half-life of less than 10 seconds, with its major degradation occurring within the vascular space. Conversion of paroxysmal supraventricular tachycardias to a sinus rhythm results in an average time of 30 seconds. The drug has negligible depressing effect on the myofibril and is therefore advantageous in patients with myocardial injury or failure.

Although adenosine is usually effective in converting or at least slowing both narrow and wide QRS supraventricular tachycardias, it may be transitory. Even so, the change in rhythm or rate is often useful for differentiating a sinus/atrial tachycardia from an A-V junctional tachycardia.

Adenosine is ineffective in the treatment of atrial flutter, atrial fibrillation, and ventricular tachycardia. It is inadvisable to use it in the presence of sinus node dysfunction and significant A-V block.

Administration. Adenosine is only effective when injected in the undiluted form as a rapid intravenous bolus. Because of its short half-life, it is important that the drug be injected directly into a vein or at least close to the entry site of an intravenous line. An isotonic saline flush will promote more complete delivery.

If unsuccessful, injections can be repeated using increasing amounts given a few minutes apart. Doses are not cumulative in the body, and excretion of active drug is independent of hepatic and renal function. Large doses, however, may cause clinically significant vasodilation resulting in a reduction in blood pressure. Experience has demonstrated a 10-fold difference among individuals in the minimum dose required for efficacy.

Side Effects. Momentary side effects may occur at the time of injection, with cutaneous symptoms (especially facial flushing) the most common. Chest discomfort and respiratory symptoms are infrequent. Complaints referable to the gastrointestinal tract (mostly nausea) and the nervous system (lightheadedness, dizziness, and paresthesias) have occasionally attended the use of intravenous adenosine.

Transient premature atrial or ventricular beats or sinus bradycardia commonly appear immediately after injection. Excessive vasodilation, more likely with higher doses, may lead to hypotension. Adenosine decreases automaticity in the sinus node, with the danger of severe bradycardia in preexisting sinus node dysfunction. Induction of A-V block is common. Occasionally ventricular pauses exceeding 2 seconds are observed.

CLASS IV: DRUGS THAT BLOCK CALCIUM CHANNELS

Drugs of Class IV (verapamil, nifedipine, diltiazem, and nicardipine) inhibit the transport of calcium through the slow channels in the membrane of excitable cells. This action inhibits impulse formation and conduction.

The calcium channel blocking agents do not affect sodium transport in the fast channels. The drugs have a particularly potent effect on cardiac cells that are predominantly or wholly dependent on the inward flux of calcium during depolarization, specifically those of the sinus node and the A-V node. It must be appreciated, however, that these agents do not block calcium channel activity absolutely; otherwise, they would bring about cessation of vital activities.

The calcium channel blocking agents have various effects at the following sites:

- Sinus node. The intrinsic rate is slowed moderately by calcium channel blockade. (Counteracting this effect is sinus node stimulation in response to drug-induced vasodilation.) In sinus node dysfunction, an exaggerated response should be anticipated, and marked bradycardia may occur.
- A-V node. Deceleration of conduction velocity and prolongation of the refractory period are the most prominent actions of calcium channel blockade. In atrial flutter and atrial fibrillation, these actions produce a modest reduction in the ventricular rate response. The drugs are also particularly effective in aborting supraventricular tachycardias that use the A-V node or an anomalous A-V connection as one limb of a reentrant pathway. In preexisting A-V block, the calcium channel blockers may precipitate more advanced impairment of impulse conduction and cause profound bradycardia.
- Ventricles. Although ventricular tachyarrhythmias often respond to calcium channel blockers, suppression is less dependable than in supraventricular tach-

ycardias. However, when the arrhythmia is triggered by acute ischemia (either from spasm or from a fixed lesion of a coronary artery), these agents can prove remarkably effective.

The calcium channel blockers have utility in tachyarrhythmias caused by digitalis, particularly those arising from Purkinje fibers. However, their potential for further increasing A-V block while inhibiting escape pacemakers limits the use of these agents in digitalis toxicity.

- Myocardium. Cardiac contraction is more dependent on relocation of sarcoplasmic calcium to unlock the myosin-actin complex than on transport of calcium across the cell membrane. Although the Class IV agents do inhibit calcium transport from the sarcoplasmic reservoirs to myosin-actin reaction sites, this effect is not prominent, and they do not impair contractility at ordinary clinical doses. At high doses, however, the intracellular action becomes more prominent, and the drugs may have a depressant myocardial action. When myocardial insufficiency is already present, further compromise of contractile function is likely at any dose.
- Blood vessels. Contraction of arterial smooth muscle depends on both calcium channel transport and on mobilization of sarcoplasmic calcium. Here, contraction is more dependent on calcium transport across the cell membrane than is the myocardium, and intracellular calcium must be continuously replenished from external sources. Consequently, the calcium channel blockers antagonize the coupling of myosin and actin in the vasculature, promoting vasodilation. It is important clinically that sympathetic reactivity is left intact.

The vasomotor relaxation is enough to induce an appreciable diminution in peripheral vascular resistance, and with it a reduction of cardiac afterload. Because the coronary arteries share the vasodilating response, myocardial blood flow is enhanced.

The various drugs described below differ largely in respect to their action on vasomotor tone, and these differences may be determined by the location of receptors within the calcium channels of blood vessels where the drugs are bound.

VERAPAMIL (CALAN, ISOPTIN). Among the calcium channel antagonists, verapamil is characterized by its relatively potent actions on various cardiac functions. It is used primarily in antiarrhythmia treatment to control reentrant supraventricular tachycardias.

Actions. Verapamil affects the cardiovascular system in the following ways:

- It terminates reentrant tachycardias of atrial origin.
- It slows conduction velocity and prolongs the refractory period in the A-V node. In atrial flutter and fibrillation, the drug reduces the ventricular rate response.
- It interrupts the reentrant circuits by its action on the A-V node, thus proving effective in tachycardias associated with ventricular preexcitation. Verapamil does not affect calcium dynamics in accessory bypass tracts but may cause dangerous acceleration of rate in ventricular preexcitation if atrial flutter or fibrillation is present.
- It reduces peripheral vascular resistance somewhat by its relatively weak vasodilating action. This mechanism probably explains the benefit of verapamil in improvement of effort-induced angina.

The His-Purkinje system is relatively resistant to the conduction-inhibiting action of verapamil. Consequently, ventricular tachycardias of the reentrant type often fail to respond. Verapamil may, in fact, lead to further hemodynamic decompensation and precipitate serious ventricular arrhythmias.

Side Effects. Verapamil is generally well tolerated by most cardiac patients. Nevertheless, these potential adversities must be anticipated:

- It may cause severe bradycardia, especially in persons with depressed cardiac automaticity or with A-V nodal conduction disorders. This possibility is increased with the coadministration of beta-blocking drugs. Verapamil is particularly hazardous when used to treat rhythms of excitation caused by digitalis toxicity. It interacts with digitalis to increase the blood level of the latter, and it works synergistically to intensify the blocking action on the A-V node.
- It depresses myocardial contractility when myocardial insufficiency is already present.
- It reduces blood pressure transiently when given rapidly by intravenous injection. Serious hypotensive reactions are more likely when the effects of other cardiodepressor drugs are superimposed.
- It may substantially accelerate heart rate—even to levels in which cardiac decompensation is precipitated—when used to treat tachycardias caused by ventricular preexcitation in the presence of atrial flutter or fibrillation. The mechanism appears to be enhanced conduction in the bypass tract due to vasodilation-induced sympathetic stimulation.

Noncardiovascular untoward reactions include the following:

- Constipation and nausea.
- Vertigo, headache, and fatigability.

Administration. After intravenous injection, verapamil reaches its maximum effect within 15 minutes; peak effect by oral dose does not occur for about 2 hours. The bioactive metabolite norverapamil gradually accumulates with continued administration, and dosage should be stepped down accordingly. Because of normal hepatic degradation, ordinary doses of verapamil may become toxic in the presence of liver dysfunction.

Oral verapamil attains peak blood levels in 1 to 2 hours. However, much slower peaks are found in supraventricular tachycardias, owing to delayed gastric emptying from the splanchnic vasoconstriction of adrenergic stimulation. Consequently, oral verapamil is not recommended when the arrhythmia is compromising cardiac output.

For long-term oral use, the drug is given three times a day with meals. A sustained-release form of verapamil is now available, permitting once-daily doses. Hepatic insufficiency dictates lower doses.

NIFEDIPINE (ADALAT, PROCARDIA). Nifedipine contrasts with verapamil in having a strong vasodilating effect and a relatively weak cardiac effect:

- Vasodilation. The potent direct action of nifedipine on smooth muscle of the arterioles is its most important property and the basis for its clinical indications. It is used in patients with hypertension, angina caused by coronary arterial spasm, Raynaud's syndrome, and other arterioconstrictive entities. Reduced cardiac afterload from diffuse vasodilation may explain the benefit of nifedipine in angina associated with fixed lesions of the coronary arteries.
- Electrophysiology. Unlike verapamil, nifedipine has little effect on cell repolarization, and it does not interfere appreciably with A-V nodal conduction. Consequently, nifedipine cannot be considered a major antiarrhythmic drug.
- Myocardium. Nifedipine has a negligible effect on myocardial contractility.

Side Effects. Vasodilation is the most common basis of nifedipine-induced reactions:

- Postural hypotension (lightheadedness, nausea).
- Dependent edema (not related to myocardial failure or to sodium/fluid retention).
- Compensatory tachycardia.
- Hot flush.
- Nasal congestion.

In addition, nifedipine may cause the following:

- Abnormal hepatic enzyme levels.
- Hyperplasia of the gums (a reaction similar to that with phenytoin) with prolonged administration.
- Gastrointestinal disturbances.

Administration. Although verapamil depends principally on hepatic excretion, nifedipine is eliminated chiefly by the kidneys. Accordingly, the dose of nifedipine must be reduced in patients with renal insufficiency.

The inconvenience of three- or four-times daily dosing and of fairly common side effects have been reduced appreciably by development of a novel form of sustained-release tablet. Based upon the mechanics of osmotic dispersion in the gastrointestinal tract, the tablet provides stable blood levels of active drug throughout a 24-hour period, thereby eliminating the prominent peaks and troughs of the ordinary preparation.

DILTIAZEM (CARDIZEM). Diltiazem stands between verapamil and nifedipine in its effects on the heart and on vascular tone:

Like verapamil, diltiazem has the following effects:

- It reduces heart rate, A-V conduction, and contractile force, although to a lesser degree than does verapamil.
- It suppresses supraventricular tachycardias having a reentrant mechanism.

Like nifedipine, diltiazem has the following effects:

- It dilates the peripheral arterial tree but to a lesser extent than does nifedipine.
- It protects against angina from coronary artery spasm.

These companion properties of diltiazem have particular utility in patients who have both angina and hypertension.

Side effects. Diltiazem may intensify any of the following conditions:

- Sinus node dysfunction.
- A-V conduction defects.
- Myocardial insufficiency.

Any of these possibilities is more likely if patients with these conditions are also taking a beta-adrenergic blocking agent.

- Postural hypotension may result from excessive vasodilation, especially in patients with conditions or on drugs that depress vascular tone.

Paradoxically, diltiazem may elevate blood pressure, accelerate heart rate, and increase premature beats if given rapidly by injection. All arise from sympathetic reflexes evoked by sudden vasodilation.

NICARDIPINE (CARDENE). One of the newer calcium channel blockers, nicardipine has a potent relaxing action on arteriolar smooth muscle, reducing peripheral vascular resistance and thereby decreasing afterload on the left ventricle. This action is at least as effective on coronary and cerebral arteries as on the peripheral vessels. Its major indications are in the treatment of hypertension and in stable and vasospastic angina.

Nicardipine has no appreciable effect on heart rate. There is no change in sinus node recovery time or in conduction in the A-V node. The effect of nicardipine on myocardial contractility is minimal, even in an ischemic heart. In fact, it is reported to improve myocardial function in left ventricular insufficiency and to increase exertional tolerance in angina. Nicardipine is especially useful when hypertension complicates acute myocardial infarction.

DIGITALIS

The digitalis compounds have complex and clinically important actions on the myocardium, vasomotor tone, and impulse formation and conduction. In the pages that follow, each of these functions is considered individually.

Myocardium

Improving the force of contraction of the failing heart is the most useful clinical property of digitalis. The mechanism is binding of the enzyme(s) that activates adenosine triphosphatase and that is responsibile for the energy-dependent sodium-potassium pump of the cell membrane. By inhibiting sodium extrusion from the resting cell, digitalis indirectly also decreases the concomitant loss of intracellular calcium from the sarcoplasmic stores. Thus, more calcium is available for the actin-myosin interaction.

By a second mechanism (and perhaps a minor one), digitalis may increase the amount of calcium moving into the cell during the slow inward current phase of depolarization. Both actions are independent of adrenergic mediation.

Vasomotor Tone

Digitalis has a mild vasoconstrictive action, probably by increasing sympathetic tone from central nervous system stimulation. This effect appears to be most important in ischemic disease of the mesenteric circulation, where the drug can exaggerate the syndrome of intestinal angina. It may have an adverse influence on the arterial nutrition of digits or on the time-to-claudication in patients with occlusive peripheral arterial disease. On the other hand, vasodilation and improved peripheral circulation may result if myocardial insufficiency (a condition associated with sympathetic-mediated vasoconstriction) is relieved by digitalis.

Electrophysiology

Digitalis affects both automaticity and conduction in all regions of the heart by its direct activity on the cell membrane. In addition, digitalis enhances parasympathetic tone and thus has indirect properties that modify the direct cellular action. Augmentation of sympathetic tone occurs as well, especially at high doses. These complex relationships will be presented at various levels of function.

IMPULSE FORMATION

SINUS NODE

Direct Effect: Inhibitory. Digitalis at high tissue concentrations depresses pacemaker activity of automatic cells in the sinus node.

Indirect Effect: Inhibitory. By enhancing parasympathetic tone, digitalis produces vagally mediated slowing of the sinus node. The acceleration of heart rate expected during exercise is blunted, an effect that can be eliminated with atropine.

These combined effects tend to cause slight slowing of sinus rate in normal individuals. Exaggerated responses include sinus arrhythmia, bradycardia, pauses, and arrest. These responses are most common and most severe in patients with sinus node dysfunction. In myocardial insufficiency with attendant tachycardia, vagally mediated sinus slowing may be a prominent and beneficial effect.

ATRIA

Direct Effect: Stimulatory. Digitalis increases the rate of Phase 4 spontaneous depolarization, increasing automaticity of latent pacemaker tissue in the atria. Atrial premature beats and atrial tachycardia are common manifestations of digitalis toxicity. These tachycardias, with onset characterized by gradual acceleration and offset by gradual deceleration, are differentiated from the suddenness of typical reentrant tachycardias. Tachycardias induced by digitalis are frequently associated with A-V block (described under Impulse Conduction, below).

Indirect effect: Inhibitory. Digitalis increases vagal tone on atrial fibers, tending to suppress atrial automaticity. This mechanism may counteract the excitatory influence on automatic firing. Thus, digitalis may be effective in abolishing spontaneous atrial ectopic beats and atrial tachycardia, most especially those triggered by sympathetic overdrive. In toxic doses, however, it may precipitate atrial tachyarrhythmias. Atrial flutter and atrial fibrillation occasionally convert to normal sinus rhythm after administration of digitalis.

The net effect of this dual action of digitalis on atrial automaticity depends on the sensitivity of the atrial fibers and the tissue levels of the drug. As blood level rises, enhancement of automatic firing dominates over the autonomic suppression. This intricate relationship has important therapeutic implications and must be considered in every patient who has atrial tachyarrhythmias and who takes digitalis.

ATRIOVENTRICULAR JUNCTIONAL TISSUE. Similar to the action on atrial fibers, digitalis has an excitatory effect on membrane activity of A-V junctional cells and an inhibitory action on their autonomic control through parasympathetic stimulation. Because spontaneous A-V nodal rhythms are much less common than atrial, nodal premature beats and nodal tachycardia in a patient taking digitalis are likely an expression of digitalis toxicity. The suspicion is further supported if runs of the tachycardia begin with gradual speeding up and end with gradual slowing, signaling an automatic mechanism.

VENTRICLES

Direct Effect: Stimulatory. Enhanced automaticity in the His-Purkinje fibers represents one of the most frequent and early signs of digitalis toxicity, an effect that is more pronounced in patients with hypokalemia. As the effective drug level and tissue sensitivity increase, ventricular premature beats become more frequent and tend to originate from multiple foci. Ventricular bigeminy is strongly suggestive of advanced digitalis toxicity. Further increases of digitalis levels are likely to lead to ventricular tachycardia (usually with multiphasic beats) and ventricular fibrillation. Similar to the supraventricular tachycardias, an accelerating beginning and decelerating ending of a run of ventricular tachycardia reflect enhanced automaticity, and digitalis etiology is highly suspect.

The mechanism responsible for ectopic automaticity from digitalis appears to involve after potential depolarization in Purkinje fibers following the major action potential. One suspected cause is the release of calcium ions from calcium-overloaded cells, resulting from inhibition of the sodium pump in the cell membrane. Enhanced adrenergic stimulation may be an additional mechanism.

Indirect Effect: Inhibitory. Under certain conditions, digitalis may depress automaticity in the ventricles. This inhibitory action is not produced by vagal reflexes (because parasympathetic innervation to the ventricles is slight if not negligible). As ventricular ectopic rhythms can be generated by metabolic abnormalities in the failing myocardium, the automaticity-suppressing effect of digitalis probably represents improved cellular metabolism and better myocardial function.

The treatment of ventricular premature beats and sustained ventricular tachyarrhythmias often involves the perplexing problem of deciding if too little or too much digitalis is being given. Unfortunately, the margin between the therapeutic dose and the toxic dose is small, and extracardiac factors (other drugs, electrolyte balance, and oxygenation) have critical roles.

IMPULSE CONDUCTION

The action of digitalis on impulse conduction parallels the functional changes in impulse formation, having a dual action on the cell membrane and on autonomic control.

SINOATRIAL JUNCTION. By increasing parasympathetic tone to the sinus node, digitalis may produce sinoatrial block or sinus standstill in persons with preexisting sinus node dysfunction.

ATRIA. The most important effect of digitalis on atrial conduction occurs in atrial flutter. By prolonging the refractory period of atrial fibers, digitalis impedes impulse propagation. At extremely rapid rates, this delay may be enough to cause microwave fronts of impulses to confront areas in the atrial wall that are at varying degrees of responsiveness and refractoriness from previous depolarizations. This heterogeneity of activity commonly converts atrial flutter to atrial fibrillation.

ATRIOVENTRICULAR NODE. Digitalis delays the conduction time of impulses in the A-V node, and several mechanisms appear to be responsible. Foremost is augmentation of vagal tone. Digitalis also appears to increase the sensitivity of the A-V node to stimulation by vagal impulses. In addition, digitalis acts directly on the cell membrane of A-V nodal fibers, prolonging the refractory period (which normally is longer than that of any other cardiac tissue). Digitalis may depress sympathetic tone and adrenergic responsiveness in A-V nodal fibers.

These several properties have both therapeutic and toxic implications.

Therapeutic Actions. By slowing conduction in the A-V node, digitalis reduces the rate of ventricular responses to supraventricular tachycardia. The effect is particularly dependable in atrial fibrillation. With the exception of treating myocardial failure, slowing the ventricles in atrial fibrillation is the most important indication for digitalis.

Contributing to the slowing of impulses through the A-V node in atrial fibrillation is the increased rate of atrial impulses (the excitatory component of digitalis). Explained by the mechanism of concealed conduction, more rapid bombardment of the A-V node increases its resistance to conduction.

In ventricular preexcitation, digitalis may break paroxysmal tachycardias or reduce the tendency for their occurrence by slowing antegrade impulses in the A-V nodal limb of the reentrant circuit. *One precautionary note:* Digitalis may shorten the refractory period in the accessory fibers; in the unusual form of the syndrome in which this pathway serves as the antegrade limb in atrial flutter or fibrillation, digitalis can lead to a tachycardia of life-endangering proportions. Therefore, the drug should not be used in these arrhythmias if an aberrant reentrant pathway is suspected unless it is given with an additional antiarrhythmic agent (such as a Class IA drug) that prolongs the refractory period of the anomalous fibers.

Toxic Effects. Lengthening of the PR interval from digitalis is almost always clinically inconsequential. However, digitalis tends to further impair conduction defects in the A-V node. For example, preexisting first-degree A-V block may be worsened to intermittent and even complete A-V block.

Complete A-V block in atrial flutter and fibrillation is assumed to be a manifestation of digitalis toxicity until another cause is established. It is identified by a *regular* ventricular rhythm in the presence of a varying FR interval in flutter or a chaotic atrial rhythm in fibrillation. If the ventricular rate is rapid and regular, coexistence of complete A-V block and a digitalis-induced A-V junctional rhythm or ventricular tachycardia is a possibility.

VENTRICLES. Digitalis slows impulse conduction in Purkinje fibers and in ventricular myofibrils. Ordinarily of no importance in a normal heart, the combined actions of digitalis to increase automaticity while decreasing conduction velocity in the ventricles predispose to reentrant tachycardia. This form of digitalis toxicity is especially threatening as a precursor to ventricular fibrillation.

Extracardiac Toxicity. Digitalis commonly produces symptoms referable to various organ systems:

- Gastrointestinal (nausea and diarrhea).
- Neurological (abnormal color vision, fatigability, malaise, and confusion).

Extracardiac reactions can occur without cardiotoxicity in some individuals, whereas in others serious arrhythmias from digitalis toxicity may be present with no extracardiac symptoms.

ASSOCIATED CONDITIONS

By altering one of several cofactors, digitalis toxicity can be precipitated in previously well-controlled cases. Hypokalemia is certainly the most important of these cofactors. Hypomagnesemia, hypercalcemia, hypothyroidism, and adrenergic enhancement may be causally associated. Hypoxia, ischemia, and myocardial insufficiency from any cause sensitize the heart to digitalis. Arrhythmias precipitated by digitalis are frequent following cardiac contusion (blunt chest trauma), open-heart surgery, and myocardial infarction.

Digoxin (Lanoxin)

For all practical purposes, digoxin is the only form of digitalis currently in general clinical use. Digoxin can be administered by the following routes:

- Intravenous injection for emergency use. It usually begins to act in 5 or 10 minutes and reaches a peak in about 1 hour. Therefore, consecutive doses can be given at relatively short intervals after maximum action from the previous doses has most likely been attained.
- Oral administration. In most patients, an effect occurs within 1 hour and reaches a peak in about 4 hours. After about 8 hours, digoxin serum levels begin to decline. Maintenance therapy can usually be achieved with once- or twice-daily administration by mouth when renal function is normal.

Binding sites on plasma and tissue proteins must be saturated before a steady-state blood level is reached with serial doses of digoxin. Therefore, initial treatment (whether parenteral or oral) requires giving a loading dose of two to five times that estimated for the total daily maintenance dose. When urgency is not an issue, an alternative method can be adopted using estimated maintenance doses daily; steady state may be reached in 1 to 3 weeks.

The kidneys are the principal pathway for clearance of digoxin. When renal insufficiency is present, the dose must be decreased accordingly. It is prudent to assume, incidentally, that all elderly patients have some degree of reduced renal function.

Blood levels of digoxin provide a useful monitor for a drug with a very narrow and complex therapeutic:toxic range. However, it cannot be overemphasized that blood levels do not identify a hypersensitive patient, and a serious arrhythmia from digoxin may be present with nontoxic blood levels. The greatest asset of blood level monitoring is in alerting clinicians of the potential danger of toxicity should the level exceed the accepted therapeutic range.

Other drugs may interact with digoxin to produce important clinical effects:

- Increases in the plasma concentrations of digoxin by displacing it from binding sites on circulating proteins (quinidine, quinine, verapamil, and amiodarone).

- Potentiation of the effect of digoxin by reducing its renal excretion and by inducing electrolyte disorders, most especially hypokalemia (thiazides, furosemide, and amphotericin B).
- Increases in the sensitivity of autoexcitable tissues to digitalis (adrenergic agents and thyroxin).
- Interference with the renal clearance of digoxin (triamterene and nifedipine).
- Synergistic action with digoxin by depressing impulse conduction, producing or intensifying sinoatrial or A-V block. The beta-adrenergic blockers are notable in this regard. Quinidine and procainamide have competing direct and indirect actions on the conduction pathways; either may potentiate or weaken the effect of digoxin on sinoatrial and A-V nodal conduction, and the result is unpredictable.

GENERAL PRECAUTIONS WHEN ADMINISTERING CARDIAC DRUGS

The dose administered is but one of many factors that determine the effect of a drug. Individual differences in alimentary absorption, binding to circulating proteins and fixed tissue, distribution in organ and tissue compartments, rate of metabolism, sensitivity of receptors, and rate of excretion all have important influences. Age, gender, pregnancy, fat:lean body composition, electrolyte patterns, acid-base balance, ischemia, and physical activity also affect individual sensitivity to drugs. The rapidly accumulating body of information on interactions between drugs is of increasing concern to clinicians. Blood level determinations now available for many agents serve as valuable guidelines for dosage, but they do not take into account most of these variables. It is well recognized (particularly in regard to the antiarrhythmic drugs) that there is no way to predict efficacy, toxicity, and proarrhythmia effect from dose alone. Furthermore, oral doses often result in wide fluctuations in the blood levels of active drug; toxicity may occur at the peak and undertreatment at the trough.

An honored dictum holds that doses, when feasible, should be started at low levels and increased gradually with sentinel alertness for desired and potentially dangerous actions. This principle is particularly appropriate in elderly patients, whose physiology changes with aging in respect to absorption, tissue distribution, and elimination of drugs and to the sensitivity of receptors for them.

Glossary*

aberrant conduction: alteration of impulse transmission from normal pathways, characterized by a change in configuration of the electrocardiographic complex. (Synonym: aberration.)

aberration: deviation of impulse conduction from normal pathways, characterized by altered configuration of the representative electrocardiographic figure. (Synonym: aberrant conduction.) (L. *ab-*, from; *errāre*, to stray.)

accelerated: refers to a rhythm of ectopic origin having a rate faster than the natural (or intrinsic) rate of that tissue. An A-V junctional rhythm with a rate above 60 beats per minute and a ventricular rhythm above 40 beats per minute are described as accelerated.

accessory: secondary. In reference to impulse conduction, the term is synonymous with *anomalous* and denotes an alternative pathway through which impulses can bypass the ordinary pathways.

Adams-Stokes syndrome (or *attacks*): also referred to as Stokes-Adams syndrome. Syncope due to pathological slowing of the heart rate. Named after Robert Adams and William Stokes, who published case histories in a Dublin medical journal in 1827 and 1846, respectively.

adrenergic: having the effect of stimulating the peripheral sympathetic nerves.

A-H interval: on the His bundle electrogram, the duration between the deflection from depolarization in the low right atrium (A) and that of the common bundle (H). Also known as the atrioventricular nodal conduction time.

anomalous: a deviation from normal. Refers to pathways of conduction that provide alternate routes from ordinary impulse conduction. (See accessory.)

A-V interval: in A-V sequential electronic pacemaker rhythms, the period between an atrial stimulus and the subsequent ventricular stimulus.

antegrade: impulse conduction in the normal (or forward) direction, usually referring to the A-V node. (Synonym: anterograde.) (L. *ante*, before.)

anterograde: (Synonym: antegrade.)

antiadrenergic: having an inhibitory effect on the peripheral sympathetic nerve activity. (Gr. *anti*, against.)

anticholinergic: having an inhibitory effect on parasympathetic nerve activity.

arrest: cessation of contractile activity of the heart, referring to either atrial or ventricular arrest. Cardiac arrest is a less specific entity and usually implies sudden

---

* A.S. = Anglo-Saxon
  Gr. = Greek
  L. = Latin
  Fr. = French

circulatory failure due either to cessation of the heartbeat or to ventricular fibrillation.

arrhythmia: variation from the normal rate and electrical sequences of cardiac activity. This term in the broadest sense has come to include abnormalities of impulse formation and conduction. (Synonym: dysrhythmia). (Gr. *a-*, without; *rhuthmos*, rhythm.)

artifact: in electrocardiography, an inscription caused by extraneous mechanical or electrical interference rather than by the electrical activity of the heart.

asynchronous electronic pacemaker: electronic power unit that continuously delivers an electrical impulse to the ventricular myocardium. (Synonym: fixed-rate electronic pacemaker.)

asystole: absence of cardiac contractions, referring to the entire heart or to a pair of chambers, such as ventricular asystole. (Gr. *a-*, without; *sustolē*, contraction.)

atrial arrest: cessation of atrial contractions. (L. *ad*, to; *restāre*, to stop.)

atrial fibrillation: turbulent, uncoordinated activity of the atria, represented by continuous, irregular deviations from the baseline of the electrocardiogram.

atrial flutter: rapid and distinct atrial depolarization (usually greater than 300 per minute) from an atrial pacemaker.

atrial premature complex: conduction initiated within the atria, occurring early in the normal cardiac cycle and resetting the sinus pacemaker cadence.

atrial tachycardia: repetitive rapid complexes arising from an ectopic focus in the atria.

atrioventricular block: a conduction defect in the A-V node or the major conduction bundles. First-degree (1°) A-V b.: excessive slowing of conduction time of sinus impulses as they pass through the A-V conduction pathway; second degree (2°) A-V b.: intermittent failure of impulses originating in the sinus node to traverse completely the A-V conduction pathways; third-degree (3°) A-V b.: complete failure of all impulses to penetrate the A-V conduction pathway; retrograde A-V b.: failure of impulses originating in the ventricles to penetrate the A-V conduction pathway and enter the atria.

atrioventricular dissociation: independent beating of the atria and ventricles, each under control of separate pacemakers.

atrioventricular node: specialized conducting fibers concentrated at the base of the atrial septum just above the ventricular septum, through which impulses pass from the atria to the ventricles.

atrium: contractile chamber of the heart. Right a. receives venous blood from the superior and inferior vena cava and ejects it into the right ventricle; left a. receives blood from the pulmonary veins and ejects it into the left ventricle. (L *ātrium*, the court or central hall of a Roman house.)

auricles: muscular pouches projecting from the right and left atrial walls. Although these structures compose only a small portion of the atrial mass, the terms auricular fibrillation and flutter have long been used synonymously with atrial fibrillation and flutter. (L. *auricula*, little ear.)

automaticity: property of self-excitatory cardiac cells in which spontaneous depolarization occurs. (Gr. *autos*, self; *-matos*, willing.)

autonomic nervous system: division of the central nervous system; it extends outward to various peripheral organs, blood vessels, and glands concerned with involuntary regulation, including the automatic, conductile, and contractile elements of the heart. Composed of two subdivisions: the sympathetic and parasympathetic systems.

axis: summation of direction of all electrical activity recorded during inscription of the component.

axis deviation: an abnormal electrical direction of a component of the cardiac cycle. Left axis deviation is present when the axis of the QRS complex is less than $-30°$

(the leftward horizontal position being reference point 0°). Right axis deviation of the QRS complex is designated greater than +120°.

beat: one complete electrical and mechanical cardiac cycle.

bigeminy: paired cardiac beats, each from a separate pacemaker in a recurring pattern. When sinus beats alternate with ectopic beats, the rhythm is designated according to the ectopic pacemaker, e.g., atrial or ventricular bigeminy. (L. *bi-*, two; *geminus*, twin.)

biphasic: In electrocardiography, an inscription both above and below the baseline. (Synonym: diphasic.)

block: delay or obstruction of impulse conduction.

bradycardia: deceleration of the cardiac rate below arbitrarily defined limits. Sinus b.: impulse formation less than 60 per minute; nodal b.: impulse formation less than 40 per minute; ventricular b.: impulse formation less than 20 per minute. (Gr. *bradus*, slow; *kardia*, heart.)

bundle: a tract of impulse conducting fibers. (See common bundle.) (Synonym: fascicle.)

bundle of His: Demonstrated in 1893 in humans and numerous animals by Wilhelm His, Jr., professor of clinical medicine in Berlin. (Synonym: common bundle.)

cadence: established rhythmicity of cardiac impulse formation.

capture: depolarization of a cardiac chamber by a stimulus, usually referring to intermittent ventricular activation by a supraventricular pacemaker in A-V dissociation or to chamber activation by an electronic pacemaker.

cardiac arrest: 1. cessation of contractile activity of the heart. 2. a general term used to describe sudden collapse from ineffective contractions of the heart; includes ventricular arrest or fibrillation.

cardioversion: process requiring delivery of electrical stimulation that is used to interrupt an abnormal rhythm allowing the sinus node to assume control of the rhythm. Can be accomplished with an electronic pacemaker activated in an overdrive mode, by an automatic implantable cardioverter-defibrillator, or by a synchronized defibrillator (termed a cardioverter).

cholinergic: having the effect of stimulating the parasympathetic nerves or simulating their activity.

chronotropic: causing change in rate of impulse formation. Positive: increases frequency of impulse formation; negative: decreases frequency of impulse formation. (Gr. *khronos*, time; *tropos*, turn, change.)

common bundle: fibers leading from the A-V node to branches in the ventricles. (Synonym: bundle of His.) Right b. branch: fibers from the common bundle that are distributed to the endocardial surface of the right ventricle; left b. branch: fibers from the common bundle that divide into an anterior (or superior) and a posterior (or inferior) branch and are distributed to the endocardial surface of the left ventricle.

compensatory pause: in sinus rhythm, a delay in ventricular systole following a premature complex; it does not interfere with the sinus cadence but does eliminate a sinus-conducted beat. The interval between R waves of the normal beats preceding and following the premature complex is twice that of the normal RR interval.

complete A-V block: absence of impulse conduction between atria and ventricles. (Synonym: complete heart block.)

concealed conduction: incomplete penetration of a propagating impulse, giving no directly observable electrocardiographic deflection, but having an effect on formation or conduction of subsequent impulses.

conduction: transmission of a depolarizing impulse through tissue. (L. *com-*, together; *dūcere*, to lead.)

connection: an accessory pathway of preferential impulse conduction between myocardial fibers.

contraction: coordinated shortening of cardiac muscle fibers resulting in a decrease in the chamber volume. (L. *com-*, together; *trahere*, to draw.)

coupling: a time relationship occurring between paired beats, referring to a constant interval between a normal beat and a subsequent premature complex.

defibrillation: process requiring discharge of an electrical stimulus that is used to interrupt ventricular fibrillation. Accomplished with an automatic implantable cardioverter-defibrillator or an external unit termed a defibrillator.

deflection: deviation of an electrocardiographic line from the baseline. Positive d.: above the baseline; negative d.: below the baseline.

delta wave: deformity of the initial portion of the QRS complex in the preexcitation syndrome. (Gr. *delta*, letter in Greek alphabet with triangular shape.)

demand mode electronic pacemaker: ventricular conduction is initiated by an electronic pacemaker when normal activation is absent. (Synonym: ventricular-inhibited electronic pacemaker.)

depolarization: process of activation of automatic, conductile, and contractile elements from the resting or polarized state. (L. *dē-*, from.)

depression: refers to any inhibitory effect on the heart that decelerates impulse formation rate or conduction velocity.

diastole: rhythmic relaxation and dilation of the cardiac chambers. (Gr. *diastolē*, dilation, separation.)

diphasic: (Synonym: biphasic.)

dissociation: separation of normally related cardiac events, applied to independent beating of the atria and ventricles. (L. *dis-*, reversal; *sociāre*, to join.)

dromotropic: causing change in velocity of conducted impulses. Positive: increases conduction velocity; negative: decreases conduction velocity. (Gr. *dromos*, running; *tropos*, turn, change.)

dysrhythmia: abnormal rhythm of the heart, generally used synonymously with *arrhythmia*. (Gr. *dus-*, faulty, diseased; *rhuthmos*, rhythm.)

echo beat: a cardiac cycle produced through a reentrant impulse from a preceding cardiac cycle. Such beats may be either atrial or ventricular. Also known as a *return extrasystole.*

ectopic: impulse originating in cardiac tissue outside the sinus node. (Gr. *ex-*, out of; *topos*, place.)

electrical mechanical dissociation: failure of mechanical contraction of the myocardium despite the presence of electrical conduction.

electrocardiogram: a recording of the electrical activity of the heart by a series of deflections that represent certain components of the cardiac cycle.

electrocardiograph: an instrument for recording the electrical activity of the heart; basically a modified galvanometer.

electrode: an electrical conducting device or terminal that completes an electrical circuit between transmitting and receiving media.

endocardial pacemaker: electronic stimulation of the myocardium is accomplished via electrodes placed within the right ventricular chamber through the central venous system.

endocardium: the inner layer of connective tissue of the heart. (Gr. *endon*, within.)

epicardial pacemaker: method for artifically stimulating the myocardium through electrodes sutured to the outer surface of the heart.

epicardium: the outer layer of connective tissue of the heart. (Gr. *epi*, over.)

escape beat: conduction originating outside the sinus node in which the ectopic pacemaker is released by depression of formation or conduction of sinus impulses.

excitability: the capacity to respond to a stimulation. (L. *ex-*, out, *cīre*, to put into motion.)

excitation: refers to any stimulating effect on the heart that accelerates impulse formation rate or conduction velocity.

exit block: failure of an impulse to conduct from its origin to adjacent tissue, as in sinoatrial block.

extrasystole: a premature beat arising from an ectopic site. (Synonyms: premature contraction or complex.) (L. *extra*, outside or additional; Gr. *sustolē*, contraction.)

fascicle: (Synonym: bundle.) (L. *fascis*, bundle.)

fibrillation: continuous disorganized electrical and contractile activity of cardiac chambers. (L. *fibrilla*, small fiber or fibril.)

fixed-rate electronic pacemaker: electronic power unit that continuously delivers an electrical impulse to the ventricular myocardium. (Synonym: asynchronous electronic pacemaker.)

flutter: extremely rapid impulse formation with coordinated activity of paired cardiac chambers. (A.S. *flot*, the sea; to float, fluctuate, or quiver.)

focus: a site within cardiac tissue with the capacity for impulse formation. [L. *focus*, fireplace, hearth (the center of the home).]

fusion beat: a cardiac complex produced by two merging depolarizing waves from impulses arriving from separate sites.

H-V interval: on the His electrogram, the time from the deflection due to depolarization in the common bundle (H) to the beginning of ventricular depolarization (V). Also known as the His-Purkinje conduction time.

hemiblock: a disruption of impulse conduction in either the anterior or the posterior branch of the left bundle. (Gr. *hemi-*, half.)

His bundle: a conduction pathway between the A-V node and the Purkinje fibers of the ventricles. Also known as the common bundle. Named after Wilhelm His, of Basel, Switzerland, who in 1893 described an embryonic rest between the atria and ventricles, forming a narrow band of muscle fibers and serving as a bridge for impulses.

His bundle electrogram: a recording of electrical activity taken from inside the heart with electrodes positioned near the common bundle (of His). This invasive technique provides information of A-V nodal conduction occurring during the isoelectric period between the end of the P wave and the beginning of the QRS complex on the standard electrocardiogram.

idio-:   prefix used with ectopic rhythms, implying self-generated impulse formation, e.g., idionodal, idioventricular. (Gr. *idios*, personal, peculiar, separate.)

infarction: area of tissue necrosis following cessation of the blood supply.

inotropic: causing change in contractile strength of muscle. Positive i.: increases contractile strength; negative i.: decreases contractile strength. (Gr. *is, inos*, fiber; *tropos*, to turn or influence.)

interference dissociation: a form of A-V dissociation in which an accelerated ventricular rhythm renders the A-V node refractory to supraventricular impulses.

interpolated: refers to ectopic premature beats that do not prevent formation of the subsequent normal beat; it thus appears as an extra beat between two normal uninterrupted beats. (L. *inter-*, between; *polīre*, to adorn.)

isorhythmic A-V dissociation: form of A-V dissociation in which the atria and ventricles beat at identical, or nearly identical, rates. (Gr. *isos*, equal.)

joule: a unit of energy equal to one watt-second. After James Prescott Joule, a British physicist (1818–1889).

junctional: refers to tissue with potential for automaticity located adjacent to the A-V node and the common bundle. Probable origin of nodal rhythms. (Synonym: A-V junctional.)

lead: arrangement of electrical conductors through which electrical activity from the body is brought to a recording device, or the recording from such a set of conductors.

Mobitz phenomenon: form of second-degree A-V block consisting of intermittent blocked sinus beats with constant PR intervals of conducted beats (also known as

Type II second-degree block). Named after Walter Mobitz of Germany, who proposed a system of classification of intermittent A-V block in 1924.

multifocal: refers to ectopic beats originating from two or more impulse-forming sites. (L. *multus*, much, many.)

multiform: varying in configuration, referring particularly to ectopic beats.

multiphasic: a waveform having several components of both upright (positive) and downward (negative) directions.

myocardium: the muscle mass of the heart. (Gr. *mus*, muscle.)

nodal accelerated rhythm: rhythm originating in the A-V junctional tissue at a rate faster than 60 beats per minute and less than 100 beats per minute.

nodal premature complex: a premature beat originating in the A-V junctional tissue. (L. *nōdus*, knob, knot.)

nodal rhythm: series of beats initiated in the A-V junctional tissue at a rate of 40 to 60 per minute. (Synonym: idionodal rhythm; A-V junctional rhythm.)

nodal tachycardia: rhythm originating in the A-V junctional tissue at a rate faster than 100 per minute. (Synonym: accelerated nodal rhythm.)

noncompensatory pause: delay in ventricular systole following a premature complex that resets the dominant sinus cadence. In contrast with a compensatory pause, in which there is no cadence change of the normal cardiac cycle.

oscilloscope: an instrument that forms a continuous visual image on the screen of a cathode-ray tube from electrical currents of an external source. (L. *ōscillare*, to swing; Gr. *skopein*, to examine.)

pacemaker: 1. cell or group of cells that depolarize spontaneously, forming impulses that propagate and initiate cardiac conduction. 2. electronic pulse generator: a. demand pacemaker: electronic pacemaker that is sensitive to spontaneous cardiac depolarization that momentarily delays the electronic pulsation; b. fixed pacemaker: electronic pacemaker that operates continuously regardless of spontaneous cardiac activity; c. synchronous pacemaker whose rate of impulses to the ventricles is governed by the rate of atrial depolarization.

parasympathetic nervous system: fibers of the autonomic nervous system derived from the brain stem and lower spinal cord. 1. motor: generally has an inhibiting effect on blood vessel tone, causing dilation, and on cardiac impulse formation rate and conduction velocity, causing deceleration. 2. sensory: relays responses from the heart and major arteries to the central nervous system. Both motor (efferent) and sensory (afferent) fibers of the cardiac parasympathetic nervous system are contained in the vagus nerve.

parasystole: complexes initiated by an ectopic pacemaker at regular intervals, unrelated to the dominant rhythm. (Gr. *para*, beside.)

paroxysmal: refers to recurring episodes of cardiac arrhythmias with sudden onset and cessation. [Gr. *para* (intensifier), beside; *oxunein*, to sharpen, goad.]

polarity: difference in electrical energy between the inner and outer surface of the cell membrane, known as the transmembrane potential; dominant direction of complex deviation from baseline.

PP interval: duration of one complete cardiac cycle.

preexcitation syndrome (PES): a clinical entity in which anomalous conductile pathways between atria and ventricles short-circuit the A-V node. (Synonym: Wolff-Parkinson-White or WPW syndrome.)

PR interval: segment of the electrocardiographic cycle measured from the beginning of the P wave to the beginning of the QRS complex.

Purkinje system (or network): conductile fibers in the subendocardial tissues of the ventricles. Described in 1839 by Johannes Purkinje, a Bohemian physiologist and pioneer in microscopic anatomy.

P wave: electrocardiographic representation of atrial depolarization.

QT interval: the time from the beginning of the QRS complex to the end of the T wave. It represents predominantly ventricular repolarization, although a small portion of the interval is taken up by ventricular depolarization.

Q wave: first negative deflection of the ventricular depolarization complex on the electrocardiogram.

reentry: a phenomenon wherein a depolarizing front enters the myocardium, which contains areas having unequal conduction velocities. Conduction is produced from the normal front, followed by conduction produced from an impulse emerging from the slower conducting area. A postulated mechanism for premature complexes.

refractory period: an interval during repolarization of automatic, conductile, and contractile tissue during which there is a decreased degree of excitability for subsequent depolarizing stimuli. 1. absolute r.p.: initial phase of repolarization in which tissue will not respond to stimuli, however intense. 2. relative r.p.: later phase of repolarization in which the tissue can respond to stimuli of greater than normal intensity. (L. *refractus*, broken off.)

repolarization: process of restoration to the normal resting electrical polarity following depolarization.

retrograde: impulse conduction in reverse or backward direction, usually referring to the A-V node. (L. *retrō*, backward.)

RR interval: distance between corresponding points of two consecutive R waves, representing the duration of one cardiac cycle.

R wave: first positive deflection of the ventricular depolarization complex on the electrocardiogram.

septum: fibrous and muscular partition that separates the right cardiac chambers from the left. (L. *sēptum*, partition, from *saepes*, hedge.)

sinoatrial block: a form of exit block wherein impulses formed in the sinus node fail to emerge from it.

sinus arrest: cessation of automaticity in the sinus node.

sinus arrhythmia: an exaggeration of the normal phasic variation in the rate of sinus impulse formation associated with ventilatory activity.

sinus bradycardia: excessive slowing of impulse formation in the sinus node to below 60 per minute.

sinus irregularity: erratic variations in the cadence of sinus impulse formation unrelated to ventilatory cycles.

sinus node: group of specialized myocardial cells located in the right atrial tissue with automatic activity. This activity results in impulse formation that is ordinarily more rapid than that of other cardiac automatic centers, so that the sinus node is the normal pacemaker of the heart. (Synonym: sinoatrial node.) [L. *sinus*, a curve (suggested by the shape of the sinus node).]

sinus pause: momentary cessation of automaticity in the sinus node.

sinus rhythm: natural cardiac rhythm directed by pacemaker activity of the sinus node, normally at 60 to 100 per minute.

sinus syndrome: markedly abnormal variability of sinus node impulse formation rate, characterized by periods of rapid and slow pacemaker activity. (Synonym: sinoatrial syndrome, bradycardia-tachycardia syndrome, sluggish sinus node syndrome, sick sinus syndrome, sinus node dysfunction.)

sinus tachycardia: impulse formation in the sinus node exceeding 100 per minute.

Stokes-Adams syndrome: see Adams-Stokes syndrome.

supraventricular: refers to a site above or proximal to the ventricles, e.g., sinus node, atria, and A-V node. (L. *suprā*, above.)

S wave: negative deflection in the electrocardiogram occurring after the R wave of the ventricular depolarizing complex.

sympathetic nervous system: fibers of the autonomic nervous system derived from the thoracolumbar spinal cord. These generally have a stimulaing effect on blood vessel tone (constriction), cardiac impulse formation rate and conduction velocity (acceleration), and myocardial contractility (increased force).

synchronous electronic pacemaker: mode of artificial myocardial stimulation that provides for ventricular activation following atrial conduction.

systole: rhythmic contractions of the cardiac chambers. (Gr. *sustolē*, contraction.)

tachyarrhythmia: abnormally accelerated heartbeat from any focus of automaticity.

tachycardia: acceleration of the cardiac rate above defined limits. Sinus t.: impulse formation faster than 100 per minute; nodal t.: impulse formation faster than 60 per minute; ventricular t.: impulse formation faster than 50 per minute. (Gr. *takhus*, swift.)

threshold: the minimal intensity of stimulation required to cause a response in automatic, conductile, and contractile tissue.

torsades de pointes: a form of wide QRS tachycardia having an undulating appearance as the waveforms change gradually in shape and amplitude (from a negative to a positive deflection) from beat to beat. (Fr., twisting around a point.)

tract: an accessory pathway extending from myocardial fibers to specialized conducting tissue.

transthoracic: inserted through the chest wall; refers to a method of placing an electronic pacemaker wire electrode into the heart. (Synonym: epicardial electronic pacemaker.)

transvenous: inserted through a vein; refers to a method of implanting an electronic pacemaker wire electrode into the heart. (Synonym: endocardial electronic pacemaker.)

trigeminy: recurring pattern of three beats, wherein the second and third beats of each group consist of premature complexes. (Gr. *tri-*, three; L. *geminus*, twin.)

T wave: electrocardiographic representation of ventricular repolarization.

unidirectional block: in a conducting tissue, a waveform may proceed in one direction but not in the reverse direction, a situation that favors development of reentrant beats.

unifocal: refers to ectopic beats originating from a single site. (L. *ūnus*, one.)

uniform: waveforms having similar configurations from beat to beat.

U wave: electrocardiographic representation of afterpotentials that normally follow ventricular repolarization.

V-A interval: in A-V sequential electronic pacemaker rhythms, the time between a ventricular stimulus and that of the subsequent atrial stimulus.

vagolytic: influence that decreases or abolishes the tone of the vagus nerve.

vagotonic: influence that increases the tone of the vagus nerve.

vagus nerve: the tenth cranial nerve; either of paired nerves of the parasympathetic nervous system with multiple branches to various visceral organs, including the heart, and containing motor and sensory fibers. [L. *vagus*, wandering (referring to its diffuse branching).]

vasovagal reflex: parasympathetic stimulation initiated by sensory impulses from the thoracic aorta and its larger branches, which are transmitted centrally to the cranial nerve nuclei and are relayed peripherally by an effector impulse in the vagus nerve, causing slowing of the sinus rate and A-V conduction and generalized vasodilation. (L. *vās*, vessel.)

vector: magnitude and direction of physical energy, such as the electrical activity of the myocardium.

ventricle: contractile chamber of the heart. Right v.: receives venous blood from the right atrium and ejects it into the pulmonary artery; left v.: major muscular chamber of the heart that receives arterial blood from the left atrium and ejects it into the aorta. (L. *ventriculus*, a swollen part, diminutive of *venter*, belly or abdomen.)

ventricular accelerated rhythm: rhythm originating in the ventricles having a rate faster than 50 beats per minute but less than 100 beats per minute.

ventricular arrest: cessation of ventricular contractions. (Synonym: ventricular standstill.)

ventricular bradycardia: slowing of an idioventricular rate to less than 20 per minute.

ventricular fibrillation: multifocal and grossly asynchronous contractions of the ventricles resulting in continuous uncoordinated twitching and cessation of circulatory flow.

ventricular flutter: extremely rapid ventricular rhythm producing an electrocardiographic pattern in which QRS complexes merge into T waves without discernible separation.

ventricular-inhibited electronic pacemaker: ventricular depolarization is initiated by an electronic pacemaker when normal activation is absent. (Synonym: demand mode electronic pacemaker.)

ventricular premature complex: beat occurring early in the normal cardiac cycle that originates from the ventricle, characterized by aberration of the QRS complex (prolonged and distorted) and the T wave.

ventricular rhythm: sustained impulse formation from a ventricular focus that paces the ventricles at a rate of 20 to 50 per minute. (Synonym: idioventricular rhythm.)

ventricular tachycardia: rhythm resulting from an accelerated firing of an automatic focus or foci within the ventricle faster than 100 per minute.

vulnerable period: interval during repolarization in which the tissue is hypersensitive to stimulation, and subthreshold stimuli may produce electrical instability. Such stimuli applied during this period have a tendency to induce sustained rhythms of excitation, e.g., tachycardia, flutter, or fibrillation. (L. *vulnus*, wound.)

V-V interval: an electronic pacemaker term, referring to the duration between successive ventricular electronic stimuli.

wandering pacemaker: impulse formation shifting from site to site within the sinus node, atria, and A-V junctional tissue, causing variation in cadence, in P wave contour, and in PR intervals.

watt-second: a unit of electrical energy, expressing the amount of current exerted over time; equal to 1 joule.

Wenckebach phenomenon: form of second-degree A-V block consisting of progressive lengthening of PR intervals in consecutive cardiac cycles until interrupted by a blocked sinus beat. Also known as Type I second-degree A-V block. Named after Karl Wenckebach of Holland, who described the forms of intermittent A-V block in 1906.

Wolff-Parkinson-White syndrome: (Synonym: WPW or preexcitation syndrome.) Named after Louis Wolff, John Parkinson, and Paul D. White, who reported in 1930 eleven cases of paroxysmal tachycardias in individuals having widened QRS complexes.

Abbreviations in Common Use

AFib	atrial fibrillation		PAT	paroxysmal atrial tachycardia
AFl	atrial flutter		PES	preexcitation syndrome
AICD	automatic implantable cardio-verter-defibrillator		RBBB	right bundle branch block
			SA	sinus arrest
APC	atrial premature complex		S-A	sinoatrial
AT	atrial tachycardia		S-AB	sinoatrial block
A-V	atrioventricular		SB	sinus bradycardia
BBB	bundle branch block		SP	sinus pause
CA-VB	complete atrioventricular block		ST	sinus tachycardia
			SVT	supraventricular tachycardia
CP	carotid pressure		VA	ventricular arrest
ECG	electrocardiogram		VB	ventricular bradycardia
EKG	electrocardiogram		VFib	ventricular fibrillation
EPM	electronic pacemaker		VFl	ventricular flutter
LAH	left anterior hemiblock		VP	ventricular pause
LBBB	left bundle branch block		VPC	ventricular premature complex
LPH	left posterior hemiblock			
MI	myocardial infarction		VT	ventricular tachycardia
NPC	nodal premature complex		WPW	Wolff-Parkinson-White syndrome
NSR	normal sinus rhythm			
NT	nodal tachycardia			

Answer Section

This section provides answers to all electrocardiograms that require a reader response and that are identified by a circled number.

Read Before Proceeding:

1. Interpretations given follow the description method. Alternate terminology may be preferred when more consistent with that used at your institution.

2. Abbreviations used are listed on page 566.

3. Cardiac rates are expressed in beats per minute. They have been determined using the three-beat ruler when feasible, beginning with the first cardiac cycle on the left unless otherwise indicated.

4. Specific electrocardiographic events are located by the distance in millimeters measured from the left-hand edge. A cardiac cycle is measured to the onset of that particular cycle (not necessarily at the maximum deflection) for consistency in identification.

5. Your measurements may vary somewhat from those provided. This is partially the result of distortions in reproduction inherent in commercial printing. However, these variations should be of minor degree and of no importance.

Good luck.

Chapter 2

1. Good monitoring lead.
2. Poor monitoring lead. R amplitude too low. Move LA electrode or reverse polarity.
3. Good monitoring lead.
4. Poor monitoring lead. R amplitude too low. Move LA electrode or reverse polarity.
5. Good monitoring lead.
6. Poor monitoring lead. T amplitude too high. Move LA electrode or reverse polarity.
7. Good monitoring lead.
8. Poor monitoring lead. R amplitude too low and T amplitude too high. Move LA electrode or reverse polarity.
9. Poor monitoring lead. P and T wave amplitude too high. Move LA electrode.

Chapter 3

10. Fastest = 74; slowest = 65.
11. Rates per minute: 78, 80, 81, 84, 86, 88, 88, 87, 85, 79.
12. Rates per minute: 82, 53, 58, 63, 75, 63, 53.

13. Rates per minute: 87, 80, 62, 75, 78, 84, 85, 84, 73.
14. Fastest = 88; slowest = 58.
15. Fastest = 82; slowest = 49.
16. Fastest = 92; slowest = 46.
17. Fastest = 93; slowest = 46.
18. Fastest = 82; slowest = 48.
19. Fastest = 72; slowest = 48.
20. Rate = 71; rate = 58.
21. Rate = 70; rate = 56.
22. Rate = 90.
23. Rate = 92; rate = 52.
24. Rate = 83.
25. Rate = 164.
26. Rate = 80.
27. Rate = 104.
28. Rate = 167.
29. Rate = 82.
30. Rate = 113.
31. Rate = 85.
32. Rate = 100.
33. Rate = 78.
34. Rate = 158.
35. Rate = 132; rate = 76.
36. Rate = 123.
37. Rate = 83.
38. Rate: ruler = 126; grid = 130; scan = 6 × 20 = 120.
39. Rate: ruler = 122; grid = 125; scan = 6 × 20 = 120.
40. Rate: ruler = 133; grid = 140; scan = 7 × 20 = 140.
41. Rate: ruler = 128; grid = 130; scan = 120.
42. Rate: ruler = 167; grid = 160; scan = 160.
43. Rate: ruler = 110; grid = 108; scan = 110.
44. Rate: ruler = 44; grid = 45; scan = 40.
45. Rate: ruler = 42; grid = 40; scan = 40.
46. Rate = 47.
47. Rate = 56 to 58.
48. Rate = 47.
49. Rate = 43.
50. Rate: shortest interval = 40; longest interval = 20.
51. Rate = 70; rate = 40.
52. Initial rate = 111; depressed rate = 71.
53. Initial rate = 45; depressed rate = 28.
54. Initial rate = 128; depressed rate = 80.
55. Initial rate = 65; depressed rate = 39.
56. Initial rate = 91; depressed rate = 27.
57. Basic rate = 61; delayed rate = 32.
58. Basic rate = 72, delayed rate = 39.
59. Basic rate = 63; delayed rate = 18. (Calculated rate: 17 large squares × 0.20 second = 3.40 seconds interval. Sixty seconds per minute divided by 3.40 = 18 per minute).
60. Rate = 45.
61. Ventricular inactivity = 6.60 seconds (33 large squares × 0.20 second).
62. Rate = 40.
63. Rate = 76.
64. Rate = 37.

65. Rate = 69; rate = 39; sinoatrial block at 140 mm.
66. Rate = 81.

Chapter 4

67. Rates: 57, 54, 51, 51.
68. Rates: 80, 67.
69. NSR, rate = 69.
70. Basic rhythm = NSR, rate = 88; ectopic beats = 3 APCs.
71. Rate = 88.
72. Basic rhythm = NSR, rate = 82; ectopic beats = 3 APCs.
73. Coupling rates: 106, 127, 107.
74. Sinus rate = 54; atrial rate = 120.
75. APCs as 16, 53, 89, 125, 160 mm.
76. APCs at 27, 80, 137 mm.
77. Basic rhythm = sinus; ectopic beats = 4 APCs; sinus/atrial ratio 1:1; interpretation: atrial bigeminy.
78. Basic rhythm = sinus; ectopic beats = 6 APCs; sinus/atrial ratio 1:1; interpretation: atrial bigeminy.
79. Basic rhythm = sinus; ectopic beats = 4 APCs; sinus/atrial ratio 1:1; interpretation: atrial bigeminy, transient.
80. Sinus rate = 47; ectopic rate = 88.
81. Sinus rate = 45; ectopic rate = 73.
82. Blocked APC at 45.5 mm.
83. Blocked APCs at 78, 114 mm.
84. Blocked APCs at 66, 158 mm.
85. Blocked APCs at 42, 158 mm.
86. Rate = 142; regular.
87. Rates = 107 slowing to 51; sinus contour; 115 beats per minute; 107 beats per minute; normal sinus rhythm.
88. Atrial rate = 135, regular; sinus rate = 82, not regular.
89. Rate = 220.
90. Rate = 62.
91. Rate = 141; PR interval = 4.5 mm (0.18 second); atrial rate = 242; A:V ratio = 2:1.
92. Equidistant; constant PR; atrial rate = 126; ventricular rate = 63.
93. Equidistant; constant PR; atrial rate = 220; ventricular rate = 110.
94. Equidistant; constant PR; atrial rate = 260; ventricular rate = 130.
95. Atrial tachycardia: rate = 136; ventricular rate = 68; 43.
96. Atrial rate = 200; ventricular rate = 100.
97. Atrial rate = 344; ventricular rate = 172.
98. Atrial rate = 207; ventricular rate = 144.
99. 5.52 seconds.
100. Atrial rate = 310; ventricular rate = 155; A:V ratio: variable.
101. Atrial rate = 292; ventricular rate = 146; A:V ratio: 2:1; FR interval = 0.12 second.
102. Atrial rate = 280; ventricular rate = 70; A:V ratio: variable (although at first it would appear to be consistent 4:1 response).
103. Atrial rate = 240; ventricular rate = 31 to 54; A:V ratio: variable.
104. Atrial rate = 320; ventricular rate = 70 to 120; A:V ratio: variable.
105. Atrial rate = 262; ventricular rate = 70 to 130; A:V ratio: variable.
106. Atrial rate = 320; ventricular rate = 80 (average); A:V ratio: variable.
107. Atrial rate = 276; ventricular rate = 69; A:V ratio: 4:1; FR interval = 0.08 second.
108. Atrial rate = 310; ventricular rate = 110 (average); A:V ratio: variable.

109. Atrial rate = 325; ventricular rate = 120 (average); A : V ratio: variable (although it appears to alternate between 3 : 1 and 2 : 1).
110. APCs at 12, 93, 174 mm.
111. APC at 50 mm.
112. Rate: three-second marks, 3.0 beats × 20 = 60.
113. Rate: three-beat ruler = 60 to 132. Three-second marks, 4.0 beats × 20 = 80.
114. Rate: three-beat ruler = 75 (average). Three-second marks, 4.0 × 20 = 80.
115. Rate: three-beat ruler = 80. Three-second marks, 4.0 × 20 = 80.
116. Rates: sinus rhythm = 77; atrial fibrillation = 50 (average).
117. Rate = 110.
118. Rate = 65.
119. Rate = 40.
120. Rate = 146; rate = 43; slower.
121. Rate = 80; rate = 39; slower.
122. Rate = 50; rate = 20; slower.
123. Rate = 126.
124. Rate = 67.
125. Rate = 140.
126. Rate = 104.
127. Rate = 88.
128. Rate = 39.
129. Rate = 96.
130. Rate = 84.
131. Ventricular rate = 130.
132. Atrial rate = 340; ventricular rate = 170.
133. Atrial rate = 325; ventricular rate = 115.

Self-Evaluation: Stage 1

134. Atrial flutter, variable A-V block, atrial rate = 300; ventricular rate = 110 (average).
135. Atrial fibrillation, average ventricular rate = 110.
136. NSR, rate = 90, with two APCs at 70 mm and 168 mm.
137. Basic rhythm = NSR, rate 70. APCs at 43 mm and 133 mm.
138. Atrial fibrillation with transition to atrial flutter and rapid ventricular rate response at 115.
139. Sinus tachycardia, rate = 125.
140. Atrial fibrillation with moderate ventricular response rate = 75 (average).
141. Sinus rhythm with atrial bigeminy, rate = 98 (average).
142. Sinus bradycardia, rate = 51.
143. Normal sinus rhythm with blocked APCs in bigeminal pattern, rate = 80.
144. Normal sinus rhythm, rate = 83. Sinus pause, rate to 23, induced by carotid pressure, followed by transient sinus bradycardia.
145. Atrial fibrillation, rapid ventricular rate response = 155 (average).
146. Sinus bradycardia, rate = 55, with APC at 87 mm.
147. Atrial fibrillation with rapid ventricular rate response = 110 (average) to sinus bradycardia, rate = 58.
148. Atrial fibrillation with moderate ventricular rate response = 85.
149. Atrial tachycardia, rate = 129, to sinus rhythm, rate = 80 for two cardiac cycles, to atrial tachycardia, rate = 140.
150. Sinus bradycardia, rate = 54.
151. Atrial tachycardia with 2 : 1 A-V block; atrial rate = 138; ventricular rate = 69.
152. Wandering atrial pacemaker, rate = 60 (average).
153. Sinus tachycardia, rate = 118.
154. Atrial tachycardia, rate = 210, to sinus tachycardia, rate = 125.

155. Sinus bradycardia, rate = 43.
156. Atrial flutter, variable A-V conduction, ventricular rate response of 70 to 140.
157. Atrial flutter with transition to atrial fibrillation, rapid ventricular rate response = 110.
158. Sinus arrhythmia, rate = 49 to 64 (average = 54).
159. Atrial flutter with constant A-V conduction (ratio 2:1); atrial rate = 264; ventricular rate = 132.
160. Basic rhythm = NSR, rate = 86; blocked APC at 150 mm.
161. Atrial flutter with constant A-V conduction (ratio 4:1); atrial rate = 332, ventricular rate = 83.
162. Sinus tachycardia, rate = 117, with sinus pause at 135 mm or possibly blocked APC at 127 mm, atrial escape beat at 142 mm; to atrial fibrillation at 155 mm, to sinus beat at 180 mm.
163. NSR, rate = 84, and development of baseline artifact (60-cycle disturbance, probably due to disconnection of right leg/ground electrode). Note that the rhythm pattern is generally discernible throughout this electrical interference. Find R spikes with calipers.
164. Sinus rhythm with atrial bigeminy, rate = 69.
165. Sinus bradycardia, rate = 36 (average).
166. Normal sinus rhythm, rate = 74 with APC at 82 mm.
167. Atrial fibrillation, ventricular rate response = 57 to 150 (average = 90).
168. Atrial fibrillation with slow ventricular rate = 32 (average).

Chapter 5

169. PR interval = 0.13 second.
170. PR interval = 0.18 second.
171. PR interval = 0.14 second.
172. PR interval = 0.18 second.
173. Rhythm: sinus, rate = 93; PR interval = 0.08 second.
174. Rate = 84; PR intervals = 0.14, 0.10 second.
175. Rate = 76; PR interval = 0.10 second.
176. Rate = 83; PR interval = 0.10 second.
177. Rate = 97.
178. Rate = 75; PR interval = 0.35 second.
179. Rate = 63; PR interval = 0.28 second.
180. Rate = 125; PR interval = 0.22 second.
181. Rate = 31; PR interval = 0.38 second.
182. Rate = 83; PR interval = 0.23 second.
183. Rate = 85; PR interval = 0.23 second.
184. Rate = 85; PR interval = 0.25 second.
185. Rate = 80; PR interval = 0.25 second.
186. Rate = 71; PR interval = 0.31 second.
187. Rate = 107; PR interval = 0.23 second.
188. Rate = 114.
189. Rate = 65; PR interval = 0.44 second.
190. Rate = 65; PR interval = 0.26 second.
191. Blocked sinus P wave at 137 mm; rate = 72; PR interval = 0.23 second.
192. Atrial rate = 76; ventricular rate = 38.
193. Blocked sinus beats occur at 33, 95, 174 mm; PR interval = 0.13 second; ratio = 5:4.
194. A:V ratio = 2:1.
195. Second-degree A-V block: PR interval = 0.14 second; A:V ratio = 2:1; sinus rate = 62; ventricular rate = 31.

196. Second-degree A-V block: prolonged PR interval = 0.24 second; A:V ratio of central group = 4:3; sinus rate = 57; ventricular rate = 40.
197. Second-degree A-V block; prolonged PR interval = 0.28 second; A:V ratio = 2:1; sinus rate = 114; ventricular rate = 57.
198. Atrial rate = 108; ventricular rate = 36; A:V ratio = 3:1; PR interval = 0.16 second.
199. Atrial rate = 108; ventricular rate = 36; A:V ratio = 3:1; PR interval = 0.14 second.
200. NSR; rate = 66; PR interval = 0.20 second.
201. Sinus rhythm with blocked sinus beats and absent ventricular action (11.88 seconds).
202. Sinus rhythm with no A-V conduction to sinus tachycardia with 2:1 A-V block.
203. Sinus rate = 106.
204. PR intervals: 0.32, 0.38, 0.40, 0.45, sinus block at 169 mm; 0.32 second.
205. PR intervals: 0.28, 0.34, 0.38, sinus block at 55 mm; 0.22, 0.28, 0.34, 0.40, sinus block at 133 mm; 0.22, 0.28, 0.36. Ratio = 5:4 in central group.
206. Sinus tachycardia. PR intervals: 0.16, 0.20, 0.23, sinus block at 33 mm; 0.16, 0.25, sinus block at 62 mm; 0.16, 0.20, 0.25, sinus block at 95 mm; 0.16, 0.23, sinus block at 103 mm; 0.16, 0.19, 0.23, sinus block at 161 mm; ratios = 4:3, 3:2, 4:3, 3:2, 4:3.
207. PR intervals: 0.23, 0.26, 0.28, 0.29, 0.30, 0.36, 0.38, sinus block at 108 mm; 0.23, 0.35, sinus block at 155 mm; 0.24, 0.34. Ratios = 8:7, 3:2.
208. Sinus block at 91 mm; PR interval: 0.12, sinus block at 121 mm, 0.12, sinus block at 150 mm; 0.12, sinus block at 180 mm. Ratios = 2:1 throughout.
209. PR intervals: 0.18, 0.28, sinus block at 38 mm, 0.18, 0.28, sinus block at 87 mm; 0.16, 0.30, sinus block at 136 mm; 0.18, 0.28, sinus block at 185 mm. Ratios = 3:2 throughout.
210. PR intervals: shortest = 0.18 second; longest = 0.24 second. A:V ratio = 9:8.
211. PR intervals: shortest = 0.22 second; longest = 0.36. A:V ratio = 8:7.
212. PR intervals: shortest = 0.26 second; longest = 0.38. A:V ratio = 5:4.
213. Prolongation of PR interval begins at 102 mm; PR intervals range from 0.14 second to 0.24 second; sinus rate slows from 95 to 62.
214. Rate = 174; A:V ratio = 1:1.
215. PR interval = 0.26 second.
216. Blocked sinus beats at 57, 153 mm.
217. A:V ratio = 2:1.

Chapter 6

218. Sinus rate = 40, 39.
219. Ventricular rate = 79, 49, 50; standardization marker at 144 mm.
220. Rate = 37; distal junctional focus.
221. Rate = 46, 39; distal junctional focus.
222. Rate = 40, 28; distal junctional focus.
223. Rate = 62; proximal junctional focus.
224. Sinus rate = 96; yes; ventricular rate = 39; yes.
225. Sinus rate = 111; A-V junctional rate = 54; no.
226. Sinus rate = 96; A-V junctional rate = 39; no; complete A-V block with junctional rhythm.
227. Atrial rate = 180; junctional rate = 79. A-V activity, unrelated; interpretation: complete A-V block with junctional rhythm.
228. Atrial rate = 108; ventricular rate = 57. A-V activity, unrelated; interpretation: complete A-V block with junctional rhythm.
229. Atrial rate = 59; ventricular rate = 37. A-V activity, unrelated; interpretation: complete A-V block with junctional rhythm.

230. Atrial rate = 52; ventricular rate = 37. A-V activity, unrelated; interpretation: complete A-V block with junctional rhythm.
231. Nodal rate = 154.
232. Sinus rate = 74.
233. Nodal tachycardia, rate = 192. Sinus tachycardia, rate = 114.
234. Atrial rate = 65; nodal rate = 66.
235. Tachycardia: rate = 190. Sinus tachycardia: rate = 126.

Self-Evaluation: Stage 2

236. Atrial tachycardia (or flutter) with 2:1 A:V ratio. Atrial rate = 288; ventricular rate = 144.
237. Second-degree A-V block with 2:1 A:V ratio. Atrial rate = 72; ventricular rate = 36.
238. Second-degree A-V block of Wenckebach type with 2:1 and 3:1 A:V ratios; PR intervals 0.15 to 0.21 second. Atrial rate = 70; ventricular rate = 40.
239. Second-degree A-V block of Wenckebach type with 5:4 and 4:3 A:V ratios: PR intervals = 0.36 to 0.60 second. Atrial rate = 70; ventricular rate = 60 (average).
240. Second-degree A-V block of Wenckebach type: 2:1 and 3:2 ratios. PR intervals = 0.14 to 0.24 second.
241. First-degree A-V block; PR interval = 0.37 seconds; sinus rate = 48.
242. Sinus irregularity with nodal escape beat at 132 mm. Rate = 60 (average).
243. Second-degree A-V block (2:1 A:V ratio) to advanced second-degree A-V block (3:1 A:V ratio). Atrial rate = 141; ventricular rate = 47.
244. Second-degree A-V block (Wenckebach) 9:8 or greater A:V ratio. PR intervals: 0.19 to 0.27 second. Atrial rate = 80; ventricular rate = 70 (average).
245. Normal sinus rhythm with NPC at 91 mm and APCs at 21 mm and 169 mm. Rate = 96.
246. Atrial tachycardia. (Possibly sinus tachycardia although strict regularity suggests atrial rhythm.) Rate = 144.
247. NSR with NPC at 40 mm. Rate = 60.
248. Nodal escape rhythm (rate = 64) to normal sinus rhythm (rate = 67).
249. NSR. NPC with delayed (aberrant ventricular conduction) at 68 mm. P wave formation and location indicate the atrial activity originated in the sinus node, which is independent from the NPC.
250. Atrial tachycardia with intermittent A-V conduction and Wenckebach phenomenon (4:3 and 3:2 A:V ratios); PR intervals: 0.14 to 0.30 second. Atrial rate = 195; ventricular rate = 132.
251. NSR to transient preexcitation rhythm (four beats) at 50 mm. Rate = 98.
252. First-degree A-V block; PR interval = 0.23 second. Rate = 61.
253. Second-degree A-V block (advanced) with 3:1 A:V ratio. Atrial rate = 108; ventricular rate = 36.
254. Sinus tachycardia with second-degree A-V block with 2:1 A:V ratio. Atrial rate = 194; ventricular rate = 97.
255. Second-degree A-V block with Wenckebach phenomenon (5:4 A:V ratio in central group); PR intervals: 0.20 to 0.30 second. Atrial rate = 57; ventricular rate = 44.
256. Sinus rhythm (rate = 92) with sinus exit block at 50 mm.
257. Complete A-V block with nodal rhythm. Atrial rate = 60; ventricular rate = 37.
258. Second-degree A-V block of Wenckebach type; PR intervals: 0.23 to 0.36 second. Atrial rate = 58; ventricular rate = 50 (average).
259. Sinus rhythm with preexcitation phenomenon. Rate = 87.
260. Accelerated nodal rhythm. Rate = 96.
261. Supraventricular tachycardia (probably atrial tachycardia or flutter). Rate = 156.
262. Sinus tachycardia (rate = 104) with blocked APC at 117 mm.

263. NSR with NPC at 132 mm. (Sinus P distorts terminal portion of QRS.) Rate = 83.
264. Second-degree A-V block of Wenckebach type with 3:2 A:V ratio in central group. Nodal escape beat at 155 mm. Atrial rate = 70; ventricular rate = 57.
265. Accelerated nodal rhythm. Rate = 62.
266. First-degree A-V block; PR = 0.28 second. Rate = 82.
267. Nodal rhythm (rate = 59) with NPC at 65 mm.
268. Sinus rhythm with blocked sinus beat at 85 mm and nodal escape beat at 104 mm. Rate = 87.
269. Atrial fibrillation. Rate = 82 to 188 (average = 120).
270. Sinus bradycardia (rate = 46) with progressive sinus slowing to nodal escape rhythm (rate = 30) (note retrograde P waves).
271. Sinus tachycardia with complete A-V block and nodal rhythm. Atrial rate = 144.
272. A-V dissociation with accelerated nodal rhythm at 87 per minute.
273. Sinus bradycardia (rate = 55) with progressive sinus slowing to sinus pause and nodal escape beat at 125 mm.
274. Nodal escape rhythm. Rate = 38.
275. Complete A-V block with nodal rhythm. Atrial rate = 75; ventricular rate = 45.
276. Second-degree A-V block (2:1 A:V ratio). Atrial rate = 104; ventricular rate = 52.
277. Sinus bradycardia (rate = 38) to nodal rhythm (rate = 37).
278. Second-degree A-V block (Wenckebach 2:1 and 3:2); PR intervals: 0.12 to 0.24 second. Atrial rate = 78; ventricular rate = 40.
279. Sinus bradycardia (rate = 27) with nodal escape beat at 115 mm.
280. Sinus rhythm (rate = 76) with sinus slowing (or sinus arrest) to nodal rhythm (rate = 69).
281. Sinus bradycardia with first-degree A-V block; PR interval = 0.27 second. Rate = 55.

Chapter 7
282. Rate = 107. PR interval = 0.12 second; QRS interval = 0.13 second.
283. Sinus rate = 106; ventricular rate = 36; QRS duration = 0.12 second.
284. Sinus tachycardia: QRS = 0.08 second; APC; QRS = 0.13 second.
285. Rate = 43 to 52; APC with RBBB at 77 mm.
286. Beats with RBBB at 6, 30, 78, 105, 138 mm.
287. PR intervals and QRS durations: 0.20, 0.11, 0.20, 0.11, 0.26, 0.14; blocked sinus beat; 0.20, 0.11, 0.23, 0.14, 0.27, 0.14.
288. PR intervals and QRS durations: 0.29, 0.14, 0.31, 0.14, 0.33, 0.14; blocked sinus beat at 70 mm; 0.20, 0.11.
289. RBBB at 1, 52, 131, 182 mm.
290. QRS duration = 0.10 second (normal). QRS duration = 0.14 second (BBB).

Chapter 8
291. QRS duration = 0.18 second.
292. Sinus arrest. Ventricular rhythm, rate = 50; QRS duration = 0.18 second (end point of QRS uncertain).
293. Sinus arrest. Ventricular rate = 41; QRS duration = 0.12 second.
294. Sinus arrest. Ventricular rate = 30; QRS duration = 0.36 second (end portion of QRS uncertain).
295. Sinus arrest. Ventricular rate = 25; QRS duration = 0.18 second.
296. Sinus rate = 75; ventricular rate = 29; QRS duration = 0.20 second.
297. Sinus rate = 34; ventricular rate = 42; QRS duration = 0.20 second.
298. Complete A-V block. Sinus rate = 102; ventricular rate = 32; QRS duration = 0.12 second.

299. Complete A-V block. Sinus rate = 128; ventricular rate = 43; QRS duration = 0.20 second.
300. Complete A-V block. Sinus rate = 96; ventricular rate = 57; QRS duration = 0.13 second.
301. VPC at 109 mm; blocked P at 114 mm.
302. VPC at 10 mm; blocked P at 14 mm (pause = 1.04 second); VPC at 88 mm; blocked P at 92 mm (pause = 1.04 second); VPC at 166 mm; blocked P at 170 mm (pause = 1.04 second).
303. VPC at 54 mm; (pause = 1.24 second); VPC at 119 mm; blocked P at 124 mm (pause = 1.16 second); VPC at 180 mm; blocked P at 185 mm.
304. VPC at 55 mm (pause = 1.08 second); VPC at 138 mm (pause = 1.16 second); blocked Ps at 59 mm, 143 mm.
305. VPC at 62 mm (pause = 0.72 second); blocked P at 64 mm.
306. APCs at 52, 163 mm; VPC at 13 mm (pause = 1.04 second); VPC at 88 mm (pause = 1.00); VPC at 125 mm (pause = 1.04 second); blocked Ps at 16, 91, and 128 mm.
307. VPC at 30 mm (pause = 1.04 second); VPC at 96 mm (pause = 1.06 second); VPC at 162 mm; blocked Ps at 34, 101, 166 mm.
308. VPC at 37 mm (pause = 1.26 second; VPC at 139 mm (pause = 1.36 second); Ps at 42, 145 mm.
309. VPC at 62 mm (pause = 1.20 second); P wave not identifiable.
310. VPC at 12 mm (pause = 0.58 second); P at 102 mm, VPC at 104 mm (pause = 0.56 second); P at 180 mm, VPC at 182 mm (pause = 0.58 second).
311. VPC at 39 mm (pause = 0.92 second); VPC at 101 mm (pause = 0.94 second); VPC at 163 mm (pause = 0.96 second). Ps at 37 mm, 99 mm, 162 mm.
312. Sinus rhythm, rate = 62; two VPCs, uniform, altered ST and T configuration.
313. Sinus rhythm, rate = 76; four VPCs, uniform, altered ST and T configuration.
314. Sinus rhythm, rate = 74; two VPCs, uniform. Ps at 40 and 160 mm.
315. Sinus tachycardia, rate = 115. Visible Ps at 40, 90, and 180 mm.
316. Sinus bradycardia with ventricular bigeminy to marked sinus slowing with nodal escape beat at 139 mm having aberrant ventricular conduction to paired ventricular premature contractions.
317. Atrial fibrillation, rate = 80. Two multiform VPCs at 69 mm and 105 mm, variable coupling intervals.
318. Normal sinus rhythm, rate = 61. Uniform VPCs in couplet at 78 mm and 93 mm and VPC with a second form at 146 mm.
319. Normal sinus rhythm, rate = 75. Multiform VPCs at 16 and 194 mm and nodal escape beat at 42 mm.
320. Normal sinus rhythm, rate = 90. VPCs = 4, uniform; coupling interval: 0.40 second, constant. (This is not ventricular trigeminy—see glossary definition.)
321. Sinus rhythm; rate = 95. Ventricular bigeminy (main stem VPCs or NPCs with aberrant ventricular conduction). Note retrograde P wave at 25 mm; this figure does not occur halfway between sinus beats and is therefore not of sinus origin.
322. NSR; rate = 80. VPCs = 4, uniform; two VPCs occur as couplet. Coupling interval: 0.42 to 0.46 second, slightly variable.
323. NSR with frequent uniform VPCs having variable coupling intervals (0.58, 0.56, 0.62 second).
324. NSR with uniform VPCs having markedly variable coupling intervals (0.40 to 0.75 second).
325. Normal sinus rhythm, rate = 80; two VPCs, uniform; fixed coupling intervals.
326. Atrial fibrillation, rate = 73. One VPC.
327. NSR, rate = 71. Two VPCs, probably uniform with varying ventricular conduction; fixed coupling intervals.

328. Sinus tachycardia, rate = 108. Ten VPCs, uniform, three couplets, one triplet; fixed coupling intervals of VPCs that follow sinus beats.
329. NSR, rate = 72; three VPCs (two uniform at 44 mm and 170 mm); one fusion beat at 109 mm; variable coupling intervals.
330. Sinus bradycardia, rate = 59; PR interval = 0.16 second; ventricular rhythm, rate = 61; PR interval, none.
331. Rate = 71. Rate = 144. Ventricular rhythm is irregular, onset is a premature beat.
332. Sinus tachycardia (rate = 106) and transient ventricular tachycardia (rate = 180 to 250), begins and ends with premature beat; apparent A-V dissociation.
333. Sinus rhythm, rate = 130. Ventricular rhythm; rate = 132.
334. Sinus rhythm, rate = 90. Ventricular rhythm; rate = 187.
335. Basic rhythm = NSR; rate = 79. Ectopic rhythm = ventricular; rate = 143. One VPC at 156 mm.
336. Sinus rhythm, rate = indeterminate. VPCs at 15 mm and 45 mm. Ventricular rhythm; rate = 170.
337. Rate = 144.
338. Ventricular rhythm; rate = 156.
339. Rate = 200.
340. Regular ventricular rhythm; rate = 130.
341. Irregular ventricular tachycardia; rate = 178.
342. Irregular ventricular tachycardia; rate = 195.
343. Irregular ventricular tachycardia; rate = 190; to ventricular rhythm; rate = 52.
344. Regular ventricular tachycardia; rate = 184.
345. Regular accelerated ventricular rhythm; rate = 76.
346. Regular accelerated ventricular rhythm; rate = 81.
347. Ventricular flutter; rate = 210; slight variance in amplitude and configuration.
348. Ventricular flutter; rate = 315; slight variance in amplitude and configuration.
349. VPCs at 51, 60, 138 mm.
350. Rate = 170. Rate = 74.
351. Rate = 39, 20.
352. Rate = 132, 36, 21.
353. Rate 49, 32, to electrical standstill; QRS duration = 0.24 second.
354. Rate = 18, 130, 18.
355. Rate = 19, 24. Multiform ventricular beats.
356. A:V ratio = 3:1; QRS interval = 0.12 second.
357. A:V ratio = 2:1; QRS interval = 0.15 second.
358. Rate = 79; QRS interval = 0.20 second.
359. Rate = 48.
360. Sinus rate = 31 (at center of tracing). Ventricular bradycardia, rate = 32.

Self-Evaluation: Stage 3
361. Complete A-V block; sinus rhythm (rate = 72) and nodal rhythm (rate = 44) with RBBB configuration.
362. Ventricular fibrillation.
363. Ventricular rhythm; rate = 30.
364. Sinus rhythm (rate = 74) with uniform (main stem bundle) bigeminal VPCs and variable coupling intervals.
365. Sinus rhythm to sinus arrest and nodal escape rhythm, then sinus rhythm; ventricular bigeminy throughout with uniform VPCs.
366. Second-degree A-V block (Wenckebach with 3:2 and 4:3 A:V ratios) and intraventricular conduction delay. Atrial rate = 66; ventricular rate = 48 (average).
367. Ventricular fibrillation.

368. A-V dissociation; sinus tachycardia and nodal rhythm with RBBB; VPC at 178 mm.
369. Sinus bradycardia (rate = 54) with interpolated uniform VPCs.
370. Normal sinus rhythm (rate = 98); four APCs with one manifesting RBBB.
371. Sinus tachycardia (rate = 104), sinus arrest (or long pause) with failure of escape mechanism and ventricular asystole.
372. NSR (rate = 80); nodal (or main stem ventricular) premature contractions with RBBB in bigeminal pattern.
373. NSR (rate = 94) with APC at 63 mm followed by a nine-beat run of ventricular tachycardia.
374. NSR with ventricular bigeminy.
375. Ventricular tachycardia (slightly varying upstroke suggests dissociated atrial activity).
376. Ventricular bradycardia (originating in main stem). Rate = 27.
377. Sinus bradycardia (rate = 50). NPC with RBBB, followed by sinus slowing (or arrest) and nodal rhythm.
378. Ventricular tachycardia exhibiting torsades de pointes pattern.
379. Sinus irregularity with APC at 98 mm followed by ventricular escape beats at 32 per minute.
380. Ventricular tachycardia to ventricular fibrillation.
381. Accelerated ventricular rhythm (rate = 86), sinus arrest or dissociated A-V activity.
382. Atrial fibrillation with moderate ventricular response (rate = 60s) and uniform VPCs having fixed coupling intervals.
383. NSR (rate = 75) with intermittent RBBB and ventricular bigeminy.
384. Sinus tachycardia (rate = 104) with uniform VPCs, some of which occur in couplets.
385. Ventricular fibrillation with asystole following electrical countershock at 38 mm reverting to ventricular fibrillation.
386. NSR (rate = 85); uniform VPCs with fixed coupling intervals.
387. Second-degree A-V block of Wenckebach type (3:2 A:V ratio). Atrial rate = 74; ventricular rate = 50 (average).
388. Ventricular rhythm (rate = 80s) with marked intraventricular conduction delay; sinus arrest.
389. Ventricular fibrillation.
390. Atrial flutter with advanced A-V block and multiform VPCs.
391. Atrial flutter with 2:1 conduction; one VPC at 95 mm. Atrial rate = 290; ventricular rate = less than 40.
392. Atrial fibrillation with slow ventricular response (average rate = 45) and one VPC at 98 mm.
393. Atrial flutter with variable A:V relationship. Atrial rate = 290; ventricular rate = 120 (average).
394. Sinus tachycardia (rate = 107) with uniform VPCs with fixed coupling intervals.
395. Atrial flutter at 290 beats per minute with variable block and ventricular response rate = 140.
396. NSR (rate = 80) with multiform VPCs, two of which occur as a couplet.
397. Atrial fibrillation with rapid ventricular rate response (rate = 150). (Because QRS durations are at upper limits of normal, ventricular tachycardia may be present.)
398. Ventricular rhythm with multiform beats. Supraventricular rhythm may be atrial fibrillation.

Chapter 9

399. Rate = 75; QRS duration = 0.16 second; supraventricular rhythm = atrial fibrillation.

400. Rate = 82; QRS duration = 0.18 second; supraventricular rhythm = indiscernible.
401. Rate = 83; QRS duration = 0.18 second; supraventricular rhythm = indiscernible.
402. Rate = 80; QRS duration = 0.14 second; supraventricular rhythm = indiscernible.
403. Rate = 70; QRS duration = 0.16 second; supraventricular rhythm = possibly sinus (note P wave deflection before fifth spike).
404. Rate = 74; QRS duration = 0.12 second; supraventricular rhythm = sinus rhythm.
405. Rate = 70; QRS duration = 0.22 second; supraventricular rhythm = indiscernible.
406. Sinus rate = 96. Complete A-V block. EPM rate = 81.
407. Sinus rate = 72. Complete A-V block. EPM rate = 76.
408. EPM rate = 76. Sinus rhythm rate = 71. A-V conduction is absent.
409. EPM rate = 90. Atrial tachycardia rate = 250. A-V conduction is absent.
410. EPM rate = 64. Atrial fibrillation. A-V conduction is absent.
411. EPM rate = 61; atrial rate = 102; ventricular rate = 30. Complete A-V block.
412. Capture failure at 70 mm. EPM rate = 70. Sinus rhythm (rate 32 to 39) with complete A-V block.
413. EPM rate = 74; sinus rate = 77.
414. Spontaneous beats with RBBB (origin not positively identified).
415. EPM rate = 72; sinus rate = 66, 75, 73, 72, 70, 68.
416. EPM rate = 71; note delay in EPM cadence after each VPC. EPM beats from right ventricle; VPCs from left ventricle. Proper on and off activity of EPM.
417. EPM rhythm (rate = 74), inhibited or demand mode to sinus tachycardia (rate = 108).
418. EPM rhythm (rate = 77), inhibited mode to NSR with RBBB (rate = 83).
419. EPM rhythm (rate = 62), inhibited mode to NSR (rate = 75).
420. Sinus pacemaker is controlling the ventricles.
421. EPM impulses at 71, 91, 110, 165 mm. Constant R to EPM = 0.80 second (800 msec). EPM to EPM = 0.78 sec (780 msec). EPM does not capture the ventricles.
422. Complete A-V block: sinus rhythm (rate = 86); EPM rhythm (rate = 69) with failure of ventricular capture in the middle of the strip.
423. Complete A-V block: sinus rhythm (rate = 86); EPM rhythm (rate = 69) with frequent failure of ventricular capture and long period of ventricular asystole (5.8 seconds).
424. Complete A-V block: sinus tachycardia (rate = 120), EPM (rate variable due to frequent resetting by spontaneous beats) with complete failure of ventricular capture and nodal pacemaker (rate = 29) with RBBB.
425. Complete A-V block: sinus tachycardia (rate = 155); EPM activity with no ventricular capture (rate variable), nodal rhythm (rate = 53).
426. Complete A-V block: intermittent atrial tachycardia (rate = 120, irregular), accelerated ventricular rhythm of multiform beats (rate = 90).
427. Complete A-V block: sinus tachycardia (rate = 166), nodal rhythm (rate = 41), EPM impulses with complete lack of ventricular capture. The sensor turn-off mechanism is not operating (EPM impulses formed immediately after some nodal beats.)
428. Sinus bradycardia (rate = 45) with RBBB and frequent blocked APCs. EPM impulses with failure of ventricular capture and sensor turn-off mechanism.
429. Complete A-V block: atrial flutter with nodal rhythm (rate = 53) with RBBB. (Regular ventricular rate in presence of variable FR intervals indicates absence of A-V conduction and independent pacemakers.) Nonstimulating EPM impulses.

430. Irregular atrial tachycardia or flutter with A-V dissociation and nodal tachycardia (rate = 170) and variable aberrant ventricular conduction.
431. Atrial flutter with A-V dissociation (variable FR intervals) and nodal tachycardia (rate = 135), and aberrantly conducted ventricular beats to marked bradycardia.
432. Atrial flutter, possibly with complete A-V block, and nodal rhythm (rate = 35) with RBBB.
433. Complete A-V block: atrial flutter with EPM rhythm (rate = 71) and complete ventricular capture. Distortion at 8 mm produced by stopping recorder momentarily.
434. Complete A-V block: sinus rhythm and EPM rhythm (rate = 75) with complete ventricular capture; unable to determine adequacy of sensing mechanism as no intrinsic beats are present.

Self-Evaluation: Stage 4
435. Atrial fibrillation with slow ventricular rate response (rate 46). VPCs at 47 mm and 157 mm.
436. Ventricular fibrillation to ventricular arrest.
437. Sinus rhythm (rate = 80) with first-degree A-V block (PR = 0.24 second) and APCs at 34 mm and 180 mm, and VPC at 75 mm.
438. Atrial flutter, variable A-V conduction, moderate ventricular rate response (rate = 90); episode of ventricular tachycardia.
439. Sinus bradycardia with preexcitation phenomenon.
440. Fine atrial fibrillation with slow ventricular rate response (rate = 40) and ventricular bigeminy.
441. Second-degree A-V block (Mobitz II; PR intervals = 0.23 second) with nodal escape beat following the blocked sinus beat at 49 mm.
442. Sinus bradycardia with APC with RBBB at 51 mm to temporary sinus arrest and nodal escape rhythm; VPC at 101 mm.
443. Complete A-V block: atrial fibrillation, nodal rhythm with RBBB.
444. Atrial tachycardia (rate = 246) with complete A-V block (accelerated nodal rhythm with rate of 98 per minute); multiform ventricular couplet at 140 mm.
445. Sinus arrest with ventricular rhythm (rate = 42) and VPC at 164 mm.
446. Atrial fibrillation, moderate ventricular rate response (average rate = 64) with uniform VPCs at 60 mm and 170 mm.
447. Normal sinus rhythm (rate = 80) with RBBB to ventricular tachycardia.
448. Complete A-V block (sinus rate = 68; ventricular rate = 50) to ventricular asystole.
449. Ventricular fibrillation.
450. Normal sinus rhythm (rate = 85) with frequent uniform VPCs including a couplet and a four-beat run of ventricular tachycardia.
451. Ventricular flutter (rate = 200).
452. NSR, blocked APC at 64 mm to atrial flutter (rate = 430) with variable A-V conduction and moderate ventricular rate response (rate = 76).
453. Second-degree A-V block (2:1 A:V ratio) to advanced second-degree (4:1 A:V ratio). Atrial rate = 60; ventricular rate = 30 to 15. PR of conducted beats = 0.28 second.
454. Sinus bradycardia (rate = 31), uniform VPCs at 68 mm and 125 mm, to NSR (rate = 75).
455. NSR (rate = 87) with RBBB, APC at 134 mm followed by sinus beat without RBBB. EPM, ventricular demand (VVI) mode, at 156 mm and 174 mm occurring simultaneously with sinus-conducted beats producing fusion beats.
456. Sinus bradycardia (rate = 48) with second-degree Wenckebach A-V block (PR intervals 0.23 to 0.42 second).

457. Sinus rhythm with atrial bigeminy and aberrant ventricular conduction of premature beats.
458. First-degree A-V block (sinus rate = 80) to sinus arrest and nodal escape rhythm.
459. NSR (rate = 79); uniform VPCs with fixed coupling intervals, each followed by a nodal escape beat.
460. NSR (rate = 63) with RBBB. Periods of sinus slowing and intermittent appearance of EPM rhythm, ventricular demand mode (VVI).
461. Atrial flutter or tachycardia (rate = 168) with advanced A-V block; ventricular escape beat at 120 mm.
462. Ventricular escape rhythm (rate = 37); EPM spikes at 76 per minute. Complete failure of pacemaker—no sensing and no chamber response.
463. Complete A-V block: sinus tachycardia (rate = 125); junctional rhythm = 75.
464. Complete A-V block: sinus rhythm = 110; VVI electronic pacemaker rhythm with complete ventricular capture (rate = 70).
465. Sinus bradycardia (rate = 48) with first-degree A-V block (PR 0.22 second) and periods of sinus slowing with nodal escape beats.
466. Sinus irregularity (rate range = 38 to 71) with RBBB; EPM impulses of ventricular demand mode (VVI) with complete failure of cardiac stimulation.
467. Atrial tachycardia (rate = 178), to atrial escape beat, to atrial standstill, to sinus bradycardia (rate = 58).
468. Sinus rhythm (rate = 56) to ventricular asystole.
469. Sinus rhythm with DDD pacemaker: sinus rate = 92; P to V spike 0.16 second. Failure to sense P wave and respond at 38 mm and 118 mm reveals V-A interval = 1.04 second and A-V interval = 0.14 second of DDD function.
470. Second-degree A-V block: sinus rhythm (rate = 80); 2:1 A:V ratio, prolonged PR (0.58 second) of conducted beats. Nonconducted APC at 116 mm and ventricular escape at 146 mm.
471. DDD electronic pacemaker in complete control: rate = 70 per minute; A-V interval = 0.16 second; V-A interval = 0.64 second.
472. Sinus tachycardia (rate = 130) with RBBB; APCs at 59 mm and 96 mm; VPCs at 15 mm and 122 mm (uniform with fixed coupling intervals); to atrial tachycardia (rate = 238) with variable A-V conduction.
473. EPM-initiated ventricular beats at 0.02 mm, 44 mm, 83 mm, 112 mm, 152 mm, 181 mm. Multiform VPCs and ventricular tachycardia. VPC at 50 mm and ventricular tachycardia are of the same form as EPM beats. VPCs at 21 mm and 63 mm of different form.
474. DDD electronic pacemaker rhythm: sinus rate = 80. P to V spike = 0.20 second.
475. Isorhythmic A-V dissociation with junctional rate = 71 per minute, and sinus rate = 71 to 73 per minute.

Index

Note: Page numbers in *italics* refer to illustrations; page numbers followed by (t) refer to tables.

A
a waves, 384
Abbreviations, 566
Aberrant conduction, Ashman phenomenon and, 421, *421*
  atrial beats and, 412–414, *414*
  atrial fibrillation and, *424*, 424–425, *425*
  bundle branch block vs., *416*, 416–417, *417*
  captured beats and, 420, *420*
  definition of, 411
  drugs and, 423
  ECG leads and, 411–412
  fusion beats and, *420*, 420–421, *421*
  hyperkalemia and, *415*, 415–416
  pauses and, 418–419, *419*
  preexcitation syndrome and, 423–424
  QRS complex prolonged by, 414–416, *415*, 419, *419*
  supraventricular tachycardia vs., 306–309, *307*, *308*
  T wave reversal in, *421*, 421–422
  tachycardia onset and, 419, *419*
  vagal stimulation and, *422*, 422–423
Aberration. See *Aberrant conduction.*
Accelerated rhythms, A-V junctional, 288
  nodal, 562
  ventricular, 378, 557
Accessory pathway(s), atrio-His bypass as, 225, *225*, *234*, 234(t)
  A-V bypass as, *228–233*, 228–234
  A-V junctional tachycardia and, 304–305
  intranodal, 220–224, *221–224*, 234(t)
  nodoventricular bypass as, 225–227, *226*, 234(t), 304–305
  short refractory period in, 308–309
  variant bypass as, 309–310
  ventricular preexcitation and, 225–227, *226*, *227*, 234(t)
Acetylcholine, 94, *94*, *95*
Actin, *14*, 14–16, *15*

Action potential, 16
  in atria, *130*, *145*
  in A-V node, *213*
  in His-Purkinje system, 322–323, *323*
  in sinus node, 82–84, *83*
  in ventricles, 340
  membrane permeability and, 17–21, *18*
  phases of, 18–21, *19*, *83*, 83–84
  refractory period and, 142–146, *145*, 563
Adams, Robert, 557
Adams-Stokes syndrome, 557
Adenosine triphosphate, 14–16
Adrenaline. See *Epinephrine.*
Adrenergic antagonists, 159
Adrenergic (excitatory) influences, 557
  anticholinergic agents as, 101–102, *102*, *103*
  physiology of, 93–96, *94–96*, *96*
  sinus tachycardia and, 96–102, *97–99*, *101–105*
Adrenergic inhibition, 96
AFib. See *Atrial fibrillation (AFib).*
AFl. See *Atrial flutter (AFl).*
Age, heart rate variations and, *84*, 84–87
AH interval, 217–218, *218*, 557
AICD. See *Automatic implantable cardioverter-defibrillator.*
Angina pectoris, 11
Anions. See *Electrolytes.*
Anomalous conduction. See *Accessory pathway(s).*
Anterograde conduction, 557
  in atria, 134–135, *135*
  in A-V junction, 271, *272*, 283
Aortic valve, embryology of, 4, *5*
APC. See *Atrial premature complex (APC).*
Arrhythmia(s). See also *Bradycardia; Tachycardia.*
  atherosclerosis and, 11–12
  compound, 329, *329*
  definition of, 1, 558
  sinus nodal, 87–91, *87–91*, 563
Artifacts. See under *Electrocardiography (ECG).*
Ashman phenomenon, 421, *421*

Asynchronous pacemakers. See under *Electronic pacemaker(s) (EPM)*.
Asystole, 558
AT. See *Atrial tachycardia (AT)*.
Atherosclerosis, 11–12
ATP, 14–16
Atria, 129–211
  action potential in, *130, 145*
  anatomy of, *1, 2, 6–8, 13*
  arrest of, 558
  auricles of, 558
  automaticity in, 129–130, *130,* 132
  bigeminy in, 141, *141,* 172
  cardiac cycle and, 25, *27*
  conduction in, 134–135, *135*
  depolarization of, 25, *27*
  embryology of, 1–5, *3–5*
  enlargement of, 60–61, *61*
  escape beats in, 130–133, *131, 132*
  fibrillation in. See *Atrial fibrillation (AFib)*.
  flutter in. See *Atrial flutter (AFl)*.
  functioning of, *1, 5, 5–6,* 558
  impulse formation in, 129–133, *130, 131, 134, 135*
  pacemakers and, electronic. See *Electronic pacemaker(s)*.
    endogenous, 130, *131, 132,* 132–133, *135*
  premature complex in. See *Atrial premature complex (APC)*.
  reentry and, *163,* 163–164. See also *Atrial tachycardia (AT), reentrant*.
  tachycardia in. See *Atrial tachycardia (AT)*.
  wandering pacemaker of, *132,* 133, 565
Atrial enlargement, 60–61, *61*
Atrial fibrillation (AFib), A-V node and, *189,* 189–190
  conduction and, aberrant, *424,* 424–425, *425*
    concealed, 190, 599
  digitalis and, 298–203, *299*
  ECG leads in, 187–188, *188*
  effects of, 193–194, *194*
  electric shock therapy in, 196–198, *196–198*
  etiology of, *191,* 191–192, *192*
  f waves in, 187–188, 191, *191*
  mechanisms of, *187,* 187–190
  pulse deficit in, 194
  treatment of, *195–199,* 195–205
Atrial flutter (AFl), A-V block in, 173, *176,* 176–177
  A-V ratios in, 178, *178–180*
  bundle branch block and, 332, *332*
  carotid pressure in, 181–183, *181–183*
  digitalis and, *185,* 186
  ECG leads in, 172–176
  electric shock therapy in, *184,* 184–185, *185*
  F wave in, 172–173, *173–175*
  mechanisms of, 172
  treatment of, 183–186, *183–186*
Atrial premature complex (APC), 558
  bigeminy and, 141, *141*
  blocked, 142–146, *142–146*
  frequency of, 138–141, *138–141*
  identification of, 135–137, *136, 137*
  impulse formation in, 133–135, *134*
  laddergram of, 134–135, *135, 146*

Atrial premature complex (APC) (*Continued*)
  multifocal, *146,* 146–147
  retrograde conduction and, 134–135, *135*
Atrial tachycardia (AT), 558
  A-V block and, 166–172, *167–171*
  carotid pressure in, *157,* 157–159, *158, 162*
  drug therapy in, 159–162, *160–162*
  electric shock therapy in, 153–154, 164–166, *165, 166*
  enhanced automaticity and, 147–150, *147–150*
  paroxysmal, 152–161, *154, 155, 160*
  reentrant, characteristics of, 153–155
    electrophysiology of, 147, 150–159, *150–159*
    intraatrial, *163,* 163–164
    mechanisms of, 150–153, *151–153*
    sinus node and, 162, *162*
Atriofascicular bypass tract, 303–304, *304.* See also *Accessory pathway(s)*.
Atrio-His bypass, 225, *225, 234,* 234(t). See also *Accessory pathway(s)*.
Atrioventricular (A-V) block, 558
  advanced, *249,* 249–250
  atrial flutter and, 173, *176,* 176–177
  atrial tachycardia and, 166–172, *167–171*
  A-V junctional rhythms and, 275–283, *276–282*
  carotid pressure and, *169,* 169–170
  complete, *262–264, 212–265,* 558
  digitalis and, *170,* 170–171
  electrogram in, *243, 244*
  electronic pacemaker and, *446,* 446–447, *447*
  first-degree, 558
    atropine and, 242, *242*
    causes of, 242–244
    ECG in, 236, *236, 237*
    electrogram in, *243*
    laddergram of, *264*
    sleep effect on, 241, *241*
    vagal stimulation and, 242, *242*
  second-degree, 558
    electrogram in, *244*
    electronic pacemaker and, *446,* 446–447, *447,* 504–506
    isoproterenol in, *251,* 251–252
    laddergram of, *264*
    Type I, 252–257, *252–257, 264*
    Type II, 259–262, *259–262, 264*
    vagal stimulation and, *245,* 245–246
    Wenckebach phenomenon in, *253–259,* 254–259, *264*
  third-degree, *262–264,* 262–265, 558
  vagal stimulation and, *242,* 242–246, *245*
  ventricular pacing and, 346–348, *346–348*
Atrioventricular (A-V) dissociation, 292–296, *293, 294,* 558. See also *Dissociation*.
Atrioventricular (A-V) junction, 266–320
  accelerated rhythms and, 288
  automaticity in, 266–267, *267*
    enhanced, 288–291, *289*
  block and, A-V nodal, 275–283, *276–282*
    retrograde, *286,* 286–287, *287*
  conduction and, anterograde, 271, *272*
    retrograde, 271–273, *271–273*
  digitalis toxicity and, 289–291, *290*
  dissociation in, 292–296, *293, 294*

Atrioventricular (A-V) junction (*Continued*)
  escape beats and, in A-V nodal block, 275–283, *276–282*
    in depressed sinus node function, 268–274, *268–275*
  impulse formation in, 266–267, *267*, 283
  laddergram and, *272*, *285*, *286*
  pacemaker role of, in A-V nodal block, 275–283, *276–282*
    in depressed sinus node function, *268–275*, 275–283
Atrioventricular (A-V) junctional premature complex
  characteristics of, 283–284
  laddergram of, *285*, *286*
  retrograde block and, *286*, 286–287, *287*
Atrioventricular (A-V) junctional tachycardia, accelerated rhythms and, 288
  accessory pathways and, A-V bypass, 305–306, *306*
    nodoventricular bypass, 304–305
    short refractory, 308–309
    variant bypass, 309–310
  A-V block and, 291–292, *292*
  digitalis toxicity and, 289–291, *290*
  dissociation and, A-V, 292–296, *293*, *294*
    isorhythmic, *293*, 293–295, *294*
  drug therapy in, *299*, *300*, 300–302
  electric shock therapy in, 302, *302*, 312
  electrolytes and, 290, *290*
  enhanced automaticity in, 288–291, *289*
  heart rate in, 288
  mechanisms of, 287
  nonparoxysmal, 299
  paroxysmal, 299–300
  reentry and, atrio-His, 302–304, *303*, *304*
    A-V, 305–306
    intranodal, *294–302*, 297–302
    nodoventricular, 304–305
  treatment of, *299*, *300*, 300–302, 310–312
  vagal stimulation in, 300–301, *301*, 311
Atrioventricular (A-V) node, 212, 265, 558
  accessory pathways in, 225–234, *225–234*
  action potential in, *213*
  anatomy of, 214–215, *215*, 244
  block in. See *Atrioventricular (A-V) block.*
  blocked atrial premature complex and, 142–146, *142–146*
  cardiac cycle role of, 28, *28*, *29*
  conduction in, 220–225, *220–225*
  ECG and, 215, *216*, *218*, *230*
  electrogram and, 217–218, *218*
  embryonic myofibril rests in, 221, 228
  functions of, 212–214
  impulse velocity in, 212–214, *214*
  reentry impulses in, 233, *234*
  refractory period of, 142–146
  ventricular preexcitation and. See *Ventricular preexcitation.*
Atropine, 101–102, *102*, *103*
  A-V block and, 242, *242*
Auricles, atrial, 558
Automatic implantable cardioverter-defibrillator, *513*, 513–515, *514*, 560

Automaticity, 83, 558
  in atria, 129–130, *130*, 132
    tachycardia and, 147–150, *148–150*
  in A-V junction, 288–291, *289*
  in sinus node, 83–84
  in ventricles, 340–341, *341*, 362
Autonomic nervous system, 558. See also *Carotid pressure (CP)*; *Vagal stimulation*
  physiology of, 93–94, *95*
  regulatory mechanisms of, 95–96, *96*
  sinus node and, 91(t), 91–96, *92*, *95*
  structure of, 91(t), 91–93, *92*, 558
A-V interval, 489–490, *490*, 557
Axis. See *QRS axis*

B
Bachman's bundle, 163
BBB. See *Bundle branch block (BBB).*
Beat, of heart. See *Cardiac cycle.*
Bethanechol (Urecholine), 94
Bifascicular block, 337
Bigeminy, 559
  atrial, 141, *141*, 172
  ventricular, 363, *363*, *364*
Biscupid valve, 4, 5
Block(s), 559
  A-V. See *Atrioventricular (A-V) block.*
  bundle branch. See *Bundle branch block (BBB).*
  retrograde, *286*, 286–287, *287*
  sinoatrial, *123–126*, 123–127, 563
  sinus exit, 124, *124*
  unidirectional, 564
Blood flow, cardiac, 5–6, *8*, *9*
Bradycardia, 559
  sinus node and, 105–109, *105–109*
  vasovagal reflex and, 114–115, *115*
  ventricular. See *Ventricular bradycardia (VB).*
Bundle branch block (BBB). See also *Bundle branch(es).*
  aberrant conduction vs., *416*, 416–417, *417*
  bifascicular, *337*, 337–338
  hemiblock as, 335–336, *336*
  left, 325
    anterior hemiblock and, 335–336, *336*
    depolarization sequence in, 332–334, *333*
    ECG and, 332–334, *333–335*
    posterior hemiblock and, 335–336, *336*
    vs. right ventricular beat, *417*, *417*
  mechanisms of, 324, *325*
  right, 325
    atrial flutter and, 332, *332*
    depolarization sequence in, 326–327
    ECG and, 326–328, *326–329*
    intermittent, 330–332, *331*
    vagal stimulation and, 330–331, *331*
    vs. left ventricular beat, *416*, *416*
  trifascicular, *338*, 338–339
Bundle branch(es). See also *Bundle branch block (BBB).*
  anatomy of, 321–322, *322*
  ECG and, 323–324, *324*
  impulse conduction in, 321–324, *322*

Bundle branch(es) (*Continued*)
  left, 28, 321–322, *322*
  right, 28, 321–322, *322*
Bundle of His. See *His bundle.*
Bundle(s), 321–339, 559
  Bachman's, 163
  branches of. See *Bundle branch(es)*
  common. See *His bundle.*
  of His. See *His bundle.*
  of Kent, 228

C
Cadence, 559
Calcium. See *Electrolytes.*
Calcium channel blockers, 110–111, *111*
  atrial tachycardia and, 159
Cannon waves, 384
Captured beats. See *Electronic pacemaker(s)*
  (EPM), capture by.
Cardiac arrest, *410*, 410–411, *411*
Cardiac cycle, autonomic control of, 91(t), 91–96
  contraction sequence of, 5–6, *8, 9, 44,* 44(t)
  ECG components and, 32–42, *32–44,* 44(t)
  embryology of, 1–2
  laddergrams of, 127–128, *128*
  physiology of, 13–21, *14–19*
  rate determination for, 45–51, *45–52,* 49(t)
  rate variations of, normal, *84–86,* 84–91, *84–91*
  respiration effect on, 84–86, *85*
Cardiac monitoring, 72–79, *73–79,* 78(t)
Cardiac output, calculation of, 6, 10
  influences on, 1
Cardioversion. See *Electric shock therapy.*
Cardioverter-defibrillator, automatic implantable,
  513–515, *513, 514,* 560
Carotid hypersensitivity, 115–116, *116*
Carotid pressure (CP). See also *Vagal stimulation.*
  atrial flutter and, 181–183, *181–183*
  atrial tachycardia and, *157,* 157–159, *158*
  A-V block and, *169,* 169–170
  cholinergic effect of, 102, *103,* 109, *109, 110*
  hypersensitivity to, 115–116, *116*
Catecholamines, 96
Cations. See *Electrolytes.*
Cellular suppressors, 159
Cholinergic (depressant) influences, 559
  antiadrenergic agents as, 102, *103, 108,* 108–109,
    159
  calcium channel blockers as, 110–111, *111*
  carotid artery pressure as, 102, *103,* 109, *109,*
    110
  carotid hypersensitivity as, 115–116, *116*
  physiology of, 94–96, *95, 96*
  sinus arrest and, *113,* 113–114, *114*
  sinus bradycardia and, 105–109, *105–109*
  sinus pause and, 111–112, *112*
  vagal stimulation as, 109, *109*
Cholinergic inhibition, 96
Cholinergic stimulators, 159
Code system, for pacemaker nomenclature, 476–
  478, *477,* 512–513, *513*
Common bundle. See *His bundle.*

Compensatory pause. See under *Pause(s).*
Complete block. See *Atrioventricular (A-V) block,*
  third-degree.
Complete ventricular capture, 440, *440*
Compound arrhythmia, 329, *329*
Conduction, 559. See also *Action potential.*
  aberrant. See *Aberrant conduction.*
  anomalous. See *Accessory pathway(s).*
  anterograde. See *Anterograde conduction.*
  concealed, 190, 559
  connections and, 226, 559
  in A-V junction, 271–273, *271–273,* 283
  in A-V node, 220–225, *220–225*
  in His-Purkinje system, 321–324, *324*
  in sinus node, 80–84, *81, 83*
  retrograde. See *Retrograde conduction.*
  unidirectional, 310
  velocity of, in Purkinje fibers, 322
Connections, 226, 559
Contraction, 13–15, *14,* 560. See also *Cardiac*
  cycle; Sarcomere.
Coronary arteries, anatomy of, 10–12, *10–12*
  sinus node and, 81–82, *82*
Coupling, *369,* 369–373, *370, 374,* 560
CP. See *Carotid pressure (CP).*

D
Defibrillator, 164–165, 401, 560. See also *Electric*
  shock therapy.
  automatic implantable, *513,* 513–515, *514,* 560
Deflection, 560
Delta wave, 225, *227,* 228–229, *229,* 560
Demand mode pacemakers. See under *Electronic*
  pacemaker(s) (EPM).
Depolarization, 560. See also *Action potential.*
  in atria, 25, *27*
  in left bundle branch block, 332–334, *333*
  in right bundle branch block, 326–327
  in sinus node, 82–84, *83*
  in ventricles, 28, *30,* 31, *31*
  in ventricular premature complex, 368–369
  phases of, 18–19, *19*
  refractory period following, 142–146, *145*
  slow channel role in, 21, 83–84
Depression. See *Cholinergic (depressant)*
  influences.
Diastole, 6, *9,* 560
Diazepam (Valium), 165–166
Digitalis, 102, *103*
  atrial fibrillation and, 198–203, *199*
  atrial flutter and, 186, *186*
  atrial tachycardia and, 149–150, *150*
  A-V block and, *170,* 170–171
  A-V junction and, 289–291, *290*
  toxicity of, 289–291, *290*
Dissociation, 560
  A-V, 292–296, *293, 294*
  electromechanical, 474
  in A-V node, 220
  interference, 561
  isorhythmic, *293,* 293–295, *294,* 561
  longitudinal, 220
  myocardium and, 474

Dissociation (*Continued*)
  ventricular preexcitation and, 220
  ventricular tachycardia and, 380, *381*
Drugs. See also specific drugs.
  differential diagnosis and, 423
  in atrial tachycardia, 159–162, *160–162*
  in torsades de pointes, 392
  in ventricular tachycardia, 388–389, *388–390*, 392
  side effects of, 300–302, 386
Dysrhythmia. See *Arrhythmia(s)*.

E
ECG. See *Electrocardiography (ECG)*.
Echo beat, 560
Ectopic beats, 560
  atrial, 130
  A-V junction and, 283
  interpolated, 561
  multifocal, 562
  unifocal, 564
  ventricular. See *Aberrant conduction*.
Edrophonium (Tensilon), 159–161, *160*
EKG. See *Electrocardiography (ECG)*.
Electric shock therapy, 164–166, *165, 166*
  automatic implantable defibrillator and, *513,*
    513–515, 514
  complications of, 166
  in atrial fibrillation, 196–198, *196–198*
  in atrial flutter, *184,* 184–185, *185*
  in A-V junctional tachycardia, 302, *302,* 312
  in reentrant tachycardias, 164–166, *165, 166*
  in ventricular fibrillation, 401–403, *402, 404*
  in ventricular tachycardia, 393–397, *393–397*
  synchronization of discharge in, 164–166, *165,*
    166
Electrocardiography (ECG), 22–79, 560
  abnormalities in, types of, 60–70, *61, 63, 64, 66–*
    70
  amplification in, 42
  artifacts in, 70–72, *70–73, 181,* 558
  atrial depolarization and, 25, *27*
  A-V node silence in, 28, *28*
  axis deviations and, 67–70, *67–70*
  baseline in, 22–23, *23,* 42
  cardiac cycle components and, 32–42, *32–42,*
    44(t)
  electrodes in. See *Leads, ECG*.
  electrolyte balance and, 67, *67*
  exercise stress test, *62–64, 62–65*
  heart rate determination in, 45–51, *45–52,* 49(t)
  instrumentation for, 22–24, *23*
  isoelectric line in, 22–23, *23,* 42
  laddergram in, 127–128, *128*
  leads for. See *Leads, ECG*.
  negative deflection in, 22–23, *23*
  P wave, formation of, 25, *27*
    identification of, 34–35, *37*
  paper tracings in, grid system for, 24, *24, 25*
    heart rate determination and, 47–51, *47–52,*
      49(t)
    speed of, 22–24, *23–25,* 45
  positive deflection in, 22–23, *23*

Electrocardiography (ECG) (*Continued*)
  PR interval, formation of, 28, *28*
    normal range of, 36, *38*
  Q wave, formation of, 34, *34*
  QRS axis and, 67–70, *68–70*
  QRS complex, formation of, 28, *30*
    identification of, 32–42, *32–42*
  QS wave, formation of, 34, *36*
  QT interval, *389,* 391–393, *392, 393*
  R wave, formation of, 34, *35, 36, 36*
  rate rulers in, 45–47, *45–47*
  R-on-T phenomenon in, *386,* 386–388, *387*
  S wave, formation of, 34, *35, 36*
  sinus node silence in, 25
  ST segment, analysis of, 29, *30, 39, 39*
    deviations in, 61–65, *63, 64*
    exercise stress test and, *62–64, 62–65*
    formation of, 29, *30*
  standardization markers in, 42, *44, 45*
  stylus in, 22–23, *23*
  T wave, formation of, 29–31, *31*
    identification of, 39, *40, 41*
  U wave, formation of, 31, *31*
    identification of, 39–40, *41*
  vectors in, 69–70, *70,* 323–324, *324*
  ventricular depolarization and, 28, *30, 31, 31*
Electrode(s), 560
  for ECG. See *Leads, ECG*.
  for electronic pacemakers. See under *Electronic*
    pacemaker(s) (EPM).
  paddle, 164
Electrogram, His bundle, 217–218, *218*
  of A-V block, *243, 244*
  of ventricular premature complex, 350, *351*
Electrolytes, aberrant conduction and, *415,* 415–
    416
  atrial tachycardia and, 149
  A-V tachycardia and, 290, *290*
  extracellular, 17–21, *18*
  intracellular, 17–21, *18*
  sinus node impulse and, 83–84
  T wave changes and, 67, *67*
Electromechanical dissociation, 474, 560. See also
    Dissociation.
Electronic pacemaker(s) (EPM), 433–522, 562
  asynchronous, 453–456, *453–456,* 474–475, *475*
  atrial overdrive by, *510,* 510–512
  atrial synchronous, 480–485, *481–485*
  atrial-inhibited, 478–479, *479, 480*
  automatic implantable defibrillator as, *513,* 513–
    515, *514*
  A-V interval of, 489–490, *490,* 557
  A-V sequential, 488–496, *489–496*
  bradycardic indications for, 445–447, *446, 447*
  capture by, 559
    complete ventricular, 440, *440*
    failure to, *448–451,* 448–452
  code system for, 476–478, *477,* 512–513, *513*
  committed, 493–495, *494, 495*
  competitive rhythms and, *453,* 453–456
  components of, 435–437, *436–437*
  defibrillator as, 513–515, *513, 514*
  demand mode, 456–476, *456–476,* 560
  ECG spike produced by, 437, *437*

Electronic pacemaker(s) (EPM) (*Continued*)
  electrodes for, 436–438, *436*, *437*
    bipolar, 436–437, *437*
    damage to, 452
    misplaced, and QRS complex, 452, *453*
    myocardial interface with, 452
    stabilizer tips on, 442–443, *443*
    unipolar, 436, *437*
  endocardial, 442–443, *443*, 560
  epicardial, *443*, 443–444, *444*
  escape interval of, 465, *465*
  external, 435, *436*, 444–445, *445*
  failure to capture by, *448–451*, 448–452
  failure to sense by, 467–468, *468*, *475*, 475–476, *476*
  fusion beats and, *462*, 462–465, *463*
  hysteresis in, 465, *465*
  implantation of, 442–444, *443*, *444*
  impulse information from, 434–435, *435*
  interference and, 465–467, *466*, *467*
  magnet effect on, 469, *470*, 502–503, *503*
  motion responsive, 486–488, *486–488*
  myocardial interface with, 452
  nomenclature code system for, 476–478, *477*, 512–513, *513*
  noncommitted, *495*, 495–496
  overdrive mode for, *510*, 510–512, *511*
  oversensing in, 465, 465–467, *466*
  power failure in, *448–451*, 448–452
  pseudofusion beats and, *494*, 494–495, *495*
  pulse generator for, 435
    reduced power from, *448–451*, 448–452
  PV interval and, 480, *482*
  rate limits and, 501–503, *501–503*
  rhythm of, fixed, 437–441, *437–442*
  safety window and, 494–495, *495*
  syndrome of, 478
  tachycardia mediated by, *507*, 507–508
  tachycardic indications for, *510–514*, 510–515
  testing of, 468–470, *469*, *470*
  transthoracic route of entry for, *443*, 443–444, *444*
  transvenous route of entry for, 442–443, *443*
  types of, 508, *509*
  universal, 496–506, *497–505*
  V-A interval of, 489, *489*, 564
  ventricular-inhibited, 456–457, 565
  V-V interval of, 490, *490*, 565
  Wenckebach phenomenon and, *504*, 504–506, *506*
Embryology, of heart, 1–5, *3–5*
Endocardium, 560. See also *Myocardium*.
  anatomy of, *13*
  blood supply to, 11, *11*
Enzymes, in cardiac muscle, 14–16
Epicardium, 560. See also *Myocardium*.
  anatomy of, *13*
  blood supply to, 11, *11*
Epinephrine, 93–96, *94–96*
EPM. See *Electronic pacemaker(s) (EPM)*.
Escape beats, 560
  atrial, 130–133, *131*, *132*
  A-V junctional, *268–282*, 268–283
  ventricular, 341–344, *341–344*
Excitation, 560. See also *Adrenergic (excitatory) influences.*

Exercise stress test, ECG and, *62–64*, 62–65
  tachycardia and, *98*, 98–100, *99*
Exit block, 124, *124*, 561. See also *Block(s).*
Extrasystole, 352, 561. See also *Atrial premature complex (APC)*; *Ventricular premature complex (VPC).*

F
F wave, 172–173, *173–175*
  f waves, 187–188, 191, *191*
Failure to capture. See under *Electronic pacemaker(s) (EPM).*
Fascicle. See *Bundle(s).*
Fast channels, 18–19
Fast tract, 220
Fetal heart development, 1–5, *3–5*
Fetal heart rate, 87
Fibrillation, 561. See also *Atrial fibrillation (AFib)*; *Ventricular fibrillation (VFib).*
Fixed-rate pacemakers. See *Electronic pacemaker(s) (EPM), asynchronous.*
Flutter, 561. See also *Atrial flutter (AFl)*; *Ventricular flutter (VFl).*
Focus, 561
Force of contraction, 14
Fusion complex, 561
  aberrant conduction and, *420*, 420–421, *421*
  electronic pacemakers and, *462*, 462–465, *463*
  in ventricular preexcitation, 229
  in ventricular premature complex, 229, 359–361, *360*
  pseudofusion vs., *494*, 494–495, *495*

G
Grid system, in ECG tracings, dimensions of, 24, *24*, *25*
  heart rate determination and, 47–51, *47–52*, 49(t)

H
H wave, 217–218, *218*
Heart, anatomy of, 1–2, 5–12, *5–13*
  beat of. See *Cardiac cycle.*
  blood flow through, 5–6, *8*, *9*
  cell physiology of, 13–21, *14–19*
  chambers of, 1–2, *2*
  contraction sequence of, 5–6, *8*, *9*. See also *Cardiac cycle.*
  embryology of, 1–5, *3–5*
  functioning of, 5–6, *8*, *9*
  innervation of, *91*
  muscle, *11*, 11–13, *13*. See also *Sarcomere.*
  rate, determination of, 45–51, *45–52*, 49(t)
    fetal, 87
    in infants, *84*, 84–85
    variations in, normal, 84–91, *84–91*
Heart block. See *Atrioventricular (A-V) block.*
Heartbeat. See *Cardiac cycle.*
Hemiblock, 335–336, *336*. See also *Bundle branch block (BBB).*

Hexaxial system, 68, *68*. See also *QRS axis.*
His, Wilhelm, 559
His bundle, 561
  anatomy of, 214–215, *215*
  branches of. See *Bundle branch(es).*
  cardiac cycle role of, 28, *29*
His bundle electrogram, 217–218, *218*. See also
  Electrogram.
His-Purkinje system, 321–323, *323*, *324*. See also
  Purkinje fibers.
HV interval, 217–218, *218*, 561
Hyperkalemia. See also *Electrolytes.*
  aberrant conduction and, *415*, 415–416
  A-V tachycardia and, 290, *290*
  T wave changes and, 67, *67*

I
Idioventricular rhythm, 344–345, *344–346*, 565
Inderal (propanolol), *108*, 108–109
Infarction, 561. See also *Myocardial infarction
  (MI).*
Intranodal tract, *220*, 220–225, *221*
Intraventricular conduction. See *Aberrant
  conduction.*
Ions. See *Electrolytes.*
Ischemia, 11, 61–65, *63*, *64*
Isoelectric line, 22–23, *23*, *42*
Isoproterenol, *251*, 251–252
Isorhythmic dissociation, *293*, 293–295, *294*. See
  also *Dissociation.*

J
Joule, James Prescott, 164
Joules (watt/seconds), 164, 561
Jugular vein, pulse in, 384
Junctional premature complex. See
  *Atrioventricular (A-V) junctional premature
  complex.*

K
Kent bundles, 228

L
Laddergrams, 127–128, *128*
  A-V junction and, *272*, *285*, *286*
  of atrial premature complex, 134–135, *135*, *146*
  of A-V block, *264*
  of ventricular premature complex, *355*
Lanoxin. See *Digitalis*
Leads, ECG, bipolar, 51–55, *54*, *55*, *59*, 60(t)
  central terminal, 56, 60(t)
  exploring, 2
  ground, 51–53
  indifferent, 52, 60(t)
  intraesophageal, 412
  oscilloscope monitoring and, *73*, 74–76, *75–79*,
    78(t)
  precordial, 52–53, 57, *58*, 60(t)
  unipolar, *56*, 56–57, *58*, *59*, 60(t)

Lidocaine (Xylocaine), *388*, 388–389, *390*
Longitudinal dissociation, 220. See also
  Dissociation.
Lown-Ganong-Levine syndrome, *234*, 296
Lyme disease, 500

M
Membrane permeability, 17–21, *18*
MI. See *Myocardial infarction (MI).*
Microcircuit, 305
Mitral valve, 4, *5*
Mobitz, Walter, 252
Mobitz phenomenon, 561–562. See also
  Atrioventricular (A-V) block, second-degree.
Monitoring, cardiac, 72–79, *73–79*, 78(t)
Myocardial infarction (MI), atherosclerosis and, 11
  Q wave changes in, 65–66
  T wave changes in, 67, *67*
  ventricular tachycardia and, 404–405, *405*
Myocardial insufficiency, 11, *11*
Myocardial ischemia, 61–65, *63*, *64*
Myocardium. See also *Sarcomere.*
  anatomy of, *13*
  blood supply to, 11, *11*, 61–65, *63*, *64*
  electromechanical dissociation in, 474
  electronic pacemaker interface with, 452
  functioning of, 12–13
Myofibrils, *14*, *15*
Myosin, *14*, 14–16, *15*

N
N fibers, 214
Nervous system, autonomic. See *Autonomic
  nervous system.*
Neurohumoral transmitters, 93
Nodal accelerated rhythm, 288, 562
Nodal approach zone, 214
Nodal premature complex. See *Atrioventricular
  (A-V) junctional premature complex.*
Nodal rhythm, 562
Nodal tachycardia. See *Atrioventricular (A-V)
  junctional tachycardia.*
Nodoventricular bypass, 225–227, *226*, 234(t). See
  also *Accessory pathway(s).*
Nomenclature code system, for pacemakers, 476–
  478, *477*, 512–513, *513*
Noncompensatory pause. See under *Pause(s).*
Nonparoxysmal tachycardia, 299
Nonrespiratory sinus arrhythmia, 90–91, *91*
Noradrenaline. See *Norepinephrine.*
Norepinephrine, 93, *94–96*, *96*
Normal phasic rate changes, *85*, 85–86
Normal sinus rhythm (NSR), 84–91, *84–91*

O
One-beat rulers, *45*, 45–46, *46*
Oscillatory afterpotentials, 289
Oscilloscope, 72–79, *73–79*, 78(t), 562

P

P cells, automaticity in, 83
  pacemaker role of, 80–82, *81*
  spontaneous diastolic depolarization of, 82–84
P wave, 562
  formation of, 25, *27*
  identification of, 34–35, *35*
  in atrial enlargement, 60, *61*
Pacemaker(s), 562
  electronic. See *Electronic pacemaker(s) (EPM).*
  endogenous, 562
    atrial, 130, *131, 132,* 132–133, *135*
    A-V junctional, *268–275,* 275–283
    P cell role as, 80–82, *81*
    sinus nodal, 25, 80–82, *81*
    ventricular, 341–343, 346–348, *346–348*
    wandering, *132,* 133, 565
Paddle electrodes, 164
Paper tracings, ECG, 22–24, *23–25*
  grid system of, 47–51, *47–52,* 49(t)
  heart rate determination and, 47–51, *47–52,* 49(t)
Parasympathetic nervous system, 91(t), 91–95, *92,*
  562
Parasystole, 374–376, *374–376,* 562
Parkinson, John, 229
Paroxysmal atrial tachycardia (PAT), 152–161, *154,*
  155, 160. See also *Atrial tachycardia (AT).*
Pause(s), compensatory, 350–356, *351–355,* 418,
  559
  noncompensatory, 354–356, *355, 356,* 562
  sinus, 111–112, *112*
  ventricular, 409
PES (preexcitation syndrome), 220, 562
Polarity. See *Transmembrane potential.*
Potassium. See *Electrolytes.*
PP interval, 562
PR interval, 562
  analysis of, 28, *28,* 36
  normal range of, 215, *216*
Preexcitation, ventricular. See *Ventricular*
  preexcitation.
Preexcitation syndrome (PES), 220, 562
Premature complexes. See *Atrial premature*
  complex (APC); Atrioventricular (A-V)
  junctional premature complex; Ventricular
  premature complex (VPC).
Procainamide, 388, 391
Pronestyl, 388, 391
Propranolol (Inderal), *108,* 108–109
Pulmonary arterial system, 1
Pulmonary blood flow, 5–6, *8*
Pulmonary valve, 4, *5*
Pulmonary venous system, 1
Pulse, venous, 194
  a waves in, 384
  cannon waves in, 384
  deficit in, 194
  jugular, 384
Pulse generator, external, 435
  for automatic defibrillator, *513,* 513–515, *514*
  internal, 435
  reduced power in, *448–451,* 448–452
Purkinje, Johannes, 562

Purkinje fibers, 562
  action potential in, *323*
  cardiac cyle role of, 28, *29*
  conduction velocity in, 322
  in bundle branches, 322
PV interval, 480, *482*

Q

Q wave, 563
  formation of, 34, *34*
  myocardial infarction and, 65, *66*
QRS axis, 67–70, *68–70*
  deviations in, 67–70, *70,* 558
  in infants, *68,* 68–69
  vectors and, 67–70, *68*
QRS complex, aberrant conduction and, 414–416,
  415, 419, *419*
  formation of, 28, *30*
  identification of, 32–42, *32–42*
  pacemaker reversal of, 452, *453*
QS wave, 34, *36*
QT interval, *389,* 391–393, *392, 393,* 563
Quinidine, atrial fibrillation and, 196, *196*
  ventricular tachycardia and, 388, 391

R

R wave, 34, *35, 36,* 563
Rate changes, normal phasic, *85,* 85–86
Rate determinations, cardiac cycle, 45–51, *45–52,*
  49(t)
Rate limits, electronic pacemakers and, 501–503,
  501–503
  for bradycardias, 559
  for nodal accelerated rhythm, 288, 562
  for ventricular tachycardia, 377–378, 565
Rate rulers, 45–47, *45–47*
Rate variations, in cardiac cycle, 84–91, *84–91*
Reentry, 563. See also *Atrial tachycardia (AT),*
  reentrant
  A-V junctional tachycardia and, 296–306, *297–*
  303
  A-V node and, 233, *234,* 296–306, *297–303*
  microcircuit in, 305
  refractory period and, 152
  sinus tachycardia and, *162,* 162–163
  ventricular premature complex and, 362–363
Refractory period, 563
  absolute, 144, *145,* 563
  blocked atrial premature complex and, 144–146,
  145
  in A-V node, 144–146, *145*
  reentry phenomena and, 152
  relative, 145, *145,* 563
  short duration, 308–309
Repolarization, *19,* 20–21, 563
  in sinus node, 84
Respiration, heart rate variations and, 84–86, *85*
  sinus arrhythmia and, 87–90, *87–90*
Retrograde block, *286,* 286–287, *287.* See also
  Block(s).

Retrograde conduction, in atrial premature complex, 134–135, *135*
 in A-V junction, 271–273, *272, 273,* 283
 in A-V junctional premature complex, 283–286, *284–286*
 in ventricular premature complex, 377
Reverse potential, 19, *19*
R-on-T phenomenon, *386,* 386–388, *387*
RR interval, 563
Rulers, rate determination, 45–47, *45–47*

S

S wave, 34, *35, 36,* 563
SA. See *Sinus arrest (SA).*
S-AB. See *Sinoatrial block (S-AB).*
Sarcomere, activated, 17–20, *18, 19*
 resting, *16,* 16–17, *17*
 structure of, 13–16, *14, 15*
SB. See *Sinus bradycardia (SB).*
Septa, 563
 anatomy of, *13*
 embryology of, 2, *4*
Sick sinus syndrome, 120
Sinoatrial block (S-AB), *123–126,* 123–127. See also *Block(s).*
Sinus arrest (SA), *113,* 113–114, *114,* 563
Sinus arrhythmia, 563. See also *Sinus bradycardia (SB); Sinus tachycardia (ST).*
 nonrespiratory, 90–91, *91*
 respiratory, 87–90, *87–90*
Sinus bradycardia (SB), 105–109, *105–109,* 563. See also *Bradycardia.*
Sinus exit block, 124, *124.* See also *Block(s).*
Sinus node, 80–128
 action potential in, 82–84, *83*
 adrenergic (excitatory) influences on, 96–102, *97–99, 101–105*
  mechanisms of, 93, *94–96,* 96
 automaticity in, 83–84
 autonomic nervous system and, 91(t), 91–96, *92, 95*
 block in, sinoatrial, *123–126,* 123–127
 blood supply to, 81–82, *82*
 bradycardia and. See *Sinus bradycardia (SB).*
 cholinergic (depressive) influences on, 105–116, *105–116*
  mechanisms of, 93, *94–96,* 96
 conduction in, 80–84, *81, 83*
 depolarization in, *83,* 83–84
 dysfunction of, 118–127, *120–126*
 impulse formation in, 25, *26, 27,* 80–84, *81, 83*
 pacemaker role of, 25, 80–82, *81*
 pause and, 111–112, *112*
 recovery time of, 122
 reentry in, *162,* 162–163
 rhythm of, *84–86,* 84–91, *88–91,* 563
 silence of, in ECG, 25
 spontaneous diastolic depolarization of, 82–84
 tachycardia and. See *Sinus tachycardia (ST).*
Sinus pause (SP), 111–112, *112,* 563
Sinus rhythm, *84–86,* 84–87, 563
Sinus syndrome, 120, 563

Sinus tachycardia (ST), 96–102, *97–99, 101–105,* 563
 reentry and, 162–163, *163*
Slow channels, depolarization role of, 20, 83–84
Slow tract, 220
Sodium. See *Electrolytes.*
SP. See (sinus pause), 111–112, *112,* 563
Spike potential, 19, *19*
Spontaneous diastolic depolarization, 82–84
ST. See *Sinus tachycardia (ST).*
ST segment, analysis of, 29, *30,* 39, *39*
 deviations in, 61–65, *63, 64*
 exercise stress test and, *62–64,* 62–65
 formation of, 29, *30*
Stenosis, 11–12, *12*
Stokes, William, 557
Stokes-Adams syndrome, 557
Stress test. See *Exercise stress test.*
Stroke volume, 6, 10
Supraventricular tachycardia (SVT), 306–309, *307, 308*
Sympathetic nervous system, 91(t), 91–95, *92,* 563–564
Synchronous pacemakers. See *Electronic pacemaker(s) (EPM), atrial synchronous.*
Syncope, mechanism of, 115
Syncytia, cardiac, 13–14, *15*
Systemic venous system, 1
Systole, 6, *9,* 564

T

T cells, 81
T wave, 564
 deviations in, 65–67, *67*
 formation of, 29–31, *31*
 identification of, 39, *40, 41*
 reversal of, *421,* 421–422
Tachyarrhythmia, 564
Tachycardia, 564
 atrial. See *Atrial tachycardia (AT).*
 A-V junctional. See *Atrioventricular (A-V) junctional tachycardia.*
 drug induced, 101–102, *101–103*
 exercise stress test and, *98,* 98–100, *99*
 pacemaker mediated, *507,* 507–508
 paroxysmal. See *Paroxysmal atrial tachycardia (PAT).*
 sinus node and, 96–102, *97–99, 101–105*
 supraventricular, 306–309, *307, 308*
 vagal stimulation and, 109, *109*
 ventricular. See *Ventricular tachycardia (VT).*
Tensilon (edrophonium), 159–161, *160*
Three-beat rulers, *46,* 46–47, *47*
Threshold, 564
Torsades de pointes, 391–393, *392, 393,* 564
Tract(s), 564. See also *Accessory pathway(s).*
 fast, 220
 intranodal, *220,* 220–225, *221*
 slow, 220
Tranquilizers, 159, 165–166
Transmembrane potential, electrolytes and, 17–21, *18*
 measurement of, *16,* 16–17, *17*

Transmembrane potential (*Continued*)
  mechanisms of, 17–21, *19*
  potassium leakage and, 17
  resting, 17, *17, 19*, 21
Tricuspid valve, 4, *5*
Trifascicular block, 337. See also *Block(s)*
Trigeminy, 364, *364*, 564

U
U wave, formation of, 31, *31*
  identification of, 39–40, *41*
Unidirectional block, 564. See also *Block(s)*.
Urecholine (bethanechol), 94

V
VA (ventricular arrest), 410–411, *410, 411,* 565
V-A interval, pacemaker and, 489, *489*, 564
Vagal stimulation. See also *Carotid pressure (CP)*.
  aberrant conduction and, *422*, 422–423
  A-V block and, 242, *242, 245*, 245–246
  A-V junctional tachycardia and, 300–301, *301*,
    311
  bundle branch block and, 330–331, *331*
  cholinergic effect of, 109, *109*
  pacemaker testing and, 468–469, *469*
  tachycardia and, 109, *109*
Vagal tone, 94–95, 158, *158*
Vagus nerve, 92–93, 564
Valium (diazepam), 165–166
Valsalva maneuver, 109, 112, *112*, 158. See also
    Vagal stimulation.
  atrial tachycardia and, 158
Valves, cardiac, anatomy of, *5, 13*
  embryology of, 2–4, *4, 5*
  functioning of, 5–6, *9*
Variant bypass, 309–310. See also *Accessory
    pathways*
Vasovagal reflex, 114–115, *115*, 564
VB. See *Ventricular bradycardia (VB)*.
Vectors, 564
  QRS axis and, 67–70, *68*
  ventricular ECG and, 323–324, *324*
Ventricle(s), 340–432, 564
  action potential in, 340
  anatomy of, 5–9, 5–12, *13*
  arrest of. See *Ventricular arrest (VA)*.
  automaticity in, 340–341, *341*, 362
  A-V block effect on, 346–348, *346–348*
  bigeminy in, 363, *363, 364*, 559
  bradycardia in. See *Ventricular bradycardia
    (VB)*.
  cardiac cycle role of, 28, *30*, 31, *31*
  conduction in, 321–324. See also *Aberrant
    conduction*.
  depolarization of, 28, *30*, 31, *31*
  embryology of, 1–5, *3–5*
  enlargement of, 60–61, *61*
  escape beats in, 341–344, *341–344*
  fibrillation in. See *Ventricular fibrillation (VFib)*.
  flutter in. See *Ventricular flutter (VFl)*.
  functioning of, 5–6, *8, 9*

Ventricle(s) (*Continued*)
  impulse formation in, 340–341, *341*, 348, *349*,
    405, *406*
  pacemakers and, electronic. See *Electronic
    pacemaker(s) (EPM)*.
    endogenous, 341–343, 346, 346–348, *346–348*
  pause in, 409
  preexcitation of. See *Ventricular preexcitation*.
  premature complex in. See *Ventricular
    premature complex (VPC)*.
  rhythms in, accelerated, 378, 565
    idioventricular, 344–345, *344–346*
  tachycardia in. See *Ventricular tachycardia
    (VT)*.
  trigeminy in, 364, *364*
  vulnerable period in, *386*, 386–388, *387*
Ventricular accelerated rhythm, 378, 565
Ventricular arrest (VA), *410*, 410–411, *411*, 565
Ventricular bradycardia (VB), 405–409, *406–409*,
    565
Ventricular fibrillation (VFib), 565
  electric shock therapy in, 401–403, *402, 404*
  mechanisms of, 399, *399–402*
  primary, 401–403, *403*
  secondary, 403, *404*
Ventricular flutter (VFl), 398, *398, 399*, 565
Ventricular pause (VP), 409
Ventricular preexcitation, aberrant conduction and,
    423–424
  accessory pathways and, *219*, 219–221, *220*,
    234(t)
    atrio-His bypass, 225, *225, 234*, 234(t)
    atrioventricular bypass, *228–233*, 228–234,
      234, 234(t)
    intranodal, 220–224, *221–224*, 234(t)
    nodoventricular bypass, 225–227, *226, 227*,
      234(t)
  definition of, 219–220, *219–220*
  delta wave in, 225, *227*, 228–229, *229*
  fusion complex in, 229
  N fibers and, 214
  nodal approach zone and, 214
  reentry and, 233, *234*
Wolff-Parkinson-White syndrome and, 229, 234(t)
Ventricular premature complex (VPC), 565
  bigeminy and, 363, *363, 364*
  bundle branch block vs., 376–377
  characteristics of, 349–350
  compensatory pause in, 350–356, *351, 355*, 418,
    559
  coupling in, 560
    fixed, 369–370, *369–370*
    variable, *370*, 370–373, *374*
  ECG and, 350–356, *350–356*, 368–359
  electrogram of, 350, *351*
  etiology of, 361–363
  fusion beats and, 359–361, *360, 361*
  impulse formation in, 349–350, *350*
  interpolated beat in, 352–353, *353*
  laddergram of, *355*
  multiform, *367*, 367–368
  noncompensatory pause in, 354–356, *355, 356*,
    562
  parasystole and, 374–376, *374–376*, 562

Ventricular premature complex (VPC) (*Continued*)
  QRS complex in, 376–377
  reentry and, 362–363
  sinoatrial isolation from, 350–353, *352*
  site of origin of, *368*, 368–369, *369*
  timing of, 356–359, *356–360, 362*
  torsades de pointes and, 391–393, *392, 393*
  trigeminy and, 364, *364*
  uniform, 364, *365,* 366, *366*
  VH interval in, 350, *351*
Ventricular rhythm. See *Idioventricular rhythm.*
Ventricular tachycardia (VT), a waves and, 384
  aberrant conduction and. See *Aberrant
    conduction.*
  accelerated rhythms and, 378, 557
  angina and, 384, *384–386*
  cardiac output and, 384
  characteristics of, 377–384, *378–384*
  coronary artery insufficiency and, 384, *384–386*
  definition of, 377–378, 565
  drug induced, 299–302
  drug therapy in, *388–390,* 388–393
  electric shock therapy in, 393–397, *393–397*
  etiology of, 386, 404
  heart rate in, 377–378, 565
  myocardial infarction and, 404–405, *405*
  pacemaker mediated, *507,* 507–508
  QT interval in, *389,* 391–393, *392, 393*
  R-on-T phenomenon and, *386,* 386–388, *387*
  supraventricular vs., 306–309, *307, 308*
  torsades de pointes, 391–393, *392, 393*
  vulnerable period and, *386,* 386–388, *387*

Ventricular-inhibited pacemakers, 456–457, 565.
    See also *Electronic pacemaker(s) (EPM).*
Verapamil, 161, *161, 162*
VFib. See *Ventricular fibrillation (VFib).*
VFl. See *Ventricular flutter (VFl).*
VH interval, 350, *351*
VP (ventricular pause), 409
VPC. See *Ventricular premature complex (VPC).*
VT. See *Ventricular tachycardia (VT).*
Vulnerable period, *386,* 386–388, *387,* 565
V-V interval, 490, *490,* 565

W
Wandering pacemaker, 565
  atrial, *132,* 133
Watt/seconds (joules), 164, 565
Wenckebach, Karl, 565
Wenckebach phenomenon, *253–259,* 254–259, *264,*
  565
  pacemakers and, 504–506, *504–506*
White, Paul D., 229
Wolff, Louis, 229
Wolff-Parkinson-White syndrome, 229, 234(t), 565

X
Xylocaine (lidocaine), *388,* 388–389, *390*